A GOOD-SENSE GUIDE

Guide to the Foods You Eat

A GOOD-SENSE GUIDE

Guide to the Foods You Eat

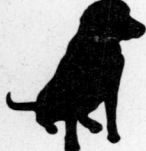

BLACK DOG & LEVENTHAL PUBLISHERS

NEW YORK

Published by

Black Dog & Leventhal Publishers Inc.
151 West 19th Street
New York, New York 10011

Distributed by

Workman Publishing Company
708 Broadway
New York, NY 10003

Special thanks to N-Squared Computing who provided nutritive value information and nutrition evaluation capabilities with their Nutritionist IV™ database.

N-Squared Computing
3040 Commercial Street SE—Suite 240
Salem Oregon 97302

Manufactured in the United States of America

ISBN: 0-9637056-2-8

CONTENTS

FOREWORD

The *Guide to the Foods You Eat* is the first in the series of Good-Sense Guides. What makes this food value encyclopedia so complete is, in addition to its nutritive value charts, its informative and useful chapters such as: an introduction by restaurant critic Gael Greene talking about healthful trends in eating out; nutritional information and guidelines to healthy eating; an FDA labeling chapter; and a dining out chapter containing popular sample menus and their nutritional values.

The nutritive value charts contain the largest compilation of data (calories, protein, fat, saturated fat, monounsaturated fat, polyunsaturated fat, carbohydrates, dietary fiber, calcium, iron, potassium, sodium, cholesterol, vitamins A, C, B_1, B_2, B_3, omega-3 fatty acids, lactose, magnesium, zinc, and percentage of calories from fat) for generic foods, brand names, and fast food restaurant chains.

The book is organized to roughly correspond with the USDA's Food Guide Pyramid (see dividers and back cover) which suggests healthy dietary guidelines. Each tabbed section contains foods from one of the four levels of the food pyramid. The data was compiled from the United States Government's Department of Agriculture (USDA) , the Canadian Nutrient File (CNF), Nutritionist IV (a nutritional analysis database), processors and producers of brand names, and restaurant chains.

Throughout the charts the terms USDA or CNF may appear next to a food to give you the specific resources for analytical comparisons. In the third section containing fish, poultry, and meats, the descriptive term "moist heat" appears. This refers to braising or simmering cooking methods. "Dry heat" means roasting or baking. Very often a value of 0.0, or 0.00 appears. This means that the value obtained from analysis was zero or the closest possible obtainable value to zero. Some foods have a blank space where a value would appear. This means that data was lacking for those foods' nutrients.

When comparing foods, pay attention to the "amount" of a food. If you need to convert a measure to a smaller or larger amount, refer to the weight conversion tables on page 432. The food amount "1 serving" refers to a portion of a particular food type typically consumed.

This compilation contains the most accurate information currently available. Please keep in mind that variables such as seasons and regions may affect the nutritional value of foods. The "normal" serving size in a restaurant is generally much greater than you might prepare at home. In the Dining Out chapter we have scaled the menu items to accurately reflect this difference. This means we erred on the side of "more" than "less" when it came to butter, oil, mayonnaise, cheese, salad dressing, meat portion, and pasta serving size.

INTRODUCTION by Gael Greene

I have long been a closet convert to healthy-eating. Not a fanatic, but a believer, a mostly quiet zealot. As New York Magazine's restaurant reviewer I've created an image of delicious excess. There is truth behind my sobriquet, The Insatiable Critic. I've often written that too much of a good thing is just barely enough. And in an essay called "The Confessions of a Sensualist," I declared that I had long ago committed myself to . . . slow death by mayonnaise. My stance as a sybarite means that I celebrate appetite, the leaping off cliffs into puddles of truffle oil, the complexity of the dish that makes one weep. At times, I've sneered at prudence or moderation.

Except for occasional safaris to spas — brief, inspirational, mostly focused on the kitchen and riddled with fantasies of food, I lyracize. A reader might well imagine that I begin my day with caviar and crème fraîche and end it, sans recrimination after a night-cap of chocolate velvet.

But long before cholesterol was invented, decades before fat was saturated or not and no one had dreamed that broccoli might extend one's life, I was already loving vegetables. An early trip to France and the emergence of great Chinese restaurants certainly helped. Mom's frozen string beans and over-cooked carrots paled beside celeri root timbale, turnip cake and Szechuan string beans. I had always suspected that Mom was right when she urged us to "eat your veggies." I secretly believed I would get scurvy if I didn't start the day with a generous dose of vitamin C — I quickly discovered fresh-squeezed orange juice and grapefruit sorbet. And always, somewhere between lobster and champagne sauce at some haughty French restaurant, I would stop to peel a carrot and crunch away. As researchers document the curative and prophylactic power of wheat germ and cantaloupe, turnip greens and brussel sprouts, I feel smug and secure.

Never an athlete — my two sports are shopping and après-ski — I began working out at the gym as my divorce became final. Not for health, but for romance — I needed that competitive svelte. And by the time I noticed my lunchtime companions had substituted fancy mineral water for their usual three martinis, I was already sipping my new favorite aperitif — grapefruit juice and soda. Not because the New England Journal of Medicine has scared me sober but because I couldn't afford the time to nap between lunch and dinner.

Remember the oat bran exaltation? I was an eager recruit (though never once dreamed of abandoning crème brulée or risotto with mascarpone and wild mushrooms). And by the time the notion of spa cuisine was attaching in fancy restaurants in fitful rashes, I was pleased to explore and critique it. Lean cuisine is mean if it isn't delicious.

My job requires me to taste everything . . . thank heaven. My guests are sharply divided. Some, especially those in their twenties and thirties, order heart-wise, determined to pamper their arteries. Denial and fatalism feeds the defiance of many older friends. They butter their bread and demolish a pound of porterhouse as if to proclaim: I've come this far on scrambled eggs and bacon . . . ."Every day science invents a new villian," they reason, "tomorrow we'll wake up and discover chocolate and caffeine and butter-fat cures everything." I polish off the swiss chard and leave them to their delusions.

Happily, chefs are discovering they have arteries to protect too. Folks who never ate fish two decades ago because it was frozen, boring and cooked to cardboard, are discovering the delights of the lowliest junkfish elevated to transcendence by the alchemy of a gifted cook (with spice rubs and per-fumed broths, salsas and exotic vinaigrettes). Venison has emerged, the red meat for the Nineties, lower in fat than chicken. And three-star chefs every-where give new dazzle to vegetables, from following Alice Waters' lead in growing their own and encouraging boutique farming to doing magic with beets and fennel, baby pumpkins and seaweed and beans nobody I know ever dreamed of in my childhood. At times I find myself thinking, pass me the beta-carotene. Mostly I'm marveling, What an amazing thing to do with carrots. Or, I never imagined mere squash could be so delicious. At Lespinasse in the St. Regis Hotel in Manhattan and at Charlie Trotter's in Chicago, you will find vegetable tasting dinners — six or seven courses of vegetables transformed by genius. And you don't have to be a vegetarian to be seduced by a plate that gathers vegetable side dishes or garnishes at your request anywhere if the chef is good.

Alas, some professional cooks knew nothing about nutrition or food val-ues and their idea of low-fat is three-quarters of a cup of extra virgin olive oil. I have seen little hearts (signifying "healthy") on dishes "with no butter or cream" but loaded with cheese, and once even on lamb chops ("But we broiled them with butter.") Yes, olive oil seems to have positive effects on your cholesterol balance but it has just as many calories as butter and is one hundred percent fat.

And except in pasta or a stir-fry, most chefs don't dare follow the portion control advanced by the government's new Food Pyramid. Customers would scream "larceny" if all that appeared on the $50 blue plate special were three ounces of salmon or veal. Ignorance and outright chicanery are rampant. Now that many newspapers and magazines include calorie counts and nutri-tional information after each recipe, you and I and even Paul Prudhomme can no longer escape in blissful ignorance. Still its not an irreversible tragedy that our favorite pasta with eggplant, sun-dried tomatoes, mozzarella and parmesan delivers a healthy fat allowance for the day. An informed cook can skinny it. And then you and I can share it.

That's why the Good-Sense Guide arrives in the nick of time. Though many home-cooks, including me, long ago stopped cooking with butter and cream, we can no longer pretend avocadoes and toasted walnuts and coconut milk are not loaded with fat. Now I'll use them sparingly at home and be wary at the mercy of a fat-loving menu.

Anyone can share dishes, as we do at reviewing meals — one-fourth of a fat-happy Caesar salad or a spoonful of eggnog ice cream can be wondrously satisfying. The menu guide and dining tips will prep you for dangerous confrontations. And if you're trying to take the new Food Pyramid seriously, the simple facts you need are brilliantly organized in this book, more nutrtional information than has ever been gathered in one volume before.

Does it make you crazy trying to decode the nutritional mysteries of supermarket labels? I'm usually too rushed to be vigilant but with this book as your guide you can specify the most wholesome brand names on your shopping list in the serenity of your own home where blinding lights and clever displays aren't designed to lead you astray.

Knowing critics and a savvy public can push reluctant chefs to think twice about the food they offer us. Manufacturers who banish the fat and bombard us with salt are already on notice. And once the great chefs of the world get the faith, they can lead us to strawberry fields. Beyond sprouts. Beyond tofu. Beyond cottage cheese. To the glorious food even non-obsessed foodniks crave, the healthful food we deserve.

GUIDELINES FOR
A HEALTHY DIET

The United States Department of Agriculture (USDA) has developed a food guidance system that goes beyond the old familiar "four basic food groups." The new dietary guidelines take the form of the Food Guide Pyramid. The Pyramid is based on research on what foods Americans eat, what nutrients these foods contain, and how to make the best choices for a healthy diet.

The Pyramid will help you choose what and how much to eat from each food category to get the nutrients you need without too many calories, too much fat, sodium and cholesterol. The USDA reports that most Americans' diets are too high in fat. The old guidelines recommended high meat consumption for protein intake, and did not acknowledge the benefits of carbohydrates. The old guidelines were not only out of date, but unhealthy as well.

The Food Guide Pyramid represents a complete reworking of dietary guidelines and has updated nutritional ideas to meet the needs of Americans. A good diet should get no more than 30 percent of its calories from fat and should contain no more than 200 to 250 milligrams of cholesterol and about 2,000 milligrams of sodium. A good diet should include fruits low in refined sugar and about 30 milligrams of fiber from vegetables, and whole grains.

PROTEIN

To be healthier according to the Food Guide Pyramid, Americans need to readjust the proportions of food we eat, with less dependence on red meat, fried foods, and fatty desserts. Protein requirements vary with age, sex and ideal weight. Young children should have a higher percrentage of protein than adults, but most of us need no more than two ounces of protein per day.

Protein intake is important to a healthy diet, but more is not better! Daily protein helps in producing enzymes and tissues, and in other metabolic functions. The body excretes a small amount of unneeded protein molecules and stores the rest (in the form of fat) for energy. An excess of protein results in an excess of calories.

FAT

Health authorities such as the National Cancer Institute, and the American Heart Association suggest that no more than 30 percent of our daily calories should be from fat with no more than one-third of those fats (10 percent of our daily calories) from saturated fat. Cutting down on fatty foods would help people lose weight without a rigorous diet. Fatty foods are high in calories because fat has more than twice as many calories per gram as do protein and carbohydrates. (Fat contains nine calories per gram; protein and carbohydrates contain four calories per gram).

To figure out the number of fat calories in a food, multiply the number of fat grams by 9. To determine the percent of total calories that come from fat, divide the number of calories from fat by the total number of calories, then multiply by 100.

$$\frac{\text{grams of fat} \times 9}{\text{total calories in food}} \times 100$$

For example, if 28 grams of a food contain 142 total calories and 6 grams of fat, the percentage of calories from fat is

$$\frac{6 \times 9}{142} \times 100 =$$

$$\frac{54}{142} \times 100 =$$

= 38 percent

The nutritive value charts in this book include a column that gives percentage of calories from fat, so there is no need for you to perform these calculations. To determine your maximum daily allowance of fat grams, multiply the total calorie intake by 0.3 (since no more than 30 percent of calories should come from fat) and divide by 9 (since each gram of fat contains nine calories).

Fats come in three types—saturated, monounsaturated, and polyunsaturated. Most saturated fats raise blood cholesterol levels, whereas mono- and polyunsaturated fats either reduce or have little effect on it. Coconut and palm kernel oils and animal fats (the fats in meat, lard and dairy products) are high in saturated fats and should be used in very small amounts.

CHOLESTEROL

Most foods from animals contain cholesterol. Americans get cholesterol from egg yolks, red meat, poultry, fish, dairy products, cooking fats and some baked goods. Our body needs cholesterol to function properly, but because our liver produces sufficient amounts, cholesterol need not necessarily be consumed.

High blood cholesterol levels are dangerous because they lead to narrowing of the arteries and heart disease. American health authorities state that consuming less cholesterol and saturated fat is the most important dietary change Americans can make. People under thirty should have levels of about 180 or lower. Those over thirty should have levels of 200 or lower. A blood cholesterol level above 240 qualifies as "high" and should be lowered.

DIETARY FIBER

Dietary fiber comes from plants. It is a kind of carbohydrate that cannot be digested by humans. Fiber passes through the body unabsorbed and therefore contains no usable calories. Some of the best sources of dietary fiber are bran, beans, fruits and vegetables. The fiber in wheat bran protects against constipation and colon cancer. Beans and oat bran have been found to aid in the control of diabetes and help lower blood cholesterol levels. The National Cancer Institute recommends a diet high in fiber with an intake of about 20 to 30 grams of fiber per day.

SODIUM

A human being needs only a small amount of sodium in the daily diet. The necessary amount is about 200 milligrams per day which equals about 1/10 teaspoon. Most Americans, however, consume 4,000 to 6,000 milligrams of sodium per day. The reason is that salt (which contains huge amounts of sodium) tastes good and enhances the flavors of many foods. The sodium column in the nutritive value charts will let you know which foods are naturally (or unnaturally) high in sodium.

High blood pressure afflicts one out of three Americans. It has no outward symptoms but can be easily detected. It is imperative to monitor your blood pressure, especially if it is high. People with high blood pressure are at high risk categories for heart attack, stroke and congestive heart failure.

VITAMINS AND MINERALS

There is more and more evidence these days that particular quantities of some vitamins and minerals may help fend off some chronic diseases. The *Good-Sense Guide's* nutritive value charts contain important information about the quantities of certain vitamins and minerals in the foods you eat. Therefore it is helpful to know what good these substances can do if ingested in substantial quantities.

Vitamin A is linked to good eyesight as it plays a role in the light-detection mechanism of the retina. It helps in the formation of healthy teeth and bones. **Beta-carotene**, a nutrient that the body converts to vitamin A, may help prevent cancer, as well as prevent heart attacks caused by clogged arteries. Large amounts of this yellow-orange pigment occur in dark yellow and dark green fruits and vegetables such as broccoli, spinach, collard greens, and carrots, sweet potatoes, peaches and cantaloupes.

Vitamin C is a widely recommended yet highly controversial vitamin. Some of its known benefits are that it aids the absorption of iron and the healing of open wounds and helps metabolize proteins. The role of vitamin C in the common cold is unclear. Some say it helps prevent colds, and many are convinced that taking vitamin C when a cold appears will help you feel better sooner. New evidence indicates that vitamin C may help prevent some forms of cancer. The multitude of possible benefits supports the recommendations to increase our consumption of fruits and vegetables rich in vitamin C.

Vitamin C-rich foods include citrus fruits and juices (including those from grapefruits, oranges, lemons, etc.) as well as red and green peppers, strawberries, baked potatoes, tomatoes, dark leafy greens, broccoli, Brussels sprouts and papaya.

Among minerals, **calcium** ranks at the top. Calcium is necessary for the development and strengthening of our bones and teeth, as well as for good blood coagulation and the functioning of our muscles. Proper calcium intake is known to fight off osteoporosis, a condition in which bones become brittle and porous, most often among older women. Good sources of calcium include milk and milk products, yogurt, cheese, and cottage cheese, green vegetables, and sardine and salmon bones.

Iron is another mineral essential for growth. It helps to carry oxygen from the lungs to other parts of the body. Iron absorbtion in the body depends on the form of the iron in the food. Meat, poultry and fish contain iron in a form the body can absorb readily. Iron becomes more available from eggs, beans, grains and green vegetables if they are eaten along with meat, poultry or fish.

Another mineral in the spotlight is **potassium**. A study at the University of California study showed that people with the lowest potassium intake had up to four times the risk of stroke than those with higher intake. Years ago it was found that medications that reduced blood pressure also depleted potassium from the body, so increased potassium intake was necessary. Now it seems that potassium actually plays a role in controlling blood pressure: The balance between sodium and potassium is what keeps blood pressure in check. Potassium also helps other nutrients keep nerves and muscles functioning and helps in carbohydrate storage and protein synthesis.

FOOD LABELING

On January 6, 1993, the U.S. Food and Drug Administration (FDA) revised its guidelines, in accordance with the Nutrition Labeling and Education Act of 1990. This was done in response to widespread public comment and inquiries about the FDA's labeling standards, the importance of mandatory nutrition labeling, and the need for a unified system of regulations on misbranding.

An 895-page document published in the *Federal Register* (the government's volumes of rules and regulations) amends a number of important laws about nutrition labeling for food. These revisions include:

- Requiring nutrition labeling on most foods regulated by FDA
- Revising the list of required nutrients and food components, and the conditions for declaring them in nutrition labeling
- Specifiying a new format for declaring nutrition information
- Allowing specified products to be exempt from nutrition labeling
- Prescribing a simplified form of nutrition labeling and the circumstances which simplified nutrition labeling may be used.

Manufacturers must comply with scores of rules set by the FDA. The uniformity of the labels and requirements is meant to facilitate easy understanding on the part of the consumer, as well as benefit the health and dietary needs of society. The following discussion should help demystify the labels and answer consumers' questions that are often met with confusing technical answers.

What is the reasoning behind the format of food labels?

The FDA has declared mandatory and voluntary nutrients to be arranged in order of public importance. This will assist in the selection of an overall diet that is consistent with dietary guidelines, based on what nutrients are present in a particular food and in what amounts.

The order is determined partly by the principle that nutrients whose over-consumption is related to increased risk of disease should be placed at the top of the list of required nutrients. The modified regulations stipulate that ingredients must be listed in the following order: calories, calories from fat, calories from saturated fat, total fat, saturated fat, monounsaturated fat, polyunsaturated fat, cholesterol, sodium, potassium, total carbohydrate, dietary fiber, soluable fiber, insoluable fiber, sugar, sugar alcohol, other carbohydrate, protein, vitamin A, vitamin C, calcium, iron, and other vitamins and minerals listed in another section of the regulations.

What does "enriched ingredient" mean?

When a food product is made with "enriched" flour as an ingredient, but doesn't make an "enriched" claim or use "enriched" in the name of the food, the nutrition label need not declare the enrichment nutrients. If, however, the product is made with unenriched flour and supplemented with nutrients as ingredients to achieve the equivalent of a product made with enriched flour, the enrichment nutrients must be listed on the nutrition label. Information on the amount of the enrichment nutrients is also required if an "enriched" claim is on the label or used in the name of the food.

Beta-carotene is not included in FDA's list of nutrients. More and more studies cite beta-carotene as an important vitamin in fighting cancer. How can I find a food's beta-carotene content?

There is increasing evidence linking the role of beta-carotene with cancer prevention. The FDA has established a voluntary method of listing the amount of beta-carotene in food products. The percentage of vitamin A that is present as beta-carotene may be declared to the nearest 10 percent. For example, a label may say, "Vitamin A (90 percent as beta-carotene)."

The term "U.S. RDA" always appears on nutrition labels. What does it mean?

The term "U.S. RDA" means United States Recommended Dietary Allowance. This term was developed in 1972 to suggest the link between Recommended Dietary Allowance and the label reference for values developed by the agency. Use of this term is being discontinued, because nutrient calculation will be evaluated on a different basis. The FDA wants to use values showing the percentage relationship of nutrients relative to total daily caloric intake.

Recently I have noticed a whole new format for nutrition labels on foods. What does it mean?

Studies have shown consumers' most common purposes for reading nutrition labels were:

- to calculate how high or low the product is in certain nutrients
- to get a general idea of nutritional content
- to compare different types of food products
- to help determine brand choices.

The new labeling amendments include an entirely new nutrition label format. The "Nutrition Information Per Serving" is being replaced with "Nutrition Facts." The FDA has concluded that this more succinct term clearly describes the information while enabling a larger typeface to be used so that the label will be more readily noticed and therefore more readily observed by consumers.

The term "Daily Value" will replace RDA. The FDA believes that consumers generally understand this term as a point of reference. The FDA wants to take this "referential nature" approach to labeling.

Daily Values are a set of reference values defined by regulation and derived from dietary guidance and, for certain nutrients, based on a 2,000-calorie-a-day diet. The FDA decided that a tabular graphic is the clearest and most effective format for nutrition labels. The table will show numbers for a 2,000 calorie-a-day diet, and a 2,500 calorie-a-day diet.

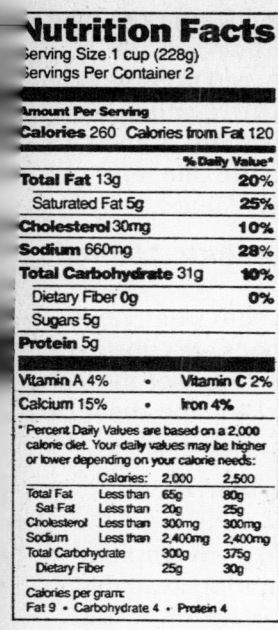

Nutrition Facts
Serving Size 1 cup (228g)
Servings Per Container 2

Amount Per Serving
Calories 260   Calories from Fat 120

	% Daily Value*
Total Fat 13g	**20%**
Saturated Fat 5g	**25%**
Cholesterol 30mg	**10%**
Sodium 660mg	**28%**
Total Carbohydrate 31g	**10%**
Dietary Fiber 0g	**0%**
Sugars 5g	
Protein 5g	

Vitamin A 4%   •   Vitamin C 2%
Calcium 15%   •   Iron 4%

* Percent Daily Values are based on a 2,000 calorie diet. Your daily values may be higher or lower depending on your calorie needs:

	Calories:	2,000	2,500
Total Fat	Less than	65g	80g
Sat Fat	Less than	20g	25g
Cholesterol	Less than	300mg	300mg
Sodium	Less than	2,400mg	2,400mg
Total Carbohydrate		300g	375g
Dietary Fiber		25g	30g

Calories per gram:
Fat 9 • Carbohydrate 4 • Protein 4

Nutrition Facts
Serving Size 1 cup (228g)
Servings Per Container 2

Amount Per Serving
Calories 260   Calories from Fat 120

	% Daily Value*
Total Fat 13g	**20%**
Saturated Fat 5g	**25%**
Cholesterol 30mg	**10%**
Sodium 660mg	**28%**
Total Carbohydrate 31g	**10%**
Dietary Fiber 0g	**0%**
Sugars 5g	
Protein 5g	

Vitamin A 4%   •   Vitamin C 2%
Calcium 15%   •   Iron 4%

*Percent Daily Values are based on a 2,000 calorie diet. Your daily values may be higher or lower depending on your calorie needs:

	Calories:	2,000	2,500
Total Fat	Less than	65g	80g
Sat Fat	Less than	20g	25g
Cholesterol	Less than	300mg	300mg
Sodium	Less than	2,400mg	2,400mg
Total Carbohydrate		300g	375g
Dietary Fiber		25g	30g

Calories per gram:
Fat 9 • Carbohydrate 4 • Protein 4

Nutrition Facts
Serv. Size 1/3 cup (56g)
Servings about 3
Calories 80
Fat Cal. 10
*Percent Daily Values (DV) are based on a 2,000 calorie diet.

Amount/serving	%DV*	Amount/serving	%DV*
Total Fat 1g	2%	**Total Carb.** 0g	0%
Sat.Fat 0g	0%	Fiber 0g	0%
Cholest. 10mg	3%	Sugars 0g	
Sodium 200mg	8%	**Protein** 17g	

Vitamin A 0% • Vitamin C 0% • Calcium 0% • Iron 6%

The above shows three possible label types, and the variations on the positioning of the tabular displays.

What is Percent DV?

Percent DV stands for percent of daily values. The FDA believes that this format improves the consumer's ability to make correct dietary judgements about a food in the context of a total daily diet. These percentages will be used with the 2,000- and 2,500 calorie-a-day tables on the labels and, it is hoped, also aid the consumers' product comparisons.

How are the percent DV's calculated?

The percent DV's and the other reference numbers on the nutrition labels are meant to help you follow and go beyond the information contained in the Food Guide Pyramid and "Dietary Guidelines for Americans." Examples include the following:

   1. Typical intakes are 1,600 to 2,200 calories for women, 2,000 to 3,000 for men, and 1,800 to 2,500 for children from four to fourteen.

   2. Use this nutrition information to help you plan your total daily diet. The Dietary Guidelines recommend that Americans:

- Eat a wide variety of foods

- Choose a diet with plenty of vegetables, fruits and grain products

- Choose a diet low in fat (30 percent or less of daily calories), saturated fat (less than 10 percent of daily calories) and cholesterol

- Use sugars, salt, and sodium in moderation

"Dietary Guidelines for Americans" explains the theory behind the new daily values and may be obtained from the federal government.

Two sets of label reference values, Daily Reference Values (DRVs, which refer to essential nutrients) and Reference Daily Intakes (RDIs, which refer to vitamins and minerals) are used to declare the nutrient content of food on its label. To avoid confusing the consumer, FDA chose to use one term on the label called Daily Values (represented as percent Daily Values).

What happens if the label doesn't follow the rules for the correct format and quantities?

Regulations are imposed on all manufacturers and those who supply food for public consumption in some sort of package form. Foods are considered "misbranded" if health claims are made on their labels that do not meet the requirements of FDA's regulations. Legal action will be taken, and the inconsistencies remedied.

What prompted fast food restaurants to begin providing nutritional information?

In 1986, McDonald's became the first chain to consent to a government agency's request to make nutrition and ingredient information available to its customers in its restaurants in New York State. In the years following, Jack-in-the-Box and KFC were the next chains to provide the data.

It was not until 1990 that the New York City Consumer Office proposed legislation that would mandate tray liners, posters and brochures with key nutrition information. Burger King then said it would provide all the necessary information in its New York outlets without waiting for the Council to act.

Many chains still refused to reveal the information, but some felt that the only way to survive in this highly competitive field they had better provide the nutritional and ingredient specifics.

What does it mean when a label makes claims like "fat free," "cholesterol free," "light," "lite," or "low sodium "?

These are called nutrient content claims, and are made on the label in order to stress a specific benefit about that particular food. The problem with these claims is that inconsistencies in the definitions of these adjectives have put the credibility of the food label into question.

The new regulations that go into effect in February 1994 regarding such circumstances have three basic objectives:

1. to make available nutrition information that can assist consumers in selecting foods that can lead to healthier diets,

2. to eliminate consumer confusion by establishing consistent nutrient content definitions, and

3. to encourage product innovation through the development and marketing of nutritionally improved foods.

One of the biggest changes is the use of a referral statement. The referral statement specifically directs the consumer to the information panel for information about other nutrients in the food in addition to the nutrient in question. For example a referral statement may read: "See side panel for information about fats and other nutrients."

The reasoning behind this statement is that if nutrient content claim is made (such as "low fat"), the label must provide the consumer with the facts that bear on the advantages asserted by the claim, with sufficient information to understand how the product fits into a total dietary regime.

What guidelines do manufacturers follow for making nutrient content claims?

One of the biggest problems for setting uniform guidelines for different products is that their serving sizes greatly vary. The FDA has figured out a method for consistent labeling. The nutrient content claims are based on the product's "reference amount" and are to be followed by a disclaimer. The disclaimer will include the equivalent household measure for each food.

The following illustrates the nutrient content claim and disclaimer: a soft drink that contains 30 milligrams of sodium per reference amount (240 milliliters) meets the criteria for "very low sodium" (less than or equal to 35 milligrams per 8 fluid ounces (240 milliliters)). A 12 fluid ounce single-serving container of this soft drink, however, contains 50 milligrams of sodium and therefore would not qualify for the "very low sodium" claim.

So the disclaimer on this 12 fluid ounce soft drink can will read "very low sodium, 35 mg or less per 240 mL (8 fl oz)." A slice of bread that meets the criteria for "high in fiber" per reference amount, but not per slice, would state "high in fiber, 20 percent or more of the Recommended Daily Intake per 50 g (about 1½ slices)."

Is a claim such as "less than 1% fat" accurate?

The regulations permit statements describing the amount and percentage of nutrients in food if they are not misleading, and if they are consistent with the terms defined by the FDA. Percent claims will help consumers identify foods that facilitate conformance to current dietary guidelines including foods that are a "good source of" or "low" or "high" in a nutrient; as well as foods that are alternatives to other reference foods (i.e. foods that are "reduced" in a nutrient).

In circumstances in which a food does not meet the criteria for a claim, an amount or percentage statement that implicitly characterizes the level of a nutrient, appearing by itself might be misinterpreted. Therefore the statement must be accompanied by a disclaimer such as, "less than 10 grams of fat, not a low fat food" or only "200 mg of sodium per serving, not a low sodium food."

The "_____% fat free" claim can only be made for "low fat" foods containing 3 grams or less of fat per serving and per 100 grams of food, or for "low fat" meal-type products(i.e. frozen dinners). A "100% fat free" claim can be made only in foods that meet the criteria for "fat free." That is they contain less then 0.5 grams of fat per 100 grams, and contain no added fat. The same is true for "saturated fat free" claims.

How can a food be labeled "sodium-free" if sodium occurs naturally in many foods?

The agency agrees that if salt (sodium chloride) or related substances such as baking soda which contains sodium, are listed in the ingredients, then a "sodium-free" claim would be inappropriate. Therefore they require that such an ingredient statement be followed by an asterisk that refers to a disclosure statement appearing below the list of ingredients. The statement reads: "adds a trivial amount of sodium," adds a negligible amount of sodium," or "adds a dietarily insignificant amount of sodium."

What do the terms "free" and "low" mean referring to fat or cholesterol?

In arriving at a definition for "free" for total fat, cholesterol, sodium, sugars, and calories, the FDA chose the level of the nutrient that is at or near the reliable limit of detection for the nutrient in food and that is dietetically trivial or psychologically inconsequential.

The FDA authorized new synonyms for free such as "no," "zero" and "without" and is changing "source" to "good source" to clarify its meaning and position in the hierarchy of descriptive terms. The FDA set limitations on when the "free" claim may not be used. They provide that a claim may not state the absence of a nutrient unless:

1. the nutrient is usually present in the food, and
2. it would assist consumers in maintaining healthy dietary practices.

Zero fat is analytically impossible to measure. Therefore, "fat free" means less than 0.5 grams of fat per serving.

The following is a list of each nutrient content claim with the corresponding required value and its relative DRV where appropriate:

NUTRIENT CONTENT CLAIM	AMOUNT PRESENT	DRV
"Low calorie"	40 calories or less	2,000 calories
"Cholesterol free"	2 milligrams or less (the food must also contain 13 grams or less of total fat per reference amount)	300 milligrams
"Low cholesterol"	20 milligrams or less	300 milligrams
"Fat free"	Less than 0.5 grams	65 grams
"Low fat"	3 grams or less per 100 grams/not more than 30 percent of calories from fat	
"Lean"	10 grams fat or less, less than 4 grams saturated fat, less than 95 milligrams of cholesterol per 100 grams reference amount	
"Extra lean"	Less than 5 grams of fat, less than 2 grams saturated fat, less than 95 milligrams cholesterol per 100 grams reference amount	
"Saturated fat free"	Less than 0.5 grams	—
"Sodium free"	Less than 5 milligrams	—
"Very low sodium"	35 milligrams or less per reference amount (amounts greater than 30 grams)	
"Sugar free"	Less than 0.5 grams	—
"High," "Rich in"	Nutrient level contains 20 percent of the RDI or DRV. (Foods claiming "high in fiber" must be "low" in fat or their labeling must disclose level of total fat in food).	
"Good source of"	10 percent to 19 percent of RDI or DRV	

How does FDA figure out "reduced" claims?

"Reduced", "light", "lite", and "less" claims are terms used for comparing the amount of a nutrient in one food with the amount of the same nutrient in another food or class of foods. Information about the foods being compared must accompany the claim. "Reduced" and "less" claims must be reduced by 75percent in sodium, 33⅓ percent in calories, and 75 percent in cholesterol.

"Light" is based on fat and calories, and a food may bear the term if it had been specifically formulated or processed to reduce its calories by at least one-third compared to the reference food with a minimum reduction of more than 40 calories per reference amount and per labeling size. "Light" may also be included as part of the name of dairy products that are altered to have one-third fewer calories and at least 50 percent less fat.

When may the term "healthy" be used?

"Healthy" may be used on a label or in the labeling of a food including a meal or main dish if:

(1) it meets the definition of "low" for fat and saturated fat

(2) neither cholesterol nor sodium is present at a level exceeding the disclosure levels for an individual food, meal product, or main dish product, and

(3) the food complies with the definitions and declaration requirements for any specific nutrient content claim

DINING OUT GUIDE

Keeping a close watch on what you eat is easy enough to do at home if you have a book such as this one, the inclination, and some time for planning. Eating out in a restaurant, however, makes it more difficult to keep track of exactly what and how much you are eating. Americans eat out, on average, about three and a half times a week, and that number is going up.

The items prepared in restaurants usually differ from processed and homemade versions in terms of ingredients, preparation, and portion size. Food items change from restaurant to restaurant, and unless an establishment represents that it is "healthy" or serves "spa cuisine" you can be sure that they don't skimp on the butter, oil, dressings, sauces, and condiments. These high-fat elements coupled with large portions of meat and cheese substantially raise the number of calories, fat and percentage of fat calories.

This Dining Out Guide gives you a general idea about the important nutritive values of your favorite and most often consumed restaurant menu items. During the course of your dining experience, a food value may be a little higher or lower, or may be the same as those in the book depending upon the amount eaten. You can make the necessary adjustments by evaluating whether the portions are smaller than our standard "generous amount" used in the Dining Out tables.

MONTEPULCIANO

NORTHERN ITALIAN CUISINE

Antipasti

Antipasto (*mozzarella and parmesan cheeses, tuna and ham, peppers, mushrooms and olives, sprinkled with olive oil*)

Stracciatella

Minestrone

Tomato and Mozzarella Salad

I Primi

Calamari Fritti

Pasta with Pesto Sauce

Spaghetti with Carbonara Sauce

Spaghettini with Red Clam Sauce

Cheese Tortellini

Risotto with Parmesan Cheese

Pasta with Alfredo Sauce

Spaghetti with Marinara Sauce

Spaghetti with Meat Balls and Red Sauce

Angel Hair Pasta with White Clam Sauce

Lasagna with Meat and Cream Sauce

Gnocchi

I Secondi

Chicken Cacciatore

Veal Scallopine

Ossobuco

Veal Parmigiana

I Dolci

Tiramisù

Cannoli

MENU ITEM	CALORIES (kcal)	CARBO-HYDRATES (g)	CHOLES-TEROL (mg)	SODIUM (mg)	PROTEIN (g)	FAT (g)	% OF CALORIES FROM FAT
Antipasti	1100	75	178	3537	87	64	52%
Stracciatella	113	6	178	3068	8	6	52%
Minestrone	278	37	18	2462	10	12	36%
Tomato & Mozzarella	589	9	87	1496	23	51	78%
Calamari Fritti	596	27	885	1040	61	25	39%
Pasta w/Alfredo Sauce	1128	65	209	4556	36	81	64%
Pasta w/Pesto	1244	73	96	2611	33	92	66%
Spaghetti w/ Marinara	447	90	76	2794	17	4	7%
Spaghetti w/ Carbonara	666	42	357	949	24	45	61%
Spag/Meatballs	1399	87	202	3345	75	84	54%
Spag/Red Clam	312	42	2	1277	12	11	31%
Angel/White Clam	351	27	0	388	4	27	65%
Cheese Tortellini	260	39	40	310	13	6	21%
Lasagna	658	57	89	2726	26	37	50%
Risotto	1391	36	49	3714	254	26	17%
Gnocchi	300	65	0	75	15	0	0%
Chicken Cacciatore	958	18	330	2456	87	57	54%
Ossobuco	1527	23	640	2440	243	44	26%
Veal Scallopine	545	18	153	455	37	32	54%
Veal Parmigiana	296	17	162	973	24	14	43%
Tiramisú	541	34	255	172	9	38	62%
Cannoli	1294	33	201	81	13	125	86%

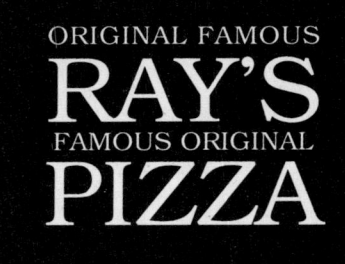

ORIGINAL FAMOUS
RAY'S
FAMOUS ORIGINAL
PIZZA

Calzone
Pizza Margherita with tomato, mozzarrella & basil
Chicken, Mushroom & Tomato Pizza
Chicken & Pineapple Pizza
Pepperoni Pizza
Shrimp, Squid & Mushroom Pizza
Cheese, Meatball & Pepper Pizza
Vegetable Pizza with onion, tomato, green pepper & mushroom
Sausage Pizza

Italian Grinder with sausage and peppers
Chicken Parmigiana Hero
Meatball Hero
Veal Cutlet Parmigiana Hero

MENU ITEM	CALORIES (kcal)	CARBO- HYDRATES (g)	CHOLES- TEROL (mg)	SODIUM (mg)	PROTEIN (g)	FAT (g)	% OF CALORIES FROM FAT
Calzone	788	75	178	2456	40	34	39%
Pizza Margherita	615	42	98	1498	33	35	51%
Pizza/Chick/Mush/Tom	608	73	0	1672	49	13	19%
Pizza/Chick/Pineapple	806	63	0	2674	42	43	48%
Pepperoni Pizza	733	79	56	1066	40	28	34%
Pizza/Shrimp/Sq/Mush	704	74	0	1602	50	23	29%
Pizza/Cheese/Meat/Pep	660	76	75	1370	47	19	26%
Pizza/Veg	455	66	0	1362	35	6	12%
Sausage Pizza	630	92	41	1512	35	14	20%
Italian Grinder	1609	160	212	4545	45	83	47%
Chick Parm Hero	1105	104	198	2560	61	49	40%
Meatball Hero	1350	122	176	3856	56	81	51%
Veal Parm Hero	1217	107	232	3631	79	51	38%

El Rincon Mexicano

Salsa Verde & Chips
Guacamole
Black Bean Soup
Ceviche—Marinated Red Snapper Cocktail

Chicken Empanandas
Refried Beans
Mexican Rice—with tomatoes, onions & garlic
Soft Tacos with Beef
Huevos Rancheros
Shrimp Tostada
Cheese Quesadilla
Red Enchiladas with Sausage
Pipán Verde de Ajonjolí—Green Chicken Fricassee with Sesame seeds
Pork Tamales
Chile Con Carne
Mole Poblano de Guajolote—Turkey in Chili & Chocolate Sauce

Flan

MENU ITEM	CALORIES (kcal)	CARBO-HYDRATES (g)	CHOLES-TEROL (mg)	SODIUM (mg)	PROTEIN (g)	FAT (g)	% OF CALORIES FROM FAT
Salsa Verde & Chips	750	87	0	1108	11	42	49%
Guacamole	203	12	0	883	3	18	72%
Black Bean Soup	699	39	115	2590	45	41	52%
Ceviche	156	11	41	461	25	2	12%
Chicken Empanadas	333	19	55	543	10	24	65%
Refried Beans	181	31	0	715	11	2	9%
Mexican Rice	230	31	9	1337	4	10	40%
Soft Tacos w/ Beef	468	26	73	736	30	27	52%
Huevos Rancheros	427	21	211	945	9	35	72%
Shrimp Tostada	576	67	230	1526	39	16	25%
Cheese Quesadilla	597	54	187	1556	25	32	48%
Red Enchiladas	673	51	233	1715	26	40	54%
Green Chick Fricassee	949	18	309	1270	84	59	56%
Pork Tamales	944	32	165	740	59	64	61%
Chile Con Carne	628	17	162	753	47	40	58%
Mole Poblano/Guajolote	1515	45	518	2338	139	88	52%
Flan	445	48	254	116	10	24	48%

HAPPY BUDDHA CHINESE RESTAURANT
CANTONESE, HUNAN AND SZECHUAN COOKING

SOUPS

Wonton Soup
Egg Drop Soup
Hot & Sour Soup

APPETIZERS

Egg Roll
Scallion Pancakes
Cold Sesame Noodles
Pork Dumplings

SEA FOOD

Shrimp Fried Rice
Shrimp Lo Mein
Sweet & Sour Shrimp
Shrimp with Lobster Sauce
Crispy Prawns with Walnuts

PORK AND BEEF

Mu Shu Pork
Barbequed Spareribs
Beef with Broccoli
Orange-Flavored Beef

POULTRY

Lemon Chicken
Crispy Roast Duck
Chicken with Peanuts

VEGETABLE

Eggplant with Garlic Sauce

MENU ITEM	CALORIES (kcal)	CARBO-HYDRATES (g)	CHOLES-TEROL (mg)	SODIUM (mg)	PROTEIN (g)	FAT (g)	% OF CALORIES FROM FAT
Wonton Soup	233	28	74	1581	16	7	25%
Egg Drop Soup	147	9	240	1778	10	8	49%
Hot & Sour Soup	434	22	301	1729	42	20	41%
Egg Roll	292	26	189	723	20	12	36%
Scallion Pancakes	399	41	0	430	5	24	54%
Cold Sesame Noodles	354	42	31	620	10	17	42%
Pork Dumplings	175	23	56	589	13	3	17%
Shrimp Fried Rice	336	28	228	379	21	15	42%
Shrimp Lo Mein	248	26	60	630	10	12	43%
Mu Shu Pork	908	62	630	901	65	43	43%
Lemon Chicken	963	34	191	1135	47	72	67%
Crispy Roast Duck	830	16	185	704	44	65	71%
Barbequed Spareribs	964	9	223	564	65	72	69%
Sweet & Sour Shrimp	467	56	262	766	24	16	32%
Beef w/ Broccoli	581	5	151	1383	45	41	64%
Chicken w/ Peanuts	377	24	63	100	22	22	52%
Eggplant w/ Garlic Sauce	257	32	0	1029	4	12	40%
Crispy Prawns w/Walnuts	770	12	113	1494	24	72	81%
Orange-Flavored Beef	415	43	40	359	31	16	33%
Shrimp w/ Lobster Sauce	160	4	193	709	21	6	36%

L'Auberge du Chien Noir
FRENCH CUISINE WITH AN ATTITUDE

LES POTAGES ET LES HORS D'OEUVRES

Cream of Leek Soup
Country Pâté
Seafood Tartare

LES VOLAILLES

Rabbit with Green Olives
Roasted Chicken with Herbs
Poulet au Vin Rouge
(Chicken in Red Wine)
Duck Braised in Red Wine & Thyme

LES POISSONS ET LES FRUITS DE MER

Noisettes of Salmon in Red Wine Sauce
Provençal Seafood Stew
Fillets of Sea Bass with Basil
& Tomatoes

LES VIANDES

Pot Au Feu
Steak Frites
Choucroute Garnie
(Garnished Saurkraut)
Cassoulet
Lamb Shanks with Lentils
Foie de Veau Lyonnaise aux Capres
(Sautéed Claf's Liver with Onions
& Capers)

LES LEGUMES

Mashed Potatoes
Ratatouille

LES DESSERTS

French Apple Tart
Crêpes Soufflé

MENU ITEM	CALORIES (kcal)	CARBO-HYDRATES (g)	CHOLES-TEROL (mg)	SODIUM (mg)	PROTEIN (g)	FAT (g)	% OF CALORIES FROM FAT
Cream of Leek Soup	211	11	66	1086	5	17	70%
Country Pate	558	7	297	1495	62	28	47%
Seafood Tartare	187	3	52	189	21	10	49%
Rabbit w/Green Olives	1278	26	390	1646	143	54	39%
Noisettes Salmon/Red	1137	21	269	1206	141	47	38%
Roasted Chicken/Herbs	1001	4	433	876	107	59	55%
Provencal Seafood Stew	322	11	51	1791	28	13	35%
Poulet/Vin Rouge	1179	19	399	1400	100	69	54%
Sea Bass w/Basil & Tom	445	10	91	168	43	25	52%
Duck Braised/Red/Thyme	1707	9	382	1015	88	136	72%
Pot Au Feu	1486	65	369	9118	121	78	48%
Steak Frites	1288	123	144	849	71	62	42%
Choucroute Garnie	965	17	298	3516	106	49	47%
Cassoulet	1246	38	277	1055	74	87	63%
Lamb Shanks w/Lentils	1196	30	565	930	173	39	30%
Calf's Liver	586	14	686	639	43	40	61%
Mashed Potatoes	453	60	59	1647	8	20	40%
Ratatouille	133	16	0	559	3	7	45%
French Apple Tart	465	83	10	408	4	14	26%
Crepes Soufflé	617	30	908	490	25	42	61%

The Hearthstone
FAMILY RESTAURANT

Chicken Noodle Soup

Ceasar Salad

Philly Cheesesteak Sandwich

Sloppy Joes

Cincinnati-Style 5-Way Chili
— with Spaghetti, chili sauce,
kidney beans, raw onions &
cheddar cheese

Tuna-Noodle Casserole

Country Chicken Stew
with Dumplings

Fried Chicken

Chicken Pot Pie

Short Ribs

Brisket

Corned Beef Hash

Roast Leg of Lamb with Rosemary
& Mint Jelly

Chopped Salsbury Steak

Spaghetti & Meatballs

Grits & Greens Spoonbread

Macaroni & Cheese

Baked Beans

Buttermilk Biscuits

Apple Crumble

MENU ITEM	CALORIES (kcal)	CARBO-HYDRATES (g)	CHOLES-TEROL (mg)	SODIUM (mg)	PROTEIN (g)	FAT (g)	% OF CALORIES FROM FAT
Chicken Noodle Soup	388	60	22	2209	15	10	23%
Ceasar Salad	771	24	279	1516	45	56	64%
Philly Cheesesteak	1088	100	135	2199	59	49	41%
Sloppy Joes	652	67	95	1208	38	24	33%
Cincinnati Chili	1173	68	186	2356	122	45	35%
Tuna-Noodle Casserole	299	24	51	1255	19	14	43%
Chicken Stew/Dumplings	1092	60	365	2108	94	51	43%
Fried Chicken	926	11	382	291	97	52	52%
Chicken Potpie	939	46	156	1134	36	69	66%
Short Ribs/BBQ Sauce	719	17	200	2342	63	44	55%
Brisket	1028	28	378	1192	129	38	34%
Corned Beef Hash	523	36	301	1707	44	21	37%
Roast Leg of Lamb	1277	28	421	661	116	75	54%
Spoonbread	735	25	1081	1753	37	54	66%
Macaroni & Cheese	250	22	16	730	12	13	46%
Baked Beans	181	31	0	715	11	1	9%
Salsbury Chopped Steak	846	8	277	2398	78	54	58%
Spaghetti and Meatballs	1399	87	202	3345	75	84	54%
Buttermilk Biscuits	314	35	22	692	5	16	48%
Apple Crumble	315	54	50	164	3	10	29%

Just for the Halibut

SHORE FOOD FOR THE EPICURE

STARTERS

New England Clam Chowder

Lobster Bisque

Crabcakes

Oysters with Spinach

Lobster Salad

Shrimp Cocktail

Crab Quiche

CRITTERS WITH SHELLS

Steamed Lobster
with Butter Sauce

Scallops with Mushrooms
& Brandy

Stuffed Mussels

CRITTERS WITH FINS

Savory Tuna Rolls

Deep Fried Fillet of Sole

Flounder in Wine
& Cream Sauce

Baked Stuffed Sardines

Swordfish Steaks in Tomato
& Black Olive Sauce

Baked Grouper with
Mushrooms & Shrimp Stuffing

Lemon & Garlic Shark Steaks

Trout A La Meunière
(Trout in Butter Sauce)

Barbequed Salmon

Mixed Seafood Au Gratin

MENU ITEM	CALORIES (kcal)	CARBO-HYDRATES (g)	CHOLES-TEROL (mg)	SODIUM (mg)	PROTEIN (g)	FAT (g)	% OF CALORIES FROM FAT
New Eng/Clam Chowder	356	34	110	1316	17	18	44%
Lobster Bisque	728	20	36	1063	85	28	34%
Crab Cakes	744	12	267	1579	25	68	81%
Oysters w/Spinach	552	28	394	1230	44	29	47%
Lobster Salad	473	9	241	1988	49	27	52%
Shrimp Cocktail	227	9	339	1906	46	0	0
Crab Quiche	964	62	224	2664	72	46	44%
Savory Tuna Rolls	599	36	43	1783	33	36	54%
Deep Fried Fillet/Sole	525	32	348	1623	48	22	37%
Flounder/Wine/Cream	563	16	177	1541	43	32	51%
Baked Stuffed Sardines	820	37	421	2415	73	43	46%
Swordfish Steaks/Tom/Blk	468	6	104	2631	51	27	51%
Baked Grouper/Stuffing	696	36	388	2067	83	19	25%
Lemon/Gar/Shark	483	2	115	1249	48	31	58%
Seafood Au Gratin	577	20	184	2948	63	25	39%
Steamed Lobster	1183	10	694	3487	163	51	40%
Scallops/Mush/Brandy	598	10	175	1845	43	38	55%
Stuffed Mussels	390	14	295	1465	41	17	41%
Trout	1108	15	195	1392	57	95	75%
Barbequed Salmon	2308	7	1068	2339	286	122	48%

Priscilla's Caboose
THE FINER DINER

BREAKFAST

Scrambled Eggs
Fried Eggs
Poached Eggs
Ham & Cheese Omelet
Spanish Omelet
Pancakes with Syrup
Waffles with Syrup
French Toast with Syrup
Hot Cereal—Cream of Wheat
Bacon
Sausage
Hash Browns
Bagel with Cream Cheese
English Muffin
Blueberry Muffin
Corn Muffin
Bran Muffin

LUNCH

Chicken & Rice Soup
Split Pea Soup
Tuna Salad Sandwich
Egg Salad Sandwich
Chicken Salad Sandwich
Ham & Cheese Sandwich
Hamburger on a Bun
Bacon Cheeseburger
Grilled Cheese
Bacon, Lettuce, & Tomato
   with Mayonnaise
Club Sandwich
Chef Salad
Greek Salad
Onion Rings—Side order
French Fries—Platter
Potato Salad
Coleslaw
Rice Pudding
Franks & Beans
Chicken & Noodles
Chicken À La King
Beef Stew with Vegetables
Bowl of Chili with Beans
Steak & Onion Sandwich

DINNER

Blue Plate Specials
Pot Roast, Potato, Peas
   with Gravy
Fried Chicken & Potatoes
   with Gravy
Meat Loaf, Potatoes & Peas
   with Gravy
Turkey, Potatoes, Peas
   with Gravy
Franks & Beans
Chicken & Noodles
Chicken À La King
Beef Stew with Vegetables
Bowl of Chili with Beans
Steak & Onion Sandwich

MENU ITEM	CALORIES (kcal)	CARBO-HYDRATES (g)	CHOLES-TEROL (mg)	SODIUM (mg)	PROTEIN (g)	FAT (g)	% OF CALORIES FROM FAT
Scrambled Eggs	390	5	826	656	26	29	67%
Fried Eggs	395	3	910	699	27	30	69%
Poached Eggs	294	2	841	556	25	20	62%
Ham/Cheese Omelet	440	3	736	989	31	33	69%
Spanish Omelet	254	12	459	2714	16	16	57%
Pancakes w/Syrup	1039	238	0	1438	12	6	5%
Waffles w/Syrup	1705	261	234	2751	28	62	33%
French Toast w/Syrup	1009	171	1	1031	23	27	24%
Cream of Wheat	134	28	0	1	4	0	0
Bacon	182	0	27	27	505	10	78%
Sausage	509	3	104	1137	21	48	82%
Hash Browns	359	17	0	56	7	33	76%
Bagel/Cream Cheese	514	63	61	778	16	22	39%
English Muffin	154	30	0	414	5	1	8%
Blueberry Muffin	158	27	17	255	3	4	21%
Corn Muffin	174	29	0	297	3	5	25%
Bran Muffin	112	17	21	168	3	5	37%
Chick/Rice Soup	127	13	12	888	12	3	22%
Split Pea Soup	189	28	8	1008	10	4	21%
Tuna Salad Sand.	514	42	25	748	38	21	37%
Egg Salad Sand.	664	33	860	814	30	46	62%
Chick. Salad Sand.	488	20	56	453	39	28	52%
Ham/Cheese Sand.	411	39	68	899	24	18	39%
Hamburger	750	72	123	680	43	32	39%
Bacon Cheeseburger	609	37	112	1044	32	37	55%
Grilled Cheese	793	35	189	2478	30	60	68%
BLT w/ Mayo	324	33	50	1404	8	18	50%
Club Sandwich	590	42	93	2601	36	21	38%
Chef Salad	417	16	98	1205	28	27	58%
Greek Salad	582	16	140	3468	33	47	68%
Onion Rings	462	43	0	425	6	30	58%
French Fries	1074	134	0	734	14	36	35%
Potato Salad	358	28	171	1323	7	21	57%
Coleslaw	157	28	28	52	3	6	30%
Rice Pudding	387	71	0	188	10	8	19%
Pot Roast/Pot/Peas/Gravy	604	39	234	2477	68	20	30%
Fried Chick/Potatoes	971	64	227	2930	63	52	48%
Meatloaf/Potatoes	716	56	147	3077	45	36	44%
Turkey Dinner	668	69	145	3282	42	22	30%
Franks & Beans	1299	135	152	3615	52	63	43%
Chicken & Noodles	690	49	181	1134	42	34	46%
Chicken A La King	870	22	344	1405	50	63	66%
Beef Stew	440	30	144	2012	32	22	44%
Chili w/Beans	300	30	50	998	20	20	47%
Steak & Onion Sandwich	653	76	101	1110	43	20	27%

THE CHOP SHOP

DINING FOR THE REST OF US

MAIN EVENTS

Fillet Mignon — 12 oz.
Porterhouse Steak — 12 oz.
London Broil — 12 oz.
T-Bone Steak — 12 oz.
Strip Steak — 12 oz.
Simmered Short Ribs — 12 oz.
Beef Tenderloin — 12 oz.

DIGRESSIONS

Creamy Coleslaw
Onion Rings
Broccoli with Butter
Creamed Spinach
Baked Potato
Scalloped Potatoes
Mashed Potatoes

MENU ITEM	CALORIES (kcal)	CARBO-HYDRATES (g)	CHOLES-TEROL (mg)	SODIUM (mg)	PROTEIN (g)	FAT (g)	% OF CALORIES FROM FAT
Creamy Coleslaw	157	28	28	52	3	6	30%
Onion Rings	462	43	0	425	6	30	58%
Broccoli w/Butter	281	14	62	1371	8	24	71%
Creamed Spinach	190	9		855	4	15	71%
Baked Potato	220	51	0	16	5	0	0
Scalloped Potatoes	90	11	30	420	3	4	39%
Mashed Potatoes	453	60	59	1647	8	20	40%
Fillet Mignon	833	0	260	232	97	46	52%
Porterhouse Steak	740	0	272	224	96	37	46%
London Broil	776	0	188	224	106	36	43%
T-Bone Steak	739	0	221	204	97	36	46%
Strip Steak	846	0	218	183	95	49	54%
Simmered Short Ribs	926	0	258	195	103	54	54%
Beef Tenderloin	680	0	284	216	96	29	41%

THE GOOD-SENSE
FOOD GUIDE PYRAMID
Your guide to daily food choices

Fats, Oils & Sweets
USE SPARINGLY

Milk, Yogurt,
Cheese Group
2-3 SERVINGS

Vegetable
Group
3-5 SERVINGS

Meat, Poultry, Fish,
Dry Beans, Eggs &
Nuts Group
2-3 SERVINGS

Fruit Group
2-4 SERVINGS

Bread, Cereal, Rice
& Pasta Group
6-11 SERVINGS

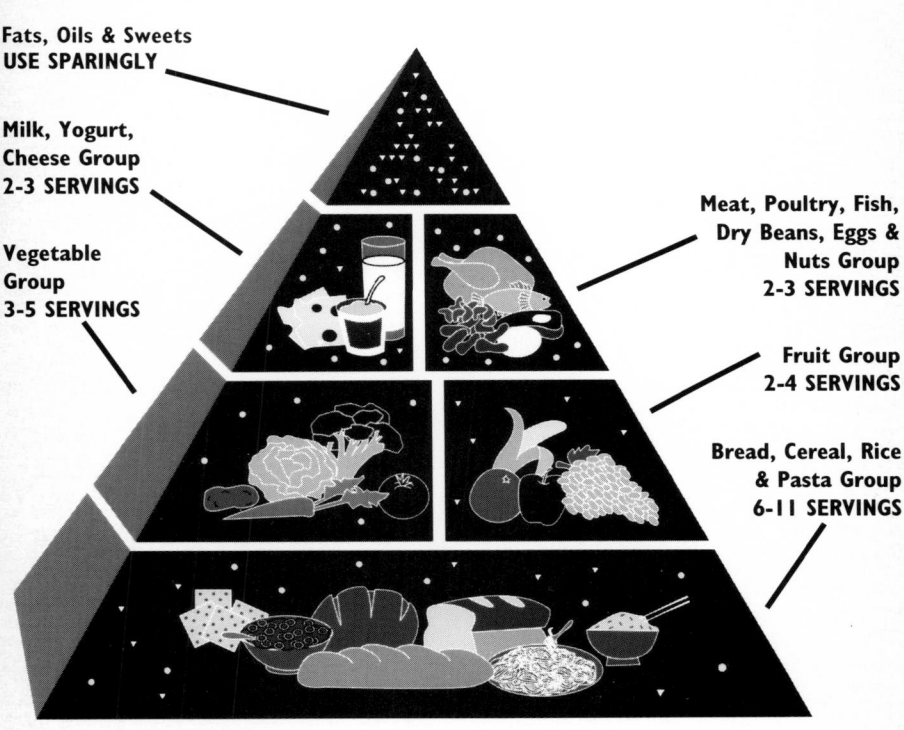

KEY ● Fat (naturally occurring and added) ▼ Sugars (added)

GRAINS, PASTAS, BREADS, BREAKFAST CEREALS, AND BABY FOOD

At the base of the Food guide Pyramid are breads, cereals, rice and pasta — all foods from grains. This section also covers baby food because it serves as the basic nutrition source for infants and toddlers. You need more servings each day from this category than from any other. These foods provide complex carbohydrates (starches), which are an important source of energy, especially in low-fat diets. They also provide vitamins, minerals and fiber.

The Food Guide Pyramid suggests six to eleven servings per day from this category. However, remember that some breakfast cereals have high sugar and sodium content. Thiamin, Riboflavin and Niacin (vitamins B_1, B_2, and B_3 respectively) help the body metabolize proteins, carbohydrates, and fats. In the Breakfast Cereal chart you will find columns for these vitamins. Breakfast cereals are a quick and easy way to get the daily vitamin B you need. A serving is one slice of bread, one ounce of ready to eat cereals, ½ a cup of cooked rice, cereal or pasta.

To get the fiber you need, choose several servings a day of foods made from whole grains, such as whole-wheat, bread, and whole-grain cereals. The term "whole-grain" refers to the entire cereal grain without the hull but with the bran and germ components intact.

CEREAL GRAINS & PASTA

FOOD	AMOUNT	CALORIES (kcal)	PROTEIN (g)	FAT (g)	SATU- RATED FAT (g)	CARBO- HYDRATES (g)	FIBER (g)
CEREAL GRAINS							
Amaranth	1 cup	729	28.18	12.69	3.24	129	7.35
Arrowroot flour	1 cup	457	0.38	0.13	0.02	113	
Barley	1 cup	651	22.97	4.23	0.89	135	5.24
Barley, pearled							
raw	1 cup	704	19.82	2.33	0.49	155	1.47
cooked	1 cup	193	3.55	0.70	0.15	44	0.37
Buckwheat	1 cup	584	22.52	5.78	1.26	122	
Buckwheat groats, roasted							
dry	1 cup	567	19.24	4.44	0.97	123	2.89
cooked	1 cup	182	6.69	1.22	0.27	39	1.04
Buckwheat flour, whole-groat	1 cup	402	15.14	3.72	0.81	85	
Bulgur							
dry	1 cup	479	17.20	1.86	0.33	106	2.50
cooked	1 cup	152	5.61	0.44	0.08	34	0.64
Corn	1 cup	605	15.64	7.88	1.11	123	4.81
Corn bran, crude	1 cup	170	6.35	0.70	0.10	65	
Corn flour, whole-grain	1 cup	422	8.11	4.52	0.64	90	
Corn flour, masa	1 cup	416	10.65	4.31	0.61	87	1.90
Corn grits							
dry	1 tbsp	36	0.90	0.10	0.02	8	0.00
cooked	¾ cup	110	2.60	0.30	0.05	24	0.10
Cornmeal							
whole-grain	1 cup	442	9.91	4.39	0.62	94	2.24
degermed	1 cup	506	11.71	2.28	0.31	107	0.86
self-rising, bolted	1 cup	408	10.10	4.15	0.58	86	1.30
self-rising, bolted, w/wheat flour added	1 cup	592	14.30	4.84	0.68	125	1.31
self-rising, degermed	1 cup	489	11.60	2.37	0.32	103	0.73
Cornstarch	1 cup	488	0.33	0.07	0.01	117	
Couscous							
dry	1 cup	692	23.47	1.17	0.22	142	1.06
cooked	1 cup	201	6.79	0.29	0.05	42	0.24
Farina							
dry	1 tbsp	40	1.20	0.10	0.01	9	0.00
cooked	¾ cup	87	2.50	0.10	0.02	19	0.10
Hominy, canned	1 cup	115	2.36	1.40	0.20	23	0.73
Millet							
dry	1 cup	756	22.03	8.44	1.45	146	2.07
cooked	1 cup	287	8.42	2.41	0.41	57	0.87
Oats	1 cup	607	26.34	10.76	1.90	103	
Oat bran, raw	½ cup	116	8.13	3.31	0.62	31	1.02
cooked	1 cup	87	7.02	1.89	0.36	25	0.81
Oats, rolled or oatmeal, dry	⅓ cup	104	4.30	1.70	0.30	18	0.30
cooked	¾ cup	108	4.50	1.80	0.31	19	0.30
Quinoa	1 cup	637	22.27	9.86	1.00	117	
Rice, brown, long-grain							
raw	1 cup	684	14.69	5.40	1.08	143	2.43
cooked	1 cup	216	5.04	1.76	0.35	45	0.67

FOOD	CALCIUM (mg)	IRON (mg)	POTAS-SIUM (mg)	SODIUM (mg)	CHOLES-TEROL (mg)	VITAMIN B6 (mg)	ZINC (mg)	% OF CALORIES FROM FAT
CEREAL GRAINS								
Amaranth	298	14.81	714	42	0	2.04	6.21	16
Arrowroot flour	51	0.42	14	2	0	0.01	0.09	0
Barley	61	6.63	831	22	0	0.59	5.10	6
Barley, pearled								
raw	57	5.00	560	18	0	0.52	4.25	3
cooked	17	2.09	145	5	0	0.18	1.29	3
Buckwheat	31	3.74	782	1	0	0.36	4.08	9
Buckwheat groats, roasted								
dry	29	4.05	525	18	0	0.58	3.97	7
cooked	14	1.58	175	8	0	0.15	1.21	6
Buckwheat flour, whole-groat	49	4.88	692		0	0.70	3.75	8
Bulgur								
dry	49	3.44	573	23	0	0.48	2.70	3
cooked	18	1.75	124	9	0	0.15	1.04	3
Corn	12	4.50	476	58	0	1.03	3.66	12
Corn bran, crude	32	2.12	33	5	0	0.12	1.18	4
Corn flour, whole-grain	8	2.78	369	6	0		2.02	10
Corn flour, masa	161	8.22	340	6	0	0.42	2.03	9
Corn grits								
dry	0	0.38	13	0	0	0.01	0.04	3
cooked	1	1.16	40	0	0	0.04	0.13	2
Cornmeal								
whole-grain	7	4.21	350	43	0	0.37	2.21	9
degermed	7	5.70	224	5	0	0.35	0.99	4
self-rising, bolted	440	7.03	311	1521	0	0.66	2.44	9
self-rising, bolted, w/wheat flour added	508	8.41	352	2242	0	0.65	2.36	7
self-rising, degermed	482	6.53	235	1860	0	0.54	1.38	4
Cornstarch	2	0.61	4	11	0		0.08	0
Couscous								
dry	44	1.99	305	18	0	0.20	1.52	2
cooked	15	0.69	104	9	0	0.09	0.46	1
Farina								
dry	2	0.41	10	0	0	0.00	0.06	2
cooked	3	0.87	22	1	0	0.02	0.12	1
Hominy, canned	15	1.00	14	336	0	0.01	1.68	11
Millet								
dry	17	6.02	390	10	0	0.77	3.37	10
cooked	8	1.51	148	5	0	0.26	2.18	8
Oats	84	7.37	669	3	0	0.19	6.19	16
Oat bran, raw	27	2.54	266	2	0	0.08	1.46	26
cooked	22	1.93	202	2	0	0.06	1.17	20
Oats, rolled or oatmeal, dry	14	1.14	95	1	0	0.03	0.83	15
cooked	15	1.19	99	1	0	0.04	0.86	15
Quinoa	102	15.73	1258		0		5.61	14
Rice, brown, long-grain								
raw	42	2.73	412	14	0	0.94	3.74	7
cooked	20	0.82	83	9	0	0.28	1.23	7

CEREAL GRAINS & PASTA

FOOD	AMOUNT	CALORIES (kcal)	PROTEIN (g)	FAT (g)	SATU- RATED FAT (g)	CARBO- HYDRATES (g)	FIBER (g)
CEREAL GRAINS (continued)							
Rice, brown, medium-grain							
raw	1 cup	687	14.25	5.09	1.02	145	1.80
cooked	1 cup	218	4.51	1.61	0.32	46	0.57
Uncle Ben's®	1 cup	220	5.00	1.82	0.46	46	2.00
Rice, white, long-grain							
chicken	1 oz	34	1.98	0.40		6	0.03
coconut milk	1 oz	48	1.19	1.62		7	0.09
fried	1 oz	55	1.39	2.15		7	0.03
regular, raw	1 cup	676	13.18	1.22	0.33	148	0.56
regular, cooked	1 cup	264	5.51	0.58	0.16	57	0.21
parboiled, dry	1 cup	686	12.57	1.03	0.28	151	0.68
parboiled, cooked	1 cup	199	4.01	0.47	0.13	43	0.29
precooked or instant, dry	1 cup	360	7.27	0.27	0.07	79	0.37
precooked or instant, prepared	1 cup	161	3.40	0.27	0.07	35	0.16
Kraft® rice & cheese							
broccoli & cheddar	1 cup	300	8.00	10.00		46	
cheddar & chicken	1 cup	300	8.00	8.00		46	
cheddar pilaf	1 cup	300	8.00	8.00		46	
Rice, white, medium-grain							
raw	1 cup	702	12.88	1.13	0.31	155	0.51
cooked	1 cup	266	4.88	0.43	0.12	59	0.19
Rice, white, short-grain							
raw	1 cup	717	13.01	1.03	0.28	158	0.57
cooked	1 cup	267	4.84	0.38	0.10	59	0.21
Rice, white, glutinous							
raw	1 cup	685	12.61	1.02	0.21	151	0.32
cooked	1 cup	234	4.86	0.47	0.09	51	0.18
Rice, white, w, pasta & seasonings							
dry	1 cup	601	15.27	3.97	0.72	123	0.88
cooked	1 cup	247	5.14	5.69	1.09	43	0.39
Rice bran, crude	1 cup	262	11.08	17.30	3.46	41	
Rice flour							
brown	1 cup	574	11.43	4.40	0.88	121	2.04
white	1 cup	578	9.40	2.24	0.61	127	
Rye	1 cup	567	24.95	4.22	0.49	118	2.53
Rye flour							
dark	1 cup	415	17.95	3.44	0.40	88	
light	1 cup	374	8.55	1.39	0.15	82	
medium	1 cup	361	9.58	1.80	0.20	79	
Semolina	1 cup	602	21.17	1.75	0.25	122	
Sorghum	1 cup	650	21.70	6.34	0.88	143	4.61
Tapioca, pearl, dry	1 cup	519	0.29	0.03		135	
Triticale	1 cup	646	25.05	4.01	0.70	139	4.99
Triticale flour, whole-grain	1 cup	440	17.14	2.36	0.41	95	1.95
Wheat							
hard red spring	1 cup	631	29.56	3.69	0.60	131	4.37
hard red winter	1 cup	628	24.20	2.95	0.52	137	4.40
soft red winter	1 cup	556	17.39	2.62	0.49	125	2.89
hard white	1 cup	656	21.71	3.28	0.53	146	

FOOD	CALCIUM (mg)	IRON (mg)	POTAS- SIUM (mg)	SODIUM (mg)	CHOLES- TEROL (mg)	VITAMIN B6 (mg)	ZINC (mg)	% OF CALORIES FROM FAT
CEREAL GRAINS (continued)								
Rice, brown, medium-grain								
raw	62	3.42	509	8	0	0.97	3.84	7
cooked	20	1.03	153	2	0	0.29	1.22	7
Uncle Ben's®	16	1.00	172	2	0	0.00		7
Rice, white, long-grain								
chicken	3	0.09	17	87	8	0.03	0.27	10
coconut milk	7	0.51	34	96	1	0.02	0.23	30
fried	6	2.15	41	126	7	0.02	0.14	35
regular, raw	52	7.98	213	8	0	0.30	2.01	2
regular, cooked	23	2.25	80	4	0	0.19	0.94	2
parboiled, dry	112	6.60	222	9	0	0.65	1.77	1
parboiled, cooked	33	1.97	66	6	0	0.03	0.53	2
precooked or instant, dry	17	3.98	17	6	0	0.04	0.92	1
precooked or instant, prepared	13	1.04	7	4	0	0.30	0.40	2
Kraft® rice & cheese								
broccoli & cheddar			200	840	10			30
cheddar & chicken			280	1180	10			24
cheddar pilaf			280	1300	10			24
Rice, white, medium-grain								
raw	17	8.50	167	2	0	0.28	2.26	1
cooked	7	3.06	60	1	0	0.10	0.86	1
Rice, white, short-grain								
raw	7	8.46	153	2	0	0.34	2.20	1
cooked	2	2.99	54	1	0	0.12	0.82	1
Rice, white, glutinous								
raw	20	2.96	142	13	0	0.20	2.21	1
cooked	4	0.34	24	13	0	0.06	0.98	2
Rice, white, w, pasta & seasonings								
dry	75	6.48	341	3041	4	0.24	1.97	6
cooked	15	1.90	85	1147	1	0.20	0.56	21
Rice bran, crude	47	15.38	1232	4	0	3.38	5.02	59
Rice flour								
brown	18	3.13	456	12	0	1.16	3.87	7
white	16	0.55	120	1	0	0.69	1.26	3
Rye	56	4.51	446	10	0	0.50	6.30	7
Rye flour								
dark	72	8.26	934	2	0	0.57	7.19	7
light	21	1.84	238	2	0	0.24	1.78	3
medium	24	2.16	347	3	0	0.27	2.03	4
Semolina	29	7.28	311	2	0	0.17	1.75	3
Sorghum	54	8.45	672		0			9
Tapioca, pearl, dry	31	2.40	17	1	0	0.01	0.18	0
Triticale	72	4.93	637	10	0	0.27	6.63	6
Triticale flour, whole-grain	45	3.37	605	3	0	0.52	3.46	5
Wheat								
hard red spring	48	6.92	653	4	0	0.65	5.34	5
hard red winter	56	6.12	697	4	0	0.58	5.08	4
soft red winter	46	5.39	667	4	0	0.46	4.41	4
hard white	62	8.76	829		0	0.71	6.39	5

CEREAL GRAINS & PASTA

FOOD	AMOUNT	CALORIES (kcal)	PROTEIN (g)	FAT (g)	SATU- RATED FAT (g)	CARBO- HYDRATES (g)	FIBER (g)
CEREAL GRAINS (continued)							
Wheat (continued)							
soft white	1 cup	571	17.96	3.34	0.62	127	
durum	1 cup	650	26.27	4.73	0.87	137	
Wheat bran, crude	½ cup	65	4.67	1.28	0.19	19	2.16
Wheat germ							
crude	1 cup	414	26.62	11.18	1.91	60	3.24
toasted	1 cup	431	32.90	12.10	2.07	56	2.60
Wheat flour							
whole-grain	1 cup	407	16.44	2.24	0.39	87	2.52
white, all-purpose	1 cup	455	12.91	1.22	0.19	95	0.31
white, bread	1 cup	495	16.42	2.27	0.34	99	
white, cake	1 cup	395	8.94	0.94	0.14	85	
white, self-rising	1 cup	442	12.36	1.21	0.19	93	0.28
white, tortilla mix	1 cup	449	10.72	11.80	4.55	75	0.20
Wheat, sprouted	1 cup	214	8.09	1.37	0.22	46	
Wild rice							
raw	1 cup	571	23.57	1.72	0.25	120	2.31
cooked	1 cup	166	6.54	0.56	0.08	35	0.54
PASTA							
Amaranth, 100% organic, Health Valley®	28.35 g	85	3.49	0.50		16	4.39
Agnolotti, fresh, Contadina®	85 g	270	13.00	7.00	2.00	38	
Cannelloni							
Bernardi® beef	1 oz	70	4.00	4.00		5	0.24
Chef Boyardee® mini	1 serving	230	9.00	7.00	1.00	33	5.00
Lean Cuisine®							
beef & pork	1 serving	260	17.00	10.00	4.00	32	2.29
cheese sauce	1 item	270	23.00	8.00		27	
cheese, tomato	1 serving	260	21.00	10.00	5.00	22	1.32
Corn							
dry	1 cup	375	7.83	2.18	0.31	83	
cooked	1 cup	176	3.68	1.03	0.14	39	
Fettuccine, cooked	1 cup	176	3.68	1.03		39	
Bernardi® raw	1 oz	80	3.00	1.00		15	
Budget Gourmet® chicken	1 serving	400	23.00	21.00		29	
Healthy Choice® alfredo	1 item	240	10.00	7.00		36	1.31
alfredo, quick meal	1 serving	240	10.00	7.00		36	
beef & broccoli	1 item	290	19.00	3.00		46	
chicken entree	1 item	240	22.00	4.00		29	
Lean Cuisine®							
alfredo	1 item	280	14.00	7.00		41	
primavera	1 item	260	14.00	8.00		32	
Stouffers® alfredo, frozen	1 item	270	8.00	18.00		19	
Ultra Slim Fast® chicken	1 item	400	31.00	10.00		46	6.45
Fresh-refrigerated, plain							
as purchased	4.5 oz	368	14.48	2.94	0.42	70	
cooked	2 oz	75	2.94	0.60	0.09	14	

FOOD	CALCIUM (mg)	IRON (mg)	POTAS-SIUM (mg)	SODIUM (mg)	CHOLES-TEROL (mg)	VITAMIN B6 (mg)	ZINC (mg)	% OF CALORIES FROM FAT
CEREAL GRAINS (continued)								
Wheat (continued)								
soft white	57	9.02	730		0	0.63	5.82	5
durum	66	6.75	827	3	0	0.81	7.98	7
Wheat bran, crude	22	3.17	355	1	0	0.39	2.18	18
Wheat germ								
crude	44	7.20	1026	14	0	1.50	14.13	24
toasted	50	10.28	1070	4	0	1.11	18.83	25
Wheat flour								
whole-grain	40	4.66	486	6	0	0.41	3.52	5
white, all-purpose	18	5.80	134	2	0	0.06	0.88	2
white, bread	21	6.04	136	2		0.05	1.17	4
white, cake	16	7.98	115	2	0	0.04	0.67	2
white, self-rising	422	5.84	155	1587	0	0.06	0.78	2
white, tortilla mix	228	7.83	111	751	0	0.04		24
Wheat, sprouted	30	2.32	182	18	0	0.29	1.79	6
Wild rice								
raw	34	3.13	683	12	0	0.63	9.53	3
cooked	5	0.99	166	6	0	0.22	2.20	3
PASTA								
Amaranth, 100% organic, Health Valley®	100	1.35	120	5	0	0.08	0.60	5
Agnolotti, fresh, Contadina®	158	1.80	150	230	40	0.03	0.75	23
Cannelloni								
Bernardi® beef	40	0.36	50	110	15	0.03	0.35	51
Chef Boyardee® mini	20	1.80	197	1050	14	0.12	1.31	27
Lean Cuisine®								
beef & pork	200	1.44	400	950	45			35
cheese sauce	300	0.72	400	590	25			27
cheese, tomato	300	0.72	330	910	35	0.15	1.60	35
Corn								
dry	4	0.98	309	3	0	0.22	1.88	5
cooked	2	0.34	43	1	0	0.08	0.88	5
Fettuccine, cooked	2	0.34	43	1	0			5
Bernardi® raw	0	0.36	50	5	5			11
Budget Gourmet® chicken	200	1.80		740	100			47
Healthy Choice® alfredo	127	1.70	70	370	45	0.13	0.87	26
alfredo, quick meal	100	1.80	70	460	45			26
beef & broccoli	20	1.08	360	520	20			9
chicken entree	80	1.80	190	370	45			15
Lean Cuisine®								
alfredo	250	1.44	270	570	15			23
primavera	300	1.44	400	510	45			28
Stouffers® alfredo, frozen			240	1195				60
Ultra Slim Fast® chicken	117	2.82	300	780	60	0.47	2.74	23
Fresh-refrigerated, plain								
as purchased	19	4.29	229	33	93	0.12	1.56	7
cooked	4	0.65	14	3	19	0.02	0.32	7

FOOD	AMOUNT	CALORIES (kcal)	PROTEIN (g)	FAT (g)	SATU- RATED FAT (g)	CARBO- HYDRATES (g)	FIBER (g
PASTA (continued)							
Fettuccine (continued)							
Fresh-refrigerated, spinach							
as purchased	4.5 oz	370	14.41	2.69	0.62	71	
cooked	2 oz	74	2.88	0.54	0.12	14	
Contadina®	85 g	260	12.00	4.00	1.00	45	
Homemade							
w/ egg, cooked	2 oz	74	3.01	0.99	0.23	13	0.00
w/out egg, cooked	2 oz	71	2.49	0.56	0.08	14	0.00
Gnocchi, potato dumplings, raw, Bernardi®	1 oz	60	3.00	0.00		13	0.28
Lasagna							
Bernardi®							
pasta sheets	1 oz	60	2.00	1.00		11	1.11
pasta sheets, wavy	1 oz	60	2.00	1.00		11	1.11
meat	1 oz	45	3.00	3.00		4	0.38
meat, pre-portioned	1 oz	45	3.00	3.00		4	0.38
solito	1 oz	45	3.00	2.00		4	0.43
supreme	1 oz	50	3.00	3.00		3	0.38
vegetable	1 oz	50	3.00	2.00		4	0.46
Budget Gourmet®							
3 cheese	1 serving	400	22.00	17.00	6.09	38	3.40
sausage	1 serving	284	20.00	20.00	8.96	38	3.82
Budget Gourmet Light®							
cheese, vegetable	1 item	290	15.00	9.00		36	4.82
meat sauce	1 item	300	18.00	13.00		28	3.24
Chef Boyardee® 7.5 oz	1 serving	240	8.00	8.00	5.13	31	3.19
Healthy Choice®							
meat sauce, entree	1 item	260	18.00	5.00		37	
zucchini, quick meal	1 item	250	14.00	3.00		41	
Lean Cuisine®							
meat w/sauce	1 serving	270	25.00	8.00	3.00	24	3.49
zucchini	1 item	260	20.00	7.00		28	
Le Menu®							
garden vegetable light	1 oz	25	1.05	0.76		3	
light	1 serving	290	19.00	8.00		36	1.82
meat sauce, light	1 serving	29	1.90	0.80		4	0.35
vegetable, frozen dinner	1 item	400	15.00	24.00	9.39	30	5.05
Light & Elegant® Florentine	1 item	280	24.00	5.00		34	
Mrs. Paul's® seafood, light	1 oz	31	1.47	0.84		4	
Stouffer® frozen dinner	1 item	385	28.00	14.00		36	
fiesta	1 serving	430	24.00	22.00		35	3.49
vegetable	1 serving	420	23.00	24.00		29	4.82
Swanson's® meat sauce, home-style	1 oz	38	2.48	1.43		4	0.35
Lasagna, spinach, Lean Cuisine® w/tuna	1 serving	270	17.00	10.00	2.00	29	2.20
Lasagna, whole wheat/germ, Health Valley®	1 oz	85	4.49	0.50	0.32	20	3.57

Food	CALCIUM (mg)	IRON (mg)	POTAS-SIUM (mg)	SODIUM (mg)	CHOLES-TEROL (mg)	VITAMIN B6 (mg)	ZINC (mg)	% OF CALORIES FROM FAT
PASTA (continued)								
Fettuccine (continued)								
Fresh-refrigerated, spinach								
as purchased	55	4.22	348	35	93	0.40	1.79	7
cooked	10	0.63	21	3	19	0.07	0.36	7
Contadina®	60	3.60	350	70	80	0.10	1.09	14
Homemade								
w/ egg, cooked	6	0.66	12	47	23	0.02	0.25	12
w/out egg, cooked	3	0.64	11	42	0	0.02	0.21	7
Gnocchi, potato dumplings, raw, Bernardi®	0	0.36	135	15	0	0.03	0.07	0
Lasagna								
Bernardi®								
pasta sheets	0	0.36	35	5	0	0.01	0.18	15
pasta sheets, wavy	0	0.36	35	5	0	0.01	0.18	15
meat	40	0.00	80	95	10	0.03	0.37	60
meat, pre-portioned	40	0.00	80	95	10	0.03	0.37	60
solito	40	0.36	95	95	10	0.03	0.22	40
supreme	40	0.00	70	95	10	0.03	0.37	54
vegetable	60	0.00	50	0	10	0.03	0.13	36
Budget Gourmet®								
3 cheese	500	2.70	437	760	65	0.16	1.84	38
sausage	400	2.70	591	950	80	0.28	3.74	63
Budget Gourmet Light®								
cheese, vegetable	283	3.03	420	780	15	0.32	1.39	28
meat sauce	208	2.82	400	760	40	0.28	2.85	39
Chef Boyardee® 7.5 oz	0	1.80	414	1010	18			30
Healthy Choice®								
meat sauce, entree	100	2.70	500	420	20			17
zucchini, quick meal	250	2.70	830	400	15			11
Lean Cuisine®								
meat w/sauce	200	1.80	550	970	60	0.29	2.71	27
zucchini			570	1050	20			24
Le Menu®								
garden vegetable light	14	0.17		48	2			28
light	195	2.39	518	510	30			25
meat sauce, light	15	0.36	66	51	3	0.03	3.04	25
vegetable, frozen dinner	296	3.18	519	1135	39	0.34	1.45	54
Light & Elegant® Florentine	280	3.60	720	975				16
Mrs. Paul's® seafood, light	26	0.15		79	6			25
Stouffer® frozen dinner	410	3.15	580	1200				33
fiesta	250	1.80	520	960	50	0.16	1.88	46
vegetable	600	1.08	380	970	37	0.32	1.39	51
Swanson's® meat sauce, home-style	48	0.26	66	102	5	0.03	0.30	34
Lasagna, spinach, Lean Cuisine® w/tuna	250	1.44	440	890	35			33
Lasagna, whole wheat/germ, Health Valley®	10	2.25	120	5	0	0.03	0.23	5

CEREAL GRAINS & PASTA

FOOD	AMOUNT	CALORIES (kcal)	PROTEIN (g)	FAT (g)	SATU- RATED FAT (g)	CARBO- HYDRATES (g)	FIBER (g)
PASTA (continued)							
Linguini							
Budget Gourmet Light® scallops, clams	1 item	290	15.00	11.00		32	3.62
Linguini (continued)							
Healthy Choice® shrimp, tomato	1 item	230	12.00	2.00		40	3.54
Lean Cuisine® clam sauce	1 item	280	17.00	8.00		36	
Stouffer® clam sauce, dinner	1 item	285	17.00	8.00		36	
Macaroni							
dry	1 cup	389	13.42	1.66	0.24	78	0.28
cooked	1 cup	197	6.67	0.93	0.13	40	0.13
cheese, baked, home recipe	1 cup	430	16.80	22.20		40	
cheese, canned	1 cup	228	9.36	9.60		26	
cheese, canned, enriched	1 cup	230	9.00	10.00		26	1.44
cheese, enriched, home recipe	1 cup	430	17.00	22.00		40	1.20
Chef Boyardee® macaroni shells	1 serving	150	6.00	1.00	0.33	31	1.69
Franco American® cheese	1 oz	23	0.81	0.81	0.41	3	0.26
Healthy Choice®							
beef, quick meal	1 item	200	12.00	3.00		32	
cheese, quick meal	1 item	280	12.00	6.00		45	
nacho cheese, quick meal	1 item	280	13.00	5.00		44	
Lean Cuisine® cheese	1 item	290	15.00	9.00		37	
Light & Elegant® macaroni & cheese	1 item	300	15.00	9.00		37	
Microquick® cheese	1 serving	200	5.00	9.00		23	1.00
Stouffers®							
beef & tomatoes	1 serving	170	11.00	7.00		15	
cheese	1 serving	250	12.00	13.00		22	2.12
Swanson's®							
beef dinner	1 oz	31	1.00	1.25		4	0.16
cheese dinner	1 oz	30	1.06	1.22		4	0.26
cheese, home-style	1 oz	39	1.70	1.90		4	0.26
cheese potpie	1 oz	29	1.00	1.14		3	0.40
Macaroni, protein-fortified							
dry	1 cup	348	18.47	2.07	0.31	63	0.79
cooked	1 cup	188	9.29	0.25	0.04	36	0.29
Macaroni, vegetable (tricolor type which contains spinach & tomato powders)							
dry	1 cup	308	11.04	0.88	0.13	63	
cooked	1 cup	171	6.07	0.14	0.02	36	
Macaroni, whole-wheat							
dry	1 cup	365	15.37	1.47	0.27	79	3.13
cooked	1 cup	174	7.46	0.75	0.14	37	1.39
Manicotti							
Bernardi®							
4.25" cheese	1 oz	50	3.00	2.00		5	0.16
5" cheese	1 oz	50	3.00	2.00		5	0.16
Budget Gourmet® cheese, meat	1 serving	450	20.00	26.00	11.10	33	2.39
Healthy Choice® cheese	1 item	220	15.00	3.00		34	

FOOD	CALCIUM (mg)	IRON (mg)	POTAS-SIUM (mg)	SODIUM (mg)	CHOLES-TEROL (mg)	VITAMIN B6 (mg)	ZINC (mg)	% OF CALORIES FROM FAT
PASTA (continued)								
Linguini								
Budget Gourmet Light® scallops, clams	173	21.40	270	710	45	0.49	2.53	34
Linguini (continued)								
Healthy Choice® shrimp, tomato	93	13.20	280	390	55	0.24	2.05	8
Lean Cuisine® clam sauce	40	2.70	90	560	30			26
Stouffer® clam sauce, dinner			115	1010				25
Macaroni								
dry	19	4.05	170	8	0	0.11	1.27	4
cooked	10	1.96	44	1	0	0.05	0.74	4
cheese, baked, home recipe	362	1.60	240	1086	68			46
cheese, canned	199	0.96	139	730	24			38
cheese, canned, enriched	199	1.00	139	729	42			39
cheese, enriched, home recipe	362	1.80	240	1086	42			46
Chef Boyardee® macaroni shells	0	1.44	129	930	0	0.15	0.83	6
Franco American® cheese	11	0.15	38	118	6	0.02	0.27	32
Healthy Choice®								
beef, quick meal	40	1.80	530	420	15			14
cheese, quick meal	150	1.80	220	520	20			19
nacho cheese, quick meal	200	1.44	420	560	20			16
Lean Cuisine® cheese	250	1.44	160	550	30			28
Light & Elegant® macaroni & cheese	238	2.00	210	1015				27
Microquick® cheese	241	1.47	150	690	4	0.08	1.32	41
Stouffers®								
beef & tomatoes	40	1.44	300	810				37
cheese	250	0.36	140	730	16	0.12	0.91	47
Swanson's®								
beef dinner	8	0.15	53	78	13	0.05	0.65	37
cheese dinner	20	0.22	38	87	6,016		0.27	36
cheese, home-style	45	0.18	38	115	6	0.02	0.27	44
cheese potpie	21	0.15	43	106	16	0.03	0.18	36
Macaroni, protein-fortified								
dry	36	3.86	187	8	0	0.17	1.67	5
cooked	12	0.83	48	6	0	0.07	0.58	1
Macaroni, vegetable (tricolor type which contains spinach & tomato powders)								
dry	29	3.60	240	36	0	0.11	0.64	3
cooked	15	0.66	42	9	0	0.03	0.58	1
Macaroni, whole-wheat								
dry	42	3.81	226	8	0	0.23	2.49	4
cooked	21	1.49	61	4	0	0.11	1.13	4
Manicotti								
Bernardi®								
4.25" cheese	20	0.00	30	80	15	0.01	0.30	36
5" cheese	20	0.00	30	80	15	0.01	0.30	36
Budget Gourmet® cheese, meat	450	2.70	484	920	50	0.23	2.29	52
Healthy Choice® cheese	150	2.70	590	310	30			12

CEREAL GRAINS & PASTA

FOOD	AMOUNT	CALORIES (kcal)	PROTEIN (g)	FAT (g)	SATU-RATED FAT (g)	CARBO-HYDRATES (g)	FIBER (g)
PASTA (continued)							
Manicotti (continued)							
Le Menu® cheese, frozen dinner	1 item	310	18.00	13.00		29	1.90
3 cheeses	1 oz	33	1.62	1.28		4	0.16
Noodles, egg	1 cup						
dry	1 cup	145	5.33	1.60	0.34	27	0.13
chicken, home recipe	1 cup	365	22.00	18.00		26	1.30
cooked	1 cup	212	7.59	2.35	0.50	40	0.20
Bernardi® home-style, raw	1 oz	80	3.00	1.00		15	
Budget Gourmet Light® beef Stroganoff	1 item	290	19.00	12.00		27	1.30
Le Menu® beef Stroganoff	1 oz	43	2.60	2.40		3	0.15
Light & Elegant® beef Stroganoff dinner	1 item	260	24.00	6.00		27	1.34
Stouffers®							
beef Stroganoff	1 serving	390	24.00	20.00	8.35	28	1.78
chicken, home-style	1 serving	310	23.00	15.00		21	2.38
meatballs & noodles	1 item	475	25.00	27.00		33	
Romanoff, frozen dinner	1 item	170	6.00	9.00		16	
tuna noodle casserole, dinner	1 item	200	10.00	9.00		18	0.49
Swanson's® chicken dinner	1 oz	27	0.67	0.76		4	
Noodles, egg, spinach							
dry	1 cup	145	5.55	1.73	0.40	27	
cooked	1 cup	211	8.06	2.51	0.58	39	
Noodles, Chinese							
cellophane or long rice, dehydrated	1 cup	492	0.22	0.08	0.02	121	0.09
chow mein	1 cup	237	3.77	13.84	1.97	26	
La Choy ® chow mein, canned	1 cup	300	6.00	16.00	2.59	32	1.70
meatless	1 cup	69	2.40	0.30		15	0.21
rice noodles	1 cup	260	4.00	8.00	1.21	42	1.14
vegetable, frozen	1 cup	135	4.20	4.80		22	0.63
Noodles, chicken chow mein							
canned	1 cup	95	7.00	0.00		18	0.90
home recipe	1 cup	255	31.00	10.00		10	0.50
Healthy Choice®	1 item	249	20.00	5.00		29	
La Choy® frozen	1 cup	228	17.70	9.00		19	0.45
canned	1 cup	132	6.90	5.70		15	0.63
Lean Cuisine® dinner	1 item	250	14.00	5.00		36	
Le Menu® light	1 serving	260	18.00	4.00		37	1.45
Noodles, Japanese							
soba, dry	8 oz	764	32.64	1.61	0.31	169	
soba, cooked	1 cup	113	5.77	0.11	0.02	24	
somen, dry	8 oz	809	25.76	1.83	0.26	168	0.82
somen, cooked	1 cup	230	7.04	0.31	0.04	48	0.40
Pasta							
Chef Boyardee®							
ABC's & 123's in sauce	1 serving	160	5.00	1.00	0.33	31	3.00
ABC's & 123's, meatballs	1 serving	240	8.00	9.00	2.07	33	
beef-o-getti	1 serving	220	7.00	9.00		27	
beef-a-roni	1 serving	220	8.00	8.00		29	

FOOD	CALCIUM (mg)	IRON (mg)	POTAS-SIUM (mg)	SODIUM (mg)	CHOLES-TEROL (mg)	VITAMIN B6 (mg)	ZINC (mg)	% OF CALORIES FROM FAT
PASTA (continued)								
Manicotti (continued)								
Le Menu® cheese, frozen dinner	348	2.99	434	840	146	0.22	2.68	38
3 cheeses	43	0.23	26	74	24	0.01	0.30	35
Noodles, egg								
dry	12	1.73	89	8	36	0.05	0.61	10
chicken, home recipe	26	2.20	149	600	96			44
cooked	19	2.55	45	11	53	0.06	1.00	10
Bernardi® home-style, raw	0	0.36	50	5	5			11
Budget Gourmet Light® beef Stroganoff	90	3.51	280	570	85			37
Le Menu® beef Stroganoff	10	0.27	61	98	9			50
Light & Elegant® beef Stroganoff dinner	45	3.00	230	785	84			21
Stouffers®								
beef Stroganoff	60	2.70	300	1090	78			46
chicken, home-style	150	1.08	430	1090	50			44
meatballs & noodles			395	1620				51
Romanoff, frozen dinner	88	0.80	95	675				48
tuna noodle casserole, dinner	98	1.15	210	670				41
Swanson's® chicken dinner	8	0.14		71				26
Noodles, egg, spinach								
dry	21	1.60	135	27	36	0.16	0.69	11
cooked	30	1.74	59	20	52	0.18	1.01	11
Noodles, Chinese								
cellophane or long rice, dehydrated	35	3.03	14	14	0			0
chow mein	9	2.13	54	197	0	0.05	0.63	53
La Choy ® chow mein, canned	12	1.98	41	440	0	0.05	0.62	48
meatless	41	10.50	219	999	0	0.24	3.27	4
rice noodles	9	0.19	14	820	0	0.02	0.20	28
vegetable, frozen	36			768	0			32
Noodles, chicken chow mein								
canned	45	1.30	418	722	98			0
home recipe	58	2.50	473	717	98			35
Healthy Choice®	20	1.44	290	530	45			18
La Choy® frozen	37			360	47			36
canned	48	3.15	491	999	18	0.44	2.38	39
Lean Cuisine® dinner			270	1030	25			18
Le Menu® light	38	2.48	274	830	50			14
Noodles, Japanese								
soba, dry	80	6.13	571	1798	0	0.55	3.88	2
soba, cooked	4	0.55	40	68	0	0.05	0.14	1
somen, dry	52	2.99	373	4177	0	0.11	1.03	2
somen, cooked	14	0.92	51	284	0	0.02	0.39	1
Pasta								
Chef Boyardee®								
ABC's & 123's in sauce	0	1.44	341	830	2	0.18	0.64	6
ABC's & 123's, meatballs	0	1.80		920	18	0.17	1.68	34
beef-o-getti	0	1.80		1240	20			37
beef-a-roni	0	1.80		1070	19			33

CEREAL GRAINS & PASTA

FOOD	AMOUNT	CALORIES (kcal)	PROTEIN (g)	FAT (g)	SATU-RATED FAT (g)	CARBO-HYDRATES (g)	FIBER (g)
PASTA (continued)							
dinosaurs, 7.5 oz	1 serving	160	4.00	1.00	0.33	33	3.00
dinosaurs, mini meatballs	1 serving	230	7.00	8.00	3.91	32	1.75
mini bites	1 serving	260	8.00	12.00	2.00	30	1.00
pac man, chicken sauce	1 serving	170	6.00	7.00		22	
pac man, tomato sauce	1 serving	150	6.00	1.00	0.33	30	
pac man, meatballs	1 serving	230	7.00	9.00	3.00	32	5.00
roller coaster	1 serving	230	7.00	10.00	3.00	28	3.00
sharks	1 serving	170	5.00	1.00	0.33	34	
sharks, meatballs	1 serving	230	8.00	7.00	3.42	32	1.75
smurf	1 serving	150	6.00	1.00		29	3.00
smurf, meatballs	1 serving	240	8.00	9.00	2.00	31	2.00
tic tac toes, 7.5 oz	1 serving	160	5.00	1.00	0.33	31	3.00
tic tac toes, meatballs	1 serving	240	8.00	9.00		31	
zooroni, meatballs	1 serving	240	8.00	8.00		33	
Franco American®							
circus-o's, cheese sauce	1 oz	23	0.68	0.27	0.16	4	0.35
circus-o's, meatballs	1 oz	29	1.22	1.08	0.47	3	0.40
sporty-o's, cheese	1 oz	23	0.67	0.27		4	
sporty-o's, meatballs, sauce	1 oz	29	1.22	1.08	0.47	3	0.40
teddy-o's, cheese sauce	1 oz	23	0.67	0.27	0.15	4	0.35
teddy-o's, meatballs	1 oz	29	1.22	1.08		3	
Healthy Choice®							
chicken cacciatore	1 item	310	26.00	3.00		47	
chicken stir fry	1 item	300	23.00	5.00		42	
chicken teriyaki	1 item	350	24.00	3.00		58	
Italiano	1 item	350	16.00	5.00		59	
Italiano, quick meal	1 item	220	7.00	1.00		46	
primavera dinner	1 serving	280	11.00	3.00		51	2.30
shrimp & vegetables	1 item	270	16.00	4.00		44	
Kraft® pasta & cheese							
cheddar, broccoli	1 cup	720	24.00	32.00		76	0.91
fettucine alfredo	1 cup	180	7.00	9.00		19	0.92
herb & garlic	1 cup	360	12.00	16.00		38	0.93
Parmesan	1 cup	360	12.00	16.00		38	0.91
vegetable, 3 cheese	1 cup	360	12.00	16.00		38	3.67
Lean Cuisine® angel hair	1 item	240	10.00	5.00		38	
Light Balance®							
beef Bordeaux	1 item	180	12.00	1.00		31	1.50
garden vegetable	1 item	190	6.00	1.00		41	5.38
Pasta Perfect® bowties, vegetables	1 cup	220	10.00	2.00		38	
Right Course® beef dijon, vegetables	1 serving	290	20.00	9.00	2.00	31	
Stouffers®							
carbonara	1 serving	620	19.00	45.00	5.50	34	3.84
casino	1 serving	300	9.00	10.00	2.67	44	1.94
Mexicali	1 serving	490	16.00	31.00		36	
Oriental	1 serving	300	8.00	14.00	0.43	35	10.90
primavera	1 serving	270	7.00	21.00	0.23	13	5.89
Ultra Slim Fast® primavera	1 item	340	18.00	9.00		52	4.21

FOOD	CALCIUM (mg)	IRON (mg)	POTAS-SIUM (mg)	SODIUM (mg)	CHOLES-TEROL (mg)	VITAMIN B6 (mg)	ZINC (mg)	% OF CALORIES FROM FAT
PASTA (continued)								
dinosaurs, 7.5 oz	20	1.08		790	1			6
dinosaurs, mini meatballs	0	1.80	326	960	19	0.26	3.46	31
mini bites	20	1.80		1020	17			42
pac man, chicken sauce	0	1.44		905				37
pac man, tomato sauce	20	1.08		830	2			6
pac man, meatballs	0	1.44		880	17			35
roller coaster	0	1.80		1070	19			39
sharks	20	1.08		780	2			5
sharks, meatballs	0	1.80	326	890	15	0.26	3.46	27
smurf	20	1.44		830	2			6
smurf, meatballs	0	1.08	707	900	19	0.35	5.47	34
tic tac toes, 7.5 oz	0	1.08		870	1			6
tic tac toes, meatballs	0	2.00		1000	18			34
zooroni, meatballs	0	1.80		970	17			30
Franco American®								
circus-o's, cheese sauce	3	0.15	45	117	1	0.02	0.11	11
circus-o's, meatballs	3	0.24	79	129	13	0.05	0.82	34
sporty-o's, cheese	3	0.14		115				11
sporty-o's, meatballs, sauce	3	0.24	79	129	13	0.05	0.82	34
teddy-o's, cheese sauce	5	0.19	45	120	1	0.02	0.11	11
teddy-o's, meatballs	3	0.24		129				34
Healthy Choice®								
chicken cacciatore	40	2.70	660	430	35			9
chicken stir fry	20	0.72	290	550	30			15
chicken teriyaki	60	2.70	390	370	45			8
Italiano	60	3.60	540	530	30			13
Italiano, quick meal	40	4.50	380	330				4
primavera dinner	53	369	340	360	15	0.11	1.55	10
shrimp & vegetables	60	1.80	320	490	50			13
Kraft® pasta & cheese								
cheddar, broccoli	69	1.63	440	2480	120			40
fettucine alfredo	70	1.65	85	590	30			45
herb & garlic	71	1.67	200	1100	60			40
Parmesan	69	1.63	220	1260	60			40
vegetable, 3 cheese	150	1.95	240	1260	50	0.17	0.95	40
Lean Cuisine® angel hair	100	2.70	500	410	10			19
Light Balance®								
beef Bordeaux	15	1.80	462	660	25			5
garden vegetable	53	1.80	415	650	0	0.24	0.92	5
Pasta Perfect® bowties, vegetables	40	2.88	340	110	0			8
Right Course® beef dijon, vegetables	40	2.70	270	580	40			28
Stouffers®								
carbonara	300	1.08	280	780	127	0.29	1.88	65
casino	80	1.80	260	800	19	0.09	1.31	30
Mexicali	300	1.80	280	1020				57
Oriental	40	1.80	180	760	0	0.06	1.73	42
primavera	150	0.36	150	580	0	0.03	0.93	70
Ultra Slim Fast® primavera	122	3.29	440	730	25	0.29	1.30	24

FOOD	AMOUNT	CALORIES (kcal)	PROTEIN (g)	FAT (g)	SATU-RATED FAT (g)	CARBO-HYDRATES (g)	FIBER (g)
PASTA (continued)							
Ravioli							
Bernardi®							
beef, meat sauce	1 oz	60	3.00	2.00		7	·0.30
beef, jumbo round	1 oz	60	3.00	2.00		7	
beef, red sauce	1 oz	60	2.00	2.00		8	0.30
beef, square	1 oz	60	3.00	2.00		7	0.21
breaded beef	1 oz	60	3.00	2.00		8	
breaded, espanol	1 oz	60	2.00	2.00		8	0.24
cheese, jumbo round	1 oz	50	3.00	2.00		6	0.19
cheese, square	1 oz	50	3.00	2.00		6	0.19
Chef Boyardee®							
beef ravioli, meat sauce	1 serving	220	8.00	5.00	1.95	35	2.27
beef ravioli, sauce, 8 oz	1 serving	220	8.00	5.00	1.95	35	2.42
cheese, beef sauce	1 serving	200	7.00	3.00	1.42	34	1.78
cheese, sauce	1 serving	200	7.00	5.00	1.00	33	4.00
chicken	1 serving	180	7.00	4.00		29	
mini ravioli, beef, 7.5 oz	1 serving	210	7.00	5.00	2.20	31	1.54
mini ravioli, chicken	1 serving	220	7.00	8.00		29	
smurf ravioli, sauce	1 serving	230	9.00	5.00		38	6.34
Contadina®							
beef, fresh	1 serving	270	13.00	11.00	6.00	30	
cheese, fresh	1 serving	270	13.00	11.00	3.00	30	
chicken, fresh	1 serving	260	11.00	10.00	2.00	32	
Franco American®							
ravioli-o's, canned, meat sauce	1 oz	28	1.14	0.57		4	0.23
raviolios, beef, meat sauce	1 oz	33	1.33	1.07		5	
Healthy Choice® cheese	1 serving	250	14.00	2.00		44	
Lean Cuisine® cheese w/tomato sauce	1 item	240	13.00	8.00		30	
Ravioletti, Bernardi®							
beef, square	1 oz	60	3.00	2.00		10	
cheese, square	1 oz	70	3.00	3.00		8	0.19
spinach, square	1 oz	70	3.00	3.00		8	0.25
Rigatoni							
Contadina® fresh	65.2 g	200	9.00	3.00	0.50	34	
Healthy Choice®							
chicken & vegetables	1 item	360	31.00	4.00		50	
meat sauce quick meal	1 item	260	16.00	6.00		34	
Lean Cuisine® meat sauce, cheese	1 serving	260	18.00	10.00	3.00	25	
Rotini							
Bernardi®							
veggie	1 oz	50	2.00	1.00		9	
wheat	1 oz	40	2.00	0.00		8	
Mrs. Paul's® seafood light	1 oz	27	1.33	0.67		4	
Pasta Perfect®							
spinach, vegetables	1 cup	200	8.00	0.00	0.00	38	
vegetables	1 cup	220	10.00	2.00	0.12	40	5.22
Ultra Slim Fast® chicken, vegetables	1 item	310	25.00	3.00		49	5.08

FOOD	CALCIUM (mg)	IRON (mg)	POTAS-SIUM (mg)	SODIUM (mg)	CHOLES-TEROL (mg)	VITAMIN B6 (mg)	ZINC (mg)	% OF CALORIES FROM FAT
PASTA (continued)								
Ravioli								
Bernardi®								
beef, meat sauce	0	0.36	50	105	15	0.03	0.38	30
beef, jumbo round	20	0.36	35	105	30			30
beef, red sauce	0	0.36	45	55	10	0.03	0.38	30
beef, square	20	0.36	35	105	30	0.04	0.63	30
breaded beef	0	0.36	35	310	25			30
breaded, espanol	20	0.36	30	310	15	0.02	0.24	30
cheese, jumbo round	40	0.36	30	75	15	0.01	0.23	36
cheese, square	40	0.36	30	75	15	0.01	0.23	36
Chef Boyardee®								
beef ravioli, meat sauce	0	1.80	437	1120	15	0.25	2.84	20
beef ravioli, sauce, 8 oz	0	1.80	465	1190	15	0.26	3.02	20
cheese, beef sauce	20	1.80	352	1205	11	0.18	1.83	14
cheese, sauce	60	1.80	337	990	5	0.16	1.22	23
chicken	60	1.80		1100	13			20
mini ravioli, beef, 7.5 oz	0	1.80	327	1140	12	0.27	4.70	21
mini ravioli, chicken	40	1.80		1090				33
smurf ravioli, sauce	0	2.70	407	1160	11	0.23	2.45	20
Contadina®								
beef, fresh	40	2.70	200	250	75	0.11	2.21	37
cheese, fresh	200	1.44	160	360	75	0.03	0.82	37
chicken, fresh	20	1.80	150	310	80	0.09	0.88	35
Franco American®								
ravioli-o's, canned, meat sauce	5	0.31	46	131				19
raviolios, beef, meat sauce	3	0.24		123				29
Healthy Choice® cheese	250	2.70	590	420	20			7
Lean Cuisine® cheese w/tomato sauce	200	1.44	380	590	55			30
Ravioletti, Bernardi®								
beef, square	0	0.36	35	120	20			30
cheese, square	40	0.36	25	100	15	0.01	0.23	39
spinach, square	40	0.36	25	100	15	0.02	0.23	39
Rigatoni								
Contadina® fresh	20	1.80	115	25	85	0.03	7.11	14
Healthy Choice®								
chicken & vegetables	100	1.80	510	430	60			10
meat sauce quick meal	150	2.70	700	540	30			21
Lean Cuisine® meat sauce, cheese	200	1.80	530	870	40			35
Rotini								
Bernardi®								
veggie	0	0.00	10	10	0			18
wheat	0	0.36	10	10	0			0
Mrs. Paul's® seafood light	22	0.20		63	2			22
Pasta Perfect®								
spinach, vegetables	0	2.16	300	30	0			0
vegetables	40	2.88	340	120	0	0.24	0.89	8
Ultra Slim Fast® chicken, vegetables	135	3.29	350	640	15	0.84	3.27	9

FOOD	AMOUNT	CALORIES (kcal)	PROTEIN (g)	FAT (g)	SATU-RATED FAT (g)	CARBO-HYDRATES (g)	FIBER (g
PASTA (continued)							
Shells							
Bernardi®							
cheese stuffed, 2¼ oz	1 oz	50	3.00	3.00		3	0.18
cheese stuffed, 3 oz	1 oz	50	3.00	3.00		3	0.18
Florentine	1 oz	40	3.00	2.00		4	
Healthy Choice® tomato sauce	1 item	330	24.00	3.00		53	
Le Menu® cheese stuffed, light	1 oz	28	1.70	0.80		3	0.18
Pasta Perfect® seashells, vegetables	1 cup	260	12.00	2.00		50	
Stouffers®							
beef & spinach	1 item	290	19.00	11.00		28	
cheese, meat sauce	1 item	320	19.00	14.00	6.58	30	1.92
cheese, tomatoes	1 item	330	17.00	15.00		32	3.24
chicken pasta, dinner	1 item	400	26.00	22.00	2.53	24	2.96
Spaghetti, dry	8 oz	842	29.02	3.59	0.51	170	0.61
canned, tomato, meat	1 cup	260	12.00	10.00		29	2.75
canned, tomato sauce, cheese	1 cup	190	6.00	2.00		39	2.50
canned, tomato sauce, meatballs	1 cup	257	12.20	10.20		29	7.75
cheese, meat	1 oz	29	3.69	0.09		3	0.26
chicken, mushroom, sauce, cheese	1 oz	25	4.71	0.06		1	0.03
cooked	1 cup	197	6.67	0.93	0.13	40	0.13
cooked, tomato sauce, meatballs	1 cup	332	18.60	11.70		39	
cooked, tomato sauce, cheese	1 cup	260	8.75	8.75		37	
shrimp, mushroom, cheese	1 oz	26	5.05	0.03		1	0.00
tomato, cheese, home recipe	1 cup	260	9.00	9.00		37	2.50
tomato, meat, home recipe	1 cup	330	19.00	12.00		39	2.73
vegetable, sauce, cheese	1 oz	28	3.80	0.11		3	0.34
Chef Boyardee®							
beef, sauce	1 serving	240	7.00	9.00	2.77	30	3.61
meatballs, 7.5 oz	1 serving	230	8.00	9.00	3.90	27	2.99
meatballs, 7.8 oz	1 serving	240	7.00	10.00		30	3.10
meatballs, 8.5 oz	1 serving	250	8.00	11.00	4.00	30	4.00
Franco American®							
meatballs, sauce	1 oz	30	1.36	1.08	0.47	4	0.40
sauce, cheese	1 oz	11	0.68	0.27		5	
spaghettio's, cheese sauce	1 oz	23	0.67	0.27		4	
spaghettio's, meatballs	1 oz	30	1.22	3.39	0.24	0	2.71
spaghettio's, sliced franks	1 oz	30	1.08	1.22	0.48	4	0.28
Health Valley® 100% organic	1 oz	85	4.49	0.50	0.02	16	3.57
Healthy Choice®							
meat sauce	1 item	310	16.00	6.00		48	3.92
meat sauce, quick meal	1 item	280	14.00	6.00		42	
turkey tetrazzini	1 item	340	23.00	6.00		49	
Lean Cuisine® beef & mushroom	1 item	280	15.00	7.00		38	
Le Menu® light	1 serving	280	12.00	6.00		45	3.49
beef sauce, light	1 oz	31	1.33	0.67		5	
Light & Elegant®	1 item	290	16.00	8.00		40	
Stouffers®							
meatballs	1 serving	380	20.00	15.00		42	
meat sauce	1 serving	370	18.00	11.00		49	

FOOD	CALCIUM (mg)	IRON (mg)	POTAS-SIUM (mg)	SODIUM (mg)	CHOLES-TEROL (mg)	VITAMIN B6 (mg)	ZINC (mg)	% OF CALORIES FROM FAT
ASTA (continued)								
hells								
Bernardi®								
cheese stuffed, 2¼ oz	60	0.00	30	95	10	0.01	0.29	54
cheese stuffed, 3 oz	60	0.00	30	95	10	0.01	0.29	54
Florentine	60	0.00	45	100	10			45
Healthy Choice® tomato sauce	400	2.70	640	470	35			8
Le Menu® cheese stuffed, light	25	0.18	26	69	3			26
Pasta Perfect® seashells, vegetables	40	3.60	400	130	0			7
Stouffers®								
beef & spinach			485	1315				34
cheese, meat sauce	146	3.44	465	1310	169	0.26	3.13	39
cheese, tomatoes	350	1.08	450	850	8	0.22	1.00	41
chicken pasta, dinner	59	3.71	350	1060	165			50
Spaghetti, dry	41	8.76	367	17	0	0.24	2.75	4
canned, tomato, meat	53	3.30	245	1220	39			35
canned, tomato sauce, cheese	40	2.80	303	955	4			9
canned, tomato sauce, meatballs	53	3.25	245	1220	23	0.88	1.37	36
cheese, meat	3	0.20	57	99	8	0.04	0.29	3
chicken, mushroom, sauce, cheese	3	0.43	17	92	3	0.03	0.29	2
cooked	10	1.96	44	1	0	0.05	0.74	4
cooked, tomato sauce, meatballs	124	3.72	665	1009	74	0.31		32
cooked, tomato sauce, cheese	80	2.25	407	955	8			30
shrimp, mushroom, cheese	3	0.37	10	77	28	0.02	0.30	1
tomato, cheese, home recipe	80	2.30	408	955	4			31
tomato, meat, home recipe	124	3.70	665	1009	75			33
vegetable, sauce, cheese	4	0.31	52	84				4
Chef Boyardee®								
beef, sauce	0	1.80	929	1120	18	0.45	2.92	34
meatballs, 7.5 oz	0	1.80	594	970	19	0.40	6.14	35
meatballs, 7.8 oz	0	1.80	616	1140	19	0.41	6.37	38
meatballs, 8.5 oz	0	1.80	672	1210	19	0.45	6.95	40
Franco American®								
meatballs, sauce	3	0.24	79	118	13	0.05	0.82	33
sauce, cheese	3	0.20		114				23
spaghettio's, cheese sauce	3	0.14		115				11
spaghettio's, meatballs	0	49.50	129	2		0.02	0.20	102
spaghettio's, sliced franks	3	0.20	49	136	3	0.03	0.18	37
Health Valley® 100% organic	10	2.25	120	5	0	0.01	0.11	5
Healthy Choice®								
meat sauce	133	4.17	510	440	15	0.44	2.87	17
meat sauce, quick meal	60	3.60	540	480	20			19
turkey tetrazzini	100	1.80	510	490	40			16
Lean Cuisine® beef & mushroom			580	1450	20			23
Le Menu® light	40	3.25	640	450	15	0.31	2.56	19
beef sauce, light	4	0.04		0	2			19
Light & Elegant®	100	6.00	273	700				25
Stouffers®								
meatballs	100	2.70	690	1510				36
meat sauce	100	2.70	690	1510				27

CEREAL GRAINS & PASTA

FOOD	AMOUNT	CALORIES (kcal)	PROTEIN (g)	FAT (g)	SATU- RATED FAT (g)	CARBO- HYDRATES (g)	FIBER (g)
PASTA (continued)							
Spaghetti (continued)							
turkey Tetrazzini	1 item	240	12.00	14.00		17	
Swanson's®							
meatballs, dinner	1 oz	31	1.12	1.36		4	0.34
meatballs, home-style	1 oz	38	1.77	1.38		5	0.40
Ultra Slim Fast® beef, mushroom	1 item	370	19.00	9.00		59	4.59
Spaghetti, protein-fortified, dry	8 oz	850	45.08	5.06	0.74	153	1.92
cooked	1 cup	229	11.31	0.30	0.04	44	0.35
Spaghetti, spinach							
dry	8 oz	845	30.32	3.57	0.51	170	7.22
cooked	1 cup	183	6.41	0.88	0.13	37	1.65
Health Valley® 100% organic	1 oz	85	4.49	0.50		16	3.57
Spaghetti, whole-wheat							
dry	8 oz	790	33.22	3.18	0.59	170	6.77
cooked	1 cup	174	7.46	0.75	0.14	37	1.39
Tortellini							
Bernardi®							
cheese	1 oz	45	2.00	1.00		7	
meat filled, frozen	1 oz	50	2.00	1.00		8	0.44
meat, raw	1 oz	80	4.00	2.00		13	0.17
meat sauce	1 oz	60	2.00	2.00		7	0.44
red sauce	1 oz	50	2.00	1.00		8	
spinach, cheese	1 oz	50	3.00	2.00		8	0.42
tomato, cheese	1 oz	60	3.00	2.00		9	0.26
Contadina®							
fresh, cheese	1 serving	260	13.00	6.00	2.00	39	
fresh, meat	1 serving	260	13.00	6.00	2.00	39	
Le Menu®							
cheese, light	1 oz	23	1.00	0.60		4	0.26
cheese sauce, light	1 oz	31	1.38	1.00		4	
Stouffers®							
beef	1 serving	360	18.00	12.00		45	2.33
cheese, alfredo	1 serving	600	28.00	40.00		32	2.27
cheese, tomato sauce	1 serving	360	18.00	16.00		37	2.46
cheese, vinaigrette	1 serving	400	15.00	27.00		24	1.23
Tortelloni							
Bernardi®							
beef	1 oz	70	3.00	2.00		9	
cheese	1 oz	70	4.00	2.00		9	0.26
spinach, cheese	1 oz	70	4.00	2.00		9	
Contadina® fresh, sausage	1 serving	260	11.00	7.00	2.00	37	
Vermicelli, Lean Cuisine® chicken vegetable	1 serving	270	20.00	8.00	2.00	29	3.97

FOOD	CALCIUM (mg)	IRON (mg)	POTAS-SIUM (mg)	SODIUM (mg)	CHOLES-TEROL (mg)	VITAMIN B6 (mg)	ZINC (mg)	% OF CALORIES FROM FAT
PASTA (continued)								
Spaghetti (continued)								
turkey Tetrazzini	72	0.60	200	620				53
Swanson's®								
meatballs, dinner	8	0.22	50	88	2	0.02	0.20	39
meatballs, home-style	8	0.42	79	72	13			33
Ultra Slim Fast® beef, mushroom	57	3.28	710	740	25	0.37	3.48	22
Spaghetti, protein-fortified, dry	88	9.42	457	19	0	0.40	4.07	5
cooked	14	1.01	58	7	0	0.09	0.70	1
Spaghetti, spinach								
dry	132	4.84	855	82	0	0.73	6.26	4
cooked	42	1.46	81	20	0	0.13	1.51	4
Health Valley® 100% organic	10	2.25	120	5	0			5
Spaghetti, whole-wheat								
dry	92	8.23	489	18	0	0.51	5.39	4
cooked	21	1.49	61	4	0	0.11	1.13	4
Tortellini								
Bernardi®								
cheese	20	0.00	15	50	5			20
meat filled, frozen	0	0.36	20	80	10	0.03	0.20	18
meat, raw	20	0.72	45	140	15	0.03	0.32	23
meat sauce	0	0.36	45	90	10	0.03	0.20	30
red sauce	0	0.36	40	45	5			18
spinach, cheese	40	0.36	20	75	15	0.03	0.19	36
tomato, cheese	20	0.36	20	70	10	0.02	0.16	30
Contadina®								
fresh, cheese	150	1.80	125	310	40	0.02	0.67	21
fresh, meat	60	1.80	180	380	45	0.09	1.39	21
Le Menu®								
cheese, light	10	0.27	45	46	2	0.02	0.16	23
cheese sauce, light	10	0.34		60	2			29
Stouffers®								
beef	100	2.70	580	780	96	0.50	5.96	30
cheese, alfredo	500	1.44	270	930	161	0.19	1.45	60
cheese, tomato sauce	300	1.44	420	860	175	0.21	1.57	40
cheese, vinaigrette	250	1.08	190	540	170	0.09	1.33	61
Tortelloni								
Bernardi®								
beef	20	1.08	30	95	15			26
cheese	40	0.36	25	90	15			26
spinach, cheese	40	0.36	25	90	15			26
Contadina® fresh, sausage	40	1.44	160	290	65	0.08	1.01	24
Vermicelli, Lean Cuisine® chicken vegetable	100	1.44	400	980	45			27

BREADS

FOOD	AMOUNT	CALORIES (kcal)	PROTEIN (g)	FAT (g)	CARBO-HYDRATES (g)	FIBER (g)	CALCIUM (mg)
Bagel							
cinnamon raisin, 3.5"	71 g	194	7.00	1.20	39		13
egg, 3.5"	71 g	197	7.60	1.50	38		9
oatbran, 3.5"	71 g	181	7.60	0.80	38		9
onion, 3.5"	71 g	195	7.50	1.10	38		53
plain, 3.5"	71 g	195	7.50	1.10	38		53
plain, 3.5", toasted	66 g	195	7.50	1.10	38		53
sesame seed, 3.5"	71 g	195	7.50	1.10	38		53
water, 3" diameter	55 g	163	6.02	1.41	31	1.16	23
BISCUIT							
buttermilk	35 g	127	2.20	5.80	17		17
buttermilk, dry mix	1 cup	514	9.60	18.50	76		215
buttermilk, dry, prepared	57 g	191	4.20	6.90	28		105
buttermilk, home recipe	60 g	212	4.20	9.80	27		141
mixed grain	41 g	125	2.90	2.70	23		8
plain	35 g	127	2.20	5.80	17		17
plain, dry mix	1 cup	514	9.60	18.50	76		215
plain, dry, prepared	57 g	191	4.20	6.90	28		105
plain, home recipe	60 g	212	4.20	9.80	27		141
refrigerated, prepared, high fat	27 g	93	1.80	4.00	13		5
refrigerated, prepared, low fat	21 g	63	1.60	1.10	12		4
Pillsbury®	35.5 g	140	2.50	7.50	16	2.70	10
ballard oven-ready	21.2 g	50	1.00	1.00	10	0.22	0
ballard oven-ready, buttermilk	21.2 g	50	1.00	1.00	10	0.22	20
butter	21.2 g	50	1.00	1.00	10	0.22	0
buttermilk	21.2 g	50	1.00	1.00	10	0.22	0
buttermilk, heat & eat	25.9 g	85	2.00	2.50	14	0.36	10
buttermilk, tender	21.2 g	50	1.00	1.00	9	0.21	0
country	21.2 g	50	1.00	1.00	10	0.22	0
good n buttery, fluffy	28.3 g	90	1.00	5.00	11	0.44	0
heat n eat, big premium	35.5 g	140	2.50	7.50	16	2.70	10
Pillsbury Big Country®							
butter tastin	34 g	100	2.00	4.00	14	0.36	0
buttermilk	34 g	100	2.00	4.00	14	0.36	0
southern	21.2 g	50	1.00	1.00	10	0.23	0
Pillsbury Hungry Jack®	28.3 g	90	2.00	4.00	13		0
butter tastin	28.3 g	90	2.00	4.00	11	0.30	0
buttermilk, extra	21.1 g	50	1.00	1.00	9	0.22	0
buttermilk, flaky	28.3 g	90	2.00	4.00	12	0.30	0
buttermilk, fluffy	28.3 g	90	2.00	4.00	12	0.30	0
flaky	21.1 g	50	1.00	1.00	9	0.22	0
honey	28.3 g	90	2.00	4.00	13		0
Pillsbury 1869®	31.1 g	100	2.00	5.00	12	0.33	0
butter tastin	31.1 g	100	2.00	5.00	12	0.33	0
buttermilk	31.1 g	100	2.00	5.00	12	0.33	0
Roman Meal® honey nut, oat bran	43 g	130	2.00	5.00	20		
Biscuit, baking powder	28.4 g	105	2.00	5.00	13	0.60	34
from home recipe	1 cup	229	4.59	10.50	28	1.30	75

FOOD	IRON (mg)	POTAS-SIUM (mg)	SODIUM (mg)	CHOLES-TEROl (mg)	SUGAR (gms)	% OF CALORIES FROM FAT
Bagel						
cinnamon raisin, 3.5"	2.70		229	0.00		6
egg, 3.5"	2.83	48	359	17.00		7
oatbran, 3.5"	2.19		360	0.00		4
onion, 3.5"	2.53	72	379	0.00		5
plain, 3.5"	2.53	72	379	0.00		5
plain, 3.5", toasted	2.52	72	379	0.00		5
sesame seed, 3.5"	2.53	72	379	0.00		5
water, 3" diameter	1.46	41	198	0.00		8
BISCUIT						
buttermilk	1.15	78	368			41
buttermilk, dry mix	3.33	195	1531			32
buttermilk, dry, prepared	1.17	107	544			33
buttermilk, home recipe	1.74	73	348	2.00		42
mixed grain	1.31	217	319	0.00		19
plain	1.15	78	368			41
plain, dry mix	3.33	195	1531			32
plain, dry, prepared	1.17	107	544			33
plain, home recipe	1.74	73	348	2.00		42
refrigerated, prepared, high fat	0.70	42	324	0.00		39
refrigerated, prepared, low fat	0.65	39	305	0.00		16
Pillsbury®	0.72	37	305	0.00		48
ballard oven-ready	0.36	105	180	0.00		18
ballard oven-ready, buttermilk	0.36	105	180	0.00		18
butter	0.36	105	180	0.00		18
buttermilk	0.36	105	180	0.00		18
buttermilk, heat & eat	0.54	28	265	0.00		26
buttermilk, tender	0.36	100	170	0.00		18
country	0.36	105	180	0.00		18
good n buttery, fluffy	0.72	75	270	0.00		50
heat n eat, big premium	0.72	38	305	0.00		48
Pillsbury Big Country®						
butter tastin	0.72	90	320	0.00		36
buttermilk	0.72	90	320	0.00		36
southern	0.36	105	180	0.00		18
Pillsbury Hungry Jack®	0.72	15	290	0.00		40
butter tastin	0.36	15	280	0.00		40
buttermilk, extra	0.36	100	180	0.00		18
buttermilk, flaky	0.36	15	300	0.00		40
buttermilk, fluffy	0.36	15	280	0.00		40
flaky	0.36	100	180	0.00		18
honey	0.72	15	290	0.00		40
Pillsbury 1869®	0.72	30	310	0.00		45
butter tastin	0.72	25	300	0.00		45
buttermilk	0.72	30	310	0.00		45
Roman Meal® honey nut, oat bran		170	280	0.00		35
Biscuit, baking powder	0.40	33	175	0.00	1.23	43
from home recipe	1.32	73	388	0.62	2.88	41

BREADS

FOOD	AMOUNT	CALORIES (kcal)	PROTEIN (g)	FAT (g)	CARBO-HYDRATES (g)	FIBER (g)	CALCIUM (mg)
BISCUIT (continued)							
Biscuit, baking powder (continued)							
from mix with milk	1 cup	201	4.40	5.76	32	0.68	4.
self rising flour	1 cup	231	4.40	10.80	29	0.80	13
Pillsbury 1869®	31.1 g	100	2.00	5.00	12	0.33	
BREAD							
Apple cinnamon							
quick bread mix	36.9 g	140	2.00	1.00	30	0.33	2
Keebler® elfin loaves	60 g	180	3.00	4.00	31		
Banana, home recipe, margarine	60 g	195	2.60	6.30	33		1
home recipe, shortening	60 g	203	2.60	7.10	33		1
quick bread mix	33 g	120	2.00	1.00	27	0.29	
Keebler® elfin loaves	60 g	190	3.00	7.00	29		
Blueberry, quick bread mix	36 g	130	2.00	1.00	29	0.32	2
Keebler® elfin loaves	56 g	170	3.00	4.00	30		
Boston brown, canned	45 g	88	2.40	0.70	20		3
Carrot, elfin loaves, Keebler®	60 g	210	3.00	10.00	27	0.79	
Cracked wheat, enriched	25 g	65	2.20	1.00	12		1
toasted	23 g	65	2.20	1.00	12		1
Newfoundland®	28.4 g	75	2.47	0.62	15	1.51	4
toasted	28.4 g	88.7	2.95	0.74	18	1.82	5
Cranberry, quick bread mix	36.9 g	140	2.00	1.00	30		
Keebler® elfin loaves	60 g	160	3.00	6.00	31	5.00	2
Date, quick bread mix	39.2 g	140	2.00	1.00	31	0.35	
Egg	40 g	115	3.80	2.40	19		3
toasted	37 g	117	3.90	2.40	19		3
French	25 g	69	2.20	0.80	13		1
toasted	23 g	69	2.20	0.80	13		1
Newfoundland® French/Vienna	28.4 g	82.2	2.58	0.85	16	0.80	2
toasted	28.4 g	95.8	3.01	0.99	18	0.91	2
Pepperidge® enriched, baked	28.4 g	75	2.50	1.00	14	0.25	2
twin, enriched	28.4 g	80	3.00	1.00	15	0.00	2
Pillsbury® crusty, loaf	23.9 g	60	2.00	1.00	11	0.77	
High calcium, dark	18 g	39	1.60	0.40	8		13
dark, toasted	16 g	39	1.60	0.40	8		13
light	18 g	41	1.50	0.40	8		13
light, toasted	16 g	40	1.50	0.40	8		12
Indian Fry	90 g	96	6.40	8.60	48		21
Irish Soda, home recipe	60 g	174	4.00	3.00	34		4
Italian	30 g	81	2.60	1.10	15		2
toasted	27 g	80	2.60	1.10	15		2
Newfoundland®	28.4 g	78.2	2.58	0.23	16	0.77	
Pepperidge Farm® brown, enriched	28.4 g	80	2.00	1.00	14	0.00	2
Melba toast, plain	4.67 g	16	1.00	0.00	3	0.29	
wheat, unsalted	4.67 g	16	1.00	0.00	3	0.35	
wheat	4.67 g	16	1.00	0.00	3	0.35	
Mixed grain	26 g	65	2.60	1.00	12		2
toasted	22 g	65.6	2.54	0.95	12	0.87	2

56

FOOD	IRON (mg)	POTAS-SIUM (mg)	SODIUM (mg)	CHOLES-TEROl (mg)	SUGAR (gms)	% OF CALORIES FROM FAT
BISCUIT (continued)						
Biscuit, baking powder (continued)						
from mix with milk	1.37	72	603	0.62		26
self rising flour	1.43	40	409	0.62	2.88	42
Pillsbury 1869®	0.72	30	310	0.00		45
BREAD						
Apple cinnamon						
quick bread mix	0.72	30	160	0.00		6
Keebler® elfin loaves	0.72	85	260	20.00		20
Banana, home recipe, margarine	0.84	81	181	26.00		29
home recipe, shortening	0.84	78	119	26.00		31
quick bread mix	0.36	20	190	0.00		8
Keebler® elfin loaves	1.08	55	260	0.00		33
Blueberry, quick bread mix	0.36	20	160	0.00		7
Keebler® elfin loaves	1.08	60	220	15.00		21
Boston brown, canned	0.94	143	284			7
Carrot, elfin loaves, Keebler®	1.08	75	170	25.00		43
Cracked wheat, enriched	0.70	44	135			14
toasted	0.70	44	135			14
Newfoundland®	0.70	38	150	0.00	1.10	8
toasted	0.83	45	179	0.00		7
Cranberry, quick bread mix	0.36	25	150	0.00		6
Keebler® elfin loaves	0.36	85	220	0.00		34
Date, quick bread mix	0.36	60	140	0.00		6
Egg	1.21	46	197	20.00		19
toasted	1.23	47	200	21.00		18
French	63.00	28	152	0.00		10
toasted	0.63	28	152	0.00		10
Newfoundland® French/Vienna	0.70	26	164	0.00		9
toasted	0.83	30	191	0.00		9
Pepperidge® enriched, baked	0.72	26	160	0.00		12
twin, enriched	0.72	26	160	0.00		11
Pillsbury® crusty, loaf	0.72	15	120	0.00		15
High calcium, dark	0.63	36	92	0.00		9
dark, toasted	0.62	36	91	0.00		9
light	0.64	34	124	0.00		9
light, toasted	0.63	34	123			9
Indian Fry	3.24	67	625	0.00		81
Irish Soda, home recipe	1.61	160	239	11.00		16
Italian	0.88	33	175	0.00		12
toasted	0.87	33	173	0.00		12
Newfoundland®	0.70	21	166	0.00		3
Pepperidge Farm® brown, enriched	0.72	21	150	0.00		11
Melba toast, plain	0.09	11	30	0.00		0
wheat, unsalted	0.10	11	5	0.00		0
wheat	0.10	11	30	0.00		0
Mixed grain	0.90	53	127	0.00		14
toasted	0.83	56	105	0.00	1.01	13

BREADS

FOOD	AMOUNT	CALORIES (kcal)	PROTEIN (g)	FAT (g)	CARBO-HYDRATES (g)	FIBER (g)	CALCIUM (mg)
BREAD (continued)							
Nut, quick bread mix	36.4 g	150	3.00	3.00	27	0.11	2
Oat, Pepperidge Farm® hearty slice	38 g	90	4.00	2.00	17	1.00	
Oat bran	30 g	71	3.10	1.30	12		1
low cal	23 g	46	1.80	0.70	10		1
low cal, toasted	19 g	45	1.80	0.70	9		1
toasted	27 g	70	3.10	1.30	12		1
Keebler® oat bran fiber, elfin loaves	60 g	170	4.00	6.00	30	5.00	4
Monterey® no cholesterol	45.4 g	99	4.10	1.20	18	3.30	
Oatmeal	27 g	73	2.30	1.20	13		1
low cal	23 g	48	1.70	0.80	10		2
low cal, toasted	19 g	48	1.70	0.80	10		2
with raisins, quick bread mix	39.2 g	140	3.00	2.00	30	0.35	2
toasted	25 g	73	2.30	1.20	13		1
Oatmeal Goodness® oatmeal & bran	35.5 g	90	4.00	2.00	15	1.00	4
Pepperidge Farm®	34 g	90	3.00	1.00	17	1.00	
Pilot, Alaska	25 g	416	8.50	10.10	73	0.05	9
Pita, white	60 g	165	5.40	0.70	33		5
Pita, whole wheat	64 g	170	6.30	1.70	35		1
Protein, gluten	19 g	47	2.30	0.40	8		2
toasted	17 g	46	2.30	0.40	8		2
Pumpernickel	32 g	80	2.80	1.00	15		2
toasted	29 g	80	2.80	1.00	15		2
Newfoundland®	28.4 g	69.7	2.58	0.34	15	1.68	4
Pumpkin, home recipe	60 g	198	2.40	7.70	31		1
Raisin	26 g	71	2.10	1.10	14		1
toasted	24 g	71	2.10	1.20	14		1
Newfoundland®	28.4 g	74.3	1.87	0.79	15	1.08	3
toasted	28.4 g	89.6	2.27	0.96	18	1.08	4
Rice bran	27 g	66	2.40	1.20	12		1
toasted	25 g	66	2.40	1.20	12		1
Rye	32 g	83	2.70	1.10	16		2
American, light	25 g	65.5	2.12	0.91	12	1.55	2
low cal	23 g	47	2.10	0.70	9		1
low cal, toasted	19 g	46	2.10	0.60	9		1
toasted	29 g	82	2.70	1.10	15		2
Newfoundland® ⅓ rye flour	28.4 g	68.9	2.58	0.31	15	1.76	3
toasted	28.4 g	79.9	3.01	0.37	17	2.04	4
Sourdough	25 g	69	2.20	0.80	13		1
toasted	23 g	69	2.20	0.80	13		1
Vienna	25 g	69	2.20	0.80	13		1
toasted	23 g	69	2.20	0.80	13		1
Wheat	25 g	65	2.30	1.00	12	0.11	2
low cal	23 g	46	2.10	0.50	10		1
low cal, toasted	19 g	45	2.10	0.50	10		1
toasted	23 g	65	2.30	1.00	12		2

FOOD	IRON (mg)	POTAS-SIUM (mg)	SODIUM (mg)	CHOLES-TEROL (mg)	SUGAR (gms)	% OF CALORIES FROM FAT
BREAD (continued)						
Nut, quick bread mix	0.72	45	180	0.00		18
Oat, Pepperidge Farm® hearty slice			140	0.00		20
Oat bran	0.94		122	0.00		16
low cal	0.71	24	81	0.00		14
low cal, toasted	0.71	23	79	0.00		14
toasted	0.93		121	0.00		17
Keebler® oat bran fiber, elfin loaves	1.08	170	160	0.00		32
Monterey® no cholesterol			204	0.00		11
Oatmeal	0.73	38	162			15
low cal	0.53		89			15
low cal, toasted	0.52	88	0			15
with raisins, quick bread mix	0.36	20	160	0.00		13
toasted	0.73	39	163			15
Oatmeal Goodness® oatmeal & bran	1.08	64	140	0.00		20
Pepperidge Farm®			200	0.00		10
Pilot, Alaska	4.84	229	569			22
Pita, white	1.57	72	322	0.00		4
Pita, whole wheat		108	340	0.00		9
Protein, gluten	0.79		104	0.00		8
toasted	0.78		102	0.00		8
Pumpernickel	0.92	66	215	0.00		11
toasted	0.91	66	214	0.00		11
Newfoundland®	0.73	129	161	0.00		4
Pumpkin, home recipe	0.99	55	188	27.00		35
Raisin	0.75	59	101	0.00		14
toasted	0.76	59	102	0.00		15
Newfoundland®	0.73	66	103	0.00		10
toasted	0.88	80	125	0.00		10
Rice bran	0.97		119	0.00		16
toasted	0.98		119	0.00		16
Rye	0.90	53	211	0.00		12
American, light	0.68	51	174	0.00	2.58	13
low cal	0.71	23	93	0.00		13
low cal, toasted	0.70	22	92	0.00		12
toasted	0.90	53	210	0.00		12
Newfoundland® 1/3 rye flour	0.65	41	158	0.00		4
toasted	0.78	48	184	0.00		4
Sourdough	0.63	28	152	0.00		10
toasted	0.63	28	152	0.00		10
Vienna	0.63	28	152	0.00		10
toasted	0.63	28	152	0.00		10
Wheat	0.83	50	132	0.00		14
low cal	0.68		117			10
low cal, toasted	0.67		115			10
toasted	0.83	50	132	0.00		14

BREADS

FOOD	AMOUNT	CALORIES (kcal)	PROTEIN (g)	FAT (g)	CARBO-HYDRATES (g)	FIBER (g)	CALCIU (m
BREAD (continued)							
Wheat bran	36 g	89	3.20	1.20	17		2
toasted	33 g	90	3.20	1.20	17		2
Wheat germ	28.4 g	74	2.70	0.80	14		2
toasted	25 g	73	2.70	0.80	14		2
Pillsbury® pipin hot loaf	28.3 g	70	2.00	2.00	12	0.81	
White, commercially prepared	25 g	67	2.10	0.90	12		2
commercially prepared, toasted	23 g	67	2.10	0.90	13		2
firm, enriched	23 g	61.4	1.90	0.90	11	0.60	2
firm, enriched, toasted	20 g	65	2.00	1.00	12	0.50	2
home recipe, 2% milk	42 g	120	3.30	2.40	21		2
home recipe, 2% milk, toasted	38 g	119	3.30	2.40	21		2
home recipe, n/f dry milk	44 g	120	3.40	1.20	24		1
home recipe, whole milk	38 g	110	3.00	2.40	19		2
home recipe, whole milk, toasted	35 g	111	3.00	2.40	19		2
low cal	23 g	48	2.00	0.60	10		2
soft, toasted	22 g	67.3	2.07	0.99	12	0.59	3
soft, enriched, cubes	30 g	80.1	2.48	1.18	15	0.81	3
soft, enriched, crumbs	45 g	120	3.73	1.76	22	1.22	5
1–2% skim milk powder	40 g	108	3.48	1.28	20	0.76	2
3–4% skim milk powder	28.4 g	76.5	2.47	0.91	14	0.54	2
5–6% skim milk powder	28.4 g	78	2.55	1.08	14	0.54	2
Newfoundland®	28.4 g	76.5	2.47	0.91	14	0.54	3
toasted	28.4 g	89	2.86	1.05	17	0.71	3
Pillsbury® pipin' hot loaf	28.3 g	70	3.00	2.00	12	0.71	
Whole wheat, commercially prep	28.4 g	70	2.70	1.20	13		2
commercially prepared, toasted	25 g	69	2.70	1.20	13		2
firm, enriched	25 g	61.3	2.41	1.09	11	2.83	1
home recipe	46 g	128	3.90	2.50	24		1
home recipe, toasted	42 g	128	3.90	2.50	24		1
soft, enriched	28.4 g	68.6	2.69	1.22	13	3.17	2
Newfoundland®	28.4 g	68.9	2.98	0.85	14	1.32	4
toasted	28.4 g	81.9	3.54	1.02	16	1.62	5
Bread crumbs, dry, grated, enriched	36.9 g	140	2.00	1.00	30	0.33	2
dry, plain	108 g	426	13.50	5.80	78		24
seasoned	120 g	441	17.10	3.10	85		1
Bread sticks, plain	6 g	25	0.70	0.60	4		
salt, regular type	48 g	184	5.76	1.39	36	0.96	
salt, Vienna bread type	48 g	146	4.56	1.49	28		4
Vienna type	35 g	106	3.30	1.10	20	1.02	
Keebler®							
garlic	3.75 g	15	0.50	0.00	3	20.40	
onion	3.75 g	15	0.50	0.00	3	0.07	
plain	3.75 g	15	0.50	0.00	3	0.06	
sesame	3.75 g	15	0.50	0.50	3	0.06	
Pillsbury® soft	38.8 g	100	3.00	2.00	17	0.98	
Cornbread, dry mix, prepared	60 g	189	4.30	6.00	29		
home recipe, 2% milk	65 g	173	4.30	4.60	28		1
home recipe, whole milk	65 g	176	4.30	5.00	28		1
Ballard®	33.7 g	120	2.00	2.00	24	0.65	

OD	IRON (mg)	POTAS-SIUM (mg)	SODIUM (mg)	CHOLES-TEROI (mg)	SUGAR (gms)	% OF CALORIES FROM FAT
READ (continued)						
Wheat bran	1.10	82	175			12
toasted	1.11	82	176	0.00		12
Wheat germ	0.98	72	157			10
toasted	0.97	71	155			10
Pillsbury® pipin hot loaf	0.72	20	170	0.00	1.00	26
White, commercially prepared	0.76	30	135	0.00		12
commercially prepared, toasted	0.77	30	136	0.00		12
firm, enriched	0.65	26	118	0.00	0.90	13
firm, enriched, toasted	0.60	28	117	0.00	0.82	14
home recipe, 2% milk	1.25	61	151	1.00		18
home recipe, 2% milk, toasted	1.24	61	150	1.00		18
home recipe, n/f dry milk	1.40	49	148	0.00		9
home recipe, whole milk	1.13	55	136	2.00		20
home recipe, whole milk, toasted	1.14	56	138	2.00		19
low cal	0.73	18	104	0.00		11
soft, toasted	0.72	28	129	0.00	0.90	13
soft, enriched, cubes	0.85	34	154	0.00	1.17	13
soft, enriched, crumbs	1.28	50	231	0.00	1.76	13
1–2% skim milk powder	0.99	34	203	1.20	1.00	11
3–4% skim milk powder	0.70	30	144	0.28	1.00	11
5–6% skim milk powder	0.70	34	140	1.13	1.00	12
Newfoundland®	0.70	30	144	0.28	1.00	11
toasted	0.83	35	167	0.28	1.00	11
Pillsbury® pipin' hot loaf	0.72	15	170	0.00	1.00	26
Whole wheat, commercially prep	0.94	71	149			15
commercially prepared, toasted	0.93	71	148			16
firm, enriched	0.86	44	159	0.00	1.00	16
home recipe	1.42	144	159	0.00		18
home recipe, toasted	1.43	145	160			18
soft, enriched	0.96	49	178	0.00	1.12	16
Newfoundland®	0.85	77	149	0.14	1.10	11
toasted	1.02	92	178	0.14	1.10	11
Bread crumbs, dry, grated, enriched	0.72	30	160	0.00		6
dry, plain	6.61	239	930			12
seasoned	3.82	324	3180			6
Bread sticks, plain	0.26	7	39	0.00		22
salt, regular type	0.43	44.1	803	1.44		7
salt, Vienna bread type	0.38	45.1	751	1.44		9
Vienna type	0.30	33	548	0.00		9
Keebler®						
garlic	0.18	7.5	10	0.00		0
onion	0.18	7.5	12.5	0.00		0
plain	0.18	7.5	15	0.00		0
sesame	0.18	7.5	15	0.00		30
Pillsbury® soft	1.08	20	230	0.00		18
Cornbread, dry mix, prepared	1.14	77	467	37.00		29
home recipe, 2% milk	1.62	96	428	26.00		24
home recipe, whole milk	1.62	95	428	28.00		26
Ballard®	1.08	45	560	0.00		15

BREADS

FOOD	AMOUNT	CALORIES (kcal)	PROTEIN (g)	FAT (g)	CARBO-HYDRATES (g)	FIBER (g)	CALCIU (m
BREAD (continued)							
Cornbread (continued)							
Pillsbury® twists	20.4 g	70	1.00	4.00	8	0.39	
Robin Hood Gold® mix, white	29.5 g	120	2.00	3.00	21		
mix, yellow	30.7 g	120	2.00	3.00	22		
CRACKERS							
American, Manischewitz®	28.4 g	115	2.90	0.09	22	0.82	
Animal, Ralston®	1.9 g	8.67	0.13	0.20	1	0.03	
Barge Pilot Biscuits	89.5 g	351	9.04	5.50	64	2.86	1
Bran thins, toasted, Nabisco®	14 g	60	1.00	3.00	9	1.00	
Butter, American Classic®	14.2 g	70	1.00	3.00	9	0.14	1
Flutters® original butter flavor	21 g	100	2.00	4.00	15	0.21	2
Pepperidge Farm® original butter	28.4 g	133	2.67	5.33	20	0.28	
Cheese	1 g	5	0.10	0.30	1		
low salt	1 g	5	0.10	0.30	1		
Cheddar Wedges® crispy cheese Ralston®	14 g	70	1.00	3.00	9	0.06	4
cheddar snacks	1.6 g	7.22	0.14	0.26	1	0.06	1
cheese snacks	1.13 g	5.6	0.11	0.26	1	0.03	1
cheese & chives	1.6 g	7.22	0.08	0.28	1	0.06	1
Club, Keebler®	3.25 g	15	0.00	1.00	2	0.07	0
low sodium	28.3 g	122	1.47	3.03	22	0.00	13
Daily thin tea, Manischewitz®	25.5 g	103	3.00	0.30	22	0.74	
Garden	21 g	100	2.00	4.00	14		
Health Valley® 7 grain vegetable	8.4 g	110		4.00	18	3.80	0
Flutters® tiny garden herb	21 g	100	2.00	4.00	14		
Pepperidge Farm® garden herb	28.4 g	133	2.67	5.33	19		0
Goldfish, Pepperidge Farm®							
cheese	28.4 g	120	4.00	4.00	19	1.00	95
pretzel	28.4 g	110	3.00	3.00	20	1.00	6
Graham	7 g	30	0.50	0.70	5		2
chocolate coated	14 g	68	0.80	3.20	9		8
cinnamon	7 g	30	0.50	0.70	5		2
plain	7 g	30	0.50	0.70	5		2
sugar, honey	7 g	30.1	0.52	0.73	5	0.12	3
Health Valley® honey	28.4 g	130	3.00	5.00	17	3.50	0
amaranth	28.4 g	100	2.50	1.67	18	2.58	1
oat bran	28.4 g	103	2.59	2.59	17	3.88	0
rye bran	28.4 g	100	3.00	3.00	15	1.00	0
Keebler® graham							
honey bulk	7.5 g	35	0.50	1.00	6	0.20	0
honey fiber	7.33 g	30	0.67	0.33	5	0.13	7
kitchen rich	6.5 g	30	0.50	1.00	5	0.21	0
Harvest Crisps, Nabisco®							
five grain	14 g	9.86	0.16	0.33	2	0.16	
oat	14 g	9.86	0.16	0.33	2	0.16	
Herb stoned wheat, Health Valley®	28.4 g	110	2.00	4.00	18	3.80	0
Matzo	28.4 g	112	2.80	0.40	24		4
egg	28.4 g	111	3.50	0.60	22		11

	IRON (mg)	POTAS-SIUM (mg)	SODIUM (mg)	CHOLES-TEROI (mg)	SUGAR (gms)	% OF CALORIES FROM FAT
FOOD						
BREAD (continued)						
Cornbread (continued)						
Pillsbury® twists	0.36	15	150	0.00		51
Robin Hood Gold® mix, white	0.72	30	470			23
mix, yellow	0.72	30	480			23
CRACKERS						
American, Manischewitz®	1.02	52	1	0.00		1
Animal, Ralston®	0.06	2	8	0.00	0.43	21
Large Pilot Biscuits	3.81	107	984	0.00		14
Bran thins, toasted, Nabisco®	0.56	30	70	0.00		45
Butter, American Classic®	0.50	15	140	2.00		39
Flutters® original butter flavor	0.74	42	150	5.00		36
Pepperidge Farm® original butter	0.00 ·	57	200	6.67		36
Cheese	0.05	1	10	0.00		54
low salt	0.05	1	5	0.00		54
Cheddar Wedges® crispy cheese	0.49	15	240	2.00		39
Ralston®						
cheddar snacks	0.07	2	14		0.05	33
cheese snacks	0.05	2	10	0.50	0.36	42
cheese & chives	0.07	2	14		0.05	35
Club, Keebler®	0.00	5	38	0.00		60
low sodium	0.51	31	149	0.00		22
Daily thin tea, Manischewitz®	1.00	34		0.00		3
Garden			190	0.00		36
Health Valley® 7 grain vegetable	.720	150	60	0.00		33
Flutters® tiny garden herb			190	0.00		36
Pepperidge Farm® garden herb	0.00		253	0.00		36
Goldfish, Pepperidge Farm®						
cheese	0.99	31	130	5.00		30
pretzel	1.28	37	160	0.00		25
Graham	0.26	9	42	0.00		21
chocolate coated	0.50	29	41	0.00		42
cinnamon	0.26	9	42	0.00		21
plain	0.26	9	42	0.00		21
sugar, honey	0.18	12	33	0.00	0.49	22
Health Valley® honey	0.72	60	90	0.00		35
amaranth	1.50	71	92	0.00		15
oat bran	2.33	73	39	0.00		23
rye bran	1.08	150	50	0.00		27
Keebler® graham						
honey bulk	0.18	13	43	0.00		26
honey fiber	0.24	10	37	0.00		10
kitchen rich	0.18	15	28	0.00		30
Harvest Crisps, Nabisco®						
five grain		5	22	0.00		30
oat		6	22	0.00		30
Herb stoned wheat, Health Valley®	0.72	150	60	0.00		33
Matzo	0.90	32	0	0.00		3
egg	0.77	43	6			5

BREADS

FOOD	AMOUNT	CALORIES (kcal)	PROTEIN (g)	FAT (g)	CARBO-HYDRATES (g)	FIBER (g)	CALCIU (m
CRACKERS (continued)							
Matzo (continued)							
egg, onion	28.4 g	111	2.80	1.10	22		1
Manischewitz® matzo meal	135 g	514	13.00	1.40	109	3.92	3
Melba toast	5 g	19	0.60	0.20	4		
pumpernickel	5 g	19	0.60	0.20	4		
rye	5 g	19	0.60	0.20	4		
wheat	5 g	19	0.60	0.10	4		
Keebler®							
garlic	2.5 g	12.5	0.50	0.00	2		
long	4.55 g	15	0.50	0.00	4		
onion	2.5 g	12.5	0.50	0.00	2		
plain	2.5 g	12.5	0.50	0.00	2		
sesame	2.5 g	12.5	0.50	0.00	2		
Milk	12 g	55	0.90	1.90	8		2
Munchems® original, Keebler	14.2 g	70	1.00	3.00	9	1.54	
Organic, wheat, Health Valley®							
cheese	28.4 g	80	2.00	2.00	18	3.80	
herb	28.4 g	80	2.00	2.00	18	3.80	
onion	28.4 g	80	2.00	2.00	18	3.80	
vegetable	28.4 g	80	2.00	2.00	18	3.80	
whole wheat	28.4 g	80	2.00	2.00	18	3.80	
Oyster, Keebler®	9 g	40	1.00	1.00	7	0.18	
Ralston®	.45 g	1.85	0.04	0.05	0	0.01	
Pita crisps	28.4 g	114	2.00	6.00	14		
poppy seed, onion	28.3 g	120	1.76	2.78	22	0.00	
Prawn	3.2 g	15.6	0.21	0.68	2	0.11	
Rich & Crisp, Ralston®	3.33 g	18	0.23	0.97	2	0.11	
Ritz®	6.5 g	22.5	1.00	0.00	5	1.05	
Rye, crispbread	10 g	37	0.80	0.10	8		
rye wafers	6.5 g	22.5	1.00	0.00	5	1.05	
Ralston Ry Krisp®							
natural	2.1 g	7.5	0.25	0.03	2	0.34	
seasoned	2.2 g	8.33	0.23	0.17	2	0.36	
sesame	2.5 g	8.33	0.28	0.23	2	0.41	
Ralston® rye snacks	1.9 g	8.67	0.14	0.36	1	0.31	
Saltine	3 g	13	0.30	0.40	2		
low salt	3 g	13	0.30	0.40	2		
Keebler® Zesta	2.9 g	12.5	0.00	0.50		0.09	
unsalted	2.9 g	12.5	0.00	0.50	2	0.06	
Nabisco® premium, no fat	14.2 g	50	1.00	0.00	12		
Sandwich, cheese filling	7 g	33	0.70	1.50	4		
cheese/peanut butter	7 g	34	0.90	1.60	4		
peanut butter filling	7 g	34	0.80	1.70	4		
wheat/cheese filling	7 g	35	0.70	1.70	4		
wheat/peanut butter filling	7 g	35	0.90	1.90	4		
Keebler® peanut butter/cheese	14.2 g	70	2.00	3.00	9	0.16	
Sesame	1.9 g	8.67	0.15	0.37	1	0.18	
Flutters® tiny golden sesame	21 g	110	2.00	5.00	13		
Pepperidge Farm® golden sesame	28.4 g	147	2.67	6.67	17		

FOOD	IRON (mg)	POTAS-SIUM (mg)	SODIUM (mg)	CHOLES-TEROl (mg)	SUGAR (gms)	% OF CALORIES FROM FAT
CRACKERS (continued)						
Matzo (continued)						
egg, onion	1.24	24	81			9
Manischewitz® matzo meal	4.10	149	3	0.00		2
Melba toast	0.19	10	41	0.00		9
pumpernickel	0.18	10	45	0.00		9
rye	0.18	10	45	0.00		9
wheat	0.22	7	42	0.00		5
Keebler®						
garlic	0.18	5	18	0.00		0
long	0.00	6	5	0.00		0
onion	0.18	5	15	0.00		0
plain	0.18	5	15	0.00		0
sesame	0.18	5	18	0.00		0
Milk	0.43	14	71			31
Munchems® original, Keebler	0.49	10	230	0.00		39
Organic, wheat, Health Valley®						
cheese	0.72	150	160	0.00		23
herb	0.72	150	160	0.00		23
onion	0.72	150	160	0.00		23
vegetable	36.00	150	60	0.00		23
whole wheat	0.72	150	160	0.00		23
Oyster, Keebler®	0.36	13	88	0.00		23
Ralston®	0.02	1	5	0.00	0.14	25
Pita crisps		30	269	0.00		47
poppy seed, onion	0.31		213			21
Prawn	0.09	3	21	0.00	0.10	39
Rich & Crisp, Ralston®	0.10	3	32	0.00		48
Ritz®	0.25	39	57	0.00	0.21	0
Rye, crispbread	0.24	32	26	0.00		2
rye wafers	0.25	39	57	0.00	0.21	0
Ralston Ry Krisp®						
natural	0.09	10	19	0.00	0.07	4
seasoned	0.08	11	27	0.00	7.00	18
sesame	0.09	12	29	0.00	0.08	25
Ralston® rye snacks	0.07	3	14	0.00	0.06	37
Saltine	0.16	4	39	0.00		28
low salt	0.16	22	19	0.00		28
Keebler® Zesta	0.00	5	38	0.00		36
unsalted	0.00	5	18	0.00		36
Nabisco® premium, no fat			15	150.00	0.00	0
Sandwich, cheese filling	0.17	30	98	0.00		41
cheese/peanut butter	0.20	17	69	0.00		42
peanut butter filling	0.21	16	66			45
wheat/cheese filling	0.18	21	64	1.00		44
wheat/peanut butter filling	0.19	21	57	0.00		49
Keebler® peanut butter/cheese	0.51	30	120	0.00		39
Sesame	0.08	4	17	0.00	0.06	38
Flutters® tiny golden sesame			150	0.00		41
Pepperidge Farm® golden sesame	0.00		200	0.00		41

BREADS

FOOD	AMOUNT	CALORIES (kcal)	PROTEIN (g)	FAT (g)	CARBO-HYDRATES (g)	FIBER (g)	CALCIUM (mg)
CRACKERS (continued)							
Snack	3 g	15	0.20	0.80	2		4
low salt	3 g	15	0.20	0.80	2		4
Stoned wheat, no salt, Health Valley®	28.4 g	110	2.00	4.00	18	3.80	0
Toasted							
Keebler®							
bacon snack	3.15 g	15	0.00	1.00	2		0
onion snack	3.15 g	15	0.00	1.00	2		0
pumpernickel	3.15 g	15	0.00	1.00	2		0
rye snack	3.15 g	15	0.00	1.00	2	0.06	0
sesame snack	3.15 g	15	0.00	1.00	2		0
wheat snack	3.15 g	15	0.00	1.00	2	0.06	0
Pepperidge® wheat	28.4 g	147	2.67	6.67	17	0.06	0
cheese	28.4 g	80	2.00	2.00	18	3.80	0
Triscuits®	4.5 g	21	0.40	0.75	3	0.16	1
Waldorf, sodium free, Keebler®	3.2 g	15	0.00	0.50	3		0
Wheat, low salt	2 g	9	0.20	0.40	1		1
wheat	2 g	9	0.20	0.40	1		1
wheat thins	1.8 g	9	0.13	0.35	1	0.10	
American Classic® cracked wheat	14.2 g	70	1.00	4.00	8	0.78	5
Flutters® tiny toasted wheat	14.2 g	70	1.00	4.00	8	0.78	5
Keebler®							
harvest wheats	13 g	15.2	0.25	0.76	2	0.72	4
sun toasted wheats	14 g	7	0.10	0.40	1	0.28	4
wheatables, ranch	13 g	70	1.00	3.00	8	0.72	4
wheatables, white cheddar	13 g	70	1.00	4.00	8	0.26	4
whole grain wheat	3.65 g	15	0.50	0.50	3	0.20	0
Whole wheat	4 g	18	0.40	0.70	3		2
low salt	4 g	18	0.40	0.70	3		2
low sodium	7.53 g	30	1.00	0.00	7	2.80	2
sodium free	7.53 g	30	1.00	0.00	7	2.80	2
Cracker meal	1 cup	440	10.60	2.00	93		27
Croissant	28.4 g	115	2.57	6.07	13	0.47	15
apple/butter	57 g	145	4.20	4.90	21		17
butter	57 g	232	4.70	12.00	26		21
cheese/margarine	57 g	236	5.20	11.90	27		30
Sara Lee®	26 g	109	2.30	6.10	11	0.56	12
frozen	28.4 g	103	2.33	5.47	11	0.05	14
Croutons	48 g	151	4.85	1.78	28	0.77	67
seasoned	40 g	186	4.30	7.30	25		38
Pepperidge Farm®							
cheddar/Romano cheese	28.4 g	120	4.00	4.00	20		40
cheese & garlic	28.4 g	140	4.00	6.00	18		40
onion & garlic	28.4 g	140	4.00	6.00	18	1.33	0
seasoned	28.4 g	140	4.00	6.00	18	1.33	40
sour cream & chive	28.4 g	140	4.00	6.00	18	0.00	40
Dumpling	28.4 g	58.4	0.85	3.15	7	2.02	11

FOOD	IRON (mg)	POTAS- SIUM (mg)	SODIUM (mg)	CHOLES- TEROI (mg)	SUGAR (gms)	% OF CALORIES FROM FAT
CRACKERS (continued)						
Snack	0.11	4	25	0.00		48
low salt	0.11	10.6	11.2	0.00		48
Stoned wheat, no salt, Health Valley®	0.72	150	60	0.00		33
Toasted						
Keebler®						
bacon snack	0.00	5	28	0.00		60
onion snack	0.00	5	35	0.00		60
pumpernickel	0.00	5	8	0.00		60
rye snack	0.00	5	35	0.00		60
sesame snack	0.00	5	33	0.00		60
wheat snack	0.00	5	30	0.00		60
Pepperidge® wheat	0.00	62	227	0.00		41
cheese	0.72	150	160	0.00		23
Triscuits®	0.15	6	24	0.00	0.14	32
Waldorf, sodium free, Keebler®	5.00	0	0			30
Wheat, low salt	0.09	4	6	0.00		40
wheat	0.09	4	6	0.00		40
wheat thins				0.00	0.06	35
American Classic® cracked wheat	0.49	25	140	0.00		51
Flutters® tiny toasted wheat	0.49	25	140	0.00		51
Keebler®						
harvest wheats	0.45	6	24	0.00		45
sun toasted wheats	0.56	2	11	0.00		51
wheatables, ranch	0.45	40	190	0.00		39
wheatables, white cheddar	0.52	40	140	0.00		51
whole grain wheat	0.00	5	35	0.00		30
Whole wheat	0.12	12	26	0.00		35
low salt	0.12	12	10	0.00		35
low sodium	0.30	33	31	0.00		0
sodium free	0.25	35	1	0.00		0
Cracker meal	5.33	132	32	0.00		4
Croissant	0.75	37	144	31.50		48
apple/butter	0.63	51	156			30
butter	1.16	67	424			47
cheese/margarine	1.23	76	316			45
Sara Lee®	1.04	40	140	28.90	2.60	50
frozen	0.58	34	144	15.70		48
Croutons	1.58	59	283	0.48		11
seasoned	1.13	72	495			35
Pepperidge Farm®						
cheddar/Romano cheese	1.44		400	0.00		30
cheese & garlic	0.72		360	0.00		39
onion & garlic	0.72	51	320	0.00		39
seasoned	0.72	51	360	0.00		39
sour cream & chive	0.72	41	340	0.00		39
Dumpling	0.09	13	138	0.91		49

BREADS

FOOD	AMOUNT	CALORIES (kcal)	PROTEIN (g)	FAT (g)	CARBO-HYDRATES (g)	FIBER (g)	CALCIUM (mg)
CRACKERS (continued)							
French toast	65 g	153	5.67	6.73	17	2.02	72
frozen	59 g	126	4.40	3.60	19		63
home recipe, 2% milk	65 g	149	5.00	7.00	16		65
home recipe, whole milk	65 g	151	5.00	7.30	16		64
with butter	67.5 g	178	5.17	9.38	18		37
French toast sticks	28.2 g	171	1.65	5.81	12		16
MUFFINS							
Almond date, fancy fruit, Health Valley®	56.6 g	140	4.00	1.00	31	8.20	40
Apple spice, fat free, Health Valley®	56.6 g	130	4.00	1.00	30	5.10	20
Banana, fat free, Health Valley®	56.6 g	130	4.00	1.00	29	4.50	20
Blueberry, commercially prepared	57 g	158	3.20	3.70	27		33
home recipe, whole milk	57 g	165	3.70	6.40	23	5.00	107
home recipe, 2% milk	57 g	163	3.70	6.10	23		108
from mix	50 g	149	2.60	4.40	24		13
toaster type	33 g	103	1.50	3.10	18		4
toaster type, toasted	31 g	103	1.50	3.10	18		4
Health Valley® fancy fruit	56.6 g	140	4.00	1.00	32	7.50	60
fat free, twin	56.6 g	140	4.00	1.00	32	5.00	60
oat bran	57 g	140	4.00	4.00	27	4.70	27
Sara Lee® free & light	64 g	120	3.00	0.00	28	0.87	90
Lovin' Lites® from mix	35.7 g	100	2.00	1.00	21	2.52	40
Bran, from home recipe	40 g	112	2.96	5.08	17	2.52	54
Carrot, fat free, twin, Health Valley®	56.6 g	130	4.00	1.00	30	5.00	20
Corn	40 g	125	3.00	4.00	19	0.95	42
commercially prepared	57 g	174	3.40	4.80	29		42
degermed cornmeal	28.4 g	89	2.01	2.86	14		30
home recipe, 2% milk	57 g	180	4.00	7.00	25		148
home recipe, whole milk	57 g	183	4.00	7.40	25		147
from mix	50 g	160	3.70	5.10	25		37
from mix with egg & milk	91.8 g	297	6.33	9.73	46	5.00	221
toaster type	33 g	114	1.70	3.70	19	6.00	6
toaster type, toasted	31 g	114	1.70	3.70	19		6
English, apple/cinnamon	57 g	138	4.30	1.50	28		84
apple/cinnamon, toasted	52 g	137	4.30	1.50	28		83
granola	66 g	155	6.00	1.20	31		129
granola, toasted	61 g	156	6.00	1.20	31		130
mixed grain, toasted	61 g	156	6.00	1.20	31		130
plain	56 g	133	4.43	1.00	26	1.68	91
raisin/cinnamon	57 g	138	4.30	1.50	28		84
raisin/cinnamon, toasted	52 g	137	4.30	1.50	28		83
sourdough	57 g	134	4.40	1.00	26		99
sourdough, toasted	52 g	133	4.40	1.00	26		99
toasted	53 g	154	5.13	1.26	30	1.49	105
wheat	57 g	127	4.90	1.10	26		101
wheat, toasted	52 g	126	4.90	1.10	25		100
whole wheat	66 g	134	5.80	1.40	27		175

FOOD	IRON (mg)	POTAS-SIUM (mg)	SODIUM (mg)	CHOLES-TEROI (mg)	SUGAR (gms)	% OF CALORIES FROM FAT
CRACKERS (continued)						
French toast	1.34	86	257	0.32		40
frozen	1.31	79	292	48.00		26
home recipe, 2% milk	1.09	87	311	75.00		42
home recipe, whole milk	1.09	86	311	76.00		44
with butter	0.95	89	256	58.50		47
French toast sticks	2.96	25	100	14.80		31
MUFFINS						
Almond date, fancy fruit, Health Valley®	3.60	210	80	0.00		6
Apple spice, fat free, Health Valley®	1.44	250	110	0.00		7
Banana, fat free, Health Valley®	1.44	530	110	0.00		7
Blueberry, commercially prepared	0.92	70	255	17.00		21
home recipe, whole milk	1.29	70	251	23.00		35
home recipe, 2% milk	1.29	70	251	21.00		34
from mix	0.57	39	219	23.00		27
toaster type	0.17	27	158			27
toaster type, toasted	0.17	27	158			27
Health Valley® fancy fruit	4.50	210	100	0.00		6
fat free, twin	4.50	210	100	0.00		
oat bran	1.40	260	95	0.00		26
Sara Lee® free & light	1.31	76	140	0.00		0
Lovin' Lites® from mix	0.36	70	160	20.00		9
Bran, from home recipe	1.26	99	168	21.00		41
Carrot, fat free, twin, Health Valley®	1.44	250	110	0.00		7
Corn	0.70	54	192	21.00		29
commercially prepared	1.60	39	297			25
degermed cornmeal	0.48	38	136	14.70		29
home recipe, 2% milk	1.49	83	334	24.00		35
home recipe, whole milk	1.49	82	333	25.00		36
from mix	0.97	65	397	31.00		29
from mix with egg & milk	1.55	101	439	53.00		29
toaster type	0.49	30	142			29
toaster type, toasted	0.48	30	142			29
English, apple/cinnamon	1.38	119	255			10
apple/cinnamon, toasted	1.37	118	253	0.00		10
granola	2.00	103	275	0.00		7
granola, toasted	2.00	103	276	0.00		7
mixed grain, toasted	2.00	103	276	0.00		7
plain	1.58	314	358	0.00	1.96	7
raisin/cinnamon	1.38	119	255			10
raisin/cinnamon, toasted	1.37	118	253	0.00		10
sourdough	1.42	75	265	0.00		7
sourdough, toasted	1.41	74	262	0.00		7
toasted	1.83	364	414	0.00	2.01	7
wheat	1.63	106	218	0.00		8
wheat, toasted	1.62	105	216	0.00		8
whole wheat	1.62	139	420	0.00		9

BREADS

FOOD	AMOUNT	CALORIES (kcal)	PROTEIN (g)	FAT (g)	CARBO-HYDRATES (g)	FIBER (g)	CALCIUM (mg)
MUFFINS (continued)							
English (continued)							
whole wheat, toasted	61 g	135	5.80	1.40	27		176
Thomas® oat bran	57 g	120	4.00	1.00	24	2.00	58
Mix, blueberry	28.4 g	104	1.40	2.80	18		7
Creamy Deluxe®							
apple cinnamon	29.2 g	100	1.00	3.00	17		0
banana nut	29.5 g	110	1.00	4.00	17	0.40	20
cinnamon struesel	38.3 g	190	2.00	8.00	27		20
oat bran	37.2 g	170	3.00	7.00	24	2.04	40
wild blueberry	30.7 g	100	1.00	3.00	17	0.42	20
Gold Medal Robin Hood®							
applesauce	33.2 g	140	2.00	4.00	25		0
banana	31.9 g	140	2.00	4.00	24		0
blueberry	33.2 g	149	2.60	4.40	24	0.08	0
caramel	30.7 g	140	1.00	4.00	24	0.40	0
corn	33 g	130	2.00	2.00	25	0.42	0
honey bran	33.1 g	140	3.00	4.00	24	1.68	20
Light Deluxe® wild blueberry	26.2 g	70	1.00	1.00	16	0.36	0
Oat bran	57 g	154	4.00	4.20	28		36
Oatmeal Goodness® honey	56.7 g	140	5.00	2.00	26	2.00	83
Plain, from home recipe	40 g	120	3.00	4.00	17	0.85	42
home recipe, 2% milk	57 g	169	3.90	6.50	24		114
home recipe, whole milk	57 g	172	3.90	6.80	24		113
Raisin, Health Valley®	56.6 g	140	3.00	4.00	31	7.70	40
oat bran	57 g	140	5.00	3.00	31	5.20	33
fancy fruit	56.6 g	140	4.00	1.00	31	7.70	40
spice, fat free	56.6 g	130	4.00	1.00	30	5.00	20
Raspberry, fat free, twin, Health Valley®	56.6 g	130	4.00	1.00	30	5.00	20
Soy	40 g	119	3.90	4.40	17	0.84	35
Wheat bran	28.4 g	112	2.00	3.40	21		16
raisins, toaster type	34 g	107	1.90	3.20	19		13
home recipe, 2% milk	57 g	161	4.10	7.00	24		106
home recipe, whole milk	57 g	164	4.00	7.30	24		106
from mix	50 g	138	3.30	4.60	23		16
Pancakes, blueberry	38 g	84	2.30	3.50	11		78
Pancakes, buckwheat	73 g	169	5.18	5.11	25	0.92	74
Pancakes, buttermilk	38 g	86	2.60	3.60	11		60
frozen	36 g	83	1.90	1.20	16		22
Pancakes, microwave, original, Pillsbury®							
blueberry	108 g	230	5.00	4.00	47	1.00	80
buttermilk	108 g	260	5.00	4.00	51	1.00	80
oat bran	108 g	230	6.00	4.00	45	3.00	80
wheat	108 g	240	6.00	4.00	48	4.20	80
whole wheat	73 g	146	4.96	6.64	17		16
Pancake mix, buckwheat	122 g	415	13.30	3.30	87		580
buttermilk	112 g	398	11.20	1.90	82		387
buttermilk- milk/egg/oil	130 g	489	13.10	6.40	93		313

70

FOOD	IRON (mg)	POTAS-SIUM (mg)	SODIUM (mg)	CHOLES-TEROl (mg)	SUGAR (gms)	% OF CALORIES FROM FAT
MUFFINS (continued)						
English (continued)						
whole wheat, toasted	1.62	139	422	0.00		9
Thomas® oat bran	2.07	127	210	0.00		8
Mix, blueberry	0.36	24	155	0.00		24
Creamy Deluxe®						
apple cinnamon	0.36	20	130	0.00		27
banana nut	0.72	45	130	0.00		33
cinnamon struesel	1.08	50	220	0.00		38
oat bran	1.44	125	220	0.00		37
wild blueberry	0.36	45	140	0.00		27
Gold Medal Robin Hood®						
applesauce	0.72	30	220			26
banana	0.72	50	220			26
blueberry	0.36	20	220	0.41		27
caramel	0.36	20	220	14.40		26
corn	0.36	25	230	15.40		14
honey bran	1.08	85	220	0.00		26
Light Deluxe® wild blueberry	0.36	20	135	0.00		13
Oat bran	2.39	289	224	0.00		25
Oatmeal Goodness® honey	1.09	68	160	0.00		13
Plain, from home recipe	0.60	50	176	21.00	1.52	30
home recipe, 2% milk	1.36	69	266	22.00		35
home recipe, whole milk	1.36	68	266	24.00		36
Raisin, Health Valley®	3.60	190	90	0.00		26
oat bran	1.70	290	100	0.00		19
fancy fruit	3.60	190	90	0.00		
spice, fat free	1.44	250	110	0.00		7
Raspberry, fat free, twin, Health Valley®	1.44	250	110	0.00		7
Soy	0.90		0	1.52		33
Wheat bran	1.02	57	198	0.00		27
raisins, toaster type	0.96	60	179	0.00		27
home recipe, 2% milk	2.39	181	335	19.00		39
home recipe, whole milk	2.39	181	335	20.00		40
from mix	1.20	73	233	34.00		30
Pancakes, blueberry	0.65	52	157	21.00		38
Pancakes, buckwheat	1.23	90	310	38.70		27
Pancakes, buttermilk	0.64	55	198	22.00		38
frozen	1.25	26	183	3.00		13
Pancakes, microwave, original, Pillsbury®						
blueberry	1.80	85	550	10.00		16
buttermilk	1.80	85	590	10.00		14
oat bran	10.00	135	580	10.00		16
wheat	1.44	170	420	68.30		15
whole wheat	0.95	179	339	48.20		41
Pancake mix, buckwheat	5.78	385	1692	0.00		7
buttermilk	3.42	213	1467	0.00		4
buttermilk- milk/egg/oil	3.90	443	1580			12

BREADS

FOOD	AMOUNT	CALORIES (kcal)	PROTEIN (g)	FAT (g)	CARBO-HYDRATES (g)	FIBER (g)	CALCIUM (mg)
Pancake mix (continued)							
low sodium/no sucrose	22 g	44	1.10	0.20	9		13
plain	112 g	398	11.20	1.90	82		383
plain-milk/egg/oil	130 g	489	13.10	6.40	93		313
whole wheat	140 g	481	17.90	2.10	100		628
Bisquick®							
apple cinnamon	66.2 g	240	6.00	3.00	47		100
blueberry	70.9 g	270	6.00	3.00	54	0.91	100
buttermilk	66.2 g	250	6.00	3.00	49	0.66	100
Betty Crocker® buttermilk	47.2 g	170	4.00	1.00	36	0.47	80
complete buttermilk	56.7 g	210	5.00	3.00	41	0.56	100
Gold Medal Robin Hood® buttermilk	22.1 g	90	3.00	2.00	15		20
Hungry Jack®							
blueberry	68 g	170	3.00	1.00	38	0.87	40
buttermilk	36 g	120	3.00	0.00	26		0
buttermilk complete	53.4 g	180	5.00	1.00	38		
Pancakes, plain	38 g	86	2.40	3.70	11		83
frozen	36 g	83	1.90	1.20	16		22
from mix	38 g	83	3.00	2.90	11		82
Pancakes, soy bean, 25% soy flour	45 g	68	2.90	1.90	10	0.51	26
Pancake/waffle mix							
buckwheat/other, dry	141 g	502	12.10	2.54	107	4.37	634
made w/egg & milk	73 g	164	5.26	5.33	24	0.80	157
plain, buttermilk, dry	73 g	147	4.45	4.09	23	0.80	161
plain, buttermilk, egg/milk	108 g	230	6.00	4.00	46	3.00	80
plain, buttermilk, milk	73 g	147	4.45	4.09	23	0.80	161
Phyllo dough	19 g	57	1.40	1.10	10		2
Pizza crust	30.7 g	110	3.00	1.00	22		0
Gold Medal Robin Hood® mix	35.4 g	90	3.00	1.00	16		0
Pillsbury® all ready	35.4 g	90	3.00	1.00	16		0
Roll, brown & served, enriched	26 g	100	1.50	4.20	14	0.57	8
Rolls/bun, raisin, ready to serve	53.1 g	146	3.66	1.54	30	2.02	40
Roll, cinnamon	26 g	100	1.50	4.20	14	0.57	8
Pepperidge Farm® 2-pack	28.4 g	124	1.78	6.22	15	0.45	9
Roll, cloverleaf	28.4 g	85	2.00	2.00	15	1.06	21
pan, commercial, enriched	35 g	120	3.00	3.00	20	1.33	16
from home recipe	35 g	120	3.00	3.00	20	1.33	16
Roll, dinner, crescent	27 g	93	1.80	4.00	13		5
commercially prepared	28.4 g	85	2.40	2.10	14		34
egg	35 g	107	3.30	2.20	18		21
home recipe, 2% milk	35 g	111	3.00	2.50	19		21
home recipe, whole milk	35 g	112	3.00	2.70	19		21
Pillsbury®							
butterflake	47.2 g	140	3.00	5.00	20	0.90	0
crescent	28.3 g	100	2.00	6.00	11	0.59	0
Roll, dough, baked	40 g	124	3.40	2.16	22	0.76	16
Roll, dough, un-risen, frozen	28.4 g	76	2.13	1.42	13		9
Roll, hamburger, low calorie	43 g	84	3.60	0.80	18		26

FOOD	IRON (mg)	POTAS- SIUM (mg)	SODIUM (mg)	CHOLES- TEROI (mg)	SUGAR (gms)	% OF CALORIES FROM FAT
Pancake mix (continued)						
low sodium/no sucrose	0.38	85	58	0.00		4
plain	3.42	213	1467	0.00		4
plain-milk/egg/oil	3.92	443	1580			12
whole wheat	11.00	623	1987	0.00		4
Bisquick®						
apple cinnamon	1.80	110	880	0.00		11
blueberry	1.80	100	840	0.00		10
buttermilk	1.80	95	880	0.00		11
Betty Crocker® buttermilk	1.44	75	760	2.72		5
complete buttermilk	1.44	150	500	37.50		13
Gold Medal Robin Hood® buttermilk	0.72	20	260			20
Hungry Jack®						
blueberry	1.08	50	780	0.00		5
buttermilk	0.72	45	530	0.00		0
buttermilk complete	1.08					5
Pancakes, plain	0.69	50	167	23.00		39
frozen	1.25	26	183	3.00		13
from mix	0.49	76	192	27.00		31
Pancakes, soy bean, 25% soy flour	0.60			0.00		25
Pancake/waffle mix						
buckwheat/other, dry	3.87	228	2020	0.00		5
made w/egg & milk	0.78	112	412	54.00		29
plain, buttermilk, dry	0.58	114	329	8.03		25
plain, buttermilk, egg/milk	1.80	140	560	10.00		16
plain, buttermilk, milk	0.58	114	329	8.03		25
Phyllo dough	0.61	14	92	0.00		17
Pizza crust	1.08	40	220			8
Gold Medal Robin Hood® mix	1.08	20	170	0.00		10
Pillsbury® all ready	1.08	20	170	0.00		10
Roll, brown & served, enriched	0.49	36	96	0.00		38
Rolls/bun, raisin, ready to serve	1.65	130	204	0.00		9
Roll, cinnamon	0.49	36	96	0.00		38
Pepperidge Farm® 2-pack	0.48	35	84	9.37		45
Roll, cloverleaf	0.80	27	155	0.00	1.12	21
pan, commercial, enriched	0.70	41	193	0.00	1.40	23
from home recipe	0.70	41	193	0.00	1.40	23
Roll, dinner, crescent	0.70	42	324	0.00		39
commercially prepared	0.89	38	148	0.00		22
egg	1.23		191			19
home recipe, 2% milk	1.04	53	145	12.00		20
home recipe, whole milk	1.04	53	145	13.00		22
Pillsbury®						
butterflake	1.08	30	530	0.00		32
crescent	0.36	65	230	0.00		54
Roll, dough, baked	1.06	38	224	2.00		16
Roll, dough, un-risen, frozen	0.65	23	137	1.42		17
Roll, hamburger, low calorie	1.28	34	190	0.00		9

BREADS

FOOD	AMOUNT	CALORIES (kcal)	PROTEIN (g)	FAT (g)	CARBO-HYDRATES (g)	FIBER (g)	CALCIUM (mg)
Roll, hard	57 g	167	5.70	2.40	30		54
Newfoundland®	28.4 g	88.5	2.78	0.91	17	0.45	23
Roll, hot, from mix, Pillsbury®	28.3 g	120	4.00	2.00	22		0
Roll, hotdog, low calorie	43 g	84	3.60	0.80	18		26
mixed grain	43 g	113	41	2.60	19		41
plain	43 g	123	3.60	2.20	22		60
Roll, submarine/hoagie, enriched	40 g	120	3.60	1.80	22	0.76	22
Roll, Kaiser	57 g	167	5.70	2.40	30		54
Roll, mix, dry	40 g	136	3.28	3.48	22	0.76	19
Rusk	28.4 g	119	3.91	2.47	20		6
Ruskets, biscuits, dry, La Loma®	15 g	55	2.00	0.00	11		10
Stuffing, bread, dry mix	28.4 g	110	3.10	1.00	22		28
bread, dry mix, prep	200 g	356	6.40	17.20	43		64
bread, home recipe	232 g	390	8.80	16.80	52		148
cornbread, dry mix	28.4 g	110	2.80	1.20	22		22
cornbread, dry mix, prep	200 g	358	5.80	17.60	44		52
General Foods® chicken	28.35 g	107	3.57	1.05	21	0.06	29
General Mills® chicken	56.8 g	220	8.00	2.00	42		40
Pepperidge Farm®							
apple & raisin	28.35 g	110	3.00	1.00	21		20
classic chicken	28.35 g	110	3.99	1.00	20	0.06	40
corn bread	28.35 g	110	3.00	0.99	22	0.56	20
country garden herb	28.35 g	120	3.99	3.99	18	0.73	40
country style	28.35 g	99.8	3.99	1.00	21		40
cube	28.35 g	110	3.00	1.00	22		40
herb seasoned	28.35 g	110	3.00	1.00	22	0.44	40
vegetable & almond	28.35 g	110	3.99	3.00	19		40
wild rice & mushroom	28.35 g	110	3.99	3.00	19		40
Stove Top®							
for beef, dry mix	29.5 g	110	4.00	1.00	21		32
chicken, rice, dry mix	30.1 g	114	4.00	1.00	22		32
chicken, flex, dry mix	29.7 g	122	4.00	3.00	20		31
corn, flex, dry mix	31.9 g	130	4.00	3.00	22		23
cornbread, dry mix	28.4 g	107	3.00	1.00	21		22
home-style, dry mix	29.7 g	122	4.00	3.00	20		33
long rice, dry mix	30.1 g	114	4.00	1.00	22		31
Waffles, buttermilk, frozen	35 g	88	2.10	2.70	14		7
frozen, toasted	33 g	87	2.00	2.70	13		7
home recipe	75 g	217	6.20	10.20	25		136
Waffles, enriched, home recipe	75 g	245	6.93	12.60	26	1.05	154
from mix, egg & milk	75 g	205	7.00	8.00	27	1.05	179
frozen	37 g	103	2.15	3.52	16	0.89	36
Waffles, oat bran, no cholesterol, Eggo®	39 g	110	3.00	4.00	16	2.00	20
Waffles, plain	72 g	201					
from home recipe	72 g	201	6.70	7.06	27	0.91	8
frozen	35 g	88	2.10	2.70	14		7
frozen, toasted	33 g	87	2.00	2.70	13		7
Wonton wrappers	8 g	23	0.80	0.10	5		

FOOD	IRON (mg)	POTAS- SIUM (mg)	SODIUM (mg)	CHOLES- TEROl (mg)	SUGAR (gms)	% OF CALORIES FROM FAT
Roll, hard	1.87	61	310	0.00		13
Newfoundland®	0.70	28	177	0.00		9
Roll, hot, from mix, Pillsbury®	0.90	58	185	12.50		15
Roll, hotdog, low calorie	1.28	34	190	0.00		9
mixed grain	1.70		197			21
plain	1.30	60	241			16
Roll, submarine/hoagie, enriched	1.03	49	125	1.60		14
Roll, Kaiser	1.87	61	310	0.00		13
Roll, mix, dry	1.06	47	112	13.20		23
Rusk	0.37	46	70	2.55		19
Ruskets, biscuits, dry, La Loma®	1.35	48				0
Stuffing, bread, dry mix	1.08	70	451			8
bread, dry mix, prep	2.18	148	1086			43
bread, home recipe	3.80	304	1068	0.00		39
cornbread, dry mix	0.92	58	364	0.00		10
cornbread, dry mix, prep	1.88	124	910	0.00		44
General Foods® chicken	1.08	77	487	14.87		9
General Mills® chicken	2.88	150	1060			8
Pepperidge Farm®						
apple & raisin	1.80		409			8
classic chicken	1.44	95	409	40.43		8
corn bread	1.08	47	319	17.17		8
country garden herb	1.80	137	300	11.18		30
country style	1.44		399			9
cube	1.44		399			8
herb seasoned	1.44	52	379	0.00		8
vegetable & almond	2.70		249			25
wild rice & mushroom	2.70		250			25
Stove Top®						
for beef, dry mix	1.00	84	516	0.00	3.40	8
chicken, rice, dry mix	1.00	81	487	0.90	2.80	8
chicken, flex, dry mix	1.00	66	524	0.80	2.40	22
corn, flex, dry mix	0.90	77	539	0.10	2.90	21
cornbread, dry mix	0.80	80	487	0.10	2.60	8
home-style, dry mix	1.30	72	462	0.70	2.50	22
long rice, dry mix	1.10	68	483	0.60	2.60	8
Waffles, buttermilk, frozen	1.49	43	262			28
frozen, toasted	1.48	42	260			28
home recipe	1.63	129	451	50.00		42
Waffles, enriched, home recipe	1.48	129	445	45.00		46
from mix, egg & milk	1.00	146	514	45.00		35
frozen	1.80	78	256	0.00		31
Waffles, oat bran, no cholesterol, Eggo®	1.80	194	220	0.00		33
Waffles, plain						0
from home recipe	1.47	104	342	90.00		32
frozen	1.49	43	262			28
frozen, toasted	1.48	42	260			28
Wonton wrappers	0.27	7	46	1.00		4

BREAKFAST CEREALS

FOOD	AMOUNT	CALORIES (kcal)	PROTEIN (g)	FAT (g)	CARBO-HYDRATES (g)	FIBER (g)	CALCIUM (mg)
All Bran®							
CNF	1 cup	162	7.95	1.32	50.0	19.9	56.3
USDA	1 cup	212	12.20	1.53	63.4	25.6	69.0
Alpen® Muesli	1 cup	453	15.50	9.54	84.4	11.1	259.0
Alpha Bits®							
CNF	1 cup	113	2.32	1.08	23.8	1.0	7.9
Post	1 cup	111	2.00	1.00	24.0	1.1	9.0
Marshmallow, Post	1 cup	110	2.00	1.00	25.0	0.9	7.0
USDA	1 cup	111	2.20	0.60	24.6	0.3	8.0
Amaranth Health Valley®							
bananas	1 oz	110	4.00	2.00	20.0	4.2	0.0
crunch, raisins	1 oz	100	3.00	1.00	20.0	2.7	0.0
Apple Cinnamon Cheerios®	1 oz	110	2.00	2.00	22.0	1.5	20.0
Apple & Cinnamon Wheats®	1 cup	236	4.74	0.65	51.9	6.0	41.0
Apple Jacks®							
CNF	1 cup	108	1.56	0.11	25.4	0.5	4.0
USDA	1 cup	110	1.50	0.10	25.7	0.2	3.0
Balance®	1 cup	212	6.59	1.26	43.9	7.7	40.1
Balance® raisins & rolled oats	1 cup	224	6.09	1.83	47.5	7.3	40.8
Cereal, bran, 100%	1 cup	162	7.59	1.03	51.9	22.5	48.2
Barbie® Ralston, sweetened	1 cup	110	1.00	1.00	25.0	0.0	5.0
Basic Four® General Mills	36.9 g	130	3.00	2.00	28.0	2.0	200.0
Batman® Ralston, sweetened	28.0 g	110	1.00	1.00	25.0	0.0	11.2
Body Buddies® natural fruit	1 oz	110	2.00	1.00	24.0	0.5	100.0
Booberry® General Mills	1 oz	110	1.00	1.00	24.0	0.5	20.0
Bran Buds®							
CNF	1 cup	214	10.10	1.34	65.8	23.8	68.9
USDA	1 cup	220	11.80	2.04	64.8	23.6	57.1
Bran Chex®	1 cup	156	5.10	1.40	39.0	7.9	29.0
Bran Flakes							
Kellogg's®	1 cup	158	5.28	0.00	40.5	7.4	
Post®	1 cup	154	5.14	1.23	37.0	7.9	28.3
Ralston®	1 cup	159	5.60	0.70	39.1	6.0	26.6
Bran Flakes & Fruit®	1 cup	179	4.37	0.74	43.5	4.7	25.6
Cap'n Crunch®							
CNF	1 cup	153	1.67	2.44	31.2	0.7	5.7
Crunchberries	1 cup	146	1.80	2.90	28.5	0.4	11.0
peanut butter	1 cup	154	2.52	4.52	26.5	0.5	7.0
USDA	1 cup	156	1.90	3.40	29.9	0.4	6.0
Cereal							
hot, oat bran	1 cup	204	11.00	4.49	29.9	10.9	44.6
hot, oat bran, dry	1 cup	446	24.20	9.81	65.5	19.4	97.7
Quaker®							
hot, w/apples & spices	34.0 g	120	4.00	2.00	26.0	3.0	
hot, raisin & cinnamon	34.0 g	120	4.00	2.00	25.0	3.0	
hot, regular flavor	28.0 g	100	6.00	2.00	17.0	4.0	
Ralston® cooked, hot	1 cup	134	5.50	0.80	28.2	4.2	14.0
Cheerios®							
CNF	1 cup	91	3.01	1.51	16.2	1.7	36.9
USDA	1 cup	89	3.42	1.45	15.7	0.9	38.8

FOOD	IRON (mg)	POTAS-SIUM (mg)	SODIUM (mg)	SUGAR (g)	THIAMIN (mg)	RIBO-FLAVIN (mg)	NIACIN (mg)	% OF CALORIES FROM FAT
All Bran®								
CNF	8.81	699	603	11.1	1.32	0.13	9.94	7
USDA	13.50	1051	961	16.5	1.11	1.28	15.00	7
Alpen® Muesli	3.43	647	245	32.0	0.40	0.33	3.30	19
Alpha Bits®								
CNF	3.77	54	149	11.3	0.57	0.00	1.36	9
Post	2.70	59	176	11.2	0.38	0.43	5.00	8
Marshmallow, Post	2.70	47	152	13.8	0.37	0.43	5.00	8
USDA	1.80	110	219	10.7	0.40	0.40	5.00	5
Amaranth Health Valley®								
bananas	1.08	110	5		0.06	0.06	0.00	16
crunch, raisins	1.08	100	30		0.00	0.00	1.60	9
Apple Cinnamon Cheerios®	4.50	70	180	10.0	0.38	0.42	5.00	16
Apple & Cinnamon Wheats®	1.84	276	29	12.3	0.08	0.05	4.51	3
Apple Jacks®								
CNF	3.77	29	122	13.3	0.57	0.02	1.36	1
USDA	4.50	23	125	15.3	0.40	0.40	5.00	1
Balance®	7.41	274	421	10.4	1.10	0.11	2.52	5
Balance® raisins & rolled oats	7.30	304	385	17.0	1.22	0.12	2.49	7
Cereal, bran, 100%	8.78	715	561	13.9	1.32	0.28	13.30	6
Barbie® Ralston, sweetened	4.44	34	70	10.0	0.37	0.25	4.94	8
Basic Four® General Mills	4.50	110	230	8.0	0.38	0.43	5.00	14
Batman® Ralston, sweetened	4.44	23	70	10.0	0.37	0.25	4.93	8
Body Buddies® natural fruit	8.10	40	280	6.0	0.38	0.43	5.00	8
Booberry® General Mills	4.50	45	210	13.0	0.38	0.43	5.00	8
Bran Buds®								
CNF	11.20	764	424	18.2	1.68	0.17	10.70	6
USDA	13.50	1425	523	10.3	1.11	1.28	15.00	8
Bran Chex®	7.80	394	455	8.2	0.60	0.26	8.60	8
Bran Flakes								
Kellogg's®	31.70	299	387	6.0	0.66	0.75	8.80	0
Post®	6.27	258	295	5.7	0.94	0.08	3.20	7
Ralston®	7.80	191	456	5.9	0.60	0.70	8.60	4
Bran Flakes & Fruit®	7.55	281	380	15.1	1.14	0.06	3.35	4
Cap'n Crunch®								
CNF	4.92	40	257		0.74	0.04	1.78	14
Crunchberries	9.04	49	243	15.5	0.59	0.67	8.13	18
peanut butter	9.11	57	268		0.60	0.70	8.97	26
USDA	9.83	48	278	14.9	0.66	0.71	8.64	20
Cereal								
hot, oat bran	4.17	316	2	0.9	0.27	0.08	1.85	20
hot, oat bran, dry	9.12	690	4	2.0	0.89	0.22	1.48	20
Quaker®								
hot, w/apples & spices		140	140					15
hot, raisin & cinnamon		170	140					15
hot, regular flavor		180	140	0.0				18
Ralston® cooked, hot	1.64	153	4	1.0	0.20	0.18	2.05	5
Cheerios®								
CNF	3.01	82	202	0.6	0.02	0.00	1.09	15
USDA	3.61	81	246	0.7	0.30	0.34	4.00	15

BREAKFAST CEREALS

FOOD	AMOUNT	CALORIES (kcal)	PROTEIN (g)	FAT (g)	CARBO-HYDRATES (g)	FIBER (g)	CALCIUM (mg)
Cinnamon & Raisin Nature Valley®	1 oz	120	2.00	4.00	20.0	1.0	0.0
Cinnamon Toast Crunch®	1 oz	120	1.00	3.00	22.0	1.0	40.0
	1 cup	153	1.88	3.90	27.9	0.7	19.5
Clusters® General Mills	1 oz	110	2.00	2.00	22.0	2.0	40.0
Coco Crunchies®	1 cup	154	2.47	0.69	34.8	0.6	6.1
Cocoa Krispies®	1 cup	139	1.90	0.50	32.0	0.2	6.0
Cocoa Pebbles®							
CNF	1 cup	128	2.04	1.88	26.9	0.7	6.8
Post	28.4 g	113	1.00	1.00	25.0	0.4	6.0
USDA	1 cup	133	1.53	1.76	27.9	0.2	5.5
Cocoa Puffs® General Mills	1 cup	108	1.91	0.63	24.3	0.2	0.0
Common Sense® Oat Bran	1 cup	177	5.82	1.23	37.1	5.4	95.1
Common Sense® Oat Bran/Raisins	1 cup	188	5.34	1.17	41.6	5.9	89.1
Cookie Crisp®	1 cup	120	1.53	1.08	26.3	0.4	5.7
Corn Bran®							
CNF	1 cup	139	2.35	1.62	28.7	6.3	5.7
USDA	1 cup	125	2.45	1.26	30.3	6.8	41.4
Corn Chex®	1 cup	111	2.00	0.10	24.9	0.5	3.0
Corn Flakes							
Kellogg's® CNF	1 cup	105	1.99	0.06	24.5	1.2	0.9
Kellogg's® USDA	1 cup	88	1.84	0.07	19.5	1.0	0.7
low sodium	1 cup	98	1.93	0.08	22.2	1.0	10.8
Ralston®	1 cup	98	1.90	0.10	21.7	1.0	2.0
Corn Grits, white							
enriched, cooked/salt	1 cup	146	3.50	0.50	31.4		1.0
enriched, dry	1 tbsp	36	0.90	0.10	7.7		0.0
unenriched, cooked/salt	1 cup	146	3.50	0.50	31.4		1.0
unenriched, dry	1 tbsp	36	0.90	0.10	7.7		0.0
Corn grits, yellow							
enriched, cooked/salt	1 cup	146	3.50	0.50	31.4		1.0
enriched, dry	1 tbsp	36	0.90	0.10	7.7		0.0
unenriched, cooked/salt	1 cup	146	3.50	0.50	31.4		1.0
unenriched, dry	1 tbsp	36	0.90	0.10	7.7		0.0
Corn Pops®	1 cup	108	1.30	0.11	25.5	0.1	1.4
Corn, shredded, added sugar	1 cup	95	2.00	0.00	22.0	1.5	1.0
Count Chocula® General Mills	1 oz	110	2.00	1.00	24.0	0.5	20.0
Country Corn Flakes® General Mills	1 oz	110	2.00	1.00	24.0		0.0
Cracklin Bran®							
CNF	1 cup	228	5.40	8.58	41.5	10.8	34.8
USDA	1 cup	229	5.50	8.80	41.1	9.1	40.0
Cracklin Oat Bran® Kelloggs	1 oz	110	3.00	4.00	20.0	2.0	20.0
Cream of Rice, cooked	1 cup	127	2.20	0.24	28.1	0.4	7.3
Cream of Wheat®							
apple/cinnamon	1 oz	22	0.37	0.05	4.9	0.2	1.6
apple/cinnamon, dry	1 oz	105	1.76	0.25	23.3	1.1	7.4
instant	1 cup	153	4.40	0.60	31.6	2.2	59.0
iron	1 oz	19	0.57	0.08	4.0	0.2	0.8
iron, dry	1 oz	105	3.06	0.45	21.5	1.1	4.1
iron, quick, cooked	1 cup	133	3.76	0.43	27.3	1.7	5.2
iron, quick, dry	1 cup	613	17.40	1.99	126.0	6.7	24.0

FOOD	IRON (mg)	POTAS-SIUM (mg)	SODIUM (mg)	SUGAR (g)	THIAMIN (mg)	RIBO-FLAVIN (mg)	NIACIN (mg)	% OF CALORIES FROM FAT
Cinnamon & Raisin Nature Valley®	0.72	80	90	6.0	0.06	0.00	0.00	30
Cinnamon Toast Crunch®	4.50	45	210	9.0	0.38	0.43	5.00	23
	4.72	54	260	11.0	0.06	0.02	6.25	23
Clusters® General Mills	4.50	105	140	7.0	0.38	0.43	5.00	16
Coco Crunchies®	5.39	43	316	12.9	0.81	0.01	1.95	4
Cocoa Krispies®	2.30	53	275	16.1	0.50	0.50	6.30	3
Cocoa Pebbles®								
CNF	4.31	72	89	13.1	0.65	0.01	1.55	13
Post	1.80	44	160	12.2	0.38	0.43	5.00	8
USDA	2.05	54	155	13.7	0.42	0.49	5.72	12
Cocoa Puffs® General Mills	3.79	47	190		0.38	0.00	1.31	5
Common Sense® Oat Bran	6.29	185	357	6.8	0.95	0.02	1.47	6
Common Sense® Oat Bran/Raisins	7.10	232	304	14.7	1.07	0.02	1.33	6
Cookie Crisp®	4.77	29	207		0.39	0.45	5.28	8
Corn Bran®								
CNF	4.79	75	321		0.72	0.06	1.73	10
USDA	12.2	70	310		0.37	0.70	10.90	9
Corn Chex®	1.80	23	271	1.3	0.40	0.07	5.00	1
Corn Flakes								
Kellogg's® CNF	3.78	31	277	1.9	0.57	0.02	1.36	0
Kellogg's® USDA	1.43	21	281	1.6	0.30	0.34	4.00	1
low sodium	0.56	18	3	1.7	0.00	0.05	0.11	1
Ralston®	0.60	22	239	1.7	0.10	0.00	1.10	1
Corn Grits, white								
enriched, cooked/salt	1.55	54	540		0.24	0.15	1.96	3
enriched, dry	0.38	13	0		0.06	0.04	0.48	3
unenriched, cooked/salt	0.48	54	540		0.05	0.02	0.48	3
unenriched, dry	0.10	13	0		0.01	0.00	0.12	3
Corn grits, yellow								
enriched, cooked/salt	1.55	54	540		0.24	0.15	1.96	3
enriched, dry	0.38	13	0		0.06	0.04	0.48	3
unenriched, cooked/salt	0.48	54	540		0.05	0.02	0.48	3
unenriched, dry	0.10	13	0		0.01	0.00	0.12	3
Corn Pops®	3.77	23	115	10.8	0.57	0.01	1.36	1
Corn, shredded, added sugar	0.60		247	.	0.33	0.05	4.40	0
Count Chocula® General Mills	4.50	60	210	13.0	0.38	0.43	5.00	8
Country Corn Flakes® General Mills	8.10	35	260	1.9	0.38	0.43	5.00	8
Cracklin Bran®								
CNF	7.98	372	303	16.8	1.20	0.07	4.02	34
USDA	3.80	355	487	17.2	0.80	0.90	10.60	35
Cracklin Oat Bran® Kelloggs	1.80	160	140		0.38	0.43	5.00	33
Cream of Rice, cooked	0.49	49	2		0.00	0.00	0.98	2
Cream of Wheat®								
apple/cinnamon	1.95	11	40	2.0	0.01	0.00	0.04	2
apple/cinnamon, dry	9.36	53	191	9.8	0.03	0.01	0.20	2
instant	12.00	48	6	1.1	0.20	0.10	1.80	4
iron	1.73	6	43	0.1	0.01	0.00	0.04	4
iron, dry	9.36	31	233	0.1	0.03	0.01	0.23	4
iron, quick, cooked	15.10	40	96	0.8	0.04	0.04	0.29	3
iron, quick, dry	69.70	184	442	1.0	0.17	0.18	1.32	3

BREAKFAST CEREALS

FOOD	AMOUNT	CALORIES (kcal)	PROTEIN (g)	FAT (g)	CARBO-HYDRATES (g)	FIBER (g)	CALCIUM (mg)
Cream of Wheat® (continued)							
iron, regular, cook	1 cup	134	3.76	0.44	27.6	2.0	5.3
iron, regular, dry	1 cup	640	18.20	2.08	132.0	7.8	25.3
packet size	1 item	132	2.50	0.40	28.9	2.0	40.0
regular, hot	1 cup	133	3.80	0.50	27.7	1.9	50.2
Crisp Rice®low sodium	1 cup	105	1.40	0.10	23.7	0.3	17.0
Crispix®	1 cup	120	2.33	0.10	27.9	0.6	5.4
Crispy Critters® Post	28.4 g	110	2.00	0.00	24.0	1.0	5.0
Crispy Rice®	1 cup	112	1.82	0.11	25.2	1.0	5.1
Crispy Wheats and Raisins®	1 cup	150	3.00	0.70	35.1	2.0	71.0
C.W. Post®							
plain	1 cup	432	8.70	15.20	69.4	2.2	47.0
w/raisins	1 cup	446	8.90	14.70	73.9	2.0	51.0
Farina							
cooked/salt	1 cup	116	3.40	0.20	24.6		4.0
enriched, dry	1 tbsp	40	1.20	0.10	8.5		2.0
unenriched, cooked/salt	1 cup	116	3.40	0.20	24.6		4.0
unenriched, dry	1 tbsp	40	1.20	0.10	8.5		2.0
Pillsbury®	22.5 g	80	2.00	1.00	17.0		0.0
Fat Free 10 Bran® Health Valley							
almond	1 oz	90	3.00	1.00	19.0	5.0	20.0
bran, apple	1 oz	90	3.00	1.00	19.0	5.0	20.0
Fibre Crunch®	1 cup	246	5.82	9.25	44.8	11.6	37.5
Fibre One® #2 General Mills	1 oz	60	2.00	1.00	23.0	13.0	65.6
Fiber 7 Flakes® Health Valley	1 oz	90	3.00	1.00	20.0	5.0	0.0
raisins	1 oz	90	3.00	1.00	20.0	5.0	0.0
Fibre Up®	1 cup	131	7.04	0.80	43.2	27.5	39.2
Fortified Oat Flakes®	1 cup	177	9.00	0.70	34.7	1.2	68.0
40% Bran Flakes							
Kellogg's®	1 cup	127	4.90	0.70	30.5	7.6	19.0
Post®	1 cup	152	5.30	0.80	37.3	9.2	21.0
Frankenberry® General Mills	1 oz	110	1.00	1.00	24.0	0.5	20.0
Froot Loops®	1 cup	111	1.59	0.54	25.0	0.5	2.8
General Mills	1 cup	111	1.70	0.50	25.0	0.3	3.0
Frosted Flakes							
Kellogg's®	1 cup	133	1.80	0.10	31.7	0.8	1.0
Ralston®	1 cup	149	2.00	0.50	34.2	0.8	4.0
Frosted Mini Wheats® Kellogg's	7.1 g	26	0.73	0.00	5.9	0.8	2.3
Frosted Rice®	1 cup	108	1.36	0.09	25.5	0.1	2.8
Frosted Rice Krispies® Kellogg's	1 cup	109	1.30	0.10	25.7	0.1	1.0
Fruit & Fiber®							
cinnamon apple crisp	1 cup	143	3.95	1.67	33.0	6.0	24.9
dates, raisins	35.4 g	120	3.00	2.00	27.0	4.7	16.0
dates, raisins, walnuts	1 cup	144	4.17	1.57	33.8	4.9	26.9
peach, raisins, almonds	1 cup	171	5.04	2.17	39.2	7.4	32.9
pineapple, banana	1 cup	161	4.27	2.69	36.0	6.5	25.0
tropical fruit	35.4 g	125	3.00	3.00	27.0	4.5	15.0
wheat bran	35.4 g	121	3.00	2.00	26.0	4.7	5.4
Fruit/Fitness® Health Valley	1 oz	110	4.50	2.00	18.5	5.4	40.0
Fruit & Nut® Nature Valley	1 oz	130	2.00	5.00	19.0	1.0	0.0

FOOD	IRON (mg)	POTAS-SIUM (mg)	SODIUM (mg)	SUGAR (g)	THIAMIN (mg)	RIBO-FLAVIN (mg)	NIACIN (mg)	% OF CALORIES FROM FAT
Cream of Wheat® (continued)								
iron, regular, cook	15.20	41	1	0.8	0.04	0.04	0.29	3
iron, regular, dry	72.80	194	5	0.6	0.17	0.21	1.38	3
packet size	8.10	55	241	0.9	0.40	0.20	5.00	3
regular, hot	10.30	43	2		0.25	0.00	1.51	3
Crisp Rice® low sodium	0.80	20	3	3.2	0.00	0.05	0.36	1
Crispix®	4.25	34	260	3.4	0.64	0.02	1.53	1
Crispy Critters® Post	8.10	54	232	3.3	0.38	0.43	5.00	0
Crispy Rice®	0.71	27	208	2.5	0.11	0.03	2.02	1
Crispy Wheats and Raisins®	6.80	174	204	15.4	0.60	0.60	7.60	4
C.W. Post®								
plain	15.40	198	167	6.6	1.30	1.50	17.10	32
w/raisins	16.40	260	160		1.30	1.50	18.10	30
Farina								
cooked/salt	1.16	30	767		0.19	0.12	1.28	2
enriched, dry	0.41	10	0		0.06	0.04	0.44	2
unenriched, cooked/salt	0.05	30	767		0.02	0.02	0.23	2
unenriched, dry	0.16	10	0		0.01	0.01	0.08	2
Pillsbury®	0.72	20	0	0.1	0.12	0.07	0.80	11
Fat Free 10 Bran® Health Valley								
almond	1.08	110	5		15.00	0.03	1.20	10
bran, apple	1.08	110	5		15.00	0.03	1.20	10
Fibre Crunch®	8.60	401	327	18.1	1.29	0.07	4.33	34
Fibre One® #2 General Mills	4.50	230	140	0.0	0.38	0.43	5.00	15
Fiber 7 Flakes® Health Valley	1.08	95	0	0.03		0.03	1.60	10
raisins	1.08	95	0		0.03	0.03	1.60	10
Fibre Up®	7.55	505	568	3.2	1.14	0.10	10.70	5
Fortified Oat Flakes®	13.70	343	429	8.8	0.60	0.70	8.40	4
40% Bran Flakes								
Kellogg's®	11.20	248	363	4.8	0.50	0.60	6.90	5
Post®	7.50	251	431	5.7	0.60	0.70	8.30	5
Frankenberry® General Mills	4.50	45	210	13.0	0.38	0.43	5.00	8
Froot Loops®	3.77	33	116	13.2	0.57	0.02	1.36	4
General Mills	4.50	26	145	13.9	0.40	0.40	5.00	4
Frosted Flakes								
Kellogg's®	2.20	22	284	13.7	0.50	0.50	6.20	1
Ralston®	1.00	24	247	15.1	0.50	0.60	6.70	3
Frosted Mini Wheats® Kellogg's	2.02	20	0	1.8	0.09	0.11	1.25	0
Frosted Rice®	3.77	21	204	11.1	0.57	0.01	1.36	1
Frosted Rice Krispies® Kellogg's	1.80	21	240	10.8	0.40	0.40	5.00	1
Fruit & Fiber®								
cinnamon apple crisp	5.71	217	224	10.7	0.86	0.06	2.06	11
dates, raisins	6.30	202	167	9.6	0.45	0.51	6.00	15
dates, raisins, walnuts	5.97	239	225	11.4	0.90	0.08	2.92	10
peach, raisins, almonds	7.05	297	249	12.5	1.06	0.09	3.45	11
pineapple, banana	6.39	279	226	11.7	0.96	0.08	3.07	15
tropical fruit	5.40	213	167	9.7	0.45	0.51	6.00	22
wheat bran	5.40	207	167	8.4	0.45	0.51	6.00	15
Fruit/Fitness® Health Valley	2.25	230	3		0.19	0.09	1.00	16
Fruit & Nut® Nature Valley	0.72	90	75	6.0	0.06	0.03	0.00	35

BREAKFAST CEREALS

FOOD	AMOUNT	CALORIES (kcal)	PROTEIN (g)	FAT (g)	CARBO-HYDRATES (g)	FIBER (g)	CALCIUM (mg)
Fruitful Bran®	1 cup	139	3.15	0.71	33.5	4.7	17.6
Fruity Marshmallow Krispies®	1 cup	106	1.79	0.11	24.8	0.2	3.1
Fruity Pebbles® Post	1 oz	115	1.13	1.47	24.4	0.2	3.4
Fruity Yummy Mummy® General Mills	1 oz	110	1.00	1.00	24.0	0.6	20.0
Golden Grahams®							
CNF	1 cup	156	2.18	1.56	33.1	0.5	14.4
USDA	1 cup	150	2.18	1.48	33.2	1.4	23.8
Granola							
homemade	1 cup	594	15.00	33.20	67.3	12.8	75.6
Nature Valley®	1 cup	503	11.50	19.60	75.5	4.2	71.0
Grape Nuts® Post	1 cup	418	14.30	1.36	91.4	13.5	46.5
CNF	28.4 g	105	3.00	0.00	23.0	2.6	10.0
USDA	1 cup	407	13.30	0.46	93.5	5.3	43.3
Grape Nuts Flakes® Post	1 cup	117	3.50	0.71	26.0	2.4	13.6
CNF	100 g	370	9.67	3.07	81.4	9.9	35.4
USDA	1 cup	116	3.48	0.36	26.6	2.9	13.0
Harvest Crunch®	1 cup	484	9.78	22.20	61.3	5.7	132.0
apples & cinnamon	1 cup	424	9.37	17.80	56.8	6.5	126.0
raisins & bran	1 cup	442	10.40	20.90	53.0	9.0	120.0
raisins & dates	1 cup	509	9.60	21.30	69.7	6.5	132.0
tropical fruit	1 cup	433	9.06	17.50	59.9	5.5	95.9
Healthy Crunch® Health Valley							
almond	1 oz	90	4.00	1.00	18.0	3.5	0.0
apple	1 oz	90	4.00	1.00	18.0	3.5	0.0
Healthy O's® Health Valley	1 oz	90	3.00	1.00	18.0	3.4	20.0
Heartand Natural® plain	1 cup	499	11.60	17.70	78.6	5.4	75.0
Hearty Grain® C.W. Post	28.4 g	128	2.00	4.00	21.2	1.4	6.0
Honey Bran®	1 cup	119	3.10	0.70	28.6	3.9	16.0
Honey Bran Crunchies®	1 cup	184	4.13	0.53	42.3	6.6	30.2
Honey Bun Oats®							
almond	28.4 g	115	2.00	3.00	22.0	1.7	14.0
roasted	28.4 g	111	2.00	2.00	23.0	1.6	9.0
Honey Comb® Post	1 cup	86	1.30	0.40	19.6	0.3	4.0
Honeycomb Crunch® Post	28.4 g	110	2.00	0.00	26.0	0.6	4.0
Honey Nut Cheerios® General Mills	1 cup	125	3.60	0.80	26.5	1.3	23.0
Honey Nut Corn Flakes®	1 cup	149	2.57	1.51	31.6	0.9	5.7
Hot-Oat Bran® Health Valley							
apple	1 oz	100	3.00	1.00	19.0	3.8	0.0
raisin	1 oz	100	3.00	1.00	19.0	3.8	0.0
Just Right®	1 cup	157	3.14	1.16	35.7	2.7	10.3
Kaboom® General Mills	1 oz	110	2.00	1.00	23.0	0.5	40.0
King Vitaman®	1 cup	85	1.09	1.16	17.8	0.3	1.7
Kix®	1 cup	74	1.70	0.44	15.6	0.3	23.6
Life®	1 cup	172	7.95	2.47	29.6	4.1	34.6
plain/cinnamon	1 cup	162	8.10	0.80	31.5	1.4	154.0
Lite-Puffed® Health Valley							
rice	1 cup	100	2.00	0.00	24.0	0.7	0.0
corn	1 cup	100	6.00	0.00	22.0	0.6	0.0
wheat	1 cup	100	4.00	0.00	22.0	2.8	0.0

FOOD	IRON (mg)	POTAS-SIUM (mg)	SODIUM (mg)	SUGAR (g)	THIAMIN (mg)	RIBO-FLAVIN (mg)	NIACIN (mg)	% OF CALORIES FROM FAT
Fruitful Bran®	5.59	227	256	9.7	0.84	0.06	2.65	5
Fruity Marshmallow Krispies®	3.78	26	223	7.3	0.57	0.01	1.36	1
Fruity Pebbles® Post	1.79	22	157		0.37	0.43	4.99	12
Fruity Yummy Mummy® General Mills	4.50	35	160	13.0	0.38	0.43	5.00	8
Golden Grahams®								
CNF	5.19	74	364		0.07	0.02	1.79	9
USDA	6.20	86	385		0.51	0.59	6.86	9
Granola								
homemade	4.84	612	12	33.4	0.73	0.31	2.14	50
Nature Valley®	3.78	389	232	30.9	0.39	0.19	0.83	35
Grape Nuts® Post	15.10	483	706	10.5	2.27	0.48	5.44	3
CNF	8.10	91	170	2.6	0.38	0.43	5.00	0
USDA	4.95	381	792	8.0	1.48	1.71	20.10	1
Grape Nuts Flakes® Post	4.31	123	178	2.8	0.65	0.03	1.55	5
CNF	28.60	305	387	10.0	1.32	1.50	17.60	7
USDA	5.17	113	250	4.2	0.42	0.49	5.72	3
Harvest Crunch®	2.42	469	64		0.31	0.31	1.42	41
apples & cinnamon	2.26	461	47		0.18	0.36	1.44	38
raisins & bran	3.74	624	58		0.31	1.26	2.65	43
raisins & dates	2.62	573	60		0.27	0.30	1.57	38
tropical fruit	2.59	382	60	23.2	0.22	0.19	1.28	36
Healthy Crunch® Health Valley								
almond	0.36	70	10		0.15	0.07	0.40	10
apple	0.36	70	35		0.15	0.07	0.40	10
Healthy O's® Health Valley	0.72	90	1	0.8	0.12	0.03	0.40	10
Heartand Natural® plain	4.33	385	294	29.9	0.36	0.16	1.61	32
Hearty Grain® C.W. Post	6.50	54	78	7.3	0.33	0.63	6.60	28
Honey Bran®	5.60	151	202	8.8	0.50	0.50	6.20	5
Honey Bran Crunchies®	6.62	242	297	9.7	0.10	0.21	3.68	3
Honey Bun Oats®								
almond	2.70	69	157	5.6	0.38	0.43	5.00	23
roasted	2.70	58	176	6.0	0.38	0.43	5.00	16
Honey Comb® Post	1.40	70	166	8.1	0.30	0.30	3.90	4
Honeycomb Crunch® Post	2.70	33	172	11.0	0.38	0.43	5.00	0
Honey Nut Cheerios® General Mills	5.20	115	299	11.8	0.40	0.50	5.80	6
Honey Nut Corn Flakes®	5.03	45	264	11.6	0.76	0.02	1.81	9
Hot-Oat Bran® Health Valley								
apple	0.72	100	10		0.06	0.00	1.20	9
raisin	0.72	100	10		0.06	0.00	1.20	9
Just Right®	5.72	93	228	2.4	0.86	0.09	2.06	7
Kaboom® General Mills	8.10	60	270	6.0	0.68	0.77	9.00	8
King Vitaman®	12.70	26	161		0.92	1.06	12.90	12
Kix®	5.41	30	226	0.8	0.25	0.28	3.33	5
Life®	5.85	284	237		0.88	0.08	2.11	13
plain/cinnamon	11.60	197	229	7.9	0.95	1.00	11.60	4
Lite-Puffed® Health Valley								
rice	0.00	90	0	0.0	0.00	0.00	0.80	0
corn	0.00	70	0		0.00	0.00	0.00	0
wheat	1.44	150	0	0.2	0.00	0.00	0.80	0

BREAKFAST CEREALS

FOOD	AMOUNT	CALORIES (kcal)	PROTEIN (g)	FAT (g)	CARBO-HYDRATES (g)	FIBER (g)	CALCIUM (mg)
Lucky Charms®							
CNF	1 cup	126	2.27	0.83	27.5	1.4	0.0
USDA	1 cup	125	2.90	1.20	26.1	0.6	36.0
Magic Crunch®	1 cup	112	1.78	0.58	24.3	0.2	10.9
Malt O Meal® cooked	1 cup	122	3.50	0.30	25.8	0.6	5.0
Maypo® cooked, hot	1 cup	170	5.80	2.40	31.8	1.2	125.0
Mini Wheats®							
brown sugar frosting	1 cup	176	4.37	0.50	41.7	4.6	22.0
frosted	1 cup	161	3.87	0.47	38.6	4.8	17.
Muffets®	1 oz	105	3.08	0.30	22.5	2.8	11.
malt flavored	1 oz	106	3.12	0.29	23.3	2.8	11.
Muslix®							
bran	1 cup	312	9.46	3.69	70.8	13.6	50.
crunchy golden	1 cup	253	6.14	5.31	48.0	6.1	39.
five-grain	1 cup	317	8.71	4.83	70.1	9.4	37.
Natural Bran Flakes® General Mills	28.4 g	88	3.00	0.00	23.0	5.7	16.
Natural Raisin Bran® General Foods	39.7 g	122	3.00	1.00	32.0	5.9	20.
Ninja Turtles® Ralston, sweetened	1 cup	110	1.00	0.00	26.0	0.0	3.
Nutri Grain®							
barley	1 cup	153	4.50	0.30	33.9	2.4	11.
corn	1 cup	160	3.40	1.00	35.5	2.6	1.
rye	1 cup	144	3.50	0.30	33.9	2.6	8.
wheat	1 cup	158	3.80	0.50	37.2	2.8	12.
Oat Bran	1 cup	162	6.83	3.09	26.7	4.5	26.
cooked	1 cup	88	7.03	1.88	25.1	1.7	21.
instant, apple cinnamon	39 g	130	3.00	2.00	30.0	5.0	3.
raisin/spice, hot	1 oz	100	3.00	1.00	19.0	3.8	16.
Kellogg's®	28.4 g	100	4.00	1.00	22.0	1.5	
Nabisco®							
instant, honey	35.4 g	110	3.00	2.00	26.0	5.0	15.
instant, regular	28.4 g	80	4.00	2.00	20.0	5.0	2.
Quaker®	1 cup	270	18.00	6.00	51.0	12.3	60.
Oat Bran Flakes® Health Valley, almond	1 oz	90	3.00	1.00	20.0	3.7	0.
Oat Bran O's® Health Valley, fruit/nut	1 oz	110	3.00	3.00	19.0	2.8	20.
Oat Chex® Ralston	1 oz	100	3.00	1.00	22.0	1.0	2.
Oat Flakes® Post	28.4 g	107	5.00	1.00	22.0	2.1	39.
Oh's® honey nut	1 cup	197	2.72	6.34	31.7	1.4	0.
Oatmeal							
cooked	1 cup	145	6.00	2.40	25.2	4.5	20.
raw	1 cup	311	13.00	5.10	54.2	4.6	42.
Oatmeal Crisp® General Mills	1 oz	110	2.00	2.00	22.0	1.0	40.
Oatmeal Raisin Crisp®	34 g	130	3.00	2.00	25.0	1.5	40.
Oats							
apple/cinnamon	1 oz	21	0.52	0.25	3.9	0.4	3.
apple/cinnamon, dry	1 oz	107	2.69	1.31	20.3	2.0	18.
cinnamon & spice	1 oz	26	0.59	0.28	5.2	1.4	3.
cinnamon & spice, dry	1 oz	107	2.47	1.19	21.7	1.7	15.
honey & graham	1 oz	20	0.50	0.25	4.0	0.3	3.

FOOD	IRON (mg)	POTAS-SIUM (mg)	SODIUM (mg)	SUGAR (g)	THIAMIN (mg)	RIBO-FLAVIN (mg)	NIACIN (mg)	% OF CALORIES FROM FAT
Lucky Charms®								
CNF	4.25	58	154		0.42	0.00	1.54	6
USDA	5.10	66	227	13.6	0.40	0.50	5.60	9
Magic Crunch®	3.70	63	170	9.6	0.56	0.00		5
Malt O Meal® cooked	9.50	31	2		0.40	0.30	5.90	2
Maypo® cooked, hot	8.40	211	9		0.70	0.80	9.40	13
Mini Wheats®								
brown sugar frosting	6.67	151	8	12.6	1.00	0.04	2.41	3
frosted	6.20	124	7	11.6	0.93	0.03	2.24	3
Muffets®	0.87	98	2		0.07	0.02	1.42	3
malt flavored	0.87	98.40	2		0.07	0.02	1.42	2
Muslix®								
bran	6.91	478	241	20.9	0.95	0.12	4.73	11
crunchy golden	6.40	249	310	10.7	0.90	0.11	2.75	19
five-grain	4.92	388	95	24.7	0.57	0.08	2.46	14
Natural Bran Flakes® General Mills	8.10	194	205	5.1	0.38	0.43	5.00	0
Natural Raisin Bran® General Foods	6.20	262	198	13.3	0.52	0.59	6.90	7
Ninja Turtles® Ralston, sweetened	1.80	21	190	11.0	0.38	0.12	5.01	0
Nutri Grain®								
barley	1.45	108	277	2.9	0.50	0.60	7.20	2
corn	0.89	98	276	2.9	0.50	0.60	7.40	6
rye	1.13	72	272	2.9	0.50	0.60	7.00	2
wheat	1.24	120	299	3.1	0.60	0.70	7.70	3
Oat Bran	7.13	183	155	6.4	0.57	0.07	2.83	18
cooked	1.93	201	2	1.6	0.35	0.07	0.32	19
instant, apple cinnamon	0.27	160	160	11.0	0.04	0.02	0.04	14
raisin/spice, hot	0.70	100	10		0.06	0.05	1.20	9
Kellogg's®	4.50	115	270	0.8	0.38	0.43	5.00	9
Nabisco®								
instant, honey	5.63	150	160	8.0	0.47	0.53	6.37	16
instant, regular	0.20	140	0	0.5	0.03	0.01	0.03	23
Quaker®	5.40	540	15		0.90	0.31	15.00	20
Oat Bran Flakes® Health Valley, almond	1.08	105	0	0.8	0.15	0.10	2.00	10
Oat Bran O's® Health Valley, fruit/nut	1.80	130	3		0.09	0.10	0.80	25
Oat Chex® Ralston	3.38	86	240	0.8	0.28	0.05	3.75	9
Oat Flakes® Post	8.10	133	127	5.8	0.38	0.42	5.00	8
Oh's® honey nut	5.75	70	210	9.5	0.86	0.39	1.99	29
Oatmeal								
cooked	1.59	132	1	0.9	0.26	0.05	0.30	15
raw	3.41	284	3	1.5	0.59	0.11	0.63	15
Oatmeal Crisp® General Mills	4.50	80	180	6.0	0.38	0.43	5.00	16
Oatmeal Raisin Crisp®	4.50	120	170	10.0	0.38	0.43	5.00	14
Oats								
apple/cinnamon	0.73	18	47		0.11	0.01	0.26	11
apple/cinnamon, dry	3.77	95	242		0.57	0.03	1.36	11
cinnamon & spice	1.79	16	62	2.2	0.28	0.01	0.74	10
cinnamon & spice, dry	7.51	67	260	9.4	1.20	0.03	3.08	10
honey & graham	1.50	10	52	1.6	0.25	0.01	0.60	11

FOOD	AMOUNT	CALORIES (kcal)	PROTEIN (g)	FAT (g)	CARBO-HYDRATES (g)	FIBER (g)	CALCIUM (mg
Oats (continued)							
honey & graham, dry	1 oz	108	2.66	1.33	21.3	1.4	16.(
instant/nonfortified, cooked	1 cup	145	6.00	2.40	25.2		20.(
instant/nonfortified, dry	1 cup	311	13.00	5.10	54.2		42.(
maple & brown sugar	1 oz	26	0.65	0.32	5.2	0.3	3.:
maple & brown sugar, dry	1 oz	108	2.67	1.32	21.4	1.3	14.:
oats & oat bran	1 oz	23	1.02	0.45	3.6	0.6	3.!
oats & oat bran, dry	1 oz	111	5.01	2.23	17.6	2.9	19.:
oats, peaches'n cream	1 oz	24	0.52	0.30	4.8	0.4	5.:
peaches'n cream, dry	1 oz	107	2.34	1.36	21.3	1.8	22.i
puffed, added sugar	1 cup	100	3.00	1.00	19.0	2.7	44.(
quick, cooked	1 cup	145	6.00	2.40	25.2		20.(
quick, dry	1 cup	311	13.00	5.10	54.2		42.(
raisin & bran	1 oz	24	0.61	0.29	4.8	0.5	4.
raisin & bran, dry	1 oz	104	2.61	1.25	20.5	2.3	18..
raisins & spice	1 oz	25	0.60	0.28	5.1	0.4	4..
raisins & spice, dry	1 oz	105	2.51	1.15	21.2	1.6	17.<
regular	1 oz	17	0.59	0.28	2.9	0.4	3.
regular, cooked	1 cup	145	6.00	2.40	25.2		20.(
regular, dry	1 oz	107	3.81	1.84	18.8	2.6	20..
regular, dry	1 cup	311	13.00	5.10	54.2		42.(
rolled, regular, quick, cooked	1 cup	145	6.08	2.34	25.3	3.7	18.
rolled, regular, quick, dry	1 cup	311	13.00	5.10	54.3	7.5	42.
Oats, Quaker®							
apple/cinnamon, packet	1 item	135	3.90	1.60	26.3	1.4	158.!
bran/raisin, packet	1 item	158	4.90	1.90	30.4	1.8	173.!
cinnamon/spice, packet	1 item	177	4.80	1.90	35.1	1.5	172.
maple/sugar, packet	1 item	163	4.60	1.90	31.9	1.4	162.
plain, instant, packet	1 item	104	4.40	1.70	18.1	1.6	163.
100% Bran®	1 cup	78	8.30	3.30	48.1	19.5	46.
100% Natural® Health Valley							
plain	1 cup	489	12.10	22.40	65.2	3.8	181.
bran, apple	1 oz	90	3.00	1.00	17.0	5.1	0.
100% Organic							
raisin bran flakes	1 oz	90	3.00	1.00	21.0	6.0	0.
sprouts 7/raisins	1 oz	90	4.00	1.00	16.0	4.7	0.
100% Organic® Health Valley							
bran/raisin	1 oz	90	4.00	1.00	15.0	5.1	0.
corn flakes	1 oz	90	3.00	1.00	19.0	4.0	0.
Orangeola® Health Valley							
almond/date	1 oz	90	3.00	1.00	19.0	3.0	20.
banana	1 oz	90	3.00	1.00	20.0	3.0	20.
Organic® Health Valley							
amaranth	1 oz	90	3.00	1.00	20.0	2.8	0.
blue corn flakes	1 oz	90	3.00	1.00	19.0	2.8	0.
crisp brown rice	1 oz	90	2.00	1.00	21.0	2.0	0
Organic Oat Bran Flakes® Health Valley	1 oz	90	3.00	1.00	20.0	3.7	0.
raisins	1 oz	90	3.00	1.00	20.0	3.7	0

FOOD	IRON (mg)	POTAS-SIUM (mg)	SODIUM (mg)	SUGAR (g)	THIAMIN (mg)	RIBO-FLAVIN (mg)	NIACIN (mg)	% OF CALORIES FROM FAT
Oats (continued)								
honey & graham, dry	7.93	55	273	8.2	1.29	0.04	3.19	11
instant/nonfortified, cooked	1.59	132	1		0.26	0.05	0.30	15
instant/nonfortified, dry	3.41	284	3		0.59	0.11	0.63	15
maple & brown sugar	0.91	17	58	0.9	0.14	0.01	0.33	11
maple & brown sugar, dry	3.77	71	239	1.8	0.57	0.03	1.36	11
oats & oat bran	0.34	26	0	0.1	0.04	0.01	0.06	18
oats & oat bran, dry	1.67	130	1	0.3	0.17	0.04	0.29	18
oats, peaches'n cream	0.84	27	46		0.13	0.01	0.30	12
peaches'n cream, dry	3.77	120	207		0.57	0.06	1.36	11
puffed, added sugar	4.00		294	0.0	0.33	0.38	4.40	9
quick, cooked	1.59	132	1		0.26	0.05	0.30	
quick, dry	3.41	284	3		0.59	0.11	0.63	15
raisin & bran	1.88	26	50	1.8	0.30	0.01	0.89	11
raisin & bran, dry	8.01	111	212	7.7	1.15	0.05	3.79	11
raisins & spice	1.79	21	48	2.3	0.26	0.01	0.70	10
raisins & spice, dry	7.51	87	202	9.4	1.09	0.04	2.95	10
regular	0.58	16	34	0.1	0.09	0.01	0.21	15
regular, cooked	1.59	132	1		0.26	0.05	0.30	15
regular, dry	3.77	104	218	0.5	0.57	0.04	1.36	15
regular, dry	3.41	284	3		0.59	0.11	0.63	15
rolled, regular, quick, cooked	1.59	131	2	1.0	0.26	0.05	0.30	15
rolled, regular, quick, dry	3.40	283	3	1.5	0.59	0.11	0.63	15
Oats, Quaker®								
apple/cinnamon, packet	6.07	107	222		0.48	0.28	5.13	11
bran/raisin, packet	7.61	236	247		0.56	0.63	8.12	11
cinnamon/spice, packet	6.65	104	280		0.56	0.34	5.66	10
maple/sugar, packet	6.35	102	280	4.7	0.53	0.32	5.35	10
plain, instant, packet	6.32	100	286	0.7	0.53	0.29	5.49	15
100% Bran®	8.12	824	457	14.7	1.60	1.80	20.90	38
100% Natural® Health Valley								
plain	3.07	514	45	22.5	0.31	0.56	2.37	41
bran, apple	0.36	80	10		0.09	0.07	4.00	10
100% Organic								
raisin bran flakes	1.44	110	5	7.6	0.15	0.03	3.00	10
sprouts 7/raisins	1.44	130	0		0.60	0.05	1.60	10
100% Organic® Health Valley								
bran/raisin	1.44	110	10	7.6	0.03	0.03	4.00	10
corn flakes	1.44	80	10	1.9	0.24	0.07	1.20	10
Orangeola® Health Valley								
almond/date	0.07	110	30		15.00	0.07	0.40	10
banana	0.72	150	30		0.15	0.07	0.40	10
Organic® Health Valley								
amaranth	1.44	65	5 -	0.02	0.00	0.00	10	
blue corn flakes	3.60	80	10	1.9	0.15	0.00	3.20	10
crisp brown rice	0.72	90	3	2.5	0.09	0.00	1.20	10
Organic Oat Bran Flakes® Health Valley	1.08	105	0	0.8	0.15	0.10	2.00	10
raisins	1.08	105	0		0.15	0.10	2.00	10

BREAKFAST CEREALS

FOOD	AMOUNT	CALORIES (kcal)	PROTEIN (g)	FAT (g)	CARBO-HYDRATES (g)	FIBER (g)	CALCIUM (mg)
Organic Oat Bran O's® Health Valley	1 oz	90	3.00	1.00	20.0	3.7	0.0
Pac Man®	1 cup	120	1.27	0.46	27.3	0.6	27.8
Pep®	1 cup	129	3.68	0.40	30.1	4.0	13.6
Pro Stars®	1 cup	95	1.49	0.78	20.0	0.9	8.8
Product 19® Kellogg's	1 cup	100	3.00	0.00	24.0	1.0	
Puffed Rice	1 cup	55	0.90	0.05	12.6	0.0	1.1
Puffed Wheats	1 cup	46	1.76	0.16	9.4	0.5	3.2
Quaker® Oat Squares	1 cup	217	7.40	3.25	39.4	4.1	32.2
Raisin Bran®	1 cup	157	3.50	0.55	39.0	5.5	19.0
California raisins	1 cup	199	5.41	1.35	48.8	8.7	35.4
California raisins/granola	1 cup	245	6.42	2.84	56.2	9.3	44.8
Raisin Wheats®	1 cup	217	4.37	0.43	49.6	6.0	23.8
Raisinut Bran	1 cup	210	5.22	3.80	42.9	6.8	36.9
Kellogg's®	1 cup	154	5.30	0.98	37.1	5.3	17.2
Post®	1 cup	174	5.28	1.08	42.9	6.0	26.7
Ralston®	1 cup	178	4.40	0.30	46.5	7.1	27.0
Raisin Grape Nuts® Post	28.4 g	102	3.00	0.00	23.0	1.6	11.0
Raisin Nut Bran® General Mills	1 oz	110	3.00	3.00	20.0	2.5	40.0
Real Oat Bran® Health Valley							
almond	1 oz	90	4.00	1.00	18.0	3.0	20.0
Hawaiian	1 oz	100	4.00	1.00	19.0	4.0	20.0
raisin	1 oz	83	3.33	0.83	15.0	3.3	16.7
Rice							
puffed, added sugar	1 cup	115	1.00	0.00	26.0	0.2	3.0
puffed, plain	1 cup	56	0.88	0.07	12.6	0.1	0.8
Rice Bran® Health Valley, almond/date	1 oz	110	2.00	3.00	19.0	2.1	0.0
Rice Chex®	1 cup	100	1.34	0.10	22.5	0.2	3.5
Rice Flakes®	1 cup	124	2.10	0.12	27.7	0.4	11.5
Rice Krispies® Kellogg's	1 cup	105	2.10	0.14	24.1	0.5	4.0
Roman meal, cooked	1 cup	147	6.60	1.00	33.0	2.3	30.0
Shredded Wheat®							
large biscuit	1 oz	102	2.78	0.33	23.6	3.2	11.6
spoon size	1 cup	170	4.75	0.56	39.3	5.3	17.2
Shredded Wheat'n Bran, Spoon Size®	1 cup	194	6.98	0.60	43.4	7.4	22.2
Shredded Wheat/Oat Bran Nabisco®	28.4 g	100	3.00	1.00	22.0	4.0	8.5
Shreddies®	51.6 g	185	4.33	0.43	43.9	5.7	20.
Shreddies & Raisins®	1 cup	208	4.88	0.49	49.0	5.6	39.
Special K® Kellogg's	1 cup	110	6.00	0.00	20.0	1.0	
S'mores Grahams® General Mills	1 oz	120	1.00	2.00	24.0	2.6	0.0
Sprouts 7/banana® Health Valley	1 oz	90	3.00	1.00	16.0	4.3	0.0
Squares							
blueberry	1 cup	187	4.54	0.57	46.0	5.1	19.
raisin	1 cup	187	4.26	0.68	45.5	4.7	19.
strawberry	1 cup	187	4.09	0.91	45.6	4.7	19.
Strawberry Wheats®	1 cup	234	5.91	0.79	50.6	5.9	33.
Sugar Crisp®	1 cup	124	2.70	0.36	28.8	1.0	20.
Sugar Smacks®	1 cup	144	3.02	0.95	31.9	0.9	6.

FOOD	IRON (mg)	POTAS-SIUM (mg)	SODIUM (mg)	SUGAR (g)	THIAMIN (mg)	RIBO-FLAVIN (mg)	NIACIN (mg)	% OF CALORIES FROM FAT
Organic Oat Bran O's® Health Valley	1.08	105	0	0.8	0.15	0.10	2.00	10
Pac Man®	4.11	20	216		0.46	0.00	1.48	3
Pep®	4.89	121	252	4.4	0.74	0.03	1.76	3
Pro Stars®	3.15	40	150	9.5	0.05	0.01	1.09	7
Product 19® Kellogg's	18.00	45	320	3.4	1.50	1.70	20.00	0
Puffed Rice	0.08	16	1	0.0	0.01	0.01	0.24	1
Puffed Wheats	0.42	43	1	0.2	0.01	0.02	0.67	3
Quaker® Oat Squares	8.68	185	265	9.1	0.76	0.08	3.69	13
Raisin Bran®	6.65	300	273	13.3	1.00	0.05	2.80	3
California raisins	8.57	369	282	17.2	1.29	0.09	4.06	6
California raisins/granola	9.93	405	315	20.8	1.49	0.10	4.78	10
Raisin Wheats®	2.20	190	22	11.8	0.09	0.08	8.16	2
Raisinut Bran	7.55	307	358	12.3	1.14	0.09	3.52	16
Kellogg's®	6.00	256	359	13.1	0.49	0.59	6.69	6
Post®	9.03	350	370	15.1	0.74	0.85	10.00	6
Ralston®	6.70	287	486	14.9	0.60	0.60	7.40	2
Raisin Grape Nuts® Post	1.80	107	141	6.2	0.38	0.43	5.00	0
Raisin Nut Bran® General Mills	4.50	140	140	8.0	0.38	0.43	5.00	25
Real Oat Bran® Health Valley								
almond	1.08	120	30		0.15	0.07	0.00	10
Hawaiian	1.08	200	30		0.23	0.07	0.40	9
raisin	0.90	133	25		0.19	0.06	0.00	9
Rice								
puffed, added sugar	0.00	43	21	11.1	0.00	0.00	0.00	0
puffed, plain	0.15	16	0	0.0	0.02	0.01	0.42	1
Rice Bran® Health Valley, almond/date	1.08	130	2		0.15	0.00	2.00	25
Rice Chex®	1.59	29	211	1.3	0.33	0.01	4.44	1
Rice Flakes®	4.24	38	284	4.9	0.64	0.07	1.53	1
Rice Krispies® Kellogg's	3.78	34	295	2.8	0.57	0.01	1.36	1
Roman meal, cooked	2.12	302	3	1.0	0.24	0.12	3.08	6
Shredded Wheat®								
large biscuit	0.91	106	5	0.5	0.09	0.08	1.30	3
spoon size	1.96	182	7	0.7	0.14	0.13	2.47	3
Shredded Wheat'n Bran, Spoon Size®	2.53	205	7	0.5	0.17	0.17	3.46	3
Shredded Wheat/Oat Bran Nabisco®	1.43	130	0	0.1	0.06	0.02	1.59	9
Shreddies®	6.86	190	429	8.1	1.03	0.18	2.47	2
Shreddies & Raisins®	8.11	235	504	16.9	1.22	0.18	2.93	2
Special K® Kellogg's	8.10	55	230	1.6	0.53	0.60	7.00	0
S'mores Grahams® General Mills	4.50	50	250	10.0	0.38	0.43	5.00	15
Sprouts 7/banana® Health Valley	1.08	170	0		0.12	0.17	2.00	10
Squares								
blueberry	7.55	162	17	11.9	1.14	0.05	2.73	3
raisin	7.55	196	9	13.1	1.14	0.05	2.73	3
strawberry	7.55	159	17	12.8	1.14	0.05	2.73	4
Strawberry Wheats®	2.18	167	19	14.6	0.09	0.06	5.24	3
Sugar Crisp®	1.15	70	29	12.7	0.66	0.00	1.58	3
Sugar Smacks®	5.03	72	45	16.7	0.76	0.07	1.81	6

89

BREAKFAST CEREALS

FOOD	AMOUNT	CALORIES (kcal)	PROTEIN (g)	FAT (g)	CARBO-HYDRATES (g)	FIBER (g)	CALCIUM (mg)
Super Golden Crisp® Post	28.4 g	104	2.00	0.00	26.0	0.4	5.0
Sugar Corn Pops® Kellogg's	1 cup	108	1.40	0.10	25.6	0.2	1.0
Sugar Smacks® Kellogg's	1 cup	141	2.65	0.72	33.0	0.5	4.2
Super Sugar Crisp® Post	1 cup	123	2.10	0.30	29.8	0.5	7.0
Swiss Breakfast® Health Valley							
raisin	1 oz	80	3.00	1.00	17.0	3.0	20.0
tropical	1 oz	80	3.00	1.00	17.0	3.0	20.0
Tasteeos®	1 cup	94	3.07	0.67	19.0	0.8	11.0
Teddy Graham Breakfast Bears®	28.4 g	120	2.00	3.00	22.0	1.0	
Team®							
CNF	1 cup	162	2.86	0.37	36.2	1.1	15.3
USDA	1 cup	164	2.70	0.70	36.0	0.4	6.0
Toasted Oat® Nature Valley	1 oz	130	2.00	5.00	20.0	1.0	0.0
Toasties®							
corn flakes	28.4 g	111	2.00	0.00	24.0	1.0	3.0
Post	1 cup	88	1.84	0.05	19.5	0.9	0.5
Total® General Mills	1 cup	116	3.30	0.70	26.0	1.0	56.0
corn flakes	1 oz	110	2.00	1.00	24.0	1.8	200.0
raisin bran	42.5 g	140	3.00	1.00	33.0	4.0	200.0
Triples® General Mills	1 oz	110	2.00	1.00	24.0		20.0
Trix® General Mills	1 cup	109	1.53	0.40	25.2	0.3	5.2
Weetabix®	1 cup	108	3.01	0.57	22.6	3.7	10.0
Wheat							
flakes, added sugar	1 cup	105	3.00	0.00	24.0	2.7	12.0
puffed, added sugar	38 g	138	5.59	0.46	30.2	2.1	10.0
puffed, plain	1 cup	44	1.76	0.14	9.6	0.4	3.0
rolled, cooked, hot	1 cup	180	5.00	1.00	41.0	2.9	19.0
shredded, biscuit	1 item	83	2.60	0.30	18.8	2.2	10.0
whole meal, cooked, hot	1 cup	110	4.00	1.00	23.0	1.6	17.0
Wheat Chex®	1 cup	169	4.50	1.10	37.8	3.4	18.0
Wheat Germ							
brown sugar/honey	1 cup	426	24.70	9.10	68.7		38.0
toasted	1 cup	431	32.90	12.10	56.1		50.0
Wheatena, cooked	1 cup	136	4.86	1.22	28.7	2.6	9.0
Wheaties®	1 cup	101	2.80	0.50	23.1	3.3	44.0
Whole Wheat Natural®	1 cup	150	4.84	0.97	33.2	2.7	16.0

OD	IRON (mg)	POTAS-SIUM (mg)	SODIUM (mg)	SUGAR (g)	THIAMIN (mg)	RIBO-FLAVIN (mg)	NIACIN (mg)	% OF CALORIES FROM FAT
uper Golden Crisp® Post	2.60	41	44	14.7	0.36	0.42	4.90	0
ugar Corn Pops® Kellogg's	1.80	17	103	13.2	0.40	0.40	5.00	1
ugar Smacks® Kellogg's	2.39	56	100	21.1	0.49	0.59	6.67	5
uper Sugar Crisp® Post	2.10	123	29	14.9	0.40	0.50	5.80	2
viss Breakfast® Health Valley								
raisin	1.08	110	20		0.12	0.07	1.20	11
tropical	0.72	150	20		0.12	0.03	1.20	11
asteeos®	3.82	71	183	0.9	0.31	0.36	4.22	6
ddy Graham Breakfast Bears®		40	135	7.0				23
am®								
CNF	5.59	74	349	5.2	0.84	0.10	2.02	2
USDA	2.57	71	259	6.6	0.50	0.60	7.40	4
asted Oat® Nature Valley	0.72	75	90	6.0	0.09	0.00	0.00	35
asties®								
corn flakes	0.40	34	310	2.0	0.38	0.43	5.00	0
Post	0.60	26	238	1.2	0.30	0.34	4.00	0
tal® General Mills	21.00	123	409	2.7	1.70	2.00	23.30	5
corn flakes	18.00	35	200	1.9	1.50	1.70	20.00	8
raisin bran	18.00	220	190	14.0	1.50	1.70	20.00	6
iples® General Mills	4.50	35	250	3.0	0.53	0.60	7.00	8
ix® General Mills	4.52	27	181	12.0	0.37	0.43	5.00	3
eetabix®	3.77	97	102	1.4	0.57	0.43	1.36	5y
heat								
flakes, added sugar	4.80	81	368	3.2	0.40	0.45	5.30	0
puffed, added sugar	1.80	132	2	17.1	0.08	0.09	4.10	3
puffed, plain	0.57	42	0	0.2	0.02	0.02	1.30	3
rolled, cooked, hot	1.70	202	535	1.0	0.17	0.07	2.20	5
shredded, biscuit	0.74	77	0	0.1	0.07	0.06	1.08	3
whole meal, cooked, hot	1.20	118	535	1.0	0.15	0.05	1.50	8
heat Chex®	7.30	174	308	2.1	0.60	0.17	8.10	6
heat Germ								
brown sugar/honey	7.71	803	3		1.41	0.70	4.73	19
toasted	10.30	1070	4		1.89	0.93	6.31	25
heatena, cooked	1.36	187	5	1.0	0.02	0.05	1.34	8
heaties®	4.60	108	363	2.4	0.40	0.40	5.10	5
hole Wheat Natural®	1.50	171	1	1.0	0.17	0.12	2.15	6

BABY FOODS

FOOD	AMOUNT	CALORIES (kcal)	PROTEIN (g)	FAT (g)	CARBO-HYDRATES (g)	FIBER (g)	CALCIUM (mg
Cereal, barley							
barley, milk	1 oz	31	1.30	0.90	4.6	3.22	6
barley, whole milk added	1 cup	231	9.61	6.66	34.3		63
dry	1 cup	137	4.26	0.88	29.0	3.14	47
mix fruit, milk	1 cup	233	10.00	7.49	32.7		58
Cereal, infantsoy							
dry	1 cup	140	11.00	0.42	22.9		55
whole milk	1 cup	228	15.30	6.09	28.1		688
Cereal, mixed							
/bananas, milk	1 cup	238	9.85	7.11	34.1		639
w/bananas, dry	1 cup	145	4.53	1.38	28.8	2.99	477
dry	1 cup	143	5.27	1.13	28.2	2.88	521
/fruit, whole milk	1 cup	239	9.80	7.27	34.0		671
w/fruit, dry	1 cup	146	4.47	1.55	28.6		513
w/milk, CNF	1 cup	236	10.50	6.89	33.5		679
Cereal, oatmeal							
dry	1 cup	149	4.72	2.21	27.7	2.53	482
prepared, w/milk	1 cup	242	10.00	7.85	33.1		643
/bananas, milk	1 cup	242	10.40	8.53	31.5	10.90	581
/bananas, dry	1 cup	149	5.10	2.95	25.9	1.99	412
Cereal, rice	1 oz	113	4.48	1.73	19.8	0.00	142
/apple, dry	1 cup	148	3.07	0.54	31.6	0.58	464
/apple, whole milk	1 cup	241	8.54	6.35	36.6	3.15	627
dry	1 cup	149	3.14	1.48	29.9	0.19	510
milk	1 oz	33	1.10	1.00	4.7	0.25	68
/strawberries, dry	1 cup	151	4.26	2.61	27.2	3.26	412
/strawberries, milk	1 cup	244	9.61	8.22	32.6		581
whole milk	1 cup	242	8.61	7.20	35.0		668
oatmeal, milk	1 oz	33	1.40	1.20	4.3	0.70	62
mixed, USDA	1 oz	32	1.30	1.00	4.5	0.25	62
Cereal, wheat, milk	1 oz	123	5.36	3.09	18.4	0.00	120
Combination foods w/vegetables							
beef	1 oz	15	0.60	0.60	2.0	0.10	3
beef, jar	1 cup	158	6.24	4.47	24.4	2.92	29
beef, strained	1 cup	129	4.30	4.73	18.1	2.56	20
beef & liver, strained	1 cup	137	6.57	3.79	20.2	2.78	51
chicken, jar	1 cup	133	4.11	3.99	21.0	3.02	45
chicken, strained	1 cup	109	4.78	2.19	18.4	2.57	32
ham, jar	1 cup	129	5.32	4.60	17.7	2.66	10
ham, strained	1 cup	127	4.89	2.73	21.6	2.91	28
lamb, jar	1 cup	122	4.60	4.07	17.7	2.66	30
lamb, strained	1 cup	130	5.16	3.88	19.5	2.84	39
macaroni, beef, jar	1 cup	156	5.45	4.36	23.2		59
spaghetti, beef, jar	1 cup	153	4.16	4.55	23.3		51
spaghetti, beef, strained	1 cup	167	4.91	4.62	25.8		67
turkey, jar	1 cup	123	3.99	4.12	18.5	2.51	66
turkey, strained	1 cup	126	4.46	4.02	19.0	2.73	40
veal, jar	1 cup	136	6.59	2.88	22.1	2.24	27
veal, strained	1 cup	115	5.28	1.50	21.0	2.20	26

FOOD	IRON (mg)	POTAS-SIUM (mg)	SODIUM (mg)	CHOLES-TEROI (mg)	SUGAR (gms)	% OF CALORIES FROM FAT
Cereal, barley						
barley, milk	3.5	54	14.0	0.0		26
barley, whole milk added	16.3	389	92.2			26
dry	18.1	137	6.7	0.0		6
mix fruit, milk	17.3	523	113.0			29
Cereal, infantsoy						
dry	19.4	283	28.8			3
whole milk	17.1	508	109.0			24
Cereal, mixed						
/bananas, milk	14.5	453	108.0			27
w/bananas, dry	16.0	207	23.8	0.0		9
dry	16.0	176	13.5	0.0		7
/fruit, whole milk	14.4	454	103.0			27
w/fruit, dry	15.9	208	18.4			10
w/milk, CNF	14.5	425	98.3			26
Cereal, oatmeal						
dry	16.8	152	4.8	0.0		13
prepared, w/milk	15.2	403	90.4			29
/bananas, milk	17.3	513	110.0	0.0		32
/bananas, dry	19.2	275	26.8	0.0		18
Cereal, rice	2.07	112	40.8	0.0		14
/apple, dry	11.5	90	3.5	0.0		3
/apple, whole milk	10.4	347	89.2	0.0		24
dry	15.7	147	3.8	0.0		9
milk	3.5	54	13.0	0.0		27
/strawberries, dry	19.2	184	29.5	0.0		16
/strawberries, milk	17.3	432	113.0			30
whole milk	14.2	399	89.6			27
oatmeal, milk	3.4	58	13.0	0.0		33
mixed, USDA	3.0	56	13.0	0.0		28
Cereal, wheat, milk	1.9	98	28.6			23
Combination foods w/vegetables						
beef	0.1	29	6.0	3.4		36
beef, jar	1.2	299	53.1	13.2		25
beef, strained	0.8	144	30.2	11.6		33
beef & liver, strained	1.5	376	45.5	45.5		25
chicken, jar	1.1	233	24.7	27.4		27
chicken, strained	2.1	75	24.5	30.3		18
ham, jar	0.5	104	38.7	12.1		32
ham, strained	0.7	136	60.9	13.2		19
lamb, jar	1.1	247	47.2	12.1		30
lamb, strained	1.0	212	40.0	15.5		27
macaroni, beef, jar	1.4	272	11.3			25
spaghetti, beef, jar	0.9	201	37.0			27
spaghetti, beef, strained	0.8	323	23.2			25
turkey, jar	1.1	80	22.8	22.8		30
turkey, strained	0.6	114	40.9	24.8		29
veal, jar	1.6	308	34.8	54.8		19
veal, strained	0.7	266	33.1	46.5		12

BABY FOODS

FOOD	AMOUNT	CALORIES (kcal)	PROTEIN (g)	FAT (g)	CARBO-HYDRATES (g)	FIBER (g)	CALCIU (m
Combination foods, meat/egg							
beef, liver, broth, strained	1 cup	319	29.80	18.30	7.0	0.00	1
beef, broth, jar	1 cup	295	33.00	16.70	0.7	0.00	1
beef, broth, strained	1 cup	311	31.20	19.00	1.7	0.00	1
chicken, broth, jar	1 cup	317	31.70	20.00	0.5	0.00	10
chicken, broth, strained	1 cup	314	30.60	19.80	1.2	0.73	15
ham, broth, jar	1 cup	281	35.60	13.80	1.2	0.00	1
ham, broth, strained	1 cup	251	31.30	12.50	1.1	0.00	1
lamb, broth, strained	1 cup	341	29.00	23.20	1.9	0.00	1
turkey, broth, jar	1 cup	335	33.60	21.20	0.0	0.00	4
turkey, broth, strained	1 cup	317	31.90	19.70	1.0	0.00	9
veal, broth, jar	1 cup	266	33.30	13.30	1.1	0.00	1
veal, broth, strained	1 cup	270	31.80	14.30	1.3	0.00	1
Cottage cheese and pineapple	1 oz	20	0.80	0.20	3.7	0.00	
Dessert, apple betty	1 oz	20	0.10	0.00	5.6	0.00	
arrowroot cookie	1 item	24	0.40	0.90	4.3	0.00	
banana & cream, jar	1 cup	187	1.69	2.42	41.9	2.88	4
bananas & cream, strained	1 cup	187	1.69	2.42	41.9	2.42	4
blueberry, jar	1 cup	156	0.52	0.26	42.3	23.90	
blueberry, strained	1 cup	154	0.51	0.26	41.6	23.50	
cherry vanilla, jar	1 cup	169	0.73	0.48	45.2	0.73	1
cherry vanilla, strained	1 cup	161	0.73	0.73	42.3	0.73	1
cookies, enriched	1 item	28	0.80	0.90	4.4	0.00	
Dutch apple	1 oz	19	0.00	0.30	4.7	0.20	
fruit, strained	1 oz	17	0.10	0.00	4.5	0.70	
orange pudding	1 oz	23	0.30	0.30	5.0	0.10	
peach cobbler, strained	1 oz	18	0.10	0.00	5.0	0.25	
peaches & cream, jar	1 cup	186	1.45	1.94	43.1	3.63	4
peaches & cream, strained	1 cup	186	1.45	1.94	43.1	3.63	4
strawberry, strained	1 cup	132	0.46	0.23	35.8		
tutti fruti, jar	1 cup	167	1.59	0.60	45.0	1.06	
tutti fruti, strained	1 cup	150	2.89	0.61	37.6	1.58	
Dessert, custard, arrowroot	1 cup	183	4.01	6.30	28.8		
banana, strained	1 cup	217	2.37	6.03	40.2	2.82	9
butterscotch	1 cup	316	2.21	18.70	36.8		
chocolate	1 oz	24	0.50	0.50	4.6	0.10	
custard, strained	1 cup	212	4.34	6.95	34.5	0.00	
vanilla	1 oz	24	0.40	0.60	4.6	0.10	
vanilla, jar	1 cup	171	4.10	6.03	38.9	0.00	1
vanilla, strained	1 cup	204	3.14	4.59	39.3	0.00	1
Dessert, fruit, & cream, jar	1 cup	195	1.69	2.18	44.5	0.87	
& cream, strained	1 cup	195	1.69	2.18	44.5		
salad, jar	1 cup	140	0.49	0.13	38.0	1.47	
salad, strained	1 cup	143	1.20	0.17	38.3	1.44	
orange, strained	1 cup	201	2.90	2.66	43.8	1.45	
pear, jar	1 cup	182	2.31	1.21	45.4		
pear, strained	1 cup	153	2.59	1.24	37.0		
strawberry, jar	1 cup	149	0.52	0.26	40.3		

94

OD	IRON (mg)	POTAS-SIUM (mg)	SODIUM (mg)	CHOLES-TEROI (mg)	SUGAR (gms)	% OF CALORIES FROM FAT
ombination foods, meat/egg						
beef, liver, broth, strained	13.8	406	179.0	910.0		52
beef, broth, jar	4.1	466	139.0	19.4		51
beef, broth, strained	3.6	492	155.0	16.9		55
chicken, broth, jar	2.3	317	98.0	38.7		57
chicken, broth, strained	2.1	311	115.0	24.2		57
ham, broth, jar	2.4	537	104.0	42.7		44
ham, broth, strained	1.9	507	253.0			45
lamb, broth, strained	1.9	479	165.0			61
turkey, broth, jar	2.1	386	135.0	33.9	0.00	57
turkey, broth, strained	2.2	404	146.0	33.9		56
veal, broth, jar	2.9	577	133.0	53.2		45
veal, broth, strained	2.1	478	154.0	46.0		48
ottage cheese and pineapple	0.0	12	15.0	2.6		9
essert, apple betty	0.1	14	3.0	0.0		0
arrowroot cookie	0.2	9	22.0	0.0		34
banana & cream, jar	0.5	177	19.4	0.0		12
bananas & cream, strained	0.5	177	19.4	0.0		12
blueberry, jar	0.8	21	23.4	0.0		2
blueberry, strained	0.8	23	20.4	0.0		1
cherry vanilla, jar	0.5	87	21.8	24.2		3
cherry vanilla, strained	0.7	102	24.2	24.2		4
cookies, enriched	0.3	33	12.0	0.0	1.51	29
Dutch apple	0.1	9	5.0	0.0		14
fruit, strained	0.1	27	4.0	0.0		0
orange pudding	0.0	24	5.7	0.0		12
peach cobbler, strained	0.0	15	2.0	0.0		0
peaches & cream, jar	0.7	254	21.8	0.0		9
peaches & cream, strained	0.7	254	21.8	0.0		9
strawberry, strained	0.5	49	18.5			2
tutti fruti, jar	0.8	159	60.9	39.8		3
tutti fruti, strained	0.5	89	42.1	39.5		4
essert, custard, arrowroot	0.5	118	75.5			31
banana, strained	0.5	128	49.7	0.0		25
butterscotch	1.0	113	140.0			53
chocolate	0.1	24	7.0	0.0	3.78	19
custard, strained	0.5	169	210.0	19.3		30
vanilla	0.1	19	8.0	0.0	4.17	23
vanilla, jar	0.5	157	62.8	19.3		32
vanilla, strained	0.5	154	65.2	19.3		20
essert, fruit, & cream, jar	0.5	271	46.0	0.0		10
& cream, strained	0.5	271	46.0			10
salad, jar	1.0	123	34.4	0.0		1
salad, strained	0.7	173	55.3	0.0		1
orange, strained	0.5	237	50.8	36.3		12
pear, jar	0.5	136	71.8			6
pear, strained	2.6	158	67.3			7
strawberry, jar	0.5	55	20.8			2

BABY FOODS

FOOD	AMOUNT	CALORIES (kcal)	PROTEIN (g)	FAT (g)	CARBO-HYDRATES (g)	FIBER (g)	CALCIU (m
Dessert, tapioca, & bananas	1 oz	16	0.10	0.00	4.3	0.70	
/mango	1 oz	23	0.10	0.10	6.1	0.00	
/papaya, apple	1 oz	20	0.10	0.00	5.4	0.10	
& plums	1 oz	20	0.00	0.00	5.6	0.25	
& prunes	1 oz	20	0.20	0.00	5.2	0.70	
Eggs, yolks	1 oz	58	2.80	4.90	0.3	0.00	2
strained	1 oz	15	0.50	0.50	2.0	0.00	
Fruit, apple							
peach, jar	1 cup	93	0.73	0.05	37.0	3.63	1
peach, strained	1 cup	88	0.73	0.24	36.8		1
raisin, jar	1 cup	186	0.52	0.50	49.9		2
raisin, strained	1 cup	180	0.50	0.40	48.7		2
raspberry, jar	1 cup	98	0.47	0.24	35.7	4.97	
raspberry, strained	1 cup	141	0.95	0.17	43.9	4.97	1
sauce, jar	1 oz	12	0.10	0.00	3.1	0.70	
sauce, strained	1 cup	108	0.35	0.38	28.9	3.99	
Fruit, apricot, jar	1 cup	200	0.92	0.13	54.3	3.96	3
strained	1 cup	179	1.11	0.23	48.1	3.69	2
Fruit, bananas, jar	1 cup	166	1.09	0.34	44.3	4.35	1
bananas, strained	1 cup	155	1.29	0.34	41.1	3.76	1
/pineapple, strained	1 cup	145	0.47	0.42	38.8	3.72	
Fruit, blueberries, jar	1 cup	147	0.24	0.24	39.9		1
strained	1 cup	149	0.24	0.24	40.6		1
Fruit							
fruit salad, jar	1 cup	95	0.48	0.07	38.2		
fruit salad, strained	1 cup	104	0.48	0.00	38.2		
mixed, jar	1 cup	126	0.74	0.47	33.1	4.69	2
mixed, strained	1 cup	111	1.07	0.31	29.2	0.95	2
Fruit, peach	1 oz	20	0.10	0.00	5.4	0.70	
jar	1 cup	123	1.14	0.24	38.5	3.80	
strained	1 cup	111	1.81	0.21	34.5	3.63	
Fruit, pear	1 oz	12	0.10	0.00	3.1	0.25	
& applesauce, jar	1 cup	158	0.47	0.14	43.2	6.23	
& applesauce, strained	1 cup	151	0.26	0.32	41.1	6.76	
& pineapple	1 oz	12	0.10	0.00	3.1	0.25	
& pineapple, jar	1 cup	107	0.95	0.31	28.2	6.19	
& pineapple, strained	1 cup	89	0.89	0.16	23.4	5.15	
Fruit, plums, jar	1 cup	195	0.75	0.50	52.3	3.00	
strained	1 cup	182	0.63	0.22	49.5	3.00	
Fruit, prunes, jar	1 cup	196	1.62	0.27	52.4	7.29	
strained	1 cup	179	2.01	0.55	46.5	6.80	
Fruit, strawberry, jar	1 cup	165	0.73	0.24	44.5		
strained	1 cup	160	0.48	0.24	34.4		
Fruit juice							
apple	1 fl oz	14	0.00	0.00	3.6	0.25	
apple blueberry	1 oz	17	0.10	0.10	4.6	0.10	
apple cherry	1 cup	106	0.38	0.15	26.4	0.25	
apple grape	1 cup	105	0.24	0.18	26.3	0.24	
apple peach	1 fl oz	13	0.00	0.00	3.2	0.25	

FOOD	IRON (mg)	POTAS-SIUM (mg)	SODIUM (mg)	CHOLES-TEROI (mg)	SUGAR (gms)	% OF CALORIES FROM FAT
Dessert, tapioca, & bananas	0.1	25	3.0	0.0		0
/mango	0.0	17	1.0	0.0		4
/papaya, apple	0.1	22	1.0	0.0		0
& plums	0.1	24	2.0	0.0		0
& prunes	0.1	50	1.0	0.0		0
Eggs, yolks	0.8	22	11.0	223.0		76
strained	0.1	11	9.0	18.0		30
Fruit, apple						
peach, jar	0.5	230	9.7	0.0		0
peach, strained	0.7	249	14.5			2
raisin, jar	1.0	551	18.0			2
raisin, strained	1.0	537	17.6			2
raspberry, jar	0.7	199	11.8	0.0		2
raspberry, strained	0.6	172	24.8	0.0		1
sauce, jar	0.1	20	1.0	0.0	2.50	0
sauce, strained	0.4	182	16.4			3
Fruit, apricot, jar	1.1	393	56.7	0.0		1
strained	1.5	346	38.2	0.0		1
Fruit, bananas, jar	0.4	228	27.2	0.0		2
bananas, strained	0.5	194	29.4			2
/pineapple, strained	0.3	109	14.0	0.0		3
Fruit, blueberries, jar	0.5	17	29.0			1
strained	1.5	15	29.0			1
Fruit						
fruit salad, jar	0.5	220	12.1	0.0		1
fruit salad, strained	0.2	210	9.7	0.0		0
mixed, jar	0.5	193	24.6	0.0		3
mixed, strained	0.7	201	28.5	0.0		2
Fruit, peach	0.1	46	2.0	0.0	4.95	0
jar	0.6	364	21.5	0.0		2
strained	0.7	327	37.5	0.0		2
Fruit, pear	0.1	37	1.0	0.0	1.74	0
& applesauce, jar	0.7	82	39.9	0.0		1
& applesauce, strained	0.8	64	30.6	0.0		2
& pineapple	0.1	33	1.0	0.0		0
& pineapple, jar	0.5	123	22.6	0.0		3
& pineapple, strained	0.5	130	24.8	0.0		2
Fruit, plums, jar	0.5	183	10.0			2
strained	0.8	216	15.0			1
Fruit, prunes, jar	1.1	478	54.0			1
strained	0.9	356	31.5			3
Fruit, strawberry, jar	0.7	70	29.0			1
strained	1.0	63	48.4			1
Fruit juice						
apple	0.2	28	1.0	0.0	3.04	0
apple blueberry	0.1	20	0.0	0.0		5
apple cherry	1.0	270	7.5	0.0		1
apple grape	1.1	171	4.8			2
apple peach	0.2	30	0.3	0.0		0

BABY FOODS

FOOD	AMOUNT	CALORIES (kcal)	PROTEIN (g)	FAT (g)	CARBO-HYDRATES (g)	FIBER (g)	CALCIUM (mg
Fruit juice (continued)							
apple pineapple	1 cup	100	0.48	0.20	24.6	0.24	1
apple plum	1 cup	124	0.25	0.25	30.9	0.25	1
apple prune	1 fl oz	23	0.10	0.00	5.6	0.50	
apple raspberry	1 cup	120	0.25	0.75	28.9	0.25	1
mixed fruit	1 fl oz	14	0.00	0.00	3.6	0.25	
orange	1 fl oz	14	0.20	0.10	3.2	0.25	
orange apple	1 fl oz	13	0.10	0.10	3.1	0.25	
orange apricot	1 fl oz	14	0.20	0.00	3.4	0.25	
orange banana	1 cup	81	1.14	0.67	18.3	0.23	1
orange pineapple	1 cup	106	1.29	0.81	24.2	0.24	2
orange prune	1 fl oz	22	0.20	0.10	5.2	0.50	
prune	1 cup	251	134.00	1.51	0.3	32.40	
Macaroni & cheese	1 oz	28	17.00	0.70	0.6	2.10	
Meat, beef	1 oz	30	3.90	1.50	0.0	0.00	
alphabet, jar	1 cup	131	4.62	2.83	21.3	2.83	4
& egg noodles, strained	1 oz	15	0.60	0.50	2.0	0.10	
w/farina, jar	1 cup	158	7.17	5.69	19.0		3
w/farina, strained	1 cup	156	8.16	4.52	20.1		4
lasagna	1 oz	22	1.20	0.60	2.8	0.10	
macaroni w/tomato	1 oz	16	0.60	0.30	2.5	0.10	
/noodle, vegetables, jar	1 cup	176	7.09	7.13	20.3	2.79	8
/noodle, vegetables, strained	1 cup	181	6.93	7.95	20.0	2.82	9
stew	1 oz	14	1.40	0.30	1.5	0.34	
stew, jar	1 cup	199	7.34	6.13	30.0	2.94	3
/vegetables, jar	1 cup	230	15.20	12.70	15.6	2.16	2
/vegetables, strained	1 cup	227	13.10	13.00	16.2	2.18	1
Meat, chicken	1 oz	37	3.90	2.20	0.0	0.00	1
& noodles	1 oz	15	0.60	0.40	2.1	0.25	
noodle w/vegetable, jar	1 cup	168	6.07	6.31	21.3	2.84	8
noodle w/vegetable, strained	1 cup	149	4.91	5.01	20.5	2.77	
rice w/vegetable, jar	1 cup	151	3.74	5.27	21.6	2.65	5
rice w/vegetable, strained	1 cup	136	5.07	4.25	19.0	2.34	6
w/rice, jar	1 cup	109	2.40	2.45	18.9		
stew, strained	1 oz	22	1.50	1.10	1.8	0.17	1
/vegetables, jar	1 cup	209	12.10	11.50	16.1	2.22	11
/vegetables, strained	1 cup	209	12.00	10.70	17.8	2.23	14
Meat, ham	1 oz	32	3.90	1.60	0.0	0.00	
& egg, vegetable, strained	1 cup	149	5.56	5.08	21.3	2.18	
& egg breakfast, jar	1 cup	122	4.21	4.80	15.1		
& egg breakfast, strained	1 cup	127	5.35	4.39	16.0		
vegetable, strained	1 cup	253	166.00	12.90	5.2	18.50	
Meat, lamb	1 oz	29	4.00	1.30	0.0	0.00	
vegetable, strained	1 cup	176	10.70	8.15	16.5	2.74	
Liver	1 oz	29	4.10	1.10	0.4	0.00	
Pork	1 oz	35	4.00	2.00	0.0	0.00	
Meat, turkey	1 oz	32	4.00	1.70	0.0	0.00	
& rice	1 oz	14	0.50	0.40	2.1	0.00	
/vegetables, jar	1 cup	176	15.10	5.68	18.0	2.22	1
/vegetables, strained	1 cup	236	13.00	14.00	16.3	2.22	

FOOD	IRON (mg)	POTAS-SIUM (mg)	SODIUM (mg)	CHOLES-TEROl (mg)	SUGAR (gms)	% OF CALORIES FROM FAT
Fruit, pear (continued)						
apple pineapple	1.0	241	4.8	0.0		2
apple plum	1.0	256	5.0	0.0		2
apple prune	0.3	46	2.0	0.0		0
apple raspberry	0.5	334	15.1	0.0		6
mixed fruit	0.1	31	1.0	0.0		0
orange	0.1	57	0.0	0.0	3.20	7
orange apple	0.1	43	1.0	0.0		7
orange apricot	0.1	62	2.0	0.0		0
orange banana	0.3	361	3.4	0.0		7
orange pineapple	0.4	344	3.5			7
orange prune	0.3	56	1.0	0.0		4
prune	30.2	1	490.0	7.5		2
Macaroni & cheese	15.0	0	13.0	21.0	1.85	32
Meat, beef	0.4	62	23.0	3.6	0.00	45
alphabet, jar	1.3	239	18.0	20.6		19
& egg noodles, strained	0.1	13	8.0	2.0		30
w/farina, jar	0.7	214	26.7			32
w/farina, strained	0.9	202	35.1			26
lasagna	0.3	35	129.0			25
macaroni w/tomato	0.1	27	5.0	1.1		17
/noodle, vegetables, jar	1.5	218	40.5	26.3		36
/noodle, vegetables, strained	1.3	190	64.1	26.7		40
stew	0.2	40	98.0	3.6		19
stew, jar	1.3	340	33.4	13.4		28
/vegetables, jar	1.3	207	64.7	43.2		50
/vegetables, strained	1.7	212	69.0	43.6		52
Meat, chicken	0.4	40	13.0		0.00	54
& noodles	0.1	11	5.0	24.1		24
noodle w/vegetable, jar	1.2	167	25.8	25.8		34
noodle w/vegetable, strained	0.9	132	37.8	25.2		30
rice w/vegetable, jar	1.3	130	18.1	24.1		31
rice w/vegetable, strained	0.8	165	29.9	41.6		28
w/rice, jar	1.2	79	12.0			20
stew, strained	0.2	26	114.0	8.13		45
/vegetables, jar	1.0	118	40.6	39.4		50
/vegetables, strained	1.7	134	85.5	39.7		46
Meat, ham	0.3	58	12.0		0.00	45
& egg, vegetable, strained	0.5	375	70.2	43.6		31
& egg breakfast, jar	2.0	67	57.0			35
& egg breakfast, strained	1.0	73	107.0			31
vegetable, strained	20.3	2	190.0	155.0	45.50	28
Meat, lamb	0.4	58	18.0	0.0	0.00	40
vegetable, strained	1.5	132	69.8	14.9		42
Liver	1.5	64	21.0	52.0	0.00	34
Pork	0.3	63	12.0	13.6	0.00	51
Meat, turkey	0.3	65	16.0		0.00	48
& rice	0.1	12	5.0	2.8		26
/vegetables, jar	1.7	235	88.9	34.6		29
/vegetables, strained	1.2	182	71.6	34.6		53

BABY FOODS

FOOD	AMOUNT	CALORIES (kcal)	PROTEIN (g)	FAT (g)	CARBO-HYDRATES (g)	FIBER (g)	CALCIUM (mg)
Meat, veal	1 oz	29	3.80	1.40	0.0	0.00	2
stew, jar	1 cup	143	6.14	2.94	24.0		136
/vegetables	1 oz	20	1.70	0.80	1.7	0.10	3
/vegetables, jar	1 cup	193	15.60	5.83	21.6	2.19	12
/vegetables, strained	1 cup	182	14.30	6.69	18.0	2.19	17
Pretzels, enriched	1 item	24	0.70	0.10	4.9	0.00	1
Soup							
cream of chicken	1 oz	16	0.70	0.50	2.4	0.31	10
vegetable, strained	1 cup	92	3.39	1.21	20.3		34
Teething biscuits	1 item	43	1.20	0.50	8.4	0.10	29
Vegetables, beets, strained	1 oz	10	0.40	0.00	2.2	0.40	4
Vegetables, beans, green	1 oz	7	0.40	0.00	1.7	0.39	11
green, strained	1 cup	52	2.81	0.22	12.1	4.27	90
green/butter, strained	1 oz	9	0.30	0.20	1.9	0.70	18
yellow, strained	1 cup	58	2.81	0.50	13.3	5.09	110
Vegetables, carrots, jar	1 cup	60	1.54	0.31	13.7	3.74	42
strained, CNF	1 cup	66	1.74	0.38	15.2	3.94	63
strained, USDA	1 oz	8	0.20	0.00	1.7	0.70	
Vegetables, creamed corn							
strained, CNF	1 cup	122	3.58	0.65	30.1	5.02	60
strained, USDA	1 oz	16	0.40	0.10	4.0	0.90	
Vegetables, garden	1 oz	11	0.70	0.10	1.9	0.70	
jar	1 cup	86	4.75	0.78	18.7	3.96	65
strained	1 cup	83	5.53	0.76	17.3	3.61	6
Vegetables, mixed	1 oz	11	0.30	0.00	2.7	0.25	
jar	1 cup	86	3.42	0.30	20.8	3.31	4
strained	1 cup	89	3.15	0.77	20.7	3.50	5
Vegetables, peas							
/carrots, strained	1 cup	91	6.47	1.21	17.8	4.39	6
creamed, strained	1 oz	15	0.60	0.50	2.5	0.70	
peas	1 oz	11	1.00	0.10	2.3	0.70	
strained	1 cup	92	8.22	1.03	17.7	4.93	3
spinach, creamed, strained	1 oz	11	0.70	0.40	1.6	1.12	2
Vegetables, squash	1 oz	7	0.20	0.10	1.6	0.70	
jar	1 cup	55	1.94	0.48	13.1	5.08	4
strained	1 cup	59	1.62	0.59	13.9	4.87	6
Vegetables, sweet potatoes	1 oz	16	0.30	0.00	3.7	0.70	
jar	1 cup	160	2.90	0.45	36.8	4.14	4
strained	1 cup	131	2.49	0.28	30.3	3.56	3
Yogurt							
apple, strained	1 cup	164	2.91	1.41	36.8		7
banana, jar	1 cup	168	3.98	1.36	37.0		7
banana, strained	1 cup	167	3.87	1.60	36.1	1.12	7
peach, jar	1 cup	184	3.15	1.17	42.4	1.69	7
peach, strained	1 cup	186	3.19	1.13	42.9	29.40	7
raspberry, jar	1 cup	146	3.63	1.45	31.2		7
raspberry, strained	1 cup	152	3.84	1.45	33.0		7
Zwieback	1 oz	120	3.03	2.49	21.1	0.71	
cookies	1 item	30	0.70	0.70	5.20	0.00	

FOOD	IRON (mg)	POTAS-SIUM (mg)	SODIUM (mg)	CHOLES-TEROl (mg)	SUGAR (gms)	% OF CALORIES FROM FAT
Meat, veal	0.4	61	18.0	11.4	0.00	43
stew, jar	1.1	310	48.1			19
/vegetables	0.2	43	7.0	6.3		36
/vegetables, jar	1.9	311	65.6	53.5		27
/vegetables, strained	1.6	245	126.0	46.2		33
Pretzels, enriched	0.2	8	16.0	0.0		4
Soup						
cream of chicken	0.1	22	5.0	1.1		28
vegetable, strained	1.5	358	43.6			12
Teething biscuits	0.4	35	40.0	0.0		10
Vegetables, beets, strained	0.1	52	24.0	0.0	1.85	0
Vegetables, beans, green	0.2	45	1.0	0.0	0.92	0
green, strained	1.7	292	48.3	0.0		4
green/butter, strained	0.4	45	1.0	0.0		20
yellow, strained	2.4	304	65.6			8
Vegetables, carrots, jar	0.4	293	78.0	0.0		5
strained, CNF	0.5	363	71.9	0.0		5
strained, USDA	0.1	56	11.0	0.0	0.91	0
Vegetables, creamed corn						
strained, CNF	0.5	249	74.1	2.4		5
strained, USDA	0.1	26	12.0	0.0	0.80	6
Vegetables, garden, garden	0.2	48	10.0	0.0		8
jar	2.1	285	34.3	0.0		8
strained	2.3	289	58.9	0.0		8
Vegetables, mixed	0.1	34	2.0	0.0		0
jar	1.2	314	51.8	0.0		3
strained	0.8	239	66.5	0.0		8
Vegetables, peas						
/carrots, strained	2.1	393	27.7	0.0		12
creamed, strained	0.2	25	4.0	0.0	0.91	30
peas	0.3	32	1.0	0.0	0.91	8
strained	2.2	280	37.6	0.0		10
spinach, creamed, strained	0.2	54	14.0	0.0	0.00	33
Vegetables, squash	0.1	51	1.0	0.0	0.56	13
jar	0.5	433	2.4	0.0		8
strained	1.0	446	23.2	0.0		9
Vegetables, sweet potatoes	0.1	75	6.0	0.0		0
jar	1.0	608	81.3	0.0		3
strained	1.0	573	47.5	0.0		2
Yogurt						
apple, strained	0.2	53	65.4			8
banana, jar	0.7	80	77.1			7
banana, strained	0.7	78	75.1	2.7		9
peach, jar	1.0	184	79.9	0.0		6
peach, strained	1.0	186	81.0	0.0		5
raspberry, jar	0.5	32	53.2			9
raspberry, strained	0.5	33	56.3			9
Zwieback	0.2	43	70.9	2.6		19
cookies	0.0	21	16.0	1.5		21

BEVERAGES

FOOD	AMOUNT	CALORIES (kcal)	PROTEIN (g)	FAT (g)	CARBO-HYDRATES (g)	FIBER (g)	CALCIUM (mg)
ALCOHOLIC BEVERAGES							
Ale, American, mild	1 cup	98	1.10	0.00	8.0		30
Beer							
regular	12 fl oz	146	0.90	0.00	13.2		18
light	12 fl oz	100	0.70	0.00	4.8		18
Budweiser®	12 fl oz	150	1.10	0.00	14.0		12
Michelob®	12 fl oz	160	1.10	0.00	15.9		12
Natural Light®	12 fl oz	100	0.40	0.00	6.0		12
Cider, fermented	1 fl oz	12	0.02	0.00	0.3		2
COCKTAILS (prepared from recipe, unless otherwise indicated)							
Bloody Mary	5 fl oz	116	0.80	0.10	4.8		10
Bourbon & soda	4 fl oz	105	0.00	0.00	0.0		4
Daiquiri	2 fl oz	111	0.00	0.00	4.1		2
Egg nog	123 g	335	3.90	15.80	18.0		44
Gin & tonic	7.5 fl oz	171	0.00	0.00	15.8		4
Highball	1 fl oz	26	0.00	0.00	0.0		1
Manhattan	2 fl oz	128	0.00	0.00	1.8		1
Martini	2.5 fl oz	156	0.00	0.00	0.2		1
Mint Julep	300 g	212	0.00	0.00	2.7		0
Old Fashioned	100 g	180	0.00	0.00	3.5		0
Pina colada	4.5 fl oz	262	0.60	2.60	39.9		11
Planters Punch	100 g	175	0.10	0.00	7.9		4
Rum sour	100 g	165	0.00	0.00	0.0		0
Scotch & soda	8 fl oz	194	0.00	0.00	0.0		7
Screwdriver	7 fl oz	174	1.20	0.10	18.4		16
Tequila sunrise	5.5 fl oz	189	0.60	0.20	14.7		10
Tom Collins	7.5 fl oz	121	0.10	0.00	3.0		10
Whiskey sour	3 fl oz	123	0.20	0.10	5.0		5
Whiskey sour mix, powder	16.7-g pkt	64	0.10	0.00	16.2		45
powder w/water & whiskey	103 g	169	0.10	0.00	16.4		47
bottled	2 fl oz	55	0.00	0.00	13.8		1
bottled prepared w/whiskey	106 g	158	0.00	0.00	13.8		1
DISTILLED SPIRITS							
Gin	1.5 fl oz	110	0.00	0.00	0.0		0
Rum, Vodka	1.5 fl oz	97	0.00	0.00	0.0		0
Whiskey	1.5 fl oz	105	0.00	0.00	0.1		0
Whiskey, Gin, Rum, Vodka-80 proof	1.5 fl oz	96	0.00	0.00	0.0		0
Whiskey, Gin, Rum, Vodka-86 proof	1.5 fl oz	104	0.00	0.00	0.0		0
Whiskey, Gin, Rum, Vodka-90 proof	1.5 fl oz	109	0.00	0.00	0.0		0
Whiskey, Gin, Rum, Vodka-94 proof	1.5 fl oz	115	0.00	0.00	0.0		0
Whiskey, Gin, Rum, Vodka-100 proof	1.5 fl oz	123	0.00	0.00	0.0		0
LIQUEUR							
Anisette	20 g	74	0.00	0.00	7.0		
Apricot Brandy	20 g	64	0.04	0.00	6.0		1

FOOD	IRON (mg)	POTAS- SIUM (mg)	SODIUM (mg)	CHOLES- TEROI (mg)	ALCOHOL (gms)	% OF AL- COHOL BY- VOLUME	% OF CALORIES FROM FAT
ALCOHOLIC BEVERAGES							
Ale, American, mild	0.20		16	0	8.90	3.9	0
Beer							
regular	0.11	89	19	0		4.5	0
light	0.12	64	10	0		4	0
Budweiser®	0.12	49	24	0	12.96	3.6	0
Michelob®	0.12	49	24	0	12.96	4	0
Natural Light®	0.12	60	24	0	14.40	4	0
Cider, fermented	0.11	36	0	0	1.57	5.2	0
COCKTAILS (prepared from recipe, unless otherwise indicated)							
Bloody Mary	0.55	216	332	0		11.7	1
Bourbon & soda		2	16	0		16.1	0
Daiquiri	0.09	13	3	0		28.3	0
Egg nog	0.70	178	75	93.8	15.00	12.2	42
Gin & tonic		12	10	0		8.8	0
Highball	0.01	1	4	0	3.77	13	0
Manhattan	0.05	15	2	0		36.9	0
Martini	0.06	13	2	0		38.4	0
Mint Julep	0.13	6	0	0	29.20	9.7	0
Old Fashioned	0.04	2	1	0	24.00	24	0
Pina colada	0.31	100	9	0		12.3	9
Planters Punch	0.10			0	21.50	21.5	0
Rum sour	0.04	2	1	0	21.50	21.5	0
Scotch & soda	0.05	5	33	0		11.2	0
Screwdriver	0.17	325	2	0		8.2	1
Tequila sunrise	0.47	178	7	0		13.5	1
Tom Collins		18	39	0		9	0
Whiskey sour	0.07	48	10	0		20.6	1
Whiskey sour mix, powder	0.07	3	46	0			0
powder w/water & whiskey	0.08	4	48	0		18	0
bottled	0.07	18	66	0			0
bottled prepared w/whiskey	0.08	19	66	0		17.4	0
DISTILLED SPIRITS							
Gin	0.00	0	1	0		45	0
Rum, Vodka	0.05	1	0	0		40	0
Whiskey	0.01	1	0	0		43	0
Whiskey, Gin, Rum, Vodka-80 proof	0.05	2	0	0	13.94		0
Whiskey, Gin, Rum, Vodka-86 proof	0.01	1	0	0	15.00		0
Whiskey, Gin, Rum, Vodka-90 proof	0.00	0	1	0	15.75		0
Whiskey, Gin, Rum, Vodka-94 proof	0.02	0	0	0	16.50		0
Whiskey, Gin, Rum, Vodka-100 proof	0.02	0	0	0	17.70		0
LIQUEUR							
Anisette				0	7.00	35	0
Apricot Brandy	0.02	11	2	0	6.00	30	0

BEVERAGES

FOOD	AMOUNT	CALORIES (kcal)	PROTEIN (g)	FAT (g)	CARBO-HYDRATES (g)	FIBER (g)	CALCIUM (mg)
ALCOHOLIC BEVERAGES (continued)							
LIQUEUR (continued)							
Benedictine	20 g	69		0.00	6.6		
Brandy, California	30 g	73		0.00			
Brandy, Cognac, Pony	30 g	73	0.00	0.00	0.0		0
Coffee, Kahlua®	1.5 fl oz	176	0.00	0.15	24.4		0
Kahlua® w/cream	1.5 fl oz	153	1.35	7.35	9.7		8
Cordials	1 fl oz	97	0.02	0.00	11.5		0
Creme de menthe	1.5 fl oz	186	0.00	0.10	20.8		0
Curacao	20 g	54		0.00	6.0		
WINE							
Dessert	2 fl oz	90	0.10	0.00	7.0		5
Table, red	3.5 fl oz	74	0.20	0.00	1.8		8
Table, rose	3.5 fl oz	73	0.20	0.00	1.5		9
Table, white	3.5 fl oz	70	0.10	0.00	0.8		9
Madeira	100 g	105	0.20	0.00	1.0		8
Muscatel/Port	100 g	158	0.20	0.00	14.0		8
California/Red	102 g	85	0.21	0.00	2.5		8
Sauterne	100 g	84	0.20	0.00	4.0		8
Sherry, dry	60 g	84	0.20	0.00	4.8		5
Vermouth, dry	100 g	105	0.00	0.00	1.0		8
Vermouth, sweet	100 g	167	0.00	0.00	12.0		8
Wine Coolers	8 fl oz	117	0.71	1.43	15.2		10
Wine Cooler, white wine & 7 Up	102 g	55	0.05	0.00	5.7		6
Champagne, domestic	120 g	84	0.20	0.00	3.0		
NONALCOHOLIC BEVERAGES, Carbonated							
Cherry-Lime Rickey, Snapple®	16 oz	110	<1	<1	56.0		
Cherry Soda, French, Snapple®	16 oz	110	<1	<1	56.0		
Club soda	12 oz	0	0.00	0.00	0.0	0.00	17
Cola	12 oz	151	0.10	0.10	38.5	0.00	9
Tab® low calorie cola	12 oz	0	0.00	0.00	0.0		
Cream soda	12 oz	191	0.00	0.00	49.3	0.00	19
Snapple® Creame Vanilla	16 oz	120	<1	<1	56.0		
Ginger ale	12 oz	124	0.10	0.00	31.9	0.00	12
Health Valley®	12 oz	154	1.00	1.00	35.0		10
Grape soda	12 oz	161	0.00	0.00	41.7	0.00	12
Lemon-lime soda	12 oz	149	0.00	0.00	38.4	0.00	9
Snapple®	16 oz	110	<1	<1	56.0		
7 Up®	12 oz	148	0.00	0.00	38.2		7
Orange soda	12 oz	177	0.00	0.00	45.8	0.00	19
Peach Melba soda, Snapple®	16 oz	120	<1	<1	56.0		
Pepper type	12 oz	151	0.00	0.40	38.2	0.00	12
Root beer	12 oz	152	0.10	0.00	39.2	0.00	19
Health Valley®							
Health Valley® Old Fashioned	12 oz	120	1.00	1.00	26.0	0	
Sarsaparilla	12 oz	154	1.00	1.00	35.0		
Snapple® Tru Root Beer	16 oz	110	<1	<1	56.0		
Wild Berry, Health Valley®	12 oz	142	1.00	1.00	33.0		
Tonic water	12 oz	125	0.00	0.00	32.2	0.00	5
Low calorie, aspartame, cola	12 oz	2	0.20	0.00	0.3	0.00	12

FOOD	IRON (mg)	POTAS-SIUM (mg)	SODIUM (mg)	CHOLES-TEROI (mg)	ALCOHOL (gms)	% OF AL-COHOL BY-VOLUME	% OF CALORIES FROM FAT
ALCOHOLIC BEVERAGES (continued)							
LIQUEUR (continued)							
Benedictine				0	6.60	33	0
Brandy, California				0	10.50	35	0
Brandy, Cognac, Pony	0.01	1	0	0	10.50	35	0
Coffee, Kahlua®	0.03	15	5	0	11.33	21.7	1
Kahlua® w/cream	0.06	15	44		6.44	13.8	43
Cordials	0.02	1	1	0	7.30	27	0
Creme de menthe	0.04	0	3	0	15.00	36	0
Curacao				0	6.00	30	0
WINE							
Dessert	0.14	54	5	0		18.8	0
Table, red	0.44	115	6	0		11.5	0
Table, rose	0.39	102	5	0		11.5	0
Table, white	0.33	82	5	0		11.5	0
Madeira	0.24	92	5	0	15.00	15	0
Muscatel/Port	1.61	75	4	0	15.00	15	0
California/Red	0.97	116	10	0	10.00	9.8	0
Sauterne	0.41	89	2	0	10.50	10.5	0
Sherry, dry	0.25	45	2	0	9.00	15	0
Vermouth, dry	0.41	75	4	0	15.00	15	0
Vermouth, sweet	0.24	92	9	0	18.00	18	0
Wine Coolers	0.65	105	19	0		4	11
Wine Cooler, white wine & 7 Up	0.19	41	7	0	4.75	4.7	0
Champagne, domestic				0	11.00	9.2	0
NONALCOHOLIC BEVERAGES, Carbonated							
Cherry-Lime Rickey, Snapple®			10				
Cherry Soda, French, Snapple®			15				
Club soda		6	75	0			
Cola	0.13	4	14	0			1
Tab® low calorie cola			45	0			
Cream soda	0.19	4	43	0			0
Snapple® Creme Vanilla			10				
Ginger ale	0.66	5	25	0			0
Health Valley®	0.61	10	30	0			6
Grape soda	0.31	3	57	0			0
Lemon-lime soda	0.25	4	41	0			0
Snapple®			30				
7 Up®	0.25	4	41	0			0
Orange soda	0.23	9	46	0			0
Peach Melba soda, Snapple®							
Pepper type	0.14	2	38	0			2
Root beer	0.18	3	49	0			0
Health Valley®							
Health Valley® Old Fashioned	0.14	22	12	0			8
Sarsaparilla		16	27	0			6
Snapple® Tru Root Beer							
Wild Berry, Health Valley®		5	27	0			6
Tonic water		1	15	0			0
Low calorie, aspartame, cola	0.11	0	21	0			0

BEVERAGES

FOOD	AMOUNT	CALORIES (kcal)	PROTEIN (g)	FAT (g)	CARBO-HYDRATES (g)	FIBER (g)	CALCIUM (mg)
NONALCOHOLIC BEVERAGES, Carbonated (continued)							
Low calorie, Nutrasweet® cola	12 oz	4	0.36	0.00	0.3		14
Low calorie, sodium saccharin	12 oz	2	0.10	0.00	0.3	0.00	14
NONALCOHOLIC BEVERAGES (See also fast food section for additional beverages)							
Apple cider	1 cup	124	0.25	0.27	34.2		15
Apple Crisp, Snapple®	10 oz	110	>1	>1	35.0		
Beef broth & tomato juice, canned	5.5 oz	61	1.00	0.20	14.3	0.20	19
Carob flavor mix, powder	3 tsp	45	0.20	0.00	11.2	0.20	
prepared w/milk	(1 cup milk)	195	8.20	8.20	22.6	0.20	291
Chocolate flavor mix, powder	2-3 tsp	75	0.70	0.70	19.5	0.20	8
prepared w/milk	(1 cup milk)	226	8.80	8.80	30.9	0.20	300
Chocolate milk	1 cup	208	7.92	8.48	25.8	0.15	280
Chocolate syrup, no added nutrients	2 tbsp	82	0.70	0.30	22.1	0.10	5
prepared w/milk	(1 cup milk)	232	8.80	8.50	33.5	0.10	297
w/added nutrients	1 tbsp	46	0.30	0.20	12.4	0.10	
Citrus fruit juice drink							
frozen concentrate	12 fl oz can	684	4.90	0.30	170.5		106
prepared w/water	1 cup	114	0.80	0.00	28.4		21
Clam & tomato juice, canned	5.5 oz	77	1.10	0.10	18.1	0.20	21
Cocoa mix, powder							
w/out added nutrients	1-oz pkt	102	3.10	1.10	22.5	0.20	96
w/added nutrients	1.1-oz pkt	120	1.90	3.00	24.1		104
reduced calorie, aspartame	0.53-oz pkt	48	3.80	0.40	8.5		90
Coconut milk	1 oz	79	0.79	8.02	0.8		3
instant	1 oz	192	3.18	16.90	6.9		5
Coconut water	1 oz	6	0.00	0.00	1.5		4
Coffee, brewed	6 fl oz	4	0.10	0.00	0.8		3
Coffee, instant, powder, regular	1 tsp	4	0.20	0.00	0.7		6
decaffeinated	1 tsp	4	0.20	0.00	0.8		6
sugar sweetened, cappuccino flavor	2 tsp	62	0.40	2.10	10.7		7
sugar sweetened, French flavor	2 tsp	57	0.50	3.40	6.6		8
sugar sweetened, mocha flavor	2 tsp	51	0.50	1.90	8.4		7
Sanka®	6 fl oz	2	0.00	0.00	1.0		5
Coffee substitute, cereal grain beverage, powder, w/water	6 fl oz	9	0.10	0.10	1.9	0.00	5
w/milk	6 fl oz	121	6.10	6.20	10.4	0.00	219
Postum® instant grain beverage, dry mix	1 oz	103	1.93	0.03	24.1		77
Cranberry-apple juice drink	6 fl oz	123	0.10	0.00	31.5		13
Cranberry-apricot juice drink	6 fl oz	118	0.30	0.00	29.9		17
Cranberry-grape juice drink	6 fl oz	103	0.30	0.20	25.8		15
Cranberry juice cocktail, bottled	6 fl oz	108	0.00	0.10	27.4		7
frozen concentrate	12 fl oz can	821	0.30	0.00	210.2		48
prepared w/water	6 fl oz	102	0.00	0.00	26.2		9
low calorie, calcium saccharin & corn sweetened, bottled	6 fl oz	33	0.00	0.00	8.5		16
Dairy drink mix, reduced calorie, aspartame sweetened	0.75-oz pkt	64	5.30	0.50	10.7		192
Eggnog, dairy	1 cup	342	9.68	19.00	34.3	0.00	330

FOOD	IRON (mg)	POTAS-SIUM (mg)	SODIUM (mg)	CHOLES-TEROI (mg)	ALCOHOL (gms)	% OF AL-COHOL BY-VOLUME	% OF CALORIES FROM FAT
NONALCOHOLIC BEVERAGES, Carbonated (continued)							
Low calorie, Nutrasweet® cola	0.11	0	21	0			0
Low calorie, sodium saccharinl	0.14	7	57	0			0
NONALCOHOLIC BEVERAGES (See also fast food section for additional beverages)							
Apple cider	1.24	295	7	0			2
Apple Crisp, Snapple®	0.02		15				
Beef broth & tomato juice, canned	0.98	162	220				3
Carob flavor mix, powder	0.55		12	0			0
prepared w/milk	0.67	370	132	33			38
Chocolate flavor mix, powder	0.68	128	45	0			8
prepared w/milk	0.80	498	165	33			35
Chocolate milk	0.60	417	149	30			37
Chocolate syrup, no added nutrients	0.79	84	36	0			3
prepared w/milk	0.91	455	156	33			33
w/added nutrients	2.55	90	29	0			4
Citrus fruit juice drink							
frozen concentrate	16.67	1660	12	0			0
prepared w/water	2.79	277	7	0			0
Clam & tomato juice, canned	1.00	149	664				1
Cocoa mix, powder							
w/out added nutrients	0.34	202	149				10
w/added nutrients	1.81	405	207				23
reduced calorie, aspartame	0.75	405	173				8
Coconut milk	0.37	113	4	0			92
instant	0.71	150	22	0			79
Coconut water	0.03	56	0	0			0
Coffee, brewed	0.72	96	4	0			0
Coffee, instant, powder, regular	0.08	64	6	0			0
decaffeinated	0.08	63	6	0			0
sugar sweetened, cappuccino flavor	0.15	119	104				30
sugar sweetened, French flavor	0.01	137					54
sugar sweetened, mocha flavor	0.24	119	36				34
Sanka®	0.06	60	0	0			0
Coffee substitute, cereal grain beverage, powder, w/water	0.12	43	7	0			10
w/milk	0.20	319	91	25			46
Postum® instant grain beverage, dry mix	1.87	896	28	0			0
Cranberry-apple juice drink	0.11	50	4	0			0
Cranberry-apricot juice drink	0.28	113	4	0			0
Cranberry-grape juice drink	0.02	44	5	0			2
Cranberry juice cocktail, bottled	0.28	34	4	0			1
frozen concentrate	1.31	213	13	0			0
prepared w/water	0.17	27	6	0			0
low calorie, calcium saccharin & corn sweetened, bottled	0.07	39	6	0			0
Dairy drink mix, reduced calorie, aspartame sweetened	1.65	479	172				7
Eggnog, dairy	0.51	420	138	149			50

BEVERAGES

FOOD	AMOUNT	CALORIES (kcal)	PROTEIN (g)	FAT (g)	CARBO-HYDRATES (g)	FIBER (g)	CALCIUM (mg)
NONALCOHOLIC BEVERAGES (continued)							
Eggnog flavor mix, powder	2 tsp	111	0.10	0.30	27.7	0.00	
prepared w/water	(1 cup water)	97	0.00	0.00	24.8		41
Fruit punch drink, canned	6 fl oz	87	0.10	0.00	22.1		14
frozen concentrate	12 fl oz can	678	0.70	0.10	173.1		33
prepared w/water	1 cup	113	0.10	0.00	28.8		9
Fruit punch juice drink							
Fruit punch juice drink, frozen	12 fl oz can	739	1.20	3.00	182.1		85
prepared w/water	1 cup	123	0.20	0.50	30.4		18
Snapple® Fruit Punch	16 oz	120	<1	<1	56.0		
Snap-up	16 oz	90	<1	<1	56.0		
Gelatin, drinking, orange flavor							
prepared w/water	4 fl oz water	67	6.20	0.20	10.5	0.00	
Grape drink, canned	6 fl oz	84	0.00	0.00	21.6		
Grape juice drink, canned	6 fl oz	94	0.20	0.00	24.2	0.00	6
Snapple® Grapeade	16 oz	120	<1	<1	56.0		
Snapple® Straight Grape	10 oz	110	<1	<1	35.0		
Instant breakfast, powder	1 cup	530	32.20	2.23	96.3		1092
made w/2% milk	1 cup	240	15.30	4.96	35.5		539
made w/skim milk	1 cup	206	15.50	0.76	33.9		543
made w/whole milk	1 cup	267	15.20	8.24	33.5		534
Carnation® instant breakfast, choc	1 item	130	7.00	1.00	23.0		100
eggnog	1 item	130	7.00	0.00	23.0		100
vanilla	1 item	130	7.00	0.00	24.0		100
Kiwi Strawberry Cocktail, Snapple®	16 oz	130	<1	<1	56.0		
Lemon Snap-up, Snapple®	16 oz	90	<1	<1	56.0		
Lemon-lime Snap-up, Snapple®	16 oz	80	<1	<1	56.0		
Lemonade flavor drink w/water	1 cup	113	0.00	0.10	28.8		29
Lemonade, powder w/water	1 cup	102	0.00	0.00	26.9		71
powder, low calorie, aspartame	0.42-oz pkt	40	0.40	0.00	10.0		369
prepared w/water	(2 qt water)	40	0.40	0.00	10.0		408
frozen concentrate	12 fl oz can	798	1.20	0.90	207.1	0.40	31
prepared w/water	1 cup	100	0.10	0.10	26.0	0.10	8
Snapple® Lemonade	16 oz	110	<1	<1	56.0		
Snapple® Pink Lemonade	16 oz	120	<1	<1	56.0		
Limeade, frozen concentrate	12 fl oz can	817	0.90	0.40	216.3		22
prepared w/water	1 cup	102	0.10	0.10	27.1		7
Malt beverage	12 fl oz	32	1.10	0.00	5.1		25
Malted milk flavor mix, powder							
chocolate, w/out added nutrients	3 tsp	79	1.10	0.80	18.4	0.00	13
prepared w/milk	(1 cup milk)	229	9.10	8.90	29.8	0.00	304
chocolate, w/added nutrients	4-5 tsp	75	1.00	0.70	17.7	0.00	93
prepared w/milk	(1 cup milk)	225	9.10	8.90	29.1	0.00	384
natural, w/out added nutrients	3 tsp	87	2.30	1.70	15.9	0.00	63
prepared w/milk	(1 cup milk)	237	10.40	9.80	27.3	0.00	354
natural, w/added nutrients	4-5 tsp	80	1.80	0.60	17.1	0.00	79
prepared w/milk	(1 cup milk)	230	9.90	8.70	28.4	0.00	370
Melon-berry, Snapple®	16 oz	120	<1	<1	56.0		
Orange flavor drink, breakfast type							
powder	3 tsp	93	0.00	0.00	23.7		46

FOOD	IRON (mg)	POTAS-SIUM (mg)	SODIUM (mg)	CHOLES-TEROl (mg)	ALCOHOL (gms)	% OF AL-COHOL BY-VOLUME	% OF CALORIES FROM FAT
NONALCOHOLIC BEVERAGES (continued)							
Eggnog flavor mix, powder	0.26		44				2
prepared w/water	0.14	2	38	0			0
Fruit punch drink, canned	0.38	47	41	0			0
frozen concentrate	1.25	184	34	0			0
prepared w/water	0.22	31	11	0			0
Fruit punch juice drink							
Fruit punch juice drink, frozen	3.38	1142	41	0			4
prepared w/water	0.57	191	12	0			4
Snapple® Fruit Punch			35				
Snap-up			35				
Gelatin, drinking, orange flavor							
prepared w/water	0.01	3	32				3
Grape drink, canned	0.31	10	12	0			0
Grape juice drink, canned	0.19	66	2	0			0
Snapple® Grapeade			5				
Snapple® Straight Grape			10				
Instant breakfast, powder	15.10	1744	644				4
made w/2% milk	3.70	769	268	35.5			19
made w/skim milk	3.66	794	271				3
made w/whole milk	3.70	762	265				28
Carnation® instant breakfast, choc	4.50	422	136				7
eggnog	4.50	266	196	0			0
vanilla	4.50	382	145	0			0
Kiwi Strawberry Cocktail, Snapple®			10				
Lemon Snap-up, Snapple®			30				
Lemon-lime Snap-up, Snapple®			35				
Lemonade flavor drink w/water	0.04	1	19	0			1
Lemonade, powder w/water	0.15	33	13	0			0
powder, low calorie, aspartame	0.68	1	1	0			0
prepared w/water	0.78	6	58	0			0
frozen concentrate	3.18	297	17	0			1
prepared w/water	0.41	38	8	0			1
Snapple® Lemonade			10				
Snapple® Pink Lemonade							
Limeade, frozen concentrate	0.44	258		0			0
prepared w/water	0.06	33	6	0			1
Malt beverage	0.05			0			0
Malted milk flavor mix, powder							
chocolate, w/out added nutrients	0.48	130	53	1			9
prepared w/milk	0.60	499	172	34			35
chocolate, w/added nutrients	3.65	251	125				8
prepared w/milk	3.77	620	244	33			36
natural, w/out added nutrients	0.15	159	103	4			18
prepared w/milk	0.27	529	223	37			37
natural, w/added nutrients	3.49	203	85				7
prepared w/milk	3.61	573	205	33			34
Melon-berry, Snapple®							
Orange flavor drink, breakfast type							
powder	0.16	40	4	0			0

BEVERAGES

FOOD	AMOUNT	CALORIES (kcal)	PROTEIN (g)	FAT (g)	CARBO-HYDRATES (g)	FIBER (g)	CALCIUM (mg)
NONALCOHOLIC BEVERAGES (continued)							
Orange flavor drink, breakfast type (continued)							
prepared w/water	6 fl oz	86	0.00	0.00	21.9		4
frozen concentrate, w/orange pulp	12 fl oz can	729	0.30	2.20	182.0		46
frozen concentrate, w/orange juice & orange pulp	12 fl oz can	669	1.60	0.10	169.9		174
Tang® orange flavor, dry	1 oz	104	0.00	0.00	26.1		71
Orange drink, canned	6 fl oz	94	0.00	0.00	24.0		12
Snapple® Snap-up	16 oz	90	<1	<1	56.0		
Snapple® Orangeade	16 oz	120	<1	<1	56.0		
Orange juice, Snapple®	10 oz	160	>1	>1	35.0		
Orange & apricot juice drink	1 cup	128	0.80	0.30	31.8	0.50	13
Ovaltine® prepared w/milk, choc	1 cup	227	9.53	8.79	29.2		392
malt flavor	1 cup	228	9.93	8.33	29.0		371
Passion Supreme, Snapple®	10 oz	120	<1	<1	35.0		
Dixie Peach, Snapple®	10 oz	160	<1	<1	35.0		
Pineapple & grapefruit juice drink, canned	1 cup	117	0.60	0.20	29.0	0.10	18
Pineapple & orange juice drink	1 cup	125	3.10	0.00	29.4	0.00	13
Raspberry Royal, Snapple®	10 oz	110	<1	<1	35.0		
Strawberry flavor mix, powder	2-3 tsp	84	0.00	0.00	21.4	0.00	
prepared w/milk	(1 cup milk)	234	8.10	8.20	32.8	0.00	292
Strawberry Royal, Snapple®	10 oz	120	<1	<1	35.0		
Sugar cane juice	1 oz	20	0.11	0.00	4.9		2
Tea, brewed	6 fl oz	2	0.00	0.00	0.4		0
Tea, brewed, decaffeinated	6 fl oz	2	0.00	0.00	0.5		0
Tea, instant, powder, unsweetened	1 tsp	2	0.10	0.00	0.4	0.00	5
unsweetened, lemon flavor	1 tsp	4	0.10	0.00	1.1	0.00	5
sugar sweetened, lemon flavor	3 tsp	87	0.10	0.10	22.1	0.00	6
low cal, saccharin, lemon flavor	2 tsp	5	0.10	0.00	1.3	0.00	5
Tea, herb, brewed	6 fl oz	1	0.10	0.00	0.3	0.00	4
Tea, Iced, Ready-to-Drink, Snapple®							
cranberry	16 oz	100	<1	<1	56.0		
decaffeinated	16 oz	110	<1	<1	56.0		
diet	16 oz	4	<1	<1	2.0		
diet, decaffeinated	16 oz	6	<1	<1	2.0		
diet, raspberry	16 oz	4	<1	<1	2.0		
mint	16 oz	110	<1	<1	56.0		
orange	16 oz	100	<1	<1	56.0		
peach	16 oz	100	<1	<1	56.0		
raspberry	16 oz	110	<1	<1	56.0		
sweetened, with lemon	16 oz	100	<1	<1	56.0		
Snap-up	16 oz	70	<1	<1	56.0		
unsweetened	16 oz	100	<1	<1	56.0		0
Thirst quencher drink, bottled	1 cup	60	0.00	0.10	15.2	0.00	0
Gatorade®	8 fl oz	60	0.00	0.00	15.2		0
Snapple® Vitamin Supreme	10 oz	100	<1	<1	35.0		0
Water, bottled, Perrier®	1 cup	0	0.00	0.00	0.0	0.00	32
Water, bottled, Poland Spring®	1 cup	0	0.00	0.00	0.0	0.00	3
Water, municipal	1 cup	0	0.00	0.00	0.0	0.00	5

FOOD	IRON (mg)	POTAS-SIUM (mg)	SODIUM (mg)	CHOLES-TEROI (mg)	ALCOHOL (gms)	% OF AL-COHOL BY-VOLUME	% OF CALORIES FROM FAT
NONALCOHOLIC BEVERAGES (continued)							
Orange flavor drink, breakfast type (continued)							
prepared w/water	0.15	37	9	0			0
frozen concentrate, w/orange pulp	1.10	1845	103	0			3
frozen concentrate, w/orange juice & orange pulp	1.13	2027	113	0			0
Tang® orange flavor, dry	0.03	81	13	0			0
Orange drink, canned	0.53	33	31	0			0
Snapple® Snap-up							
Snapple® Orangeade			10				
Orange juice, Snapple®	0.04		15				
Orange & apricot juice drink	0.25	201		0			2
Ovaltine® prepared w/milk, choc	4.77	600	228	34.2			35
malt flavor	4.49	576	201	37.4			33
Passion Supreme, Snapple®	0.02		20				
Dixie Peach, Snapple®			30				
Pineapple & grapefruit juice drink, canned	0.77	154	34	0			2
Pineapple & orange juice drink	0.67	116	9	0			0
Raspberry Royal, Snapple®	0.02		20				
Strawberry flavor mix, powder	0.09		8	0			0
prepared w/milk	0.22	370	128	33			32
Strawberry Royal, Snapple®			5				
Sugar cane juice	0.06	16	0	0			0
Tea, brewed	0.04	66	5	0			0
Tea, brewed, decaffeinated	0.04	66	5	0			0
Tea, instant, powder, unsweetened	0.04	47	8	0			0
unsweetened, lemon flavor	0.02	49	14	0			0
sugar sweetened, lemon flavor	0.05	50		0			1
low cal, saccharin, lemon flavor	0.15	41	24	0			0
Tea, herb, brewed	0.14	15	2	0			0
Tea, Iced, Ready-to-Drink, Snapple®							
cranberry			5				
decaffeinated			5				
diet			10				
diet, decaffeinated	0.02		5				
diet, raspberry			35				
mint			35				
orange							
peach	0.02		5				
raspberry	0.02						
sweetened, with lemon			10				
Snap-up			5				
unsweetened	0.02		50				
Thirst quencher drink, bottled	0.12	26	96	0			2
Gatorade®	0.12	26	96	0			0
Snapple® Vitamin Supreme	0.02		10				
Water, bottled, Perrier®	0.00	0	3	0			
Water, bottled, Poland Spring®	0.01	0	1	0			
Water, municipal	0.01	1	7	0			

THE GOOD-SENSE FOOD GUIDE PYRAMID

Your guide to daily food choices

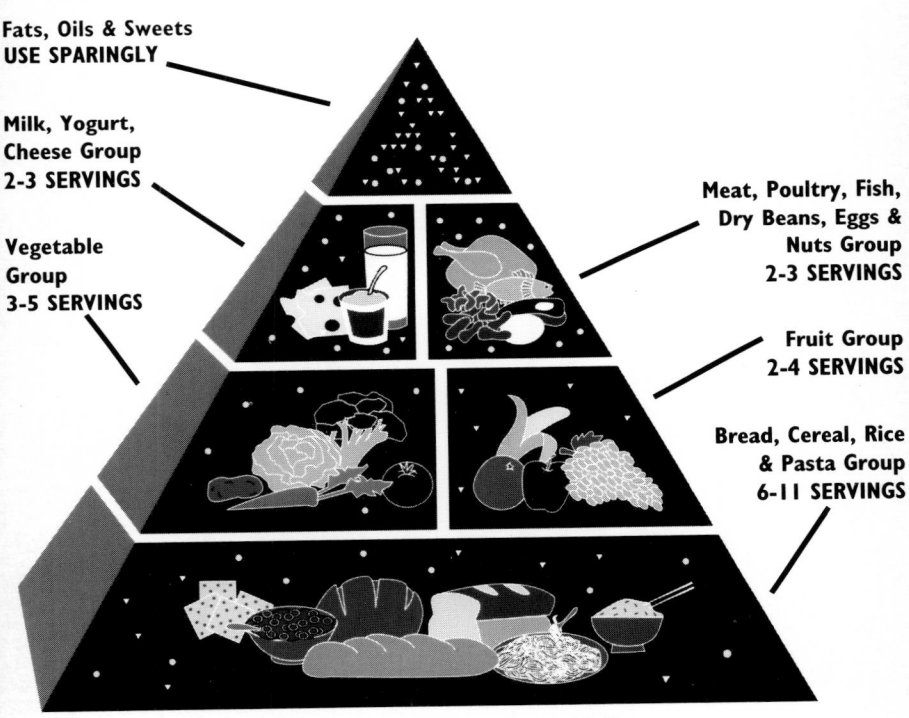

**Fats, Oils & Sweets
USE SPARINGLY**

**Milk, Yogurt,
Cheese Group
2-3 SERVINGS**

**Vegetable
Group
3-5 SERVINGS**

**Meat, Poultry, Fish,
Dry Beans, Eggs &
Nuts Group
2-3 SERVINGS**

**Fruit Group
2-4 SERVINGS**

**Bread, Cereal, Rice
& Pasta Group
6-11 SERVINGS**

KEY ● Fat (naturally occurring and added)   ▼ Sugars (added)

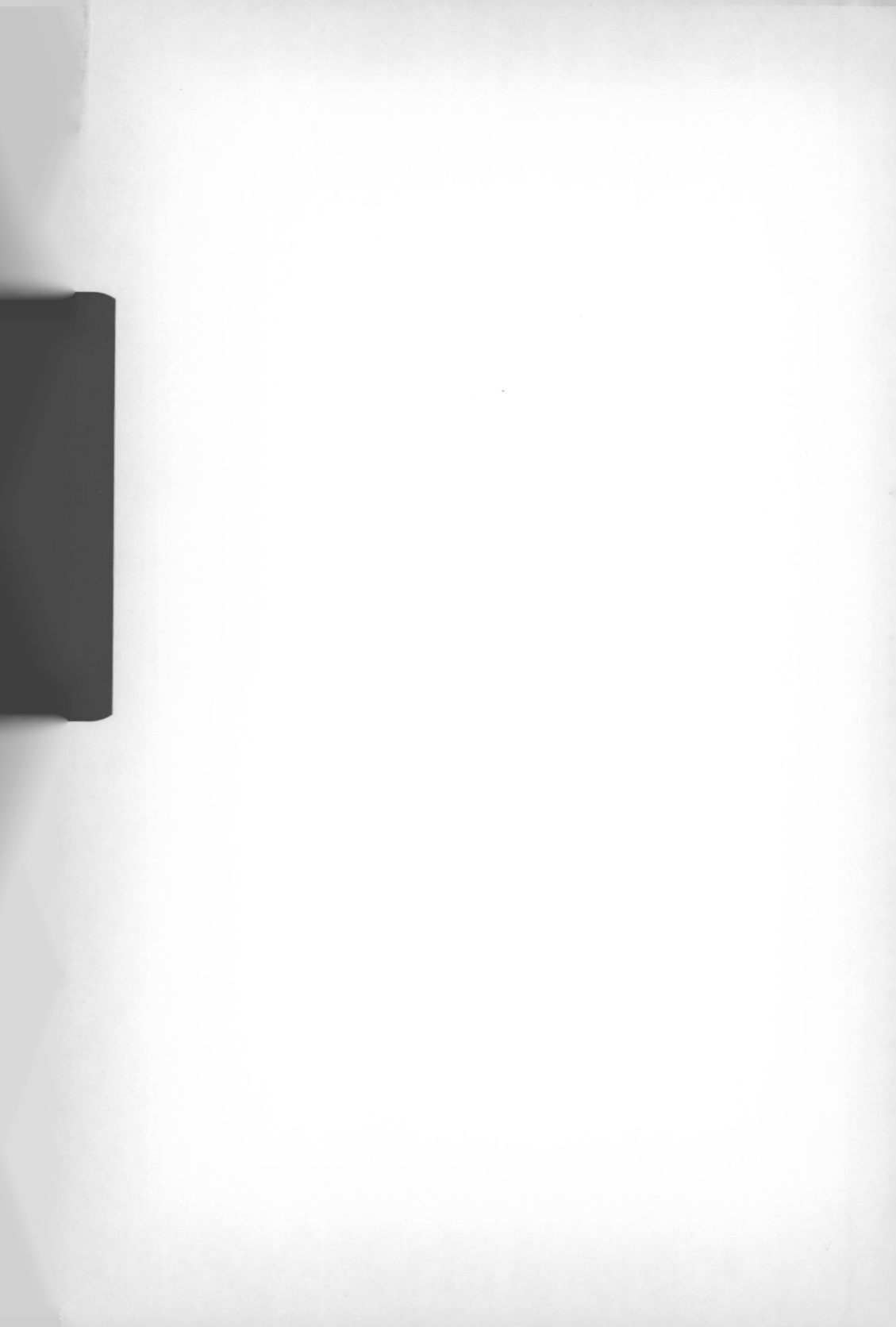

VEGETABLES, LEGUMES, FRUIT, SOUPS, SAUCES, NUTS, SEEDS, EGGS, AND DAIRY

The Food Guide Pyramid suggests three to five servings of vegetables and two to four servings of fruit per day. Vegetables provide vitamins, such as vitamins A and C and folic acid and minerals such as iron and magnesium. They are naturally low in fat and provide fiber. Fruits and fruit juices provide important amounts of vitamin A and C and potassium. They are low in fat and sodium.

Legumes, soups, sauces, nuts, and seeds are included in this section, although they are not on the same level of the Food Guide Pyramid. Legumes are in the next level of the Pyramid, with their higher content of protein, which you should eat in moderation. Nuts and seeds are high in fat, so they, too, must be eaten in moderation.

Legumes are dry beans and seeds. Raw legumes are not eaten because they may contain toxic factors. In addition, they don't taste good and are hard to digest. The usual processing or preparation, such as cooking or canning, remove these problems.

USDA standards for soups, sauces and gravies made from meat and poultry require that condensed meat soup must contain at least 10 percent meat, based on fresh uncooked weight. A meat sauce must contain 6 percent meat, and gravy must have either 6 percent meat or 25 percent meat stock. A condensed poultry soup must contain at least 4 percent poultry meats.

Eggs and dairy products appear in the next level of the Food Guide Pyramid.

Milk products provide protein, vitamins, and minerals. Milk, yogurt, and cheese are the best sources of calcium. The Pyramid suggests two servings a day for most people and three servings for teenagers, young adults up to twenty-four, and pregnant or breast-feeding women.

When eating food from this category keep in mind the following:

- Egg yolks are high in cholesterol
- Many cheeses are high in fat, especially saturated fat.

VEGETABLES & VEGETABLE PRODUCTS

FOOD	AMOUNT	CALORIES (kcal)	PROTEIN (g)	FAT (g)	CARBO-HYDRATES (g)	FIBER (g)	CALCIUM (mg)
Alfalfa seeds, sprouted, raw	1 cup	10	1.32	0.23	1	0.54	10
Amaranth, raw	1 cup	7	0.69	0.09	1	0.27	60
cooked, boiled, drained	1 cup	28	2.78	0.24	5	1.73	276
Arrowhead, raw	12 g corm	12	0.64	0.03	2	0.10	1
cooked, boiled, drained	12 g corm	9	0.54	0.01	2	0.18	1
Artichokes, raw	128 g	65	3.40	0.26	15	1.36	61
cooked, boiled, drained	120 g	53	2.76	0.20	12	1.10	47
frozen, unprepared	9-oz pkg	96	6.71	1.08	20	1.98	48
frozen, cooked, boiled, drained	9-oz pkg	108	7.46	1.20	22	2.21	50
Arugula, raw	½ cup	2	0.26	0.07	0		16
Asparagus, raw	4 spears	14	1.32	0.12	3		12
cooked, boiled, drained	4 spears	14	1.56	0.19	3	0.50	12
canned, solids & liquids	1 can	58	7.41	0.79	9	2.17	58
canned, drained solids	1 can	48	5.30	1.60	6		
frozen, unprepared	4 spears	14	1.87	0.13	2	0.51	15
frozen, cooked, boiled, drained	4 spears	17	1.77	0.25	3	0.50	14
Balsam-pear leafy tips, raw	½ cup	7	1.27	0.17	1	0.55	20
cooked, boiled, drained	½ cup	10	1.04	0.06	2	0.54	12
Balsam-pear pods, raw	1 cup	16	0.93	0.16	3	1.30	18
cooked, boiled, drained	1 cup	24	1.04	0.22	5	1.30	11
Bamboo shoots, raw	1 cup	41	3.93	0.45	8	1.06	20
cooked, boiled, drained	1 cup	15	1.83	0.26	2	0.78	14
canned, drained solids	1 cup	25	2.26	0.52	4	0.87	10
La Choy®	1 cup	25	2.26	0.53	4	2.00	11
Beans, shellie, canned, solids & liquid	1 cup	75	4.30	0.47	15	1.47	72
Beans, green, frozen, boiled, Health Valley®	1 cup	50	2.00	2.00	8	2.00	60
Beans, snap, raw	1 cup	34	2.00	0.13	8	1.21	41
cooked, boiled, drained	1 cup	44	2.36	0.36	10	1.79	58
canned, solids & liquid	1 can	68	3.71	0.45	15	2.76	104
canned, drained solids	1 can	52	3.02	0.26	12		69
canned, seasoned, solids & liquid	1 can	71	3.65	0.88	15	3.73	98
frozen, unprepared	½ cup	21	1.12	0.13	5	0.68	26
frozen, cooked, boiled, drained	½ cup	18	0.92	0.09	4	0.70	31
Bean sprouts, canned, La Choy®	1 cup	11	1.20	0.20	3	1.29	12
Beets, raw	2 beets	71	2.41	0.23	16	1.30	25
cooked, boiled, drained	2 beets	31	1.06	0.05	7	0.85	11
canned, solids & liquid	½ cup	36	1.03	0.09	8	0.75	17
canned, drained solids	½ cup	27	0.78	0.12	6		
harvard, canned, solids & liquids	½ cup	89	1.03	0.07	22		13
pickled, canned, solids & liquids	½ cup	75	0.91	0.10	19	0.71	13
Beet greens, raw	½ cup	4	0.35	0.01	1	0.25	23
cooked, boiled, drained	½ cup	20	1.85	0.14	4	0.76	82
Borage, raw	1 cup	19	1.60	0.62	3	0.82	83
Broccoli, raw	½ cup	12	1.31	0.15	2	0.49	21
cooked, boiled, drained	½ cup	23	2.32	0.22	4	0.94	89
frozen, chopped, unprepared	10-oz pkg	75	7.97	0.81	14	3.13	159
frozen, chopped, cooked, boiled, drained	½ cup	25	2.85	0.11	5	1.10	47

FOOD	IRON (mg)	POTAS- SIUM (mg)	SODIUM (mg)	VITAMIN C (mg)	THIAMIN (mg)	NIACIN (mg)	VITAMIN A (mg)	% OF CALORIES FROM FAT
Alfalfa seeds, sprouted, raw	0.32	26	2	2.70	0.03	0.16	5	21
Amaranth, raw	0.65	171	5	12.10	0.01	0.18	82	12
cooked, boiled, drained	2.98	846	28	54.30	0.03	0.74	366	8
Arrowhead, raw	0.31	111	3	0.10	0.02	0.20	0	2
cooked, boiled, drained	0.15	106	2	0.00	0.02	0.14	0	1
Artichokes, raw	2.10	434	102	13.80	0.10	0.97	24	4
cooked, boiled, drained	1.62	316	79	8.90	0.07	0.71	17	3
frozen, unprepared	1.27	632	120	13.40	0.15	2.19	39	10
frozen, cooked, boiled, drained	1.34	634	127	12.00	0.15	2.20	38	10
Arugula, raw		37	3		0.00	0.03	24	32
Asparagus, raw	0.51	158	1	7.60	0.08	0.68	34	8
cooked, boiled, drained	0.44	96	7	6.50	0.07	0.65	32	12
canned, solids & liquids	2.38	628	1432	67.40	0.22	3.50	195	12
canned, drained solids	4.55							30
frozen, unprepared	0.42	147	5	18.50	0.07	0.70	55	8
frozen, cooked, boiled, drained	0.38	131	2	14.70	0.04	0.62	49	13
Balsam-pear leafy tips, raw	0.49	146	3	21.10	0.04	0.27	42	22
cooked, boiled, drained	0.30	174	4	16.10	0.04	0.29	50	5
Balsam-pear pods, raw	0.40	275	5	78.10	0.04	0.37	35	9
cooked, boiled, drained	0.47	396	8	40.90	0.06	0.35	14	8
Bamboo shoots, raw	0.76	805	7	6.00	0.23	0.91	3	10
cooked, boiled, drained	0.29	640	5	0.00	0.02	0.36	0	16
canned, drained solids	0.42	104	9	1.40	0.03	0.18	1	19
La Choy®	0.65	654	9	1.46	0.04	0.19	0	19
Beans, shellie, canned, solids & liquid	2.43	268	819	7.50	0.08	0.50	56	6
Beans, green, frozen, boiled, Health Valley®	1.62	152	18	12.30	0.09	0.78	135	36
Beans, snap, raw	1.14	230	6	17.90	0.09	0.83	74	3
cooked, boiled, drained	1.60	373	4	12.10	0.09	0.77	83	7
canned, solids & liquid	3.85	428	1615	17.40	0.11	0.88	142	6
canned, drained solids	2.36	286	657	12.50	0.04	0.53	91	5
canned, seasoned, solids & liquid	2.08	407	1637	13.60	0.11	1.02	231	11
frozen, unprepared	0.53	115	2	8.00	0.06	0.31	30	6
frozen, cooked, boiled, drained	0.56	76	9	5.60	0.03	0.28	36	5
Bean sprouts, canned, La Choy®	0.94	220	31	29.90	0.02	0.20	3	16
Beets, raw	1.49	528	118	17.90	0.08	0.65	3	3
cooked, boiled, drained	0.62	312	49	5.50	0.03	0.27	1	1
canned, solids & liquid	0.82	175	324	4.80	0.01	0.19	1	2
canned, drained solids	1.55							4
harvard, canned, solids & liquids	0.44	201	199	2.90		0.10		1
pickled, canned, solids & liquids	0.47	169	301	2.60	0.03	0.29	1	1
Beet greens, raw	0.63	104	38	5.70	0.02	0.08	116	2
cooked, boiled, drained	1.37	654	173	17.90	0.08	0.36	367	6
Borage, raw	2.94	418	71	31.20	0.05	0.80	374	29
Broccoli, raw	0.39	143	12	41.00	0.03	0.28	68	11
cooked, boiled, drained	0.89	127	8	49.00	0.06	0.59	110	9
frozen, chopped, unprepared	2.30	602	68	160.20	0.15	1.34	587	10
frozen, chopped, cooked, boiled, drained	0.56	166	22	36.90	0.05	0.42	174	4

115

VEGETABLES & VEGETABLE PRODUCTS

FOOD	AMOUNT	CALORIES (kcal)	PROTEIN (g)	FAT (g)	CARBO-HYDRATES (g)	FIBER (g)	CALCIUM (mg)
Broccoli (continued)							
frozen, spears, unprepared	10-oz pkg	84	8.69	0.97	15	3.22	115
frozen, spears, cooked, boiled, drained	10-oz pkg	69	7.76	0.29	13	2.78	127
Health Valley® frozen, boiled	1 cup	50	6.00	2.00	10	4.00	
Brussels sprouts, raw	½ cup	19	1.49	0.13	4	0.66	18
cooked, boiled, drained	½ cup	30	1.99	0.40	7	1.07	28
frozen, unprepared	10-oz pkg	116	10.72	1.16	22	4.01	75
frozen, cooked, boiled, drained	½ cup	33	2.84	0.31	6	1.13	19
Burdock root, raw	1 cup	85	1.80	0.17	20	2.29	48
cooked, boiled, drained	1 cup	110	2.61	0.18	26	2.29	62
Butterbur (also known as Fuki), raw	1 cup	13	0.37	0.04	3	1.22	97
canned	1 cup	3	0.14	0.16	0	1.08	42
Cabbage, raw	½ cup	8	0.42	0.06	2	0.28	16
cooked, boiled, drained	½ cup	16	0.72	0.18	4	0.45	25
Cabbage, Chinese, raw	½ cup	5	0.53	0.07	1	0.21	37
cooked, boiled, drained	½ cup	10	1.32	0.14	2	0.51	79
Cabbage, Chinese, raw	1 cup	12	0.91	0.15	2	0.46	58
cooked, boiled, drained	1 cup	16	1.79	0.20	3	0.60	38
Cabbage, red, raw	½ cup	10	0.49	0.09	2	0.35	18
cooked, boiled, drained	½ cup	16	0.79	0.15	3	0.57	28
Cabbage, Savoy, raw	½ cup	10	0.70	0.04	2	0.28	12
cooked, boiled, drained	½ cup	18	1.31	0.07	4	0.51	22
Cardoon, raw	½ cup	18	0.62	0.09	4		62
Carrots, raw	1 carrot	31	0.74	0.14	7	0.75	19
cooked, boiled, drained	1 carrot	21	0.50	0.08	5	0.68	14
canned, solids & liquids	1 can	102	2.77	0.79	23	3.37	114
canned, drained solids	1 can	65	1.82	0.54	16	2.27	71
frozen, unprepared	10-oz pkg	112	3.09	0.60	26	3.02	92
frozen, cooked, boiled, drained	½ cup	26	0.87	0.08	6	0.86	21
baby, raw	1 medium	4	0.08	0.05	1		2
Carrot juice, canned	6 fl oz	73	1.74	0.27	17	1.75	44
Cauliflower, raw	½ cup	12	0.99	0.09	2	0.42	14
cooked, boiled, drained	½ cup	15	1.16	0.11	3	0.51	17
frozen, unprepared	½ cup	16	1.33	0.18	3	0.66	15
frozen, cooked, boiled, drained	½ cup	17	1.45	0.19	3	0.72	15
Vlasic®							
hot & spicy	1 oz	4	0.00	0.00	1		0
sweet	1 oz	35	0.00	0.00	9	0.60	0
Celeriac, raw	½ cup	31	1.17	0.23	7	1.01	34
Celery, raw	½ cup	9	0.40	0.07	2	0.41	22
cooked, boiled, drained	½ cup	11	0.38	0.08	3	0.49	27
Celtuce, raw	1 leaf	2	0.07	0.02	0	0.03	3
Chard, Swiss, raw	½ cup	3	0.32	0.04	1	0.14	9
cooked, boiled, drained	½ cup	18	1.65	0.07	4	0.83	51
Chayote, fruit, raw	1 cup	32	1.19	0.40	7	0.92	25
cooked, boiled, drained	1 cup	38	0.99	0.77	8	0.93	21
Chicory greens, raw	1 cup	42	3.06	0.54	8	1.44	180
Chicory roots, raw	½ cup	33	0.63	0.09	8	0.88	18

FOOD	IRON (mg)	POTAS-SIUM (mg)	SODIUM (mg)	VITAMIN C (mg)	THIAMIN (mg)	NIACIN (mg)	VITAMIN A (mg)	% OF CALORIES FROM FAT
Broccoli (continued)								
frozen, spears, unprepared	2.03	710	49	194.00	0.20	1.31	406	10
frozen, spears, cooked, boiled, drained	1.53	451	60	36.90	0.05	0.42	174	4
Health Valley® frozen, boiled		332	44		0.00			36
Brussels sprouts, raw	0.62	171	11	37.40	0.06	0.33	39	6
cooked, boiled, drained	0.94	247	17	48.40	0.08	0.47	56	12
frozen, unprepared	2.65	1052	28	210.40	0.30	1.81	231	9
frozen, cooked, boiled, drained	0.58	254	18	35.60	0.08	0.42	46	8
Burdock root, raw	0.94	363	6	3.50	0.01	0.35	0	2
cooked, boiled, drained	0.96	450	5		0.05	0.40	0	1
Butterbur (also known as Fuki), raw	0.09	616	7	29.60	0.02	0.19	5	3
canned	0.78	15	5	14.80	0.01	0.17	0	48
Cabbage, raw	0.20	86	6	16.50	0.02	0.11	4	7
cooked, boiled, drained	0.29	154	14	18.20	0.04	0.17	6	10
Cabbage, Chinese, raw	0.28	88	23	15.80	0.01	0.18	105	13
cooked, boiled, drained	0.88	315	29	22.10	0.03	0.36	218	13
Cabbage, Chinese, raw	0.23	181	7	20.50	0.03	0.30	91	11
cooked, boiled, drained	0.36	268	11	18.80	0.05	0.60	115	11
Cabbage, red, raw	0.17	72	4	20.00	0.02	0.11	1	8
cooked, boiled, drained	0.27	105	6	25.80	0.03	0.15	2	8
Cabbage, Savoy, raw	0.14	81	10	10.90	0.03	0.11	35	4
cooked, boiled, drained	0.28	134	17	12.40	0.04	0.02	65	4
Cardoon, raw	0.62	356	151	1.80	0.02	0.27	11	5
Carrots, raw	0.36	233	25	6.70	0.07	0.67	2025	4
cooked, boiled, drained	0.28	104	30	1.10	0.02	0.23	1129	3
canned, solids & liquids	2.76	784	1095	12.70	0.09	1.91	5973	7
canned, drained solids	1.82	508	684	7.70	0.05	1.57	3912	7
frozen, unprepared	1.72	515	167	12.30	0.11	1.80	6044	5
frozen, cooked, boiled, drained	0.35	115	43	2.00	0.02	0.32	1292	3
baby, raw		28	3	0.80	0.00	0.09	20	11
Carrot juice, canned	0.85	538	54	15.70	0.17	0.71	4738	3
Cauliflower, raw	0.29	178	7	35.80	0.04	0.32	1	7
cooked, boiled, drained	0.26	200	4	34.30	0.04	0.34	1	7
frozen, unprepared	0.36	127	16	32.20	0.03	0.28	2	10
frozen, cooked, boiled, drained	0.37	125	16	28.20	0.03	0.28	2	10
Vlasic®								
hot & spicy	0.36		434	0.00	0.00	0.00	0	0
sweet	0.36	76	225	0.00	0.00	0.00	0	0
Celeriac, raw	0.55	234	78	6.20	0.04	0.55	0	7
Celery, raw	0.29	170	53	3.80	0.02	0.18	8	7
cooked, boiled, drained	0.10	266	48	3.50	0.02	0.19	8	7
Celtuce, raw	0.04	26	1	1.60	0.00	0.04	28	9
Chard, Swiss, raw	0.32	68	38	5.40	0.01	0.07	59	12
cooked, boiled, drained	1.99	483	158	15.80	0.03	0.32	276	4
Chayote, fruit, raw	0.53	198	5	14.50	0.04	0.66	7	11
cooked, boiled, drained	0.35	276	1	12.80	0.04	0.67	7	18
Chicory greens, raw	1.62	756	81	43.20	0.11	0.90	720	12
Chicory roots, raw	0.36	131	23	2.30	0.02	0.18	0	2

VEGETABLES & VEGETABLE PRODUCTS

FOOD	AMOUNT	CALORIES (kcal)	PROTEIN (g)	FAT (g)	CARBO-HYDRATES (g)	FIBER (g)	CALCIUM (mg)
Chicory, witloof, raw	1/2 cup	7	0.45	0.05	1		
Chives, raw	1 tbsp	1	0.10	0.02	0		3
freeze-dried	1 tbsp	1	0.04	0.01	0	0.02	2
Chop suey vegetables, canned, La Choy®	1 cup	17	1.06	0.13	4	0.01	20
Chrysanthemum, garland, raw	1 cup	4	0.39	0.04	1	0.22	14
cooked, boiled, drained	1 cup	20	1.64	0.09	4	1.16	69
Coleslaw	1/2 cup	42	0.77	1.57	7	0.36	27
Collards, raw	1 cup	35	2.92	0.40	7	1.06	218
cooked, boiled, drained	1 cup	27	2.09	0.29	5	0.76	148
frozen, unprepared	10-oz pkg	93	7.65	1.05	18	2.78	570
frozen, cooked, boiled, drained	1 cup	61	5.04	0.69	12	1.84	357
Coriander	1/4 cup	1	0.09	0.02	0	0.03	4
Corn, sweet, raw	1 ear	77	2.90	1.06	17	0.63	2
cooked, boiled, drained	1 ear	83	2.56	0.98	19	0.46	2
canned, solids & liquid	1 can	294	9.35	2.17	71	2.36	19
canned, drained solids	1 can	242	7.82	2.97	55		
canned, cream style	1 can	349	8.40	2.02	87	2.35	15
canned, vacuum pack	1 can	270	8.19	1.71	66	2.66	16
frozen, kernels, cut off cob, unprepared	10-oz pkg	250	8.58	2.20	59	1.76	12
frozen, kernels, cut off cob, cooked, boiled, drained	10-oz pkg	231	8.57	0.21	58	1.36	6
frozen, kernels, on cob, unprep	1 ear	123	4.10	0.97	29	0.86	4
frozen, kernels, on cob, cooked, boiled, drained	1 ear	59	1.96	0.46	14	0.41	2
Health Valley® frozen, boiled	1 cup	160	6.00	2.00	2	4.00	
Corn w/red & green peppers, canned, solids & liquids	1 cup	171	5.28	1.25	41	1.41	11
Corn pudding	1 cup	271	10.99	13.29	32	0.90	100
Corn salad, raw	1 cup	12	1.12	0.22	2	0.45	1
Cress, garden, raw	1/2 cup	8	0.65	0.18	1	0.28	20
cooked, boiled, drained	1/2 cup	16	1.29	0.41	3	0.61	41
Cucumber, raw	1 cucumber	39	1.63	0.39	9	1.81	42
Dandelion greens, raw	1 cup	25	1.49	0.39	5	0.88	103
cooked, boiled, drained	1 cup	35	2.10	0.63	7	1.37	147
Dock, raw	1 cup	29	2.66	0.93	4	1.06	59
Eggplant, raw	1/2 cup	11	0.45	0.04	3	0.41	15
cooked, boiled, drained	1/2 cup	13	0.40	0.11	3	0.47	3
Endive, raw	1/2 cup	4	0.31	0.05	1	0.23	13
Eppaw, raw	1/2 cup	75	2.30	0.90	16		55
Fennel, bulb, raw	1 cup	27	1.08	0.18	6		43
Garden mix, hot & spicy, Vlasic®	1 oz	4	0.00	0.00	1		0
Garlic, raw	1 clove	4	0.19	0.02	1	0.05	5
Ginger root, raw	1/4 cup	17	0.42	0.18	4	0.25	4
Gourd, dishcloth (a.k.a. towelgourd), raw	1 cup	19	1.14	0.19	4	0.48	19
cooked, boiled, drained	1 cup	99	1.17	0.61	26	0.68	16
Gourd, white-flowered (a.k.a. calabash gourd), raw	1/2 cup	8	0.36	0.01	2	0.32	15

FOOD	IRON (mg)	POTAS-SIUM (mg)	SODIUM (mg)	VITAMIN C (mg)	THIAMIN (mg)	NIACIN (mg)	VITAMIN A (mg)	% OF CALORIES FROM FAT
Chicory, witloof, raw	0.23	82	3	4.50	0.03	0.23	0	6
Chives, raw	0.05	9	0	1.70	0.00	0.02	13	18
freeze-dried	0.04	6		1.30	0.00	0.01	14	9
Chop suey vegetables, canned, La Choy®	1.65	151	662	41.40	0.03	0.43	0	7
Chrysanthemum, garland, raw	0.78	143	13	9.30	0.01	0.22	367	9
cooked, boiled, drained	3.74	569	53	23.90	0.02	0.72	505	4
Coleslaw	0.35	109	14	19.60	0.04	0.16	49	34
Collards, raw	1.16	275	52	43.30	0.05	0.70	619	10
cooked, boiled, drained	0.78	177	36	18.60	0.03	0.45	422	10
frozen, unprepared	3.03	719	136	113.50	0.14	1.82	1623	10
frozen, cooked, boiled, drained	1.90	427	85	44.90	0.08	1.08	1017	10
Coriander	0.08	22	1	0.40	0.00	0.03	11	18
Corn, sweet, raw	0.46	243	14	6.20	0.18	1.53	25	12
cooked, boiled, drained	0.47	192	13	4.80	0.17	1.24	17	11
canned, solids & liquid	1.69	738	1220	32.30	0.13	4.53	58	7
canned, drained solids	2.55						46	11
canned, cream style	1.83	646	1376	22.20	0.12	4.63	47	5
canned, vacuum pack	1.44	632	925	27.60	0.14	3.97	82	6
frozen, kernels, cut off cob, unprepared	1.20	596	9	18.20	0.24	4.90	37	8
frozen, kernels, cut off cob, cooked, boiled, drained	0.86	394	14	7.30	0.20	3.64	71	1
frozen, kernels, on cob, unprep	0.85	367	6	9.00	0.13	2.10	31	7
frozen, kernels, on cob, cooked, boiled, drained	0.39	158	3	3.00	0.11	0.96	13	7
Health Valley® frozen, boiled		228	8					11
Corn w/red & green peppers, canned, solids & liquids	1.79	346	788	20.00	0.05	2.16	53	7
Corn pudding	1.39	402	138	7.10	1.03	2.47	89	44
Corn salad, raw								17
Cress, garden, raw	0.33	152	4	17.30	0.02	0.25	233	20
cooked, boiled, drained	0.54	240	5	15.60	0.04	0.54	524	23
Cucumber, raw	0.84	448	6	14.20	0.09	0.90	14	9
Dandelion greens, raw	1.71	218	42	19.30	0.11		770	14
cooked, boiled, drained	1.89	244	46	18.90	0.14		1228	16
Dock, raw	3.19	519	5	63.80	0.05	0.67	532	29
Eggplant, raw	0.22	90	1	0.70	0.04	0.25	3	3
cooked, boiled, drained	0.17	119	2	0.60	0.04	0.29	3	8
Endive, raw	0.21	79	6	1.60	0.02	0.10	51	11
Eppaw, raw	0.58	170	6	6.50	0.06	0.15	0	11
Fennel, bulb, raw		360	45	10.50	0.01	0.56		6
Garden mix, hot & spicy, Vlasic®	0.36		379	3.59	0.00	0.00	20	0
Garlic, raw	0.05	12	1	0.90	0.01	0.02	0	5
Ginger root, raw	0.12	100	3	1.20	0.01	0.17	0	10
Gourd, dishcloth (a.k.a. towelgourd), raw	0.34	132	3	11.40	0.05	0.38	39	9
cooked, boiled, drained	0.64	807	37	10.10	0.08	0.46	46	6
Gourd, white-flowered (a.k.a. calabash gourd), raw	0.12	87	1	5.90	0.02	0.19	0	1

VEGETABLES & VEGETABLE PRODUCTS

FOOD	AMOUNT	CALORIES (kcal)	PROTEIN (g)	FAT (g)	CARBO-HYDRATES (g)	FIBER (g)	CALCIUM (mg)
Gourd, white-flowered (a.k.a. calabash gourd) (continued)							
cooked, boiled, drained	½ cup	11	0.44	0.01	3	0.46	18
Horseradish-tree leafy tips, raw	1 cup	13	1.97	0.29	2	0.32	
cooked, boiled, drained	1 cup	25	2.21	0.39	5	0.72	
Horseradish-tree pods, raw	1 cup	37	2.10	0.20	9	1.30	30
cooked, boiled, drained	1 cup	42	2.46	0.22	10	2.17	24
Jerusalem-artichokes, raw	1 cup	114	3.00	0.02	26	1.20	21
Jew's Ear (a.k.a. Pepeao), raw	1 cup	25	0.47	0.04	7	2.11	16
dried	1 cup	72	1.16	0.11	19	7.43	27
Jute, potherb, raw	1 cup	10	1.30	0.07	2	0.34	58
cooked, boiled, drained	1 cup	32	3.20	0.17	6	1.71	184
Kale, raw	1 cup	33	2.21	0.47	7	1.01	90
cooked, boiled, drained	1 cup	41	2.47	0.52	7	1.04	94
frozen, unprepared	10-oz pkg	79	7.55	1.29	14	2.46	385
frozen, cooked, boiled, drained	1 cup	39	3.69	0.64	7	1.21	179
Kale, Scotch, raw	1 cup	28	1.88	0.40	6	0.82	137
cooked, boiled, drained	1 cup	37	2.46	0.53	7	1.11	171
Kanypo (dried gourd strips)	½ cup	70	2.32	0.15	18	2.47	76
Kohlrabi, raw	1 cup	38	2.38	0.14	9	1.40	34
cooked, boiled, drained	1 cup	48	2.97	0.18	11	1.82	41
Lamb'squarters, cooked, boiled, drained	1 cup	58	5.76	1.26	9	3.24	464
Leeks, raw	¼ cup	16	0.39	0.08	4	0.39	15
cooked, boiled, drained	¼ cup	8	0.21	0.05	2	0.21	8
freeze-dried	¼ cup	3	0.12	0.02	1	0.07	3
Lettuce, butterhead, raw	1 head	21	2.09	0.36	4		
cos or romaine, raw	½ cup	4	0.45	0.06	1	0.20	10
iceberg, raw	1 head	70	5.44	1.02	11	2.86	102
loose leaf, raw	½ cup	5	0.36	0.08	1	0.20	19
Lotus root, raw	10 slices	45	2.11	0.08	14	0.64	36
cooked, boiled, drained	10 slices	59	1.40	0.06	14	0.76	23
Mountain yam, Hawaii, raw	½ cup	46	0.91	0.07	11	0.31	18
cooked, steamed	½ cup	59	1.24	0.06	14	0.40	5
Mushrooms, raw	1 mushroom	5	0.38	0.08	1	0.13	1
cooked, boiled, drained	1 mushroom	3	0.26	0.06	1	0.10	1
canned, drained solids	1 mushroom	3	0.22	0.04	1		
Enoki, raw	1 mushroom	2	0.08	0.02	0		0
Shiitake, dried	4 mushrooms	44	1.44	0.15	11	1.73	2
Shiitake, cooked	4 mushrooms	40	1.12	0.16	10	1.41	2
Mustard greens, raw	1 cup	14	1.51	0.11	3	0.62	58
cooked, boiled, drained	1 cup	21	3.16	0.34	3	0.96	103
frozen, unprepared	10-oz pkg	58	7.06	0.76	10	2.27	329
frozen, cooked, boiled, drained	10-oz pkg	40	4.81	0.52	7	1.55	213
Mustard spinach (a.k.a. tendergreen), raw	1 cup	33	3.30	0.45	6	1.50	315
cooked, boiled, drained	1 cup	29	3.06	0.36	5	1.44	284
New Zealand spinach, raw	1 cup	8	0.84	0.11	1	0.39	32
cooked, boiled, drained	1 cup	22	2.34	0.31	4	1.10	86

FOOD	IRON (mg)	POTAS-SIUM (mg)	SODIUM (mg)	VITAMIN C (mg)	THIAMIN (mg)	NIACIN (mg)	VITAMIN A (mg)	% OF CALORIES FROM FAT
Gourd, white-flowered (a.k.a. calabash gourd) (continued)								
cooked, boiled, drained	0.18	124	1	6.20	0.02	0.29	0	1
Horseradish-tree leafy tips, raw	0.84	71	2	10.90	0.05	0.47	159	20
cooked, boiled, drained	0.97	144	4	13.00	0.09	0.84	295	14
Horseradish-tree pods, raw	0.36	461	42		0.05	0.62	7	5
cooked, boiled, drained	0.53	539	51		0.05	0.70	8	5
Jerusalem-artichokes, raw	5.10			6.00	0.30	1.95	3	0
Jew's Ear (a.k.a. Pepeao), raw	0.55	42	9	0.60	0.08	0.07	0	1
dried	1.47	170	17	0.30		0.72	0	1
Jute, potherb, raw	1.33	156	2	10.40	0.04	0.35	156	6
cooked, boiled, drained	2.73	479	9	28.70	0.08	0.77	451	5
Kale, raw	1.14	299	29	80.40	0.07	0.67	596	13
cooked, boiled, drained	1.17	296	30	53.30	0.07	0.65	962	11
frozen, unprepared	2.63	947	43	111.50	0.16	1.98	1776	15
frozen, cooked, boiled, drained	1.22	417	20	32.80	0.06	0.87	826	15
Kale, Scotch, raw	2.01	302	47	87.10	0.05	0.87	208	13
cooked, boiled, drained	2.51	356	59	68.60	0.05	1.03	259	13
Kanypo (dried gourd strips)	1.38	427	4	0.10	0.00	0.78	0	2
Kohlrabi, raw	0.56	490	28	86.80	0.07	0.56	5	3
cooked, boiled, drained	0.66	561	34	89.10	0.07	0.64	6	3
Lamb'squarters, cooked, boiled, drained	1.26			66.60	0.18	1.62	1746	20
Leeks, raw	0.55	47	5	3.10	0.02	0.10	2	5
cooked, boiled, drained	0.29	23	3	1.10	0.01	0.05	1	6
freeze-dried	0.06	19	0	0.90	0.01	0.03	0	6
Lettuce, butterhead, raw	0.49	416	8	13.00	0.10	0.49	158	15
cos or romaine, raw	0.31	81	2	6.70	0.03	0.14	73	14
iceberg, raw	2.70	852	48	21.00	0.25	1.01	178	13
loose leaf, raw	0.39	74	3	5.00	0.01	0.11	53	14
Lotus root, raw	0.94	450	33	35.60	0.13	0.32	0	2
cooked, boiled, drained	0.80	323	40	24.40	0.11	0.27	0	1
Mountain yam, Hawaii, raw	0.30	284	9	1.80	0.07	0.33	0	1
cooked, steamed	0.31	356	9	0.00	0.06	0.09	0	1
Mushrooms, raw	0.22	67	1	0.60	0.02	0.74	0	14
cooked, boiled, drained	0.21	43	0	0.50	0.01	0.54	0	18
canned, drained solids	0.10						0	12
Enoki, raw		19	0	0.60	0.00	0.18	0	9
Shiitake, dried	0.26	230	2	0.50	0.05	2.12	0	3
Shiitake, cooked	0.32	85	3	0.20	0.03	1.08	0	4
Mustard greens, raw	0.82	198	14	39.20	0.05	0.45	297	7
cooked, boiled, drained	0.98	283	22	35.40	0.06	0.61	424	15
frozen, unprepared	3.67	481	83	71.80	0.14	0.89	1464	12
frozen, cooked, boiled, drained	2.38	295	53	29.40	0.09	0.55	948	12
Mustard spinach (a.k.a. tendergreen), raw	2.25			195.00			1485	12
cooked, boiled, drained	1.44			117.00			1476	11
New Zealand spinach, raw	0.45	73	73	16.80	0.02	0.28	246	12
cooked, boiled, drained	1.19	183	193	28.80	0.05	0.70	652	13

VEGETABLES & VEGETABLE PRODUCTS

FOOD	AMOUNT	CALORIES (kcal)	PROTEIN (g)	FAT (g)	CARBO- HYDRATES (g)	FIBER (g)	CALCIUM (mg)
Okra, raw	8 pods	36	1.90	0.10	7	0.89	77
cooked, boiled, drained	8 pods	27	1.59	0.14	6	0.77	54
frozen, unprepared	10-oz pkg	85	4.80	0.70	19	2.35	231
frozen, cooked, boiled, drained	10-oz pkg	94	5.30	0.77	21	2.60	245
Onion rings (onions are breaded & par-fried in vegetable oil)							
frozen, unprepared	16-oz pkg	1170	14.30	63.96	138		208
frozen, prepared, heated in oven	2 rings	81	1.07	5.34	8	0.08	6
Onions, raw	1/2 cup	27	0.94	0.21	6	0.35	20
cooked, boiled, drained	1/2 cup	29	0.95	0.17	7	0.44	29
canned, solids & liquids	1/2 cup	21	0.95	0.10	5		51
dehydrated flakes	1/4 cup	45	1.25	0.06	12	0.64	36
frozen, chopped, unprepared	10-oz pkg	83	2.24	0.28	19	1.33	50
frozen, chopped, cooked, boiled, drained	1/2 cup	30	0.80	0.10	7	0.48	17
frozen, whole, unprepared	10-oz pkg	101	2.54	0.18	24	1.96	102
spring, raw	1/2 cup	13	0.87	0.07	3	0.42	30
Vlasic® cocktail, lightly spiced	1 oz	4	0.00	0.00	1	0.45	0
Parsley, raw	1/2 cup	11	0.89	0.24	2		41
freeze-dried	1/4 cup	4	0.44	0.07	1	0.14	2
Parsnips, raw	1/2 cup	50	0.80	0.20	12	1.34	24
cooked, boiled, drained	1/2 cup	63	1.03	0.23	15	1.72	29
Peas, edible-podded, raw	1/2 cup	30	2.02	0.14	5	1.80	31
cooked, boiled, drained	1/2 cup	34	2.62	0.18	6	0.83	33
frozen, unprepared	1/2 cup	30	2.02	0.22	5	1.73	36
frozen, cooked, boiled, drained	1/2 cup	42	2.80	0.30	7	2.40	48
Peas, green, raw	1/2 cup	63	4.22	0.31	11	1.72	19
cooked, boiled, drained	1/2 cup	67	4.28	0.17	13	1.85	22
canned, solids & liquid	1/2 cup	61	3.70	0.35	11	1.77	22
canned, drained solids	1/2 cup	59	3.76	0.29	11	1.69	17
canned, seasoned, solids & liquids	1/2 cup	57	3.52	0.31	11	1.93	18
frozen, unprepared	1/2 cup	55	3.75	0.27	10	1.51	16
frozen, cooked, boiled, drained	1/2 cup	63	4.12	0.22	11	1.71	19
Health Valley® frozen, boiled	1 cup	160	8.00	2.00	22	6.00	
Peas, mature seeds, raw	1/2 cup	77	5.28	0.41	17	1.67	21
Peas & carrots, can, solids & liquids	1/2 cup	48	2.77	0.35	11	1.46	29
frozen, unprepared	1/2 cup	37	2.38	0.33	8	1.07	19
frozen, cooked, boiled, drained	1/2 cup	38	2.47	0.34	8	1.11	18
Peas & onions, can, solids & liquids	1/2 cup	30	1.97	0.23	5	0.74	10
frozen, unprepared	1/2 cup	48	2.74	0.22	9		16
frozen, cooked, boiled, drained	1/2 cup	40	2.29	0.18	8		13
Peppers, hot chili (red & green varieties)							
raw	1 pepper	18	0.90	0.09	4	0.81	8
canned, solids & liquid	1 pepper	18	0.66	0.07	4	0.88	5
Peppers, jalapeno, canned, solids & liquid	1/2 cup	17	0.54	0.41	3	1.56	18
Vlasic® hot Mexican	1 oz	8	0.00	0.00	2	0.43	0
tiny	1 oz	6	0.00	0.00	2	0.43	0
Peppers, mild cherry, Vlasic®	1 oz	8	0.00	0.00	2		0

FOOD	IRON (mg)	POTAS-SIUM (mg)	SODIUM (mg)	VITAMIN C (mg)	THIAMIN (mg)	NIACIN (mg)	VITAMIN A (mg)	% OF CALORIES FROM FAT
Okra, raw	0.76	287	8	20.00	0.19	0.95	63	3
cooked, boiled, drained	0.38	273	5	13.90	0.11	0.74	49	5
frozen, unprepared	1.62	600	7	35.10	0.25	2.01	131	7
frozen, cooked, boiled, drained	1.71	597	8	31.10	0.25	2.00	131	7
Onion rings (onions are breaded & par-fried in vegetable oil)								
frozen, unprepared	4.21	860	1116	20.70	0.45	3.14	79	49
frozen, prepared, heated in oven	0.34	26	75	0.30	0.06	0.72	5	59
Onions, raw	0.29	124	2	6.70	0.05	0.08	0	7
cooked, boiled, drained	0.21	159	8	6.00	0.04	0.08	0	5
canned, solids & liquids	0.15	124	416					4
dehydrated flakes	0.22	227	3	10.50	0.07	0.14	0	1
frozen, chopped, unprepared	0.93	353	35	9.50	0.09	0.43	10	3
frozen, chopped, cooked, boiled, drained	0.32	114	13	2.70	0.02	0.15	4	3
frozen, whole, unprepared	1.29	402	27	22.60	0.07	0.50	7	2
spring, raw	0.94	128	2	22.50	0.04	0.10	250	5
Vlasic® cocktail, lightly spiced	0.00	43	364	0.00	0.00	0.00	0	0
Parsley, raw	1.86	166	17	39.90	0.03	0.39	0	20
freeze-dried	0.75	88	5	2.10	0.02	0.15	89	16
Parsnips, raw	0.39	251	7	11.40	0.06	0.47	0	4
cooked, boiled, drained	0.45	287	8	10.10	0.07	0.57	0	3
Peas, edible-podded, raw	1.50	144	3	43.20	0.11	0.43	10	4
cooked, boiled, drained	1.58	192	3	38.30	0.10	0.43	10	5
frozen, unprepared	1.44	139	3	15.80	0.04	0.36	10	7
frozen, cooked, boiled, drained	1.92	173	4	17.60	0.05	0.45	13	6
Peas, green, raw	1.15	190	4	31.20	0.21	1.63	50	4
cooked, boiled, drained	1.24	217	2	11.40	0.21	1.62	48	2
canned, solids & liquid	1.37	108	340	13.50	0.14	1.04	47	5
canned, drained solids	0.81	147	186	8.10	0.10	0.62	65	4
canned, seasoned, solids & liquids	1.37	139	290	13.10	0.11	0.79	49	5
frozen, unprepared	1.10	107	81	12.90	0.19	1.23	52	4
frozen, cooked, boiled, drained	1.26	134	70	7.90	0.23	1.18	53	3
Health Valley® frozen, boiled		268	140					11
Peas, mature seeds, raw	1.35	229	12	6.20	0.14	1.85	10	5
Peas & carrots, can, solids & liquids	0.97	128	332	8.40	0.10	0.74	739	7
frozen, unprepared	0.76	136	55	7.80	0.13	0.99	665	8
frozen, cooked, boiled, drained	0.75	127	55	6.50	0.18	0.92	621	8
Peas & onions, can, solids & liquids	0.52	57	265	1.80	0.06	0.77	10	7
frozen, unprepared	1.06			9.60	0.21	1.19	38	4
frozen, cooked, boiled, drained	0.84			6.20	0.14	0.94	31	4
Peppers, hot chili (red & green varieties)								
raw	0.54	153	3	109.10	0.04	0.43	35	5
canned, solids & liquid	0.37			49.60	0.02	0.58	44	4
Peppers, jalapeno, canned, solids & liquid	1.90	92	995	8.80	0.02	0.34	116	22
Vlasic® hot Mexican	0.36	96	379		0.00	0.00	10	0
tiny	0.00	96	429	1.20	0.00	0.00	0	0
Peppers, mild cherry, Vlasic®	0.36		409	5.99	0.00	0.00	10	0

VEGETABLES & VEGETABLE PRODUCTS

FOOD	AMOUNT	CALORIES (kcal)	PROTEIN (g)	FAT (g)	CARBO-HYDRATES (g)	FIBER (g)	CALCIUM (mg)
Peppers, pepperoncini, mild Greek, Vlasic®	1 oz	4	0.00	0.00	1	0.43	0
Peppers, sweet (red & green varieties)							
raw	1 pepper	18	0.63	0.33	4	0.89	4
cooked, boiled, drained	1 pepper	13	0.45	0.24	3	0.64	3
canned, solids & liquids	½ cup	13	0.56	0.21	3	0.56	28
frozen, chopped, unprepared	10-oz pkg	58	3.06	0.60	13	2.84	26
freeze-dried	¼ cup	5	0.29	0.05	1	0.26	2
Peppers, sweet, yellow, raw	1 pepper	50	1.86	0.39	12		20
Pepper rings, hot banana, Vlasic®	1 oz	4	0.00	0.00	1		0
Pickle, cucumber							
dill (including Kosher & Polish)	1 pickle	12	0.40	0.12	3	0.37	6
sour	1 pickle	4	0.12	0.07	1	0.20	0
sweet	1 pickle	41	0.13	0.09	11	0.20	1
Vlasic®							
baby dills, kosher	1 oz	4	0.00	0.00	1	0.43	0
bread & butter chips	1 oz	30	0.00	0.00	7	0.43	0
bread & butter chunks	1 oz	25	0.00	0.00	6	0.43	0
bread & butter stixs	1 oz	18	0.00	0.00	5	0.43	0
bread & butter, deli	1 oz	25	0.00	0.00	6	0.43	0
crunchy dills, kosher	1 oz	4	0.00	0.00	1	0.43	0
dill chips, low salt, kosher	1 oz	2	0.00	0.00	1	0.43	0
dill gherkins, kosher	1 oz	4	0.00	0.00	1	0.43	0
dill halves, deli	1 oz	4	0.00	0.00	1	0.43	0
dill spears, kosher	1 oz	4	0.00	0.00	1	0.43	0
dill spears, no garlic	1 oz	4	0.00	0.00	1		0
dill, low salt, kosher	1 oz	4	0.00	0.00	1	0.43	0
dill, original	1 oz	2	0.00	0.00	1	0.43	0
dill, zesty snack chunks	1 oz	4	0.00	0.00	1	0.43	0
dill, zesty, crunchy	1 oz	2	0.00	0.00	1		0
Polish snack chunks	1 oz	4	0.00	0.00	1		0
spears, dill, zesty	1 oz	4	0.00	0.00	1	0.43	0
spears, low salt, kosher	1 oz	4	0.00	0.00	1	0.43	0
sweet chip, low salt, kosher	1 oz	30	0.00	0.00	7	0.43	0
Pickle relish, hamburger	1 tbsp	19	0.09	0.08	5	0.14	1
hotdog	1 tbsp	14	0.23	0.07	4	0.13	1
sweet	1 tbsp	19	0.06	0.07	5	0.13	0
Poi	1 cup	269	0.91	0.34	65	1.30	37
Pokeberry shoots, raw	1 cup	37	4.16	0.64	6		85
cooked, boiled, drained	1 cup	33	3.80	0.66	5		87
Potatoes, raw, flesh	1 potato	88	2.32	0.11	20	0.49	8
raw, skin	1 potato	22	0.98	0.04	5	0.68	11
baked, flesh & skin	1 potato	220	4.65	0.20	51	1.33	20
baked, flesh	1 potato	145	3.06	0.16	34	0.59	8
baked, skin	1 potato	115	2.49	0.06	27	1.32	20
boiled, cooked in skin, flesh	1 potato	119	2.54	0.14	27	0.43	7
boiled, cooked in skin, skin	1 potato	27	0.97	0.03	6	1.25	15
boiled, cooked w/out skin, flesh	1 potato	116	2.31	0.14	27	0.51	10
microwaved, cooked in skin, flesh & skin	1 potato	212	4.93	0.20	49	1.64	22

FOOD	IRON (mg)	POTAS-SIUM (mg)	SODIUM (mg)	VITAMIN C (mg)	THIAMIN (mg)	NIACIN (mg)	VITAMIN A (mg)	% OF CALORIES FROM FAT
Peppers, pepperoncini, mild Greek, Vlasic®	0.36	96	449	0.00	0.00	0.00	0	0
Peppers, sweet (red & green varieties)								
raw	0.94	144	2	94.70	0.06	0.40	39	17
cooked, boiled, drained	0.64	94	2	81.30	0.04	0.27	28	17
canned, solids & liquids	0.56	102	958	32.60	0.02	0.39	11	15
frozen, chopped, unprepared	1.76	259	15	166.60	0.20	3.89	104	9
freeze-dried	0.17	51	3	30.40	0.02	0.12	10	9
Peppers, sweet, yellow, raw		393	3	341.40	0.05	1.66	44	7
Pepper rings, hot banana, Vlasic®	0.36		464	8.98	0.00	0.00	0	0
Pickle, cucumber								
dill (including Kosher & Polish)	0.35	75	833	1.30	0.01	0.04	21	9
sour	0.14	8	423	0.30	0.00	0.00	5	16
sweet	0.21	11	328	0.40	0.00	0.06	4	2
Vlasic®								
baby dills, kosher	0.36	57	210	0.00	0.00	0.00	0	0
bread & butter chips	0.00	57	160	0.00	0.00	0.00	0	0
bread & butter chunks	0.00	57	120	0.00	0.00	0.00	0	0
bread & butter stixs	0.00	57	110	0.00	0.00	0.00	0	0
bread & butter, deli	0.00	57	120	0.00	0.00	0.00	0	0
crunchy dills, kosher	0.36	57	210	0.00	0.00	0.00	0	0
dill chips, low salt, kosher	0.00	473	175	0.00	0.00	0.00	0	0
dill gherkins, kosher	0.36	57	210	0.00	0.00	0.00	0	0
dill halves, deli	0.00	57	290	0.00	0.00	0.00	0	0
dill spears, kosher	0.00	57	175	0.00	0.00	0.00	0	0
dill spears, no garlic	0.36		210	0.00	0.00	0.00	0	0
dill, low salt, kosher	0.00	473	125	0.00	0.00	0.00	0	0
dill, original	0.00	57	374	0.00	0.00	0.00	0	0
dill, zesty snack chunks	0.00	57	290	0.00	0.03	0.00	0	0
dill, zesty, crunchy	0.00		374	0.00	0.00	0.00	0	0
Polish snack chunks	0.00		300	1.20	0.00	0.00	0	0
spears, dill, zesty	0.00	57	230	0.00	0.00	0.00	0	0
spears, low salt, kosher	0.00	473	120	0.00	0.00	0.00	0	0
sweet chip, low salt, kosher	0.00	57	80	0.00	0.00	0.00	0	0
Pickle relish, hamburger	0.17	11	164	0.30	0.00	0.09	4	4
hotdog	0.19	12	164	0.10	0.01	0.08	3	5
sweet	0.13	4	122	0.10	0.00	0.04	2	3
Poi	2.11	439	28	9.60	0.31	2.64	5	1
Pokeberry shoots, raw	2.72			217.60	0.13	1.92	1392	16
cooked, boiled, drained	1.98			135.30	0.12	1.82	1436	18
Potatoes, raw, flesh	0.85	608	7	22.10	0.10	1.66	0	1
raw, skin	1.23	157	4	4.30	0.01	0.39		2
baked, flesh & skin	2.75	844	16	26.10	0.22	3.32		1
baked, flesh	0.55	610	8	20.00	0.16	2.18		1
baked, skin	4.08	332	12	7.80	0.07	1.78		0
boiled, cooked in skin, flesh	0.42	515	6	17.60	0.14	1.96		1
boiled, cooked in skin, skin	2.06	138	5	1.80	0.01	0.42		1
boiled, cooked w/out skin, flesh	0.42	443	7	10.00	0.13	1.77		1
microwaved, cooked in skin, flesh & skin	2.50	903	16	30.50	0.24	3.46		1

VEGETABLES & VEGETABLE PRODUCTS

FOOD	AMOUNT	CALORIES (kcal)	PROTEIN (g)	FAT (g)	CARBO-HYDRATES (g)	FIBER (g)	CALCIUM (mg)
Potatoes (continued)							
microwaved, cooked in skin, flesh	1 potato	156	3.28	0.16	36	0.64	8
microwaved, cooked in skin, skin	1 potato	77	2.55	0.06	17	1.79	27
canned, solids & liquid	1 can	181	6.18	0.68	39	1.07	134
canned, drained solids	½ cup	54	1.27	0.18	12	0.24	5
Potatoes, whole, frozen, unprep	1 cup	142	4.33	0.29	32	0.73	15
Potatoes, french-fried							
frozen, unprepared	10 strips	107	1.66	4.20	16	0.33	4
frozen, home-prepared, oven	10 strips	111	1.73	4.38	17	0.34	4
frozen, restaurant-prepared, fried in vegetable oil	10 strips	158	2.01	8.28	20	0.37	10
frozen, cottage-cut, unprepared	10 strips	100	1.57	3.75	16	0.33	4
frozen, cottage-cut, prepared, heated in oven	10 strips	109	1.72	4.10	17	0.36	5
frozen, extruded, unprepared	10 strips	169	1.84	9.72	20	0.37	6
frozen, extruded, prepared, oven	10 strips	163	1.78	9.36	19	0.35	6
Potatoes au gratin, home-prepared	1 cup	322	12.40	18.59	28	0.67	292
dry mix, unprepared	5-½-oz pkg	490	13.88	5.77	116	1.45	485
dry mix, prepared	5-½-oz pkg	764	18.91	33.87	106	1.40	682
General Mills® dry mix	49.6 g	200	4.00	2.00	40		120
Kraft® frozen	107 g	140	4.00	5.00	20		
w/broccoli	107 g	140	5.00	5.00	20	1.10	128
Stouffers® frozen	109 g	110	4.00	6.00	10	1.12	80
Hashed brown potatoes							
home prepared	½ cup	163	1.89	10.85	17	0.32	6
frozen, plain, unprepared	½ cup	86	2.17	0.65	19	0.37	11
frozen, plain, prepared	½ cup	170	2.46	8.97	22	0.42	12
frozen, w/butter sauce, unprep	6-oz pkg	229	3.17	11.31	31		43
General Mills® dry mix	56.8 g	220	4.00	2.00	48		0
Julienne potatoes, dry mix, General Mills®	42.4 g	180	4.00	2.00	34		80
Mashed potatoes							
home prepared, w/whole milk & table fat added	½ cup	111	1.97	4.44	18	0.32	27
home prepared, w/whole milk added	½ cup	81	2.03	0.62	18	0.33	28
dehydrated, flakes w/out milk, dry	½ cup	361	7.97	0.62	83	3.10	35
dehydrated, flakes w/out milk, prepared	½ cup	118	2.00	5.88	16	0.50	52
granules w/out milk, dry	½ cup	80	1.69	0.18	18	0.35	13
granules w/out milk, prepared	½ cup	137	2.00	6.51	18		57
granules w/ milk, dry	½ cup	358	10.90	1.10	78	1.50	142
granules w/ milk, prepared	½ cup	83	2.10	2.31	14	0.32	33
Potato buds, dry mix, Gen Mills®	39 g	140	4.00	0.00	32		0
Potatoes O'Brien, home-prepared	1 cup	157	4.57	2.49	30	0.83	70
Scalloped potatoes, home-prepared	1 cup	210	7.03	9.02	26	0.72	140
dry mix, unprepared	5-½-oz pkg	558	12.12	7.16	115	2.23	97
dry mix, prepared	5-½-oz pkg	764	17.43	35.35	105	2.22	296
General Mills® dry mix	47.2 g	180	4.00	2.00	38		0
Hormel® w/ham	28.4 g	28	1.60	1.10	3	0.60	8
Kraft® frozen	107 g	140	4.00	5.00	20	2.27	31

FOOD	IRON (mg)	POTAS-SIUM (mg)	SODIUM (mg)	VITAMIN C (mg)	THIAMIN (mg)	NIACIN (mg)	VITAMIN A (mg)	% OF CALORIES FROM FAT
Potatoes (continued)								
microwaved, cooked in skin, flesh	0.64	641	11	23.60	0.20	2.54		1
microwaved, cooked in skin, skin	3.44	377	9	8.90	0.04	1.29		1
canned, solids & liquid	4.41	1103	1367	56.20	0.15	4.03		3
canned, drained solids	1.13	206		4.60	0.06	0.82		3
Potatoes, whole, frozen, unprep	1.84	630	46	25.80	0.28	3.06		2
Potatoes, french-fried								
frozen, unprepared	0.64	219	15	6.50	0.07	1.16		35
frozen, home-prepared, oven	0.67	229	15	5.50	0.06	1.15		36
frozen, restaurant-prepared, fried in vegetable oil	0.38	366	108	5.20	0.09	1.63		47
frozen, cottage-cut, unprepared	0.68	220	21	5.50	0.06	1.16		34
frozen, cottage-cut, prepared, heated in oven	0.75	240	23	4.80	0.06	1.21		34
frozen, extruded, unprepared	0.86	280	318	4.10	0.05	1.46		52
frozen, extruded, prepared, oven	0.83	270	307	3.10	0.04	1.33		52
Potatoes au gratin, home-prepared	1.56	970	1060	24.30	0.16	2.43	93	52
dry mix, unprepared	2.54	1544	3268	24.20	0.11	6.34		11
dry mix, prepared	2.63	1800	3609	25.50	0.16	7.72		40
General Mills® dry mix	0.72	480	1040	0.00	0.00	1.60	0	9
Kraft® frozen		400	500					32
w/broccoli	0.69	420	500					32
Stouffers® frozen	0.36	260	510	2.40	0.00	0.80	0	49
Hashed brown potatoes								
home prepared	0.63	251	19	4.50	0.06	1.56		60
frozen, plain, unprepared	1.03	299	23	8.60	0.10	1.75		7
frozen, plain, prepared	1.17	340	27	4.90	0.09	1.89		47
frozen, w/butter sauce, unprep	1.28	422	130	9.80	0.09	1.93	20	44
General Mills® dry mix	0.72	860	80	0.00	0.00	3.20	0	8
Julienne potatoes, dry mix, General Mills®	0.72	580	1040	0.00	0.00	1.60	0	10
Mashed potatoes								
home prepared, w/whole milk & table fat added	0.28	303	309	6.40	0.09	1.13	21	36
home prepared, w/whole milk added	0.29	314	318	7.00	0.09	1.17	6	7
dehydrated, flakes w/out milk, dry	1.06	662	137	72.60	0.67	6.01		2
dehydrated, flakes w/out milk, prepared	0.23	245	349	10.20	0.12	0.70	22	45
granules w/out milk, dry	0.40	199	24	9.90	0.00	1.43		2
granules w/out milk, prepared	4.27	223	358	1.40	0.04	0.74	192	43
granules w/ milk, dry	3.50	1848	82	16.00	0.19	4.20	9	3
granules w/ milk, prepared	0.63	352	246	3.20	0.03	0.84	14	25
Potato buds, dry mix, Gen Mills®	0.00	360	40	0.00	0.00	2.40	0	0
Potatoes O'Brien, home-prepared	0.91	516	421	32.40	0.15	1.96	111	14
Scalloped potatoes, home-prepared	1.41	925	821	26.10	0.17	2.58	46	39
dry mix, unprepared	3.14	1412	2462	25.70	0.09	7.07		12
dry mix, prepared	3.12	1669	2803	27.10	0.16	8.46		42
General Mills® dry mix	0.72	480	1020	0.00	0.00	2.40	0	10
Hormel® w/ham	0.11	68	146	0.60	0.05	0.37	8	35
Kraft® frozen	1.20	400	490					32

VEGETABLES & VEGETABLE PRODUCTS

FOOD	AMOUNT	CALORIES (kcal)	PROTEIN (g)	FAT (g)	CARBO-HYDRATES (g)	FIBER (g)	CALCIUM (mg)
Scalloped potatoes (continued)							
Stouffers® frozen	109 g	90	3.00	4.00	11	2.31	80
Swanson® scalloped, homestyle, with ham	28.4 g	33	2.11	1.44	3	0.20	39
Potato chips (see also Snacks & Sweets)	1 oz	148	1.82	10.05	15	0.40	7
Potato chips, from dried potatoes	1 oz	164	1.59	13.06	12	0.37	6
Potato flour	1 cup	628	14.32	1.43	143	2.86	59
Potato pancakes	1 pancake	495	4.63	12.61	26	0.50	21
Potato puffs, frozen, prepared	1 puff	16	0.23	0.75	2	0.04	2
Potato salad	1 cup	358	6.70	20.50	28	0.93	48
Potato sticks	1-oz pkg	148	1.90	9.79	15	0.34	5
Pumpkin, raw	1 cup	30	1.16	0.12	8	1.28	24
cooked, boiled, drained	1 cup	49	1.76	0.17	12	2.03	37
canned	1 cup	83	2.70	0.69	20	3.96	64
Pumpkin flowers, raw	1 cup	5	0.34	0.02	1	0.21	13
cooked, boiled, drained	1 cup	20	1.46	0.11	4	1.23	50
Pumpkin leaves, raw	1 cup	8	1.23	0.16	1	0.39	15
cooked, boiled, drained	1 cup	15	1.93	0.16	2	0.75	31
Pumpkin pie mix, canned	1 cup	282	2.93	0.34	71	3.21	99
Purslane, raw	1 cup	7	0.56	0.04	1	0.34	28
cooked, boiled, drained	1 cup	21	1.71	0.22	4	0.93	90
Radicchio, raw	½ cup	5	0.29	0.05	1		4
Radishes, raw	½ cup	10	0.35	0.31	2	0.32	12
Radishes, Oriental (includes Daikon & Chinese varieties), raw	½ cup	8	0.26	0.04	2	0.28	12
cooked, boiled, drained	½ cup	13	0.49	0.18	3	0.36	12
dried	½ cup	157	4.58	0.42	37	4.85	365
Radishes, white icicle, raw	½ cup	7	0.55	0.05	1	0.35	14
Radish seeds, sprouted, raw	½ cup	8	0.72	0.48	1		10
Rutabagas, raw	½ cup	25	0.84	0.14	6	0.77	33
cooked, boiled, drained	½ cup	29	0.94	0.16	7	0.89	36
Salsify, raw	1 cup	109	4.39	0.27	25	2.39	80
cooked, boiled, drained	1 cup	92	3.68	0.22	21	2.01	64
Sauerkraut, canned, solids & liquid	1 cup	44	21.15	0.33	10	2.53	72
Vlasic® old fashioned	1 oz	4	0.00	0.00	1	0.00	0
Seaweed, agar, raw	100 g	26	0.54	0.03	7	0.45	54
agar, dried	100 g	306	6.21	0.30	81	0.70	625
Irishmoss, raw	100 g	49	1.51	0.16	12		72
kelp, raw	100 g	43	1.68	0.56	10	1.33	168
laver, raw	100 g	35	5.81	0.28	5	0.27	70
spirulina, raw	100 g	26	5.92	0.39	2	0.34	
spirulina, dried	100 g	290	57.47	7.72	24	3.64	
wakame, raw	100 g	45	3.03	0.64	9	0.54	150
Sesbiana flower, raw	1 cup	5	0.26	0.01	1	0.30	4
cooked, steamed	1 cup	23	1.18	0.05	5	1.61	23
Shallots, raw	1 tbsp	7	0.25	0.01	2	0.07	4
freeze-dried	1 tbsp	3	0.11	0.00	1	0.04	2

FOOD	IRON (mg)	POTAS-SIUM (mg)	SODIUM (mg)	VITAMIN C (mg)	THIAMIN (mg)	NIACIN (mg)	VITAMIN A (mg)	% OF CALORIES FROM FAT
Scalloped potatoes (continued)								
Stouffers® frozen	0.36	250	420	2.40	0.03	0.40	0	40
Swanson® scalloped, homestyle, with ham	0.20	94	120	0.60	0.05	0.37	8	39
Potato chips (see also Snacks & Sweets)	0.34	369	133	11.80	0.04	1.19	0	61
Potato chips, from dried potatoes	0.43	312	216	2.40	0.04	0.85		72
Potato flour	30.79	2843	61	34.00	0.75	6.09	0	2
Potato pancakes	1.21	538	388	0.40	0.10	1.61	27	23
Potato puffs, frozen, prepared	0.11	27	52	0.50	0.01	0.15	0	42
Potato salad	1.63	635	1323	24.90	0.19	2.23	82	52
Potato sticks	0.65	351	71	13.40	0.03	1.36	0	60
Pumpkin, raw	0.93	394	1	10.40	0.06	0.70	186	4
cooked, boiled, drained	1.40	564	3	11.50	0.08	1.01	265	3
canned	3.41	504	12	10.20	0.06	0.90	5404	7
Pumpkin flowers, raw	0.23	57	2	9.20	0.01	0.23	64	4
cooked, boiled, drained	1.18	142	8	6.70	0.02	0.42	232	5
Pumpkin leaves, raw	0.87	170	4	4.30	0.04	0.36	76	18
cooked, boiled, drained	2.27	311	5	0.70	0.05	0.60	176	10
Pumpkin pie mix, canned	2.87	372	561	9.50	0.04	1.01	2241	1
Purslane, raw	0.86	213	20	9.00	0.02	0.21	57	5
cooked, boiled, drained	0.89	561	51	12.10	0.04	0.53	213	9
Radicchio, raw		60	4	1.60	0.00	0.05	1	9
Radishes, raw	0.17	134	14	13.20	0.00	0.17	0	28
Radishes, Oriental (includes Daikon & Chinese varieties), raw	0.18	100	9	9.70	0.01	0.09	0	5
cooked, boiled, drained	0.11	211	10	11.20	0.00	0.11	0	12
dried	3.90	2027	161	0.00	0.16	1.97	0	2
Radishes, white icicle, raw	0.40	140	8	14.50	0.02	0.15	0	6
Radish seeds, sprouted, raw	0.16	16	1	5.50	0.02	0.54	7	54
Rutabagas, raw	0.36	236	14	17.50	0.06	0.49	0	5
cooked, boiled, drained	0.40	244	15	18.60	0.06	0.54	0	5
Salsify, raw	0.93	505	27	10.60	0.11	0.67	0	2
cooked, boiled, drained	0.74	381	21	6.20	0.08	0.53	0	2
Sauerkraut, canned, solids & liquid	3.47	401	1561	34.80	0.05	0.34	4	7
Vlasic® old fashioned	0.36	1	280	2.40	0.00	0.00	0	0
Seaweed, agar, raw	1.86	226	9	0.00	0.01	0.06	0	1
agar, dried	21.40	1125	102	0.00	0.01	0.20	0	1
Irishmoss, raw	8.90	63	67		0.02	0.59		3
kelp, raw	2.85	89	233		0.05	0.47	12	12
laver, raw	1.80	356	48	39.00	0.10	1.47	520	7
spirulina, raw		127	98	0.90	0.22	1.20		14
spirulina, dried	28.50	1363	1048	10.10	2.38	12.82		24
wakame, raw	2.18	50	872	3.00	0.06	1.60	36	13
Sesbiana flower, raw	0.17	37	3	14.60	0.02	0.09	0	2
cooked, steamed	0.58	111	11	38.50	0.05	0.26	0	2
Shallots, raw	0.12	33	1	0.80	0.01	0.02		1
freeze-dried	0.05	15	1	0.40	0.00	0.01		0

VEGETABLES & VEGETABLE PRODUCTS

FOOD	AMOUNT	CALORIES (kcal)	PROTEIN (g)	FAT (g)	CARBO-HYDRATES (g)	FIBER (g)	CALCIUM (mg)
Spinach, raw	½ cup	6	0.80	0.10	1	0.25	28
cooked, boiled, drained	½ cup	21	2.67	0.23	3	0.79	122
canned, solids & liquid	½ cup	22	2.47	0.43	3	0.80	97
canned, drained solids	½ cup	25	3.01	0.54	4		135
frozen, unprepared	10-oz pkg	68	8.29	0.89	11	2.60	314
frozen, cooked, boiled, drained	10-oz pkg	63	6.91	0.45	12	2.42	321
Health Valley® frozen, boiled	1 cup	50	6.00	2.00	10	4.00	
Spinach souffle	1 cup	218	10.99	18.35	3	0.81	230
Squash, summer, all varieties, raw	1 cup	26	1.53	0.28	6	0.78	26
cooked, boiled, drained	1 cup	36	1.63	0.56	8	1.08	48
Squash, summer, crookneck, raw	1 cup	24	1.22	0.31	5	0.72	28
cooked, boiled, drained	1 cup	36	1.63	0.56	8	1.08	48
canned, drained solids	1 can	31	1.48	0.18	7	0.91	30
frozen, unprepared	1 cup	26	1.07	0.18	6	0.86	23
frozen, cooked, boiled, drained	1 cup	47	2.46	0.37	11	1.56	38
Squash, summer, scallop, raw	½ cup	12	0.78	0.13	3	0.36	12
cooked, boiled, drained	½ cup	14	0.93	0.15	3	0.43	14
Squash, summer, zucchini, raw	½ cup	9	0.75	0.09	2	0.29	10
cooked, boiled, drained	½ cup	14	0.57	0.05	4	0.45	12
frozen, unprepared	10-oz pkg	48	3.28	0.38	10	1.58	52
frozen, cooked, boiled, drained	½ cup	19	1.28	0.15	4	0.62	19
Italian style, canned	½ cup	33	1.17	0.13	8	0.58	19
baby, raw	1 medium	2	0.30	0.04	0		2
Squash, winter, all varieties, raw	1 cup	43	1.68	0.26	10	1.62	35
cooked, baked	1 cup	79	1.81	1.29	18	1.46	28
Squash, winter, acorn, raw	1 cup	56	1.12	0.14	15	1.96	46
cooked, baked	1 cup	115	2.29	0.29	30	4.01	90
cooked, boiled, drained	1 cup	83	1.65	0.21	22	2.89	65
Squash, winter, butternut, raw	1 cup	63	1.40	0.14	16	1.96	67
cooked, baked	1 cup	83	1.84	0.18	22	2.58	84
frozen, unprepared	12-oz pkg	192	5.98	0.34	49	4.22	97
frozen, cooked, boiled	1 cup	95	2.94	0.17	24	2.07	45
Squash, winter, hubbard, raw	1 cup	47	2.32	0.58	10	1.62	16
cooked, baked	1 cup	103	5.08	1.27	22	3.57	35
cooked, boiled, mashed	1 cup	70	3.50	0.88	15	2.45	23
Squash, winter, spaghetti, raw	1 cup	33	0.65	0.58	7	1.41	23
cooked, boiled, drained, or baked	1 cup	45	1.02	0.40	10	2.17	33
Succotash, raw	100 g	99	5.03	1.02	20	1.30	18
cooked, boiled, drained	½ cup	111	4.86	0.76	23	1.29	16
canned, w/ cream style corn	½ cup	102	3.51	0.72	23	1.71	15
canned, w/ whole kernel corn, solids & liquid	½ cup	81	3.33	0.63	18	0.79	14
frozen, unprepared	½ cup	73	3.36	0.70	16	0.80	12
frozen, cooked, boiled, drained	½ cup	79	3.66	0.76	17	0.87	13
Swamp cabbage, chopped, raw	1 cup	11	1.46	0.11	2	0.62	43
cooked, boiled, drained	1 cup	20	2.03	0.24	4	0.83	53
Sweetpotatoes, raw	1 sweetpotato	136	2.14	0.38	32	1.11	29
cooked, baked in skin	1 sweetpotato	118	1.96	0.13	28	0.91	32
cooked, boiled, w/out skin	1 cup	344	5.40	0.97	80	2.79	70

FOOD	IRON (mg)	POTAS-SIUM (mg)	SODIUM (mg)	VITAMIN C (mg)	THIAMIN (mg)	NIACIN (mg)	VITAMIN A (mg)	% OF CALORIES FROM FAT
Spinach, raw	0.76	156	22	7.90	0.02	0.20	188	15
cooked, boiled, drained	3.21	419	63	8.90	0.09	0.44	737	10
canned, solids & liquid	1.85	269	373	15.80	0.02	0.32	753	18
canned, drained solids	2.46	370	29	15.30	0.02	0.42	939	19
frozen, unprepared	5.83	918	211	68.90	0.24	1.24	2203	12
frozen, cooked, boiled, drained	3.34	656	190	27.00	0.13	0.92	1712	6
Health Valley® frozen, boiled		566	164					36
Spinach souffle	1.34	202	763	2.90	0.09	0.48	675	76
Squash, summer, all varieties, raw	0.60	253	3	19.20	0.08	0.72	25	10
cooked, boiled, drained	0.64	346	2	10.00	0.08	0.92	52	14
Squash, summer, crookneck, raw	0.62	276	2	10.90	0.07	0.59	44	12
cooked, boiled, drained	0.64	346	2	10.00	0.09	0.92	52	14
canned, drained solids	1.71	231	11	6.50	0.04	1.01	29	5
frozen, unprepared	0.63	271	6	8.30	0.05	0.52	36	6
frozen, cooked, boiled, drained	0.99	485	12	13.10	0.07	0.85	37	7
Squash, summer, scallop, raw	0.26	118	1	11.70	0.05	0.39	7	10
cooked, boiled, drained	0.29	126	1	9.70	0.05	0.42	8	10
Squash, summer, zucchini, raw	0.28	161	2	5.90	0.05	0.26	22	9
cooked, boiled, drained	0.32	228	2	4.20	0.04	0.39	22	3
frozen, unprepared	1.46	619	7	15.10	0.14	1.23	137	7
frozen, cooked, boiled, drained	0.54	218	2	4.10	0.05	0.43	48	7
Italian style, canned	0.78	312	427	2.60	0.05	0.60	61	4
baby, raw		50	0	3.80	0.01	0.08	5	18
Squash, winter, all varieties, raw	0.67	406	4	14.20	0.11	0.93	471	5
cooked, baked	0.67	895	3	19.70	0.17	1.44	730	15
Squash, winter, acorn, raw	0.98	486	5	15.40	0.20	0.98	48	2
cooked, baked	1.91	896	9	22.10	0.34	1.81	88	2
cooked, boiled, drained	1.37	645	6	15.90	0.25	1.30	63	2
Squash, winter, butternut, raw	0.98	493	5	29.40	0.14	1.68	1092	2
cooked, baked	1.22	583	7	30.90	0.15	1.99	1435	2
frozen, unprepared	2.99	722	8	21.10	0.31	2.52	1629	2
frozen, cooked, boiled	1.40	320	4	8.30	0.12	1.11	801	2
Squash, winter, hubbard, raw	0.46	371	8	12.80	0.08	0.58	626	11
cooked, baked	0.96	734	16	19.50	0.15	1.14	1237	11
cooked, boiled, mashed	0.67	504	12	15.40	0.10	0.79	945	11
Squash, winter, spaghetti, raw	0.32	109	17	2.10	0.04	0.96	5	16
cooked, boiled, drained, or baked	0.52	182	28	5.50	0.06	1.26	17	8
Succotash, raw	1.83	369	4	15.10	0.21	1.59	29	9
cooked, boiled, drained	1.46	393	16	7.80	0.16	1.27	28	6
canned, w/ cream style corn	0.73	243	325	8.50	0.04	0.81	19	6
canned, w/ whole kernel corn, solids & liquid	0.68	209	283	5.90	0.04	0.82	19	7
frozen, unprepared	0.73	230	35	6.60	0.07	1.07	20	9
frozen, cooked, boiled, drained	0.76	225	38	5.00	0.06	1.11	20	9
Swamp cabbage, chopped, raw	0.94	174	63	30.80	0.02	0.50	353	9
cooked, boiled, drained	1.29	278	119	15.70	0.02	0.49	510	11
Sweetpotatoes, raw	0.76	265	17	29.60	0.09	0.88	2608	3
cooked, baked in skin	0.52	397	12	28.10	0.08	0.69	2488	1
cooked, boiled, w/out skin	1.83	602	42	55.90	0.17	2.10	5594	3

VEGETABLES & VEGETABLE PRODUCTS

FOOD	AMOUNT	CALORIES (kcal)	PROTEIN (g)	FAT (g)	CARBO-HYDRATES (g)	FIBER (g)	CALCIUM (mg)
Sweetpotatoes (continued)							
cooked, candied	1 piece	144	0.91	3.41	29	0.41	27
canned, vacuum pack	1 cup	233	4.21	0.51	54	1.80	56
canned, mashed	1 cup	258	5.05	0.51	59		76
canned, syrup pack, solids & liquid	1 cup	202	2.24	0.46	48	1.05	35
canned, syrup pack, drained solids	1 cup	213	2.51	0.62	50	1.10	32
frozen, unprepared	1 cup	169	3.00	0.32	39	1.38	66
frozen, cooked, baked	1 cup	176	3.01	0.21	41	1.36	62
Sweetpotato leaves, raw	1 cup	12	1.40	0.11	2	0.42	13
cooked, steamed	1 cup	22	1.48	0.19	5	0.84	15
Taro, sliced, raw	1 cup	112	1.56	0.21	28	0.83	45
cooked	1 cup	187	0.68	0.15	46	1.14	24
Taro chips	10 chips	110	0.47	5.86	15	0.27	10
Taro leaves, raw	1 cup	12	1.39	0.21	2	0.57	30
cooked, steamed	1 cup	35	3.95	0.59	6	0.78	124
Taro shoots, sliced, raw	½ cup	5	0.40	0.04	1	0.25	5
cooked	½ cup	10	0.51	0.06	2	0.38	9
Taro, Tahitian, sliced, raw	½ cup	25	1.73	0.60	4	1.09	80
cooked	½ cup	30	2.83	0.46	5	1.55	101
Tomatillos, raw, chopped	½ cup	21	0.64	0.68	4		4
Tomatoes, green, raw	1 tomato	30	1.48	0.25	6	0.62	16
Tomatoes, red, ripe, raw, chopped	1 cup	35	1.60	0.39	8	0.84	12
cooked, boiled	1 cup	60	2.68	0.65	14	1.84	20
cooked, stewed	1 cup	59	1.77	2.21	10	0.48	19
canned, whole	1 cup	47	2.24	0.59	10	1.09	63
canned, stewed	1 cup	68	2.37	0.36	16	1.08	84
canned, wedges in tomato juice	1 cup	67	2.07	0.42	16	1.16	68
canned, w/green chilies	1 cup	37	1.66	0.18	9	0.84	48
sun-dried	1 cup	140	7.62	1.60	30		60
Hunt's®							
crushed, Angela Mia	100 gm	30	1.19	0.19	6		30
diced, in puree	100 gm	24	0.99	0.20	5	2.30	35
diced, in tomato juice	100 gm	21	0.86	0.18	4		38
stewed	100 gm	29	0.92	0.19	7	2.05	38
Tomato juice, canned	6 fl oz	32	1.38	0.11	8	0.72	16
Campbell's®	1 oz	7	0.17	0.00	1	0.23	0
Hunt's®	100 gm	20	0.72	0.09	4	0.80	8
Mott's® Clamato, tomato and clam juice	1 cup	111	1.45	0.24	26	1.45	29
Tomato paste, canned	½ cup	110	4.95	1.17	25	1.25	46
Hunt's®	100 gm	92	3.44	0.40	19	4.30	29
Tomato puree, canned	1 cup	102	4.18	0.29	25	2.05	37
Hunt's®	100 gm	52	1.93	0.23	11	2.30	15
Tomato sauce, canned	½ cup	37	1.62	0.20	9	0.87	17
w/herbs & cheese	½ cup	72	2.59	2.36	13		45
w/mushrooms	½ cup	42	1.77	0.15	10	1.03	16
w/onions	½ cup	52	1.91	0.24	12	0.98	20
w/onions, green peppers, & celery	½ cup	50	1.15	0.91	11		16

FOOD	IRON (mg)	POTAS-SIUM (mg)	SODIUM (mg)	VITAMIN C (mg)	THIAMIN (mg)	NIACIN (mg)	VITAMIN A (mg)	% OF CALORIES FROM FAT
Sweetpotatoes (continued)								
cooked, candied	1.19	198	73	7.00	0.02	0.41	440	21
canned, vacuum pack	2.26	796	136	67.30	0.09	1.89	2036	2
canned, mashed	3.39	536	191	13.30	0.07	2.44	3858	2
canned, syrup pack, solids & liquid	1.83	423	100	23.80	0.06	1.04	1304	2
canned, syrup pack, drained solids	1.86	378	76	21.20	0.05	0.67	1403	3
frozen, unprepared	0.93	643	11	23.40	0.12	1.05	3280	2
frozen, cooked, baked	0.95	663	14	16.00	0.12	0.98	2888	1
Sweetpotato leaves, raw	0.35	181	3	3.90	0.06	0.40	36	8
cooked, steamed	0.38	305	8	1.00	0.07	0.64	59	8
Taro, sliced, raw	0.57	615	12	4.70	0.10	0.62	0	2
cooked	0.95	638	20	6.60	0.14	0.67	0	1
Taro chips	0.31	189	85		0.01	0.01	0	48
Taro leaves, raw	0.63	181	1	14.60	0.06	0.42	135	16
cooked, steamed	1.70	668	3	51.50	0.20	1.84	614	15
Taro shoots, sliced, raw	0.26	143	0	9.00	0.02	0.34	2	7
cooked	0.29	240	1					5
Taro, Tahitian, sliced, raw	0.81	376	31	59.50	0.04	0.62	127	22
cooked	1.06	423	37	25.80	0.03	0.33	120	14
Tomatillos, raw, chopped		177	1	7.70	0.03	1.22	7	29
Tomatoes, green, raw	0.63	251	16	28.80	0.07	0.62	79	8
Tomatoes, red, ripe, raw, chopped	0.86	372	15	31.60	0.11	1.08	204	10
cooked, boiled	1.44	624	25	50.30	0.17	1.72	325	10
cooked, stewed	0.78	170	374	14.80	0.07	0.75	102	34
canned, whole	1.45	529	390	36.30	0.11	1.76	145	11
canned, stewed	1.86	611	647	33.80	0.12	1.82	141	5
canned, wedges in tomato juice	1.21	655	568	38.70	0.15	1.76	151	6
canned, w/green chilies	0.63	259	966	15.00	0.08	1.54	94	4
sun-dried		1851	1131	21.20	0.29	4.89	47	10
Hunt's®								
crushed, Angela Mia	1.03		232	19.20	0.07	0.99	127	6
diced, in puree	0.70	420	330	17.80	0.06	0.75	116	7
diced, in tomato juice	0.56		331	15.90	0.06	0.63	104	8
stewed	0.61	273	260	20.20	0.06	0.76	105	6
Tomato juice, canned	1.06	400	658	33.20	0.09	1.23	101	3
Campbell's®	0.12	62	90	3.99	0.01	0.20	12	0
Hunt's®	0.74	220	325	10.40	0.04	0.66	70	4
Mott's® Clamato, tomato and clam juice	1.45	217	965	9.89	0.10	0.46	53	2
Tomato paste, canned	3.91	1221	86	55.40	0.20	4.22	323	10
Hunt's®	3.51	932	276	49.40	0.20	3.12	333	4
Tomato puree, canned	2.32	1051	49	88.20	0.18	4.29	340	3
Hunt's®	1.97	420	22	27.70	0.11	1.75	187	4
Tomato sauce, canned	0.94	452	738	16.00	0.08	1.40	119	5
w/herbs & cheese	1.06			12.30	0.09	1.48	120	30
w/mushrooms	1.08	464	552	15.10	0.09	1.54	116	3
w/onions	1.13	504	672	15.50	0.09	1.52	104	4
w/onions, green peppers, & celery	0.92			16.00	0.08	1.34	99	16

VEGETABLES & VEGETABLE PRODUCTS

FOOD	AMOUNT	CALORIES (kcal)	PROTEIN (g)	FAT (g)	CARBO-HYDRATES (g)	FIBER (g)	CALCIUM (mg)
Tomato sauce, canned (continued)							
w/tomato tidbits, canned	½ cup	39	1.61	0.47	9	1.34	13
Spanish style, canned	½ cup	40	1.76	0.32	9		20
Spaghetti sauce, canned	15-½-oz jar	479	7.99	20.94	70	4.10	124
Tree fern, cooked, chopped	½ cup	28	0.21	0.05	8	0.43	6
Turnips, raw	½ cup	18	0.59	0.07	4	0.59	20
cooked, boiled, drained	½ cup	14	0.55	0.06	4	0.55	18
frozen, unprepared	10-oz pkg	44	2.95	0.45	8	1.30	64
Turnip greens, raw	½ cup	7	0.42	0.08	2	0.22	53
cooked, boiled, drained	½ cup	15	0.82	0.16	3	0.44	99
canned, solids & liquid	½ cup	17	1.59	0.35	3	0.71	138
frozen, unprepared	½ cup	18	2.02	0.26	3	0.62	97
frozen, cooked, boiled, drained	½ cup	24	2.75	0.35	4	0.85	125
Turnip greens & turnips, frozen, unprepared	10-oz pkg	59	6.98	0.54	10	1.73	322
Vegetable juice cocktail, canned	6 fl oz	34	1.14	0.17	8	0.42	20
V8, vegetable juice, regular	1 cup	49	0.00	0.00	10	2.40	29
Campbell's®	1 oz	6	0.17	0.00	1	0.23	3
no salt	1 oz	6	0.17	0.00	1		3
spicy hot	1 oz	6	0.17	0.00	1	0.23	3
Vegetables, mixed							
canned, solids & liquid	1 cup	88	3.48	0.61	17	2.92	51
canned, drained solids	1 cup	77	4.22	0.41	15	2.14	44
frozen, unprepared	10-oz pkg	201	9.46	1.48	38	3.34	72
frozen, cooked, boiled, drained	10-oz pkg	163	7.87	0.41	36	3.22	67
Health Valley® frozen, boiled	1 cup	140	6.00	2.00	24	4.00	
La Choy® Chinese, canned	1 cup	17	1.33	0.13	3	0.33	9
Waterchestnuts, Chinese, sliced, raw	½ cup	66	0.87	0.06	15	0.50	7
canned, solids & liquid	½ cup	35	0.62	0.04	9	0.41	3
La Choy®	1 cup	75	1.35	0.15	19	3.30	6
Watercress, raw, chopped	½ cup	2	0.39	0.02	0	0.12	20
Waxgourd, cubes, raw	1 cup	17	0.53	0.26	4	0.66	25
cooked, boiled, drained	1 cup	23	0.70	0.35	5	0.88	32
Yam, cubes, raw	1 cup	177	2.29	0.26	42		25
cooked, boiled, drained	1 cup	158	2.02	0.18	38		19
Yambean, raw (tuber portion only), slices	1 cup	46	0.87	0.11	11		14

ENTREES/SIDE DISHES

FOOD	AMOUNT	CALORIES (kcal)	PROTEIN (g)	FAT (g)	CARBO-HYDRATES (g)	FIBER (g)	CALCIUM (mg)
Broccoli, in cheese sauce, Microquick®	128 g	70	4.00	3.00	7	2.30	168
Cabbage rolls, frozen dinner	227 g	168	11.00	6.00	17		49
Hormel® in tomato sauce	28.4 g	23	1.10	0.70	3		6
Lean Cuisine® stuffed w/meat	305 g	220	14.00	10.00	19	3.76	60
Corn souffle, Stouffer® frozen side dish	113 g	155	4.00	7.00	19		48
Eggplant, breaded cutlets, Bernardi®	28.4 g	60	1.00	4.00	5		0
Garden vegetable, Le Menu® light	298 g	260	11.00	8.00	35		

FOOD	IRON (mg)	POTAS-SIUM (mg)	SODIUM (mg)	VITAMIN C (mg)	THIAMIN (mg)	NIACIN (mg)	VITAMIN A (mg)	% OF CALORIES FROM FAT
Tomato sauce, canned (continued)								
w/tomato tidbits, canned	0.83	455	18	26.20	0.09	1.44	98	11
Spanish style, canned	4.25		576	10.50	0.09	1.58	120	7
Spaghetti sauce, canned	2.85	1687	2179	49.10	0.24	6.61	539	39
Tree fern, cooked, chopped	0.11	3	3	21.30	0.00	2.49	14	2
Turnips, raw	0.20	124	44	13.70	0.03	0.26	0	4
cooked, boiled, drained	0.17	106	39	9.00	0.02	0.23	0	4
frozen, unprepared	1.99	388	71	12.50	0.09	1.14	7	9
Turnip greens, raw	0.31	83	11	16.80	0.02	0.17	213	10
cooked, boiled, drained	0.57	146	21	19.70	0.03	0.30	396	10
canned, solids & liquid	1.77	165	325	18.10	0.01	0.42	420	19
frozen, unprepared	1.23	151	9	22.00	0.04	0.31	507	13
frozen, cooked, boiled, drained	1.59	184	12	17.90	0.04	0.38	654	13
Turnip greens & turnips, frozen, unprepared	4.62	233	52	73.10	0.13	1.10	1735	8
Vegetable juice cocktail, canned	0.77	351	664	50.40	0.08	1.32	213	5
V8, vegetable juice, regular	1.46	513	819	49.10	0.05	1.70	342	0
Campbell's®	0.12	55	93	4.99	0.01	0.20	37	0
no salt	0.12		7	4.99	0.01	0.20	42	0
spicy hot	0.12	55	108	5.99	0.01	0.20	42	0
Vegetables, mixed								
canned, solids & liquid	1.59	339	548	9.30	0.08	1.18	1245	6
canned, drained solids	1.71	474	243	8.20	0.08	0.94	1899	5
frozen, unprepared	2.70	603	132	29.50	0.35	3.56	1442	7
frozen, cooked, boiled, drained	2.26	464	96	8.90	0.20	2.34	1176	2
Health Valley® frozen, boiled		308	64					13
La Choy® Chinese, canned	0.84	180	55	43.90	0.03	0.45	0	7
Waterchestnuts, Chinese, sliced, raw	0.37	362	9	2.50	0.09	0.62	0	1
canned, solids & liquid	0.61	82	6	0.90	0.01	0.25	0	1
La Choy®	1.31	177	12	1.95	0.02	0.54	0	2
Watercress, raw, chopped	0.03	56	7	7.30	0.02	0.03	80	9
Waxgourd, cubes, raw	0.53	8	147	17.20	0.05	0.53	0	14
cooked, boiled, drained	0.67	10	186	18.40	0.06	0.67	0	14
Yam, cubes, raw	0.82	1224	14	25.70	0.17	1.14	0	1
cooked, boiled, drained	0.70	911	11	16.50	0.13	0.75	0	1
Yambean, raw (tuber portion only), slices	0.72	180	5	24.20	0.03	0.24	3	2
ENTREES/SIDE DISHES								
Broccoli, in cheese sauce, Microquick®	1.13	280	420	36.00	0.09	0.74	300	39
Cabbage rolls, frozen dinner	1.40	290	1026	0.00	0.09	2.70	136	32
Hormel® in tomato sauce	0.25	87	127	0.18	0.76	0.29		27
Lean Cuisine® stuffed w/meat	1.80	530	930	6.00	0.15	3.00	150	41
Corn souffle, Stouffer® frozen side dish	0.40	190	510	0.00	0.08	0.80	94	41
Eggplant, breaded cutlets, Bernardi®	0.36	45	45	0.00	0.06	0.40	0	60
Garden vegetable, Le Menu® light			500					28

VEGETABLES & VEGETABLE PRODUCTS

FOOD	AMOUNT	CALORIES (kcal)	PROTEIN (g)	FAT (g)	CARBO-HYDRATES (g)	FIBER (g)	CALCIUM (mg)
Green bean & mushroom casserole, Stouffers®	135 g	160	3.00	11.00	13		80
Mushroom Stroganoff, Light Balance®	234 g	180	7.00	5.00	28	1.23	85
Onion rings, crispy, prepared, Mrs. Paul's®	28.4 g	76	0.80	4.80	8	0.36	8
Pea pods, snow, frozen, La Choy®	114 g	48	3.19	0.23	9	4.17	49
Peas, in cream sauce, Microquick®	142 g	160	6.00	7.00	18	2.88	93
Potato, baked, Lean Cuisine®							
w/broccoli & cheddar	294 g	290	14.00	9.00	37		400
w/sour cream	294 g	230	9.00	5.00	38		200
Potatoes w/cheese							
Healthy Choice® wedges w/broccoli & cheese	269 g	240	8.00	5.00	41		100
Kraft® w/2 cheeses	107 g	140	4.00	4.00	20	1.10	128
Microquick® cheddar	128 g	160	4.00	7.00	20	1.00	
Potato casserole, garden, quick meal, Healthy Choice®	262 g	180	12	4	23		250
Ratatouille, Stouffer® frozen side dish	142 g	60	1.00	3.00	9	2.27	
Spinach, Stouffer® frozen side dish							
cream of	227 g	210	7.00	15.00	12	3.21	200
creamed	128 g	190	4.00	15.00	9		
crepes, in cheese sauce	269 g	415	16.00	25.00	30		
souffle	113 g	140	6.00	9.00	8	0.99	80
Vegetables, Birds Eye® Bavarian style	93.6 g	90	3.00	5.00	11		
La Choy® stir fry, frozen	133 g	47	1.33	0.27	9	0.33	27
Zucchini Romano, Le Menu® frozen dinner	234 g	350	17.00	19.00	27		

FOOD	IRON (mg)	POTAS-SIUM (mg)	SODIUM (mg)	VITAMIN C (mg)	THIAMIN (mg)	NIACIN (mg)	VITAMIN A (mg)	% OF CALORIES FROM FAT
Green bean & mushroom casserole, Stouffers®	0.36	220	680	2.40	0.06	0.40	40	62
Mushroom Stroganoff, Light Balance®	1.44	504	620	1.96	0.16	4.04	90	25
Onion rings, crispy, prepared, Mrs. Paul's®	0.14	40	92					57
Pea pods, snow, frozen, La Choy®	2.12	260	5	68.40	0.17	0.68	48	4
Peas, in cream sauce, Microquick®	1.34	170	360					39
Potato, baked, Lean Cuisine®								
w/broccoli & cheddar	1.44	880	590	48.00	0.23	2.00	80	28
w/sour cream	1.08	900	570	30.00	0.23	1.20	350	20
Potatoes w/cheese								
Healthy Choice® wedges w/broccoli & cheese	2.70	1010	510					19
Kraft® w/2 cheeses	0.69	400	450					26
Microquick® cheddar		320	570	12.00				39
Potato casserole, garden, quick meal, Healthy Choice®	1.08	600	360	15.00	0.23		200	20
Ratatouille, Stouffer® frozen side dish	1.00	505	1320	10.00	0.30	1.00	146	45
Spinach, Stouffer® frozen side dish								
cream of	0.36	350	1020	3.60	0.09	0.40	175	64
creamed		585	855					71
crepes, in cheese sauce		440	995					54
souffle	1.08	180	500	2.40	0.06	0.00	150	58
Vegetables, Birds Eye® Bavarian style			260					50
La Choy® stir fry, frozen			27	39.90	0.08	1.06	931	5
Zucchini Romano, Le Menu® frozen dinner			680					49

LEGUMES & LEGUME PRODUCTS

FOOD	AMOUNT	CALORIES (kcal)	PROTEIN (g)	FAT (g)	CARBO-HYDRATES (g)	FIBER (g)
Adzuki beans, raw	1 cup	649	39.13	1.04	123.9	10.37
cooked, boiled	1 cup	294	17.29	0.22	56.9	4.63
canned, sweetened	1 cup	702	11.25	0.09	162.8	4.56
yokan (sugar & bean confection)	1 slice	36	0.46	0.02	8.5	0.19
Baked beans, home-prepared	1 cup	382	14.02	13.02	54.1	1.86
canned, plain or vegetarian	1 cup	235	12.17	1.14	52.1	2.89
canned, w/beef	1 cup	321	16.96	9.18	44.9	2.80
canned, w/franks	1 cup	366	17.34	16.88	39.5	2.44
canned, w/pork	1 cup	268	13.13	3.93	50.5	3.00
canned, w/pork & sweet sauce	1 cup	282	13.42	3.69	53.1	4.33
canned, w/pork & tomato sauce	1 cup	247	13.05	2.60	49.0	2.99
Health Valley® Boston baked, fat free	1 oz	25	1.07	0.13	5.4	0.67
Beans, black, raw	1 cup	661	41.91	2.75	120.9	10.24
cooked, boiled	1 cup	227	15.24	0.92	40.7	3.49
Beans, black turtle soup, raw	1 cup	623	39.10	1.66	116.3	9.71
cooked, boiled	1 cup	241	15.13	0.64	45.0	3.76
canned	1 cup	218	14.46	0.70	39.7	2.83
Beans, cranberry, raw	1 cup	652	44.90	2.39	117.1	4.86
cooked, boiled	1 cup	240	16.53	0.82	43.3	1.78
canned	1 cup	216	14.41	0.73	39.3	2.39
Beans, French, raw	1 cup	631	34.61	3.72	117.9	6.86
cooked, boiled	1 cup	228	12.48	1.34	42.5	2.47
Beans, great northern, raw	1 cup	621	40.00	2.09	114.1	12.34
cooked, boiled	1 cup	210	14.75	0.79	37.3	5.27
canned	1 cup	300	19.31	1.01	55.0	5.96
Beans, kidney, all types, raw	1 cup	613	43.39	1.52	110.4	11.47
all types, cooked, boiled	1 cup	225	15.35	0.88	40.3	4.98
all types, canned	1 cup	208	13.30	0.80	38.0	2.47
California red, raw	1 cup	607	44.85	0.46	110.0	11.47
California red, cooked, boiled	1 cup	219	16.17	0.17	39.6	4.13
red, raw	1 cup	619	41.45	1.95	112.7	11.38
red, cooked, boiled	1 cup	225	15.35	0.88	40.3	4.98
red, canned	1 cup	216	13.43	0.88	39.9	2.38
royal red, raw	1 cup	605	46.60	0.83	107.3	11.36
royal red, cooked, boiled	1 cup	218	16.79	0.30	38.6	4.09
mature seeds, sprouted, raw	1 cup	53	7.73	0.92	7.5	
Beans, navy, raw	1 cup	697	46.44	2.67	126.1	11.48
cooked, boiled	1 cup	259	15.83	1.04	47.8	5.72
canned	1 cup	296	19.72	1.13	53.5	4.87
mature seeds, sprouted, raw	1 cup	70	6.40	0.73	13.5	2.60
Beans, pink, raw	1 cup	721	44.01	2.38	134.8	6.09
cooked, boiled	1 cup	252	15.30	0.83	47.1	2.70
Beans, pinto, raw	1 cup	656	40.31	2.17	122.3	11.59
cooked, boiled	1 cup	235	14.04	0.89	43.8	5.16
canned	1 cup	186	10.95	0.76	34.9	3.02
frozen, unprepared	10-oz pkg	484	27.83	1.42	92.3	
frozen, cooked, boiled, drained	10-oz pkg	460	26.44	1.35	87.6	

138

FOOD	CALCIUM (mg)	IRON (mg)	POTAS-SIUM (mg)	SODIUM (mg)	CHOLES-TEROI (mg)	% OF CALORIES FROM FAT
Adzuki beans, raw	130	9.81	2470	9	0	1
cooked, boiled	63	4.60	1224	18	0	1
canned, sweetened	66	3.34	353	646	0	0
yokan (sugar & bean confection)	4	0.16	6	12	0	1
Baked beans, home-prepared	155	5.04	907	1068	13	31
canned, plain or vegetarian	128	0.74	752	1008	0	4
canned, w/beef	119	4.26	851	1264	59	26
canned, w/franks	123	4.45	604	1105	15	42
canned, w/pork	133	4.31	781	1048	17	13
canned, w/pork & sweet sauce	155	4.20	673	849	17	12
canned, w/pork & tomato sauce	141	8.30	759	1113	17	9
Health Valley® Boston baked, fat free	11	0.48	95	3	0	5
Beans, black, raw	239	9.73	2877	10	0	4
cooked, boiled	47	3.60	611	1	0	4
Beans, black turtle soup, raw	294	16.01	2760	16	0	2
cooked, boiled	103	5.27	801	6	0	2
canned	84	4.56	739	922	0	3
Beans, cranberry, raw	248	9.75	2597	12	0	3
cooked, boiled	89	3.70	685	1	0	3
canned	87	4.02	675	863	0	3
Beans, French, raw	342	6.26	2421	33	0	5
cooked, boiled	111	1.92	655	11	0	5
Beans, great northern, raw	320	10.01	2538	25	0	3
cooked, boiled	121	3.77	692	4	0	3
canned	139	4.11	919	11	0	3
Beans, kidney, all types, raw	263	15.09	2587	44	0	2
all types, cooked, boiled	50	5.20	713	4	0	4
all types, canned	69	3.14	658	889	0	3
California red, raw	359	17.20	2742	21	0	1
California red, cooked, boiled	116	5.27	741	7	0	1
red, raw	153	12.31	2500	22	0	3
red, cooked, boiled	50	5.20	713	4	0	4
red, canned	62	3.22	658	873	0	4
royal red, raw	241	16.01	2477	24	0	1
royal red, cooked, boiled	78	4.90	669	8	0	1
mature seeds, sprouted, raw	31	1.49	344		0	16
Beans, navy, raw	322	13.40	2372	29	0	3
cooked, boiled	128	4.51	669	2	0	4
canned	123	4.84	755	1173	0	3
mature seeds, sprouted, raw	16	2.01	319		0	9
Beans, pink, raw	273	14.22	3073	16	0	3
cooked, boiled	88	3.89	858	3	0	3
Beans, pinto, raw	233	11.34	2563	19	0	3
cooked, boiled	82	4.47	800	3	0	3
canned	89	3.85	723	998	0	4
frozen, unprepared	165	8.52			0	3
frozen, cooked, boiled, drained	149	7.70			0	3

LEGUMES & LEGUME PRODUCTS

FOOD	AMOUNT	CALORIES (kcal)	PROTEIN (g)	FAT (g)	CARBO-HYDRATES (g)	FIBER (g)
Beans, small white, raw	1 cup	723	45.38	2.53	133.8	5.81
cooked, boiled	1 cup	253	16.05	1.15	46.2	4.30
Beans, yellow, raw	1 cup	676	43.12	5.10	118.9	5.33
cooked, boiled	1 cup	254	16.21	1.92	44.7	2.00
Beans, white, raw	1 cup	674	47.19	1.71	121.7	12.07
cooked, boiled	1 cup	249	17.41	0.63	44.9	4.45
canned	1 cup	306	19.01	0.75	57.4	1.80
Broadbeans, raw	1 cup	511	39.18	2.29	87.4	4.45
cooked, boiled	1 cup	186	12.92	0.68	33.4	1.61
canned	1 cup	183	14.00	0.56	31.7	1.08
Carob flour	1 cup	185	4.75	0.67	91.5	7.41
Chickpeas, raw	1 cup	729	38.60	12.07	121.3	8.17
cooked, boiled	1 cup	269	14.54	4.25	44.9	4.10
canned	1 cup	285	11.88	2.74	54.2	3.26
Chili w/beans, canned	1 cup	286	14.57	13.99	30.3	5.47
Cowpeas, raw	1 cup	184	13.05	1.16	31.6	2.61
cooked, boiled, drained	1 cup	179	13.37	1.32	29.9	2.93
frozen, unprepared	10-oz pkg	396	25.49	1.99	71.3	4.57
frozen, cooked, boiled, drained	1 cup	224	14.43	1.13	40.3	2.59
Cowpeas, leafy tips, raw	1 cup	10	1.48	0.09	1.7	0.47
cooked, boiled, drained	1 cup	12	2.47	0.05	1.4	1.39
Cowpeas, young pods w/seeds						
raw	½ cup	21	1.55	0.14	4.4	0.80
cooked, boiled, drained	½ cup	16	1.22	0.14	3.2	0.80
Cowpeas, mature, dry seeds, raw	1 cup	562	39.27	2.11	100.2	7.66
cooked, boiled	1 cup	198	13.21	0.90	35.5	3.94
canned, plain	1 cup	184	11.37	1.32	32.7	1.62
canned, w/pork	1 cup	199	6.59	3.83	39.6	1.63
Cowpeas, catjang, raw	1 cup	572	39.83	3.46	99.5	7.77
cooked, boiled	1 cup	200	13.90	1.21	34.7	2.71
Falafel	1 patty	57	2.26	3.03	5.4	0.18
Humus	1 cup	420	12.06	20.79	49.6	3.33
Hyacinth beans, mature, dry seed						
raw	1 cup	723	50.18	3.54	127.5	15.02
cooked, boiled	1 cup	228	15.79	1.12	40.1	4.73
Hyacinth beans, fresh, raw	1 cup	37	1.68	0.16	7.3	1.04
cooked, boiled, drained	1 cup	43	2.57	0.23	8.0	1.55
Lentils, raw	1 cup	649	53.87	1.85	109.6	9.99
cooked, boiled	1 cup	231	17.87	0.74	39.8	5.46
sprouted, raw	1 cup	81	6.90	0.43	17.0	2.35
Lima beans, large, mature, dry seeds, raw	1 cup	602	38.20	1.22	112.8	11.28
cooked, boiled	1 cup	217	14.67	0.71	39.2	5.80
canned, solids & liquids	1 cup	191	11.87	0.40	35.9	2.96
Lima beans, baby, mature, dry seeds, raw	1 cup	677	41.65	1.89	126.9	11.52
cooked, boiled	1 cup	229	14.64	0.68	42.4	6.54
frozen, unprepared	10-oz pkg	376	21.56	1.26	71.3	6.18
frozen, cooked, boiled, drained	10-oz pkg	326	20.68	0.92	60.4	

FOOD	CALCIUM (mg)	IRON (mg)	POTAS-SIUM (mg)	SODIUM (mg)	CHOLES-TEROI (mg)	% OF CALORIES FROM FAT
Beans, small white, raw	373	16.62	3316	26	0	3
cooked, boiled	131	5.09	828	4	0	4
Beans, yellow, raw	325	13.74	2042	24	0	7
cooked, boiled	110	4.39	576	8	0	7
Beans, white, raw	486	21.09	3626	32	0	2
cooked, boiled	161	6.61	1003	11	0	2
canned	191	7.84	1189	13	0	2
Broadbeans, raw	154	10.04	1593	19	0	4
cooked, boiled	62	2.54	456	8	0	3
canned	67	2.56	620	1161	0	3
Carob flour	359	3.03	852	36	0	3
Chickpeas, raw	211	12.48	1750	49	0	15
cooked, boiled	80	4.74	477	11	0	14
canned	78	3.23	413	718	0	9
Chili w/beans, canned	119	8.75	932	1330	43	44
Cowpeas, raw	38	1.60	626	6	0	6
cooked, boiled, drained	46	2.36	693	7	0	7
frozen, unprepared	73	6.69	1252	17	0	5
frozen, cooked, boiled, drained	40	3.60	638	9	0	5
Cowpeas, leafy tips, raw	23	0.69	164	2	0	8
cooked, boiled, drained	36	0.58	186	3	0	4
Cowpeas, young pods w/seeds						
raw	31	0.47	101	2	0	6
cooked, boiled, drained	26	0.33	92	1	0	8
Cowpeas, mature, dry seeds, raw	183	13.82	1858	27	0	3
cooked, boiled	42	4.29	476	6	0	4
canned, plain	48	2.34	413	718	0	6
canned, w/pork	41	3.41	427	840	17	17
Cowpeas, catjang, raw	141	16.62	2295	97	0	5
cooked, boiled	44	5.22	641	32	0	5
Falafel	9	0.58	99	50	0	48
Humus	124	3.87	427	599	0	45
Hyacinth beans, mature, dry seed						
raw	273	10.71	2594	45	0	4
cooked, boiled	77	8.88	653	13	0	4
Hyacinth beans, fresh, raw	40	0.59	201	2	0	4
cooked, boiled, drained	36	0.66	228	2	0	5
Lentils, raw	99	17.32	1738	19	0	3
cooked, boiled	37	6.59	731	4	0	3
sprouted, raw	19	2.47	248	8	0	5
Lima beans, large, mature, dry seeds, raw	144	13.36	3070	32	0	2
cooked, boiled	32	4.50	955	4	0	3
canned, solids & liquids	50	4.35	531	809	0	2
Lima beans, baby, mature, dry seeds, raw	163	12.50	2834	26	0	3
cooked, boiled	52	4.36	729	5	0	3
frozen, unprepared	98	6.28	1283	147	0	3
frozen, cooked, boiled, drained	89	6.10	1277	90	0	3

LEGUMES & LEGUME PRODUCTS

FOOD	AMOUNT	CALORIES (kcal)	PROTEIN (g)	FAT (g)	CARBO-HYDRATES (g)	FIBER (g)
Lima beans, fresh, raw	1 cup	176	10.68	1.34	31.4	2.95
cooked, boiled, drained	1 cup	208	11.58	0.54	40.1	3.54
Lima beans, fordhook						
frozen, unprepared	10-oz pkg	301	18.17	1.00	56.3	5.61
frozen, cooked, boiled, drained	10-oz pkg	312	18.87	1.04	58.4	5.82
Lupins, raw	1 cup	668	65.10	17.54	72.6	24.79
cooked, boiled	1 cup	197	25.84	4.84	16.4	1.11
Mothbeans, raw	1 cup	673	44.95	3.15	120.5	7.75
cooked, boiled	1 cup	207	13.83	0.97	37.0	2.38
Mung beans, mature, dry seeds						
raw	1 cup	719	49.39	2.39	129.6	10.92
cooked, boiled	1 cup	213	14.19	0.78	38.6	0.93
long rice, dehydrated	1 cup	492	0.22	0.08	120.5	0.09
Mung beans, mature seeds, sprouted, raw	½ cup	16	1.58	0.10	3.0	0.42
cooked, boiled, drained	½ cup	13	1.26	0.06	2.6	0.32
Mungo beans, raw	1 cup	726	51.87	3.78	126.2	9.17
cooked, boiled	1 cup	190	13.56	0.99	33.0	2.40
Peas, split (for additional information on peas & pea products, see also Vegetables & Vegetable Products), raw	1 cup	671	48.37	2.28	118.9	7.32
cooked, boiled	1 cup	231	16.35	0.76	41.3	3.86
Peanuts, all types, raw	1 cup	828	37.66	71.88	23.5	7.08
cooked, boiled	1 cup	200	8.51	13.87	13.3	1.23
oil-roasted	1 cup	837	37.94	70.99	27.2	7.68
dry-roasted	1 cup	855	34.57	72.50	31.4	7.45
Peanuts, Spanish, raw	1 cup	833	38.18	72.42	23.1	7.09
oil-roasted	1 cup	851	41.17	72.08	25.6	7.49
Peanuts, Valencia, raw	1 cup	833	36.63	69.46	30.5	3.16
oil-roasted	1 cup	848	38.94	73.79	23.4	3.25
Peanuts, Virginia, raw	1 cup	822	36.78	71.17	24.1	7.14
oil-roasted	1 cup	826	37.00	69.52	28.4	7.69
Peanut butter, smooth style	2 tbsp	188	7.87	15.99	6.6	0.77
chunk style	2 tbsp	188	7.70	15.98	6.9	0.80
Peanut flour, defatted	1 cup	196	31.32	0.33	20.8	2.43
low-fat	1 cup	257	20.28	13.14	18.7	
Pigeon peas, mature, dry seeds						
raw	1 cup	704	44.48	3.06	128.6	6.40
cooked, boiled	1 cup	204	11.36	0.63	39.0	1.84
Pigeon peas, fresh, raw	½ cup	105	5.54	1.26	18.3	2.06
cooked, boiled, drained	½ cup	86	4.59	1.05	15.0	2.23
Refried beans, canned	1 cup	270	15.77	2.70	46.8	8.03
Simulated meat products						
bacon	1 strip	25	0.85	2.36	0.5	
meat extender	1 oz	88	10.67	0.83	10.7	0.47
sausage	1 link	64	4.63	4.54	2.4	

FOOD	CALCIUM (mg)	IRON (mg)	POTAS-SIUM (mg)	SODIUM (mg)	CHOLES-TEROI (mg)	% OF CALORIES FROM FAT
Lima beans, fresh, raw	54	4.89	729	13	0	7
cooked, boiled, drained	54	4.17	969	29	0	2
Lima beans, fordhook						
frozen, unprepared	68	4.29	1357	166	0	3
frozen, cooked, boiled, drained	67	4.23	1268	164	0	3
Lupins, raw	317	7.85	1824	26	0	24
cooked, boiled	85	1.99	407	7	0	22
Mothbeans, raw	294	21.26	2333	58	0	4
cooked, boiled	6	5.56	538	17	0	4
Mung beans, mature, dry seeds						
raw	273	13.94	2579	30	0	3
cooked, boiled	55	2.83	536	4	0	3
long rice, dehydrated	35	3.03	14	14	0	0
Mung beans, mature seeds, sprouted, raw	7	0.47	77	3	0	6
cooked, boiled, drained	7	0.40	63	6		4
Mungo beans, raw	406	14.15	2121	53	0	5
cooked, boiled	95	3.14	416	13	0	5
Peas, split (for additional information on peas & pea products, see also Vegetables & Vegetable Products), raw	108	8.72	1932	30	0	3
cooked, boiled	26	2.52	710	4	0	3
Peanuts, all types, raw	134	6.69	1029	27	0	78
cooked, boiled	35	0.64	113	473	0	62
oil-roasted	126	2.63	982	624	0	76
dry-roasted	79	3.30	960	1187	0	76
Peanuts, Spanish, raw	155	5.71	1086	32	0	78
oil-roasted	147	3.35	1141	637	0	76
Peanuts, Valencia, raw	90	3.05	485	1	0	75
oil-roasted	78	2.38	881	1111	0	78
Peanuts, Virginia, raw	130	3.72	1008	15	0	78
oil-roasted	123	2.38	933	619	0	76
Peanut butter, smooth style	11	0.53	231	153	0	77
chunk style	13	0.61	239	156	0	77
Peanut flour, defatted	84	1.26	774	108	0	2
low-fat	78	2.84	815	0		46
Pigeon peas, mature, dry seeds						
raw	267	10.72	2853	34	0	4
cooked, boiled	72	1.86	644	9	0	3
Pigeon peas, fresh, raw	32	1.23	425	4	0	11
cooked, boiled, drained	27	1.02	351	3	0	11
Refried beans, canned	118	4.47	994	1071		9
Simulated meat products						
bacon	2	0.19	14	117	0	85
meat extender	57	3.36		3	0	8
sausage	16	0.93	58	222	0	64

LEGUMES & LEGUME PRODUCTS

FOOD	AMOUNT	CALORIES (kcal)	PROTEIN (g)	FAT (g)	CARBO-HYDRATES (g)	FIBER (g)
Soybeans, mature, dry seeds, raw	1 cup	774	67.88	37.08	56.1	9.23
cooked, boiled	1 cup	298	28.63	15.43	17.0	3.50
roasted	1 cup	811	60.58	43.69	57.7	7.91
dry-roasted	1 cup	775	68.08	37.19	56.2	9.26
Soybeans, green, raw	1 cup	376	33.15	17.41	28.2	5.25
cooked, boiled, drained	1 cup	255	22.23	11.52	19.8	3.33
Soybeans, mature seeds, sprouted						
raw	½ cup	43	4.58	2.34	3.3	0.80
cooked, steamed	½ cup	38	3.98	2.09	3.0	0.92
Soybean products						
miso	1 cup	565	32.47	16.70	76.9	6.79
natto	1 cup	371	31.02	19.25	25.1	2.80
tempeh	1 cup	331	31.45	12.74	28.2	4.96
Soy flour, full-fat, raw	1 cup	368	32.13	17.55	27.1	4.01
full-fat, roasted	1 cup	373	32.37	18.58	25.8	1.89
defatted	1 cup	327	51.46	1.22	33.9	4.27
low-fat	1 cup	325	44.81	5.90	29.5	3.72
Soy meal, defatted, raw	1 cup	411	60.02	2.92	43.7	7.06
Soy milk, fluid	1 cup	79	6.60	4.58	4.3	
Soy protein, concentrate	1 oz	92	17.81	0.13	7.1	1.05
isolate	1 oz	93	24.73	0.95	0.0	0.07
Soy sauce, made from soy & wheat	1 tbsp	9	0.93	0.01	1.5	0.00
made from soy	1 tbsp	11	1.89	0.02	1.0	0.00
made from hydrolyzed vegetable protein	1 tbsp	7	0.44	0.01	1.3	0.00
Tofu, raw, firm	½ cup	183	19.88	10.98	5.4	0.18
raw, regular	½ cup	94	10.02	5.93	2.3	0.09
dried-frozen	1 piece	82	8.15	5.16	2.4	0.03
fried	1 piece	35	2.23	2.62	1.3	0.02
Okara	½ cup	47	1.96	1.05	7.6	2.51
salted & fermented	1 block	13	0.90	0.88	0.5	0.03
Winged beans, mature, dry seeds						
raw	1 cup	745	53.95	29.70	75.9	12.46
cooked, boiled	1 cup	252	18.26	10.05	25.6	4.22
Winged beans, fresh, raw	1 cup	22	3.06	0.38	1.9	1.13
cooked, boiled, drained	1 cup	23	3.29	0.41	1.9	0.86
Yardlong beans, mature, dry seeds						
raw	1 cup	580	40.62	2.19	103.3	7.96
cooked, boiled	1 cup	202	14.17	0.77	36.0	2.78
Yardlong beans, fresh, raw	1 cup	43	2.55	0.36	7.6	
cooked, boiled, drained	1 cup	49	2.63	0.10	9.5	1.57

FOOD	CALCIUM (mg)	IRON (mg)	POTAS-SIUM (mg)	SODIUM (mg)	CHOLES-TEROI (mg)	% OF CALORIES FROM FAT
Soybeans, mature, dry seeds, raw	515	29.20	3343	4	0	43
cooked, boiled	175	8.84	886	1	0	47
roasted	237	6.71	2528	280	0	48
dry-roasted	465	6.79	2347	4	0	43
Soybeans, green, raw	504	9.09			0	42
cooked, boiled, drained	261	4.50			0	41
Soybeans, mature seeds, sprouted						
raw	23	0.73	169	5	0	49
cooked, steamed	28	0.62	167	5	0	50
Soybean products						
miso	183	7.52	451	10028	0	27
natto	380	15.05	1276	12	0	47
tempeh	154	3.75	609	10	0	35
Soy flour, full-fat, raw	175	5.42	2138	11	0	43
full-fat, roasted	160	4.94	1734	11	0	45
defatted	241	9.24	2384	20	0	3
low-fat	165	5.27	2262	16	0	16
Soy meal, defatted, raw	297	16.71	3038	3	0	6
Soy milk, fluid	10	1.38	338	30	0	52
Soy protein, concentrate	102	3.02	617	1	0	1
isolate	50	4.06	23	281	0	9
Soy sauce, made from soy & wheat	3	0.36	32	1029	0	1
made from soy	4	0.43	38	1005	0	2
made from hydrolyzed vegetable protein	1	0.27	27	1024	0	1
Tofu, raw, firm	258	13.19	298	17	0	54
raw, regular	130	6.65	150	9	0	57
dried-frozen	62	1.65	3	1	0	57
fried	48	0.63	19	2	0	67
Okara	49	0.79	130	6	0	20
salted & fermented	5	0.22	8	316	0	61
Winged beans, mature, dry seeds						
raw	800	24.45	1778	70	0	36
cooked, boiled	244	7.45	481	22	0	36
Winged beans, fresh, raw	37	0.66	98	2	0	16
cooked, boiled, drained	38	0.68	170	3	0	16
Yardlong beans, mature, dry seeds						
raw	230	14.37	1932	28	0	3
cooked, boiled	72	4.51	539	9	0	3
Yardlong beans, fresh, raw	46	0.42	218	4	0	8
cooked, boiled, drained	46	1.02	302	4	0	2

FRUITS

FOOD	AMOUNT	CALORIES (kcal)	PROTEIN (g)	FAT (g)	CARBOHY-DRATES (g)	FIBER (g)	CALCIUM (mg)
Acerola							
raw	1 cup	31	0.39	0.29	7.5	1.1	12.0
APPLES							
can, sweet, heated	1 cup	137	0.37	0.88	34.4	5.1	8.0
canned, sweetened	1 cup	136	0.36	1.00	34.1		9.0
cooked, no skin	1 cup	96	0.48	0.71	24.5	3.4	8.0
dehydrated, cooked	1 cup	142	0.54	0.24	38.4	3.9	8.0
dehydrated, raw	1 cup	208	0.79	0.35	56.1	1.3	12.0
green	1 oz	11	0.09	0.06	2.6	0.8	1.4
mammy, raw	846 g	431	4.23	4.23	106.0	25.4	93.0
red	1 oz	16	0.06	0.11	3.7	0.6	1.4
Tree Top® dehydrated, evaporated	100 g	262	1.00	1.60	60.8	11.0	31.0
Tree Top® dehydrated, low	100 g	334	1.40	2.00	77.5	14.1	40.0
Dried							
cooked, sugar added	1 cup	232	0.56	0.19	58.1	5.1	8.0
cooked, unsweetened	1 cup	145	0.56	0.18	39.1	3.9	7.7
uncooked	1 cup	209	0.80	0.27	56.7	8.6	12.0
Frozen							
unsweetened, heated	1 cup	97	0.60	0.67	24.7	3.9	9.0
unsweetened, unheated	1 cup	83	0.48	0.56	21.3	3.5	8.0
Raw							
peeled	128 g	73	0.19	0.40	19.0	1.9	5.0
peeled, boiled	1 cup	91	0.45	0.61	23.3	4.1	8.6
with skin	1 cup	117	0.38	0.71	30.2	3.8	13.9
with skin, 2¾ inch diameter	138 g	81	0.27	0.49	21.1	3.0	10.0
sliced, with skin	1 cup	65	0.21	0.39	16.8	2.4	8.0
without skin, sliced, boiled	1 cup	91	0.45	0.62	23.3	1.5	8.6
Applesauce, canned							
sweetened, CNF	1 cup	194	0.46	0.46	50.8	3.0	10.2
sweetened, USDA	1 cup	194	0.47	0.47	50.8	3.1	9.0
unsweetened, CNF	1 cup	105	0.42	0.12	27.5	3.7	7.3
unsweetened, USDA	1 cup	105	0.42	0.12	27.6	3.7	7.3
APRICOT							
frozen, sweetened	1 cup	237	1.69	0.24	60.7	4.1	24.0
halves, with skin, canned in water	1 oz	6	0.20	0.01	1.6	0.5	5.4
raw, without pit	35 g	17	0.49	0.18	3.9	0.7	4.9
Canned							
extra heavy syrup pack	1 cup	236	1.35	0.10	61.1	4.4	19.0
extra light syrup pack	1 cup	121	1.48	0.25	30.9	4.5	25.0
heavy syrup pack	1 cup	214	1.32	0.22	55.4	4.6	22.0
heavy syrup, with skin	1 cup	214	1.37	0.20	55.4	5.5	22.0
juice pack	1 cup	119	1.56	0.09	30.6	2.8	30.0
light syrup pack	1 cup	159	1.35	0.12	41.7	4.6	27.8
no skin	1 cup	51	1.56	0.07	12.4	4.1	19.0
water pack	1 cup	66	1.73	0.39	15.5	4.1	19.4
Dehydrated							
cooked, sulfured	1 cup	314	4.80	0.60	81.2	8.5	60.0
dehydrated, raw	1 cup	381	5.83	0.73	98.6	2.3	73.0

FOOD	IRON (mg)	POTAS-SIUM (mg)	SODIUM (mg)	CHOLES-TEROL (mg)	VITAMIN A (mg)	VITAMIN C (mg)	BETA-CAROTENE (ug)	% OF CALORIES FROM FAT
Acerola								
raw	0.20	143	7	0.0	75	1644	75.5	8
APPLES								
can, sweet, heated	0.49	142	7	0.0	11	0		6
canned, sweetened	0.46	138	7	0.0	10	1		7
cooked, no skin	0.28	159	1	0.0	7	1	3.4	7
dehydrated, cooked	0.82	263	51	0.0	4	1	3.9	2
dehydrated, raw	1.20	384	74	0.0	5	1	3.0	2
green	0.06	21	1	0.0	6	1	33.5	5
mammy, raw	5.92	398	127	0.0	195	118	195.0	9
red	0.06	24	1	0.0	7	1	41.4	6
Tree Top® dehydrated, evaporated	1.60	569	202			10		6
Tree Top® dehydrated, low	2.00	730	255	0.0	0	4	0.0	5
Dried								
cooked, sugar added	0.88	275	53	0.0	4	3	5.1	1
cooked, unsweetened	0.84	267	52	0.0	4	3	5.1	1
uncooked	1.21	387	75	0.0	0	3	0.0	1
Frozen								
unsweetened, heated	0.39	156	5	0.0	4	1	9.4	6
unsweetened, unheated	0.32	134	5	0.0	6	0		6
Raw								
peeled	0.09	144	0	0.0	6	5	6.4	5
peeled, boiled	0.32	150	2	0.0	8	0	8.6	6
with skin	0.36	228	0	0.0	10	11	9.9	5
with skin, 2¾ inch diameter	0.25	159	1	0.0	7	8		5
sliced, with skin	0.20	126	0	0.0	6	6		5
without skin, sliced, boiled	0.33	150	2	0.0	7	0		
Applesauce, canned								
sweetened, CNF	0.89	156	8	0.0	3	4	2.6	2
sweetened, USDA	0.89	156	8	0.0	3	4		2
unsweetened, CNF	0.29	183	5	0.0	7	24	7.3	1
unsweetened, USDA	0.29	183	5	0.0	7	3		1
APRICOT								
frozen, sweetened	2.18	554	10	0.0	407	22	571.0	1
halves, with skin, canned in water	0.15	44	3	0.0	51	1	36.6	1
raw, without pit	0.19	104	0	0.0	92	4		7
Canned								
extra heavy syrup pack	1.53	310	32	0.0	362	6	303.0	0
extra light syrup pack	0.74	346	5	0.0	314	10	326.0	2
heavy syrup pack	1.10	345	27	0.0	320	7	317.0	1
heavy syrup, with skin	0.77	361	10	0.0	317	8		1
juice pack	0.74	409	9	0.0	420	12	419.0	1
light syrup pack	0.99	349	10	0.0	334	7	334.0	1
no skin	1.23	350	25	0.0	411	4	279.0	1
water pack	0.78	467	7	0.0	314	8	313.0	5
Dehydrated								
cooked, sulfured	6.18	1812	13	0.0	1097	18	588.0	2
dehydrated, raw	7.51	2201	15	0.0	1508	11	311.0	2

FRUITS

FOOD	AMOUNT	CALORIES (kcal)	PROTEIN (g)	FAT (g)	CARBOHY- DRATES (g)	FIBER (g)	CALCIUM (mg)
APRICOT (continued)							
Dried							
cooked, sugar added	1 cup	305	3.16	0.40	79.0	8.3	39.0
sulfured, cooked, no sugar	1 cup	213	3.24	0.40	54.8	19.5	40.0
sulfured, uncooked	1 cup	309	4.75	0.60	80.3	10.1	59.0
Apricot nectar, canned	1 cup	141	0.93	0.23	36.1	1.5	17.6
Avocado							
raw, all varieties	1 cup	370	4.56	35.20	17.0	5.8	25.0
raw, California	173 g	306	3.64	30.00	12.0	6.8	19.0
raw, Florida	304 g	340	4.83	27.00	27.1	8.3	33.4
Avocado pear	1 oz	51	0.57	5.41	0.0	1.6	6.0
Banana							
common varieties	1 oz	29	0.37	0.11	6.7	0.1	3.1
raw	1 cup	216	2.42	1.13	55.1	4.0	14.1
raw, peeled	114 g	105	1.18	0.55	26.7	1.9	7.0
smoked	1 oz	96	1.45	0.06	22.3	0.3	6.5
Banana chips	1 oz	147	0.70	9.50	16.6	1.9	5.0
Banana flakes, dehydrated or powdered	1 tbsp	22	0.24	0.11	5.5	0.5	1.4
Blackberries							
canned, heavy syrup pack	1 cup	236	3.35	0.36	59.1	17.7	54.0
frozen, unsweetened	1 cup	97	1.78	0.65	23.7	7.6	43.8
raw	1 cup	75	1.04	0.56	18.4	8.9	46.1
Blueberries							
canned, heavy syrup pack	1 cup	225	1.67	0.85	56.5	2.8	14.0
frozen, sweetened	1 cup	187	0.91	0.31	50.5	5.3	13.0
frozen, unsweetened	1 cup	79	0.65	0.99	18.9	4.9	12.4
mixed, frozen, thawed, Alaska	1 cup	44	0.70	0.00	10.4		15.0
raw	1 cup	81	0.97	0.55	20.5	3.9	8.7
Boysenberries							
canned, heavy syrup pack	1 cup	225	2.53	0.31	57.1	5.7	46.0
frozen, unsweetened	1 cup	66	1.46	0.35	16.1	5.2	36.0
Breadfruit							
raw	384 g	396	4.11	0.88	104.0	46.8	65.3
Carambola							
raw	127 g	42	0.69	0.44	9.9	1.5	6.0
star fruit	1 oz	7	0.20	0.03	1.4	0.5	1.4
Carissa							
raw	20 g	12	0.10	0.26	2.7		2.2
Cashew apple	1 oz	12	0.17	0.06	2.7	0.2	0.9
Cherimoya							
raw	547 g	514	7.11	2.19	131.0	13.0	126.0
CHERRIES							
red, sour, canned, light syrup	1 cup	189	1.86	0.25	48.6	2.3	25.2
sweet, frozen, sweetened	1 cup	231	2.98	0.34	57.9	8.7	31.1
sweet, raw	6.80 g	5	0.08	0.07	1.1	0.1	1.0
Sour							
canned, water pack	1 cup	88	1.88	0.24	21.8	2.2	26.8
frozen, unsweetened	1 cup	71	1.43	0.68	17.1	1.9	20.2

148

FOOD	IRON (mg)	POTAS-SIUM (mg)	SODIUM (mg)	CHOLES-TEROL (mg)	VITAMIN A (mg)	VITAMIN C (mg)	BETA-CAROTENE (ug)	% OF CALORIES FROM FAT
APRICOT (continued)								
Dried								
cooked, sugar added	4.10	1195	9	0.0	578	4	579.0	1
sulfured, cooked, no sugar	4.17	1222	9	0.0	591	4		2
sulfured, uncooked	6.11	1791	13	0.0	941	3		2
Apricot nectar, canned	0.95	286	8	0.0	331	84	331.0	1
Avocado								
raw, all varieties	2.35	1378	24	0.0	141	18	140.0	86
raw, California	2.04	1097	21	0.0	106	14		88
raw, Florida	1.61	1484	15	0.0	186	24		71
Avocado pear	0.65	132	2	0.0	9	3	56.7	95
Banana								
common varieties	0.17	68	8	0.0	14	5	85.0	3
raw	0.73	931	2	0.0	19	21	18.8	5
raw, peeled	0.35	451	1	0.0	9	10		5
smoked	0.40	269	238	0.0	1	7	3.1	1
Banana chips	0.35	152	2	0.0	8	2	7.8	58
Banana flakes, dehydrated or powdered	0.07	92	0	0.0	2	0		5
Blackberries								
canned, heavy syrup pack	1.66	254	7	0.0	56	7	56.3	1
frozen, unsweetened	1.21	211	2	0.0	17	5	16.6	6
raw	0.82	282	0	0.0	24	30		7
Blueberries								
canned, heavy syrup pack	0.84	102	9	0.0	16	3	12.9	3
frozen, sweetened	0.90	137	3	0.0	10	2	18.4	1
frozen, unsweetened	0.28	84	2	0.0	13	4	12.4	11
mixed, frozen, thawed, Alaska	1.10				16	2		0
raw	0.25	129	9	0.0	15	19		6
Boysenberries								
canned, heavy syrup pack	1.10	230	9	0.0	10	16		1
frozen, unsweetened	1.12	183	2	0.0	9	4	9.2	5
Breadfruit								
raw	2.07	1882	8	0.0	15	111	15.3	2
Carambola								
raw	0.33	207	2	0.0	63	27	56.3	9
star fruit	0.09	28	2	0.0	14	7	84.8	4
Carissa								
raw	0.26	52	1	0.0	1	8		19
Cashew apple	0.09	24	3	0.0	2	40	9.9	4
Cherimoya								
raw	2.74			0.0	6	49		4
CHERRIES								
red, sour, canned, light syrup	3.33	239	18	0.0	184	5	40.3	1
sweet, frozen, sweetened	0.91	515	3	0.0	49	3		1
sweet, raw	0.03	15	0	0.0	1	0		12
Sour								
canned, water pack	3.34	239	17	0.0	184	5	39.0	3
frozen, unsweetened	0.82	192	2	0.0	135	3	116.0	9

FRUITS

FOOD	AMOUNT	CALORIES (kcal)	PROTEIN (g)	FAT (g)	CARBOHY-DRATES (g)	FIBER (g)	CALCIUM (mg)
CHERRIES (continued)							
Sour, Red							
canned, extra heavy	1 cup	297	1.85	0.24	76.3	2.4	26.0
canned in heavy syrup	1 cup	233	1.87	0.26	59.6	2.3	25.6
canned in light syrup	1 cup	189	1.86	0.24	48.6	2.3	26.0
raw	1 cup	77	1.55	0.47	18.9	1.9	24.0
Sweet, Canned							
extra heavy syrup	1 cup	267	1.54	0.39	68.5	1.8	23.0
heavy syrup pack	1 cup	213	1.55	0.39	54.7	1.8	23.0
juice pack	1 cup	135	2.28	0.05	34.5	0.6	35.0
light syrup pack	1 cup	170	1.54	0.39	43.6	1.8	23.0
water pack	1 cup	114	1.91	0.31	29.2	0.6	27.0
Coconut, dried, shredded	1 cup	466	2.68	33.00	44.3	3.9	14.0
Crabapples							
raw	1 cup	83	0.44	0.33	21.9		20.0
Cranberries							
high bush, Alaska	1 cup	29	1.10	0.20	12.3		20.0
Low bush, lingenberry, Alaska	1 cup	49	0.40	0.50	12.2		26.0
raw	1 cup	54	0.43	0.22	14.0	4.6	8.0
Cranberry sauce, canned, sweetened	1 cup	418	0.55	0.42	108.0	3.2	11.1
Currants							
european black, raw	1 cup	71	1.57	0.45	17.2	4.8	61.0
red & white, raw	1 cup	63	1.57	0.22	15.5	4.8	37.0
zante, dried	1 cup	407	5.88	0.38	107.0	9.8	124.0
Custard apple	1 oz	22	0.57	0.09	4.8	0.0	4.0
Dates							
domestic, natural and dry, chopped	1 cup	490	3.51	0.80	131.0	15.5	57.0
domestic, natural and dry, whole	8.30 g	23	0.16	0.04	6.1	0.7	2.7
dried	1 oz	84	0.71	0.00	20.3	0.5	15.6
Duku	1 oz	16	0.26	0.09	3.4	0.1	3.4
Durian	1 oz	43	0.77	0.96	7.9	0.3	11.3
fermented	1 oz	32	0.77	0.74	5.6	0.4	4.0
Durian cake	1 oz	87	0.91	0.79	19.2	0.6	3.7
Elderberries							
raw	1 cup	106	0.96	0.73	26.7	12.3	55.1
Figs							
candied	1 cup	558	6.54	0.37	138.0		235.0
Figs, candied							
extra heavy syrup pack	1 cup	280	0.98	0.26	72.7	5.7	68.0
heavy syrup pack	1 cup	228	0.99	0.26	59.3	8.9	69.0
light syrup pack	1 cup	173	0.99	0.26	45.2		69.0
water pack	1 cup	131	0.99	0.25	34.7	5.2	69.4
Figs, dried							
cooked	1 cup	279	3.33	1.27	71.4	12.4	157.0
uncooked	1 cup	507	6.07	2.33	130.0	18.5	287.0
raw	50 g	37	0.38	0.15	9.6	3.2	18.0
Fruit, spicy, pickled	1 oz	95	0.34	9.10	3.0	0.6	20.4

FOOD	IRON (mg)	POTAS-SIUM (mg)	SODIUM (mg)	CHOLES-TEROL (mg)	VITAMIN A (mg)	VITAMIN C (mg)	BETA-CAROTENE (ug)	% OF CALORIES FROM FAT
CHERRIES (continued)								
Sour, Red								
canned, extra heavy	3.30	237	18	0.0	182	5	196.0	1
canned in heavy syrup	3.33	238	18	0.0	183	5		1
canned in light syrup	3.32	238	18	0.0	183	5		1
raw	0.50	268	5	0.0	199	16	198.0	5
Sweet, Canned								
extra heavy syrup	0.90	371	7	0.0	39	9	39.2	1
heavy syrup pack	0.91	373	7	0.0	40	9	38.5	2
juice pack	1.45	328	8	0.0	31	6	32.5	0
light syrup pack	0.90	372	7	0.0	39	9	40.3	2
water pack	0.89	325	3	0.0	40	5	32.2	2
Coconut, dried, shredded	1.78	313	244	0.0	0	1		64
Crabapples								
raw	0.39	213	1	0.0	4	9		4
Cranberries								
high bush, Alaska	1.00	140	26		318	15		6
Low bush, lingenberry, Alaska	0.40				9	21		9
raw	0.22	78	1	0.0	5	15	5.5	4
Cranberry sauce, canned, sweetened	0.61	72	80	0.0	6	11		1
Currants								
european black, raw	1.72	361	2	0.0	26	203	13.4	6
red & white, raw	1.11	308	1	0.0	13	46	13.4	3
zante, dried	4.69	1285	11	0.0	10	7	10.1	1
Custard apple	0.14	78	0	0.0	0	3	0.0	3
Dates								
domestic, natural and dry, chopped	2.05	1161	5	0.0	9	0		1
domestic, natural and dry, whole	0.10	54	0	0.0	0	0		1
dried	0.23	152	1	0.0	7	0	39.7	0
Duku	0.09	40	1	0.0	0	0	0.0	5
Durian	0.54	20	11		7	7	42.5	20
fermented	0.28	133	164		3	0	19.6	21
Durian cake	0.31	134	8		0	0	0.0	8
Elderberries								
raw	2.32	406	9	0.0	87	52	87.0	6
Figs								
candied	5.60	1195	64	0.0		0		1
Figs, candied								
extra heavy syrup pack	0.72	254	3	0.0	9	3	10.4	1
heavy syrup pack	0.73	258	3	0.0	10	3	10.4	1
light syrup pack	0.73	256	3	0.0	9	3		1
water pack	0.72	255	2	0.0	10	2	9.9	2
Figs, dried								
cooked	2.44	779	12	0.0	41	12	41.4	4
uncooked	4.44	1417	22	0.0	26	2	25.9	4
raw	0.18	116	1	0.0	7	1	7.0	4
Fruit, spicy, pickled	0.31	45	420		0	0	0.0	86

FRUITS

FOOD	AMOUNT	CALORIES (kcal)	PROTEIN (g)	FAT (g)	CARBOHY-DRATES (g)	FIBER (g)	CALCIUM (mg)
Fruit bar, fat free, Health Valley®							
apple	42.50 g	140	3.00	1.00	33.0	3.7	20.0
apricot	42.50 g	140	3.00	1.00	33.0	3.7	20.0
date	42.50 g	140	3.00	1.00	33.0	3.7	20.0
raisin	42.40 g	140	3.00	1.00	33.0	3.7	20.0
Fruit bar, oat bran jumbo, Health Valley®							
date	42.50 g	140	4.00	2.00	27.0	4.0	20.0
fruit	42.50 g	140	4.00	2.00	27.0	4.0	20.0
raisin	42.50 g	140	4.00	1.00	28.0	4.0	20.0
Fruit bar, rice bran jumbo, Health Valley®	42.50 g	160	3.00	5.00	27.0	3.7	40.0
Fruit cocktail, canned	1 oz	22	0.20	0.11	5.1	0.2	1.7
extra light syrup	1 cup	110	0.98	0.18	28.6	0.0	20.0
extra heavy syrup	1 cup	230	1.01	0.18	59.5	2.9	16.0
in heavy syrup	1 cup	186	1.00	0.18	48.2	3.8	16.0
juice pack	1 cup	114	1.14	0.03	29.4	1.5	19.8
light syrup pack	1 cup	145	1.01	0.18	37.6	2.8	16.0
water, dietetic	1 oz	9	0.40	0.03	2.4	0.1	1.7
water pack	1 cup	78	1.03	0.12	20.8	1.6	12.3
Fruit leather							
bars	23 g	81	0.40	1.20	18.0	0.5	7.0
bars with cream	24 g	89	0.20	2.00	18.7	0.5	5.0
pieces	27 g	92	0.30	1.90	21.1	0.6	5.0
rollups	21 g	73	0.20	0.60	17.7	0.5	7.0
Fruit roll up							
cherry	14.40 g	50	0.00	1.00	12.0		
Fruit rollup							
Betty Crocker®							
cherry/strawberry	14.20 g	50	1.00	1.00	12.0		0.0
fruit punch	14.20 g	50	1.00	1.00	12.0		0.0
grape	14.20 g	50	1.00	1.00	12.0		0.0
raspberry	14.20 g	50	1.00	1.00	12.0		0.0
Fruit salad							
canned, extra heavy syrup	1 cup	227	0.85	0.16	59.0		17.0
canned, heavy syrup pack	1 cup	187	0.87	0.19	48.7	2.8	16.0
canned, light syrup pack	1 cup	146	0.85	0.16	38.2		17.0
tropical, canned, heavy syrup	1 cup	221	1.05	0.26	57.5		34.0
FRUIT SNACKS							
Garfield®							
Fat cat funnies	14.2 g	50	1.00	1.00	12.0		0.0
Fruit party	14.2 g	50	1.00	1.00	12.0	1.2	0.0
Punch/cat cooler	25.5 g	100	1.00	1.00	22.0		0.0
Very strawberry	25.5 g	100	1.00	1.00	22.0		0.0
Fruit by the Foot® cherry	21.2 g	80	1.00	2.00	18.0		0.0
Squeezit®							
Berry b wild	191 g	90	0.00	0.00	22.0		0.0
Chucklin cherry	191 g	90	0.00	0.00	23.0	16.1	0.0
Grumpy grape	191 g	90	0.00	0.00	23.0		0.0

FOOD	IRON (mg)	POTAS-SIUM (mg)	SODIUM (mg)	CHOLES-TEROL (mg)	VITAMIN A (mg)	VITAMIN C (mg)	BETA-CAROTENE (ug)	% OF CALORIES FROM FAT
Fruit bar, fat free, Health Valley®								
apple	2.70	280	10	0.0	0	0		6
apricot	0.90	280	10	0.0	20	0		6
date	2.70	280	10	0.0	0	0	4.7	6
raisin	3.60	280	10	0.0	0	0		6
Fruit bar, oat bran jumbo, Health Valley®								
date	1.08	200	10	0.0	0	0		13
fruit	1.08	260	10	0.0	0	0	16.1	13
raisin	1.08	210	10	0.0	0	0		6
Fruit bar, rice bran jumbo, Health Valley®	0.18	280	5	0.0	0	4		28
Fruit cocktail, canned	0.09	14	1		5	1	32.6	5
extra light syrup	0.74	256	10	0.0	57	7	7.4	1
extra heavy syrup	0.73	225	15	0.0	52	5	52.0	1
in heavy syrup	0.73	224	15	0.0	52	5		1
juice pack	0.52	236	10	0.0	76	7	76.9	0
light syrup pack	0.73	225	15	0.0	52	5	52.9	1
water, dietetic	0.14	26	1	0.0	7	1	7.1	3
water pack	0.61	230	10	0.0	61	5	75.9	1
Fruit leather								
bars	0.18	32	18	0.0	3	16	0.2	13
bars with cream	0.20	51	23	0.0	0	15	0.2	20
pieces	0.20	44	109	0.0	3	15	0.3	19
rollups	0.21	62	13	0.0	2	1	0.2	7
Fruit roll up								
cherry		45	5	0.0				18
Fruit rollup								
Betty Crocker®								
cherry/strawberry	0.00	20	40		0	0		18
fruit punch	0.00	40	40		0	0		18
grape	0.00	25	40		0	0		18
raspberry	0.00	30	40		0	0		18
Fruit salad								
canned, extra heavy syrup	0.73	207	14	0.0	165	5		1
canned, heavy syrup pack	0.72	205	14	0.0	129	6	51.0	1
canned, light syrup pack	0.73	208	14	0.0	108	6		1
tropical, canned, heavy syrup	1.33	337	5	0.0	33	45		1
FRUIT SNACKS								
Garfield®								
Fat cat funnies	0.00	30	20		0	0		18
Fruit party	0.00	40	40	0.0	0	0	34.7	18
Punch/cat cooler	0.00	30	60		0	0		9
Very strawberry	0.00	20	60		0	0		9
Fruit by the Foot® cherry	0.00	70	45		0	0		23
Squeezit®								
Berry b wild	0.00	10	0	0.0	0	0		0
Chucklin cherry	0.00	10	5	0.0	0	0	467.0	0
Grumpy grape	0.00	10	0	0.0	0	0		0

FRUITS

FOOD	AMOUNT	CALORIES (kcal)	PROTEIN (g)	FAT (g)	CARBOHY-DRATES (g)	FIBER (g)	CALCIUM (mg)
FRUIT SNACKS (continued)							
Squeezit® (continued)							
Mean green punch	191 g	90	0.00	0.00	23.0		0.0
Silly strawberry	191 g	90	0.00	0.00	23.0	16.1	0.0
Smarty arty orange	191 g	90	0.00	0.00	23.0		0.0
Thunder Jets®							
Fruit squares	25.5 g	100	1.00	1.00	24.0		0.0
Mach one	25.5 g	100	1.00	1.00	24.0		0.0
Nintendo® Super Mario/link	25.0 g	100	0.00	1.00	22.0	0.6	10.8
Shark Bites®							
berry bears	25.5 g	100	1.00	1.00	22.0		0.0
fruit punch	25.5 g	100	1.00	1.00	22.0		0.0
Surfs Up®							
Sun splash	25.5 g	100	1.00	1.00	22.0		0.0
Tutti frutti	25.5 g	100	1.00	1.00	22.0		0.0
Gooseberries							
canned, heavy syrup pack	1 cup	184	1.64	0.50	47.3	7.0	40.3
raw	1 cup	66	1.32	0.87	15.3	4.0	37.5
GRAPEFRUIT	1 oz	11	0.23	0.03	2.5	0.5	6.5
red/pink/white-raw	1 cup	74	1.45	0.23	18.6	3.2	27.0
Canned							
juice pack	1 cup	92	1.74	0.22	22.9	1.6	37.4
in light syrup	1 cup	152	1.43	0.25	39.2	1.7	36.0
water pack	1 cup	88	1.42	0.24	22.3	1.6	36.6
Pink & red							
california, raw	1 cup	86	1.15	0.23	22.3	3.2	25.0
raw	246 g	74	1.36	0.25	18.5	3.4	36.0
raw	1 cup	69	1.27	0.23	17.7	3.2	25.0
White							
raw, all areas	1 cup	85	1.78	0.26	21.6	4.6	30.9
California, raw	1 cup	84	2.02	0.23	20.9	1.4	27.0
Florida, raw	1 cup	75	1.45	0.23	18.8	1.4	35.0
raw	236 g	78	1.63	0.24	19.8	2.5	28.0
Grapes							
raw, adherent skin (European) type	160 g	114	1.06	0.92	28.4	2.6	17.0
	1 oz	19	0.23	0.00	4.6	0.3	6.0
raw, slip skin (American) type	1 cup	58	0.58	0.32	15.8	1.5	13.0
thompson, canned, water pack	1 cup	98	1.23	0.27	25.2	1.7	24.5
thompson, canned, heavy syrup pack	1 cup	187	1.23	0.26	50.3	1.7	25.0
Grape drink, canned	253 g	154	1.42	0.20	37.8	0.0	22.8
Groundcherries							
raw	1 cup	74	2.66	0.98	15.7	1.7	13.0
Guavas							
common, raw	1 oz	13	0.31	0.06	2.8	1.9	9.4
	90 g	46	0.74	0.54	10.7	5.4	18.0
strawberry, raw	6 g	4	0.04	0.04	1.0	0.4	1.3
Haws							
scarlet, flesh & skin, raw	1 oz	25	0.57	0.20	5.9	0.7	4.8

154

FOOD	IRON (mg)	POTAS-SIUM (mg)	SODIUM (mg)	CHOLES-TEROL (mg)	VITAMIN A (mg)	VITAMIN C (mg)	BETA-CAROTENE (ug)	% OF CALORIES FROM FAT
FRUIT SNACKS (continued)								
Squeezit® (continued)								
Mean green punch	0.00	5	0	0.0	0	0		0
Silly strawberry	0.00	5	0	0.0	0	0	467.0	0
Smarty arty orange	0.00	5	50	0.0	0	0		0
Thunder Jets®								
Fruit squares	0.00	25	30		0	0		9
Mach one	0.00	20	30		0	0		9
Nintendo® Super Mario/link	0.98	22	10	0.0	20	1	0.3	9
Shark Bites®								
berry bears	0.00	25	20		0	0		9
fruit punch	0.00	25	20		0	0		9
Surfs Up®								
Sun splash	0.00	20	30		0	0		9
Tutti frutti	0.00	20	20		0	0		9
Gooseberries								
canned, heavy syrup pack	0.83	194	5	0.0	35	25		2
raw	0.47	297	2	0.0	44	42	43.5	12
GRAPEFRUIT	0.06	26	1	0.0	1	11	3.7	2
red/pink/white-raw	0.20	321	1	0.0	29	79	27.6	3
Canned								
juice pack	0.52	420	19	0.0	0	84	0.0	2
in light syrup	1.02	328	4	0.0	0	54		1
water pack	1.00	322	5	0.0	0	53	0.0	3
Pink & red								
california, raw	0.17	338	1	0.0	59	88	27.6	2
raw	0.30	312	0	0.0	64	91		3
raw	0.28	296	1	0.0	59	88	27.6	3
White								
raw, all areas	0.15	381	0	0.0	3	86	30.8	3
California, raw	0.17	330	1	0.0	2	77	27.6	2
Florida, raw	0.12	345	1	0.0	2	85	27.6	3
raw	0.14	350	0	0.0	2	79		3
Grapes								
raw, adherent skin (European) type	0.41	296	3	0.0	12	17		7
	0.14	34	3	0.0	1	2	7.9	0
raw, slip skin (American) type	0.27	176	2	0.0	9	4		5
thompson, canned, water pack	2.40	262	15	0.0	16	2		2
thompson, canned, heavy syrup pack	2.41	264	14	0.0	16	3	15.4	1
Grape drink, canned	0.61	334	8	0.0	2	0		1
Groundcherries								
raw	1.40	242	4	0.0	101	15	179.0	12
Guavas								
common, raw	0.34	8	7	0.0	3	43	17.0	4
	0.28	256	3	0.0	71	165	71.1	11
strawberry, raw	0.01	18	2	0.0	1	2	4.7	8
Haws								
scarlet, flesh & skin, raw	0.86	131	69	0.0	0	4	0.0	7

FRUITS

FOOD	AMOUNT	CALORIES (kcal)	PROTEIN (g)	FAT (g)	CARBOHY-DRATES (g)	FIBER (g)	CALCIUM (mg)
Hog plum/ambarella	1 oz	9	0.20	0.03	2.0	0.7	4.8
pickled	1 oz	8	0.03	0.03	1.9	0.2	3.4
Huckleberry, Alaska	1 cup	37	0.40	0.10	8.7		15.0
Jackfruit							
raw	1 oz	27	0.42	0.09	6.8	0.5	9.6
Java							
plum, raw	1 cup	82	0.97	0.32	21.0	2.0	25.0
JUICE							
Acerola, raw	1 cup	51	0.97	0.73	11.6		24.0
Apple							
canned or bottled	1 cup	116	0.15	0.28	29.0	0.5	16.0
concentrate, undiluted	1 fl oz	58	0.18	0.13	14.5	0.0	7.2
frozen, concentrate, diluted	1 cup	118	0.35	0.25	29.1	0.3	15.1
frozen, concentrate, undiluted	1 cup	467	1.43	1.04	115.0		56.3
frozen, diluted	1 cup	112	0.34	0.24	27.6	0.6	14.3
Kraft® 100% Pure	170 g	80	0.00	0.00	20.0	0.2	0.0
Apricot nectar, canned	1 cup	141	0.92	0.22	36.1	1.5	17.0
Citrus fruit, frozen, concentrate	1 fl oz	57	0.41	0.03	14.2	0.0	8.8
Cranapple							
canned	1 cup	170	0.25	0.00	43.2	0.0	17.7
Ocean Spray®	1 fl oz	5	0.00	0.00	1.1	0.0	1.0
Cranberry							
bottled	1 cup	144	0.00	0.25	36.4	0.0	7.6
frozen	1 cup	548	0.29	0.00	140.0	0.0	31.9
frozen, water	1 cup	137	0.00	0.00	34.9	0.0	12.5
cocktail, bottled	1 cup	144	0.00	0.25	36.4	0.0	7.6
Ocean Spray®	1 fl oz	6	0.01	0.02	4.7	0.0	1.0
apple, bottled	1 cup	164	0.25	0.00	41.9	0.2	17.1
Grape							
bottled	1 fl oz	17	0.00	0.02	4.3	0.0	2.0
bottled	1 cup	137	0.49	0.25	34.3	0.1	19.6
canned & bottled	1 cup	154	1.42	0.20	37.8	0.0	22.8
frozen concentrate	216 g	387	1.40	0.67	95.8	0.6	28.1
frozen, concentrate, diluted	1 cup	125	0.47	0.22	31.3	0.2	9.8
frozen, concentrate, undiluted	1 cup	516	1.87	0.89	128.0		37.4
frozen, diluted	1 cup	128	0.47	0.23	31.9	0.0	9.0
canned	1 fl oz	16	0.00	0.00	4.0		1.0
Kraft® No sugar	170 g	104	1.00	0.00	25.0		0.0
Grapefruit							
canned, sweetened	1 cup	115	1.45	0.23	27.8	0.0	20.0
canned, unsweetened	1 cup	94	1.28	0.25	22.1	0.4	17.3
dehydrated, prepared	1 cup	100	1.00	0.00	24.0	0.0	22.0
frozen concentrate	207 g	302	4.08	0.99	71.5	0.0	56.0
frozen, diluted	1 cup	101	1.36	0.32	24.0	0.0	19.8
raw	1 cup	96	1.24	0.42	22.7	0.5	22.2
Kraft® No sugar	170 g	70	1.00	0.00	16.0		0.0
Lemon							
canned & bottled	1 cup	51	0.98	0.71	15.8	0.7	26.8

FOOD	IRON (mg)	POTAS-SIUM (mg)	SODIUM (mg)	CHOLES-TEROL (mg)	VITAMIN A (mg)	VITAMIN C (mg)	BETA-CAROTENE (ug)	% OF CALORIES FROM FAT
Hog plum/ambarella	0.96	54	1	0.0	7	6	41.1	3
pickled	0.45	147	119	0.0	41	11	249.0	3
Huckleberry, Alaska	0.30		10		8	3		2
Jackfruit								
raw	0.17	86	1	0.0	9	2	8.5	3
Java								
plum, raw	0.25	106	18	0.0	0	19	43.2	4
JUICE								
Acerola, raw	1.21	235	7	0.0	123	3872		13
Apple								
canned or bottled	0.92	296	7	0.0	0	2		2
concentrate, undiluted	0.32	158	9	0.0	0	1	0.0	2
frozen, concentrate, diluted	0.66	317	18	0.0	0	84		2
frozen, concentrate, undiluted	2.56	1260	70	0.0	0	376		2
frozen, diluted	0.62	301	17	0.0	0	1		2
Kraft® 100% Pure	0.72	210	5	0.0	0	0	0.0	0
Apricot nectar, canned	0.96	286	9	0.0	330	1		1
Citrus fruit, frozen, concentrate	1.39	138	1	0.0	5	34	1.5	0
Cranapple								
canned	0.15	68	5	0.0	0	81		0
Ocean Spray®	0.05	8	1	0.0		14		0
Cranberry								
bottled	0.38	46	5	0.0	0	57	0.0	2
frozen	0.87	142	9	0.0	9	227	0.0	0
frozen, water	0.23	35	7	0.0	3	52	0.0	0
cocktail, bottled	0.38	46	10	0.0	0	90		2
Ocean Spray®	0.05	8	1	0.0	0	14	0.0	2
apple, bottled	0.15	66	5	0.0	0	57	0.0	0
Grape								
bottled	0.00	7	1	0.0	0	10	0.2	1
bottled	0.02	59	7	0.0	0	57	1.5	2
canned & bottled	0.61	334	8	0.0	2	0		1
frozen concentrate	0.78	160	15	0.0	6	179		2
frozen, concentrate, diluted	0.25	52	5	0.0	2	37		2
frozen, concentrate, undiluted	1.04	213	20	0.0	9	173		2
frozen, diluted	0.26	53	5	0.0	2	60		2
canned	0.03	11	0	0.0	0	5		0
Kraft® No sugar	0.36	85	0	0.0	0	0		0
Grapefruit								
canned, sweetened	0.90	405	5	0.0	0	67		2
canned, unsweetened	0.49	378	2	0.0	2	72		2
dehydrated, prepared	0.20	412	2	0.0	2	91		0
frozen concentrate	1.02	1002	6	0.0	7	248		3
frozen, diluted	0.35	336	2	0.0	2	83		3
raw	0.49	400	2	0.0	2	94		4
Kraft® No sugar	0.00	280	0	0.0	0	60		0
Lemon								
canned & bottled	0.32	249	51	0.0	4	61		12

FRUITS

FOOD	AMOUNT	CALORIES (kcal)	PROTEIN (g)	FAT (g)	CARBOHY-DRATES (g)	FIBER (g)	CALCIUM (mg)
JUICE (continued)							
Lemon (continued)							
frozen, single strength	1 cup	54	1.12	0.78	15.9	0.7	19.5
raw	1 cup	61	0.93	0.00	21.1	0.7	17.1
Lime							
canned & bottled	1 cup	52	0.62	0.57	16.5	0.0	29.5
raw	1 cup	66	1.08	0.25	22.2	0.0	22.1
Limeade							
canned, frozen concentrate	218 g	410	0.00	0.00	108.0	2.2	11.0
frozen concentrate, diluted	1 cup	100	0.00	0.00	27.0	0.5	3.0
Orange							
canned	1 cup	104	1.46	0.36	24.5	0.3	21.0
canned, frozen concentrate	213 g	339	5.10	0.44	81.3	1.7	67.0
dehydrated, prepared	1 cup	115	1.00	0.00	27.0	0.0	25.0
frozen concentrate, diluted	1 cup	112	1.68	0.14	26.8	0.5	22.0
frozen, concentrate, undiluted	1 cup	452	6.79	0.60	108.0	2.3	90.9
Kraft® no sugar	170 g	80	1.00	0.00	19.0		0.0
Orange-grapefruit							
canned	1 cup	106	1.48	0.25	25.4	0.5	19.8
frozen, diluted	1 cup	110	1.00	0.00	26.0	0.0	20.0
Kraft® no sugar	170 g	80	1.00	0.00	19.0		0.0
Orange-pineapple							
raw	1 cup	111	1.74	0.50	25.8	2.0	27.0
raw, all varieties	1 cup	121	2.42	0.31	30.2	4.6	103.0
Kraft® no sugar	170 g	80	1.00	0.00	19.0		0.0
Passion fruit							
purple	1 cup	126	0.96	0.12	33.6	3.4	9.0
yellow	1 cup	148	1.65	0.45	35.7	1.3	9.9
Pineapple							
canned	1 cup	140	0.80	0.20	34.5	0.3	42.5
frozen concentrate	1 fl oz	65	0.47	0.04	15.9	0.0	14.0
frozen, diluted	1 cup	130	1.00	0.08	31.9	0.3	27.5
grapefruit, canned	1 cup	118	0.50	0.25	29.1	0.3	17.5
orange, vitamin C, canned	1 cup	125	3.26	0.00	29.6	0.4	12.5
Prune, canned & bottled	256 g	182	1.56	0.08	44.7	2.6	30.7
Raisin, concentrated, Sun Maid®	100 g	225	2.10	0.20	68.0	0.0	37.0
Tangerine							
canned, sweetened	1 cup	125	1.25	0.50	29.9	0.6	45.0
frozen, diluted	1 cup	110	1.03	0.27	26.7	0.5	18.0
frozen, sweetened	1 fl oz	57	0.53	0.14	13.9		9.5
raw	1 cup	106	1.24	0.49	25.0	0.8	44.0
Jujube							
dried	1 oz	81	1.05	0.31	20.9		22.4
raw	1 oz	22	0.34	0.01	5.7		6.0
Kiwifruit							
raw	1 oz	13	0.26	0.11	2.8	0.3	7.7
	76 g	46	0.75	0.33	11.3	2.6	19.8
Kumquats							
raw	19 g	12	0.17	0.02	3.1	1.3	8.0

FOOD	IRON (mg)	POTAS-SIUM (mg)	SODIUM (mg)	CHOLES-TEROL (mg)	VITAMIN A (mg)	VITAMIN C (mg)	BETA-CAROTENE (ug)	% OF CALORIES FROM FAT
JUICE (continued)								
Lemon (continued)								
frozen, single strength	0.29	217	2	0.0	3	77		13
raw	0.07	303	2	0.0	5	112		0
Lime								
canned & bottled	0.57	185	39	0.0	4	16		10
raw	0.07	268	2	0.0	3	72		3
Limeade								
canned, frozen concentrate	0.20	129	2	0.0	0	26		0
frozen concentrate, diluted	0.00	32	2	0.0	0	6		0
Orange								
canned	1.10	436	6	0.0	44	86		3
canned, frozen concentrate	0.74	1435	7	0.0	59	294		1
dehydrated, prepared	0.50	518	2	0.0	50	109		0
frozen concentrate, diluted	0.24	474	2	0.0	19	97		1
frozen, concentrate, undiluted	0.99	1914	9	0.0	80	433	72.3	1
Kraft® no sugar	0.00	310	0	0.0	0	60		0
Orange-grapefruit								
canned	1.14	390	7	0.0	29	72		2
frozen, diluted	0.20	439	2	0.0	27	102		0
Kraft® no sugar	0.00	340	0	0.0	0	60		0
Orange-pineapple								
raw	0.50	496	2	0.0	50	124		4
raw, all varieties	0.26	466	0	0.0	54	137	54.0	2
Kraft® no sugar	0.00	280	0	0.0	0	42		0
Passion fruit								
purple	0.59	687	15	0.0	177	74	387.0	1
yellow	0.89	687	15	0.0	595	45	387.0	3
Pineapple								
canned	0.65	335	3	0.0	1	27		1
frozen concentrate	0.32	170	1	0.0	2	15	0.4	1
frozen, diluted	0.75	340	3	0.0	3	30	2.5	1
grapefruit, canned	0.78	153	35	0.0	10	83	1.3	2
orange, vitamin C, canned	0.68	115	8	0.0	133	57	22.5	0
Prune, canned & bottled	3.02	707	10	0.0	1	11		0
Raisin, concentrated, Sun Maid®	3.00	110	25	0.0	1	4	0.0	1
Tangerine								
canned, sweetened	0.50	443	2	0.0	105	55		4
frozen, diluted	0.23	273	2	0.0	138	58	96.2	2
frozen, sweetened	0.12	142	1	0.0	72	30		2
raw	0.49	440	2	0.0	104	77	98.6	4
Jujube								
dried	0.51	151	3	0.0		4		3
raw	0.14	71	1	0.0	1	20		0
Kiwifruit								
raw	0.11	51	1		2	25	11.9	8
	0.31	252	4	0.0	13	75	13.7	6
Kumquats								
raw	0.07	37	1	0.0	6	7	5.7	2

FRUITS

FOOD	AMOUNT	CALORIES (kcal)	PROTEIN (g)	FAT (g)	CARBOHY-DRATES (g)	FIBER (g)	CALCIUM (mg)
Lemon							
lemon peel, raw	1 tbsp	4	0.09	0.02	1.0	0.0	8.0
raw, unpeeled	108 g	22	1.30	0.32	11.6	1.0	65.9
raw, without peel	58 g	17	0.64	0.17	5.4	0.6	15.1
Lemonade							
canned, frozen concentrate	219 g	425	0.00	0.00	112.0	5.6	9.0
frozen concentrate, diluted	1 cup	105	0.00	0.00	28.0	0.6	2.0
Lime							
raw	67 g	20	0.47	0.13	7.1	0.4	22.1
Loganberries							
frozen	1 cup	81	2.23	0.46	19.1	7.1	38.2
Longans							
dried	1 oz	81	1.39	0.11	21.0		12.8
raw	3.2 g	2	0.04	0.00	0.5		0.0
Loquats							
raw	9.9 g	5	0.04	0.02	1.2	0.3	1.6
Lychee							
dried	1 oz	79	1.08	0.34	20.0	0.6	9.4
raw	9.6 g	6	0.08	0.04	1.6	0.0	0.5
Mango							
raw	207 g	135	1.06	0.57	35.2	4.8	21.0
	1 oz	20	0.60	0.14	4.0	0.1	5.4
candied	1 oz	91	0.14	0.11	22.3	0.1	10.8
pickled	1 oz	28	0.09	0.03	7.0	0.2	0.9
Mangosteen	1 oz	10	0.17	0.28	1.6	1.5	2.0
MELONS							
Cantaloupe	1236 g	392	10.90	1.36	97.9	14.3	160.0
raw	1 cup	56	1.40	0.45	13.3	1.1	17.5
raw, cubed pieces	1 cup	56	1.41	0.45	13.4	1.1	17.6
Casaba, raw	1 cup	44	1.53	0.17	10.5	2.0	8.5
Honeydew, raw, cubed pieces	1 cup	60	0.78	0.17	15.6	1.5	10.2
Melon balls, frozen	1 cup	57	1.45	0.43	13.7	2.6	17.3
Mixed fruit							
canned, heavy syrup pack	1 cup	184	0.94	0.26	47.8	2.9	3.0
frozen, sweetened	1 cup	245	3.54	0.46	60.6	3.0	18.0
Mulberries							
raw	1 cup	60	2.02	0.55	13.7	2.4	54.6
Nutmeg, pickled	1 oz	68	0.06	0.06	16.7	0.5	0.3
Nectarines							
raw	136 g	67	1.28	0.63	16.0	1.6	6.8
Oheloberries							
raw	1 cup	39	0.53	0.31	9.6	3.6	10.0
Olive							
olive	1 oz	25	0.31	1.56	2.4	2.0	38.8
ripe, canned, large	4.4 g	5	0.04	0.47	0.3	0.1	4.0
Orange							
orange	1 oz	14	0.20	0.14	3.0	0.2	11.3
Florida, raw	1 cup	84	1.30	0.39	21.3	3.5	80.0

FOOD	IRON (mg)	POTAS-SIUM (mg)	SODIUM (mg)	CHOLES-TEROL (mg)	VITAMIN A (mg)	VITAMIN C (mg)	BETA-CAROTENE (ug)	% OF CALORIES FROM FAT
Lemon								
lemon peel, raw	0.05	10	0	0.0	0	8		5
raw, unpeeled	0.76	157	3	3.2	83	3		14
raw, without peel	0.35	80	1	0.0	2	31		9
Lemonade								
canned, frozen concentrate	0.40	153	4	0.0	4	66		0
frozen concentrate, diluted	0.10	40	0	0.0	1	17		0
Lime								
raw	0.40	68	1	0.0	1	20	0.7	6
Loganberries								
frozen	0.94	213	1	0.0	5	23	5.9	5
Longans								
dried	1.53	187	14	0.0	0	8		1
raw	0.00	9	0	0.0		3		1
Loquats								
raw	0.03	26	0	0.0	15	0		4
Lychee								
dried	0.48	315	1	0.0	0	52	0.0	4
raw	0.03	16	0	0.0	0	7	0.0	6
Mango								
raw	0.26	322	4	0.0	806	57	805.0	4
	0.06	31	2	0.0	0	6	0.0	7
candied	0.45	6	57	0.0	1	2	5.4	1
pickled	0.28	4	106	0.0	1	1	4.0	1
Mangosteen	0.28	13	2	0.0	0	1	0.0	26
MELONS								
Cantaloupe	2.60	2947	249	0.0	4696	461	28.6	3
raw	0.33	491	14	0.0	511	67	512.0	7
raw, cubed pieces	0.34	494	14	0.0	516	68		7
Casaba, raw	0.68	357	20	0.0	5	27	5.1	3
Honeydew, raw, cubed pieces	0.12	461	17	0.0	7	42		3
Melon balls, frozen	0.50	484	54	0.0	307	11	306.0	7
Mixed fruit								
canned, heavy syrup pack	0.92	214	10	0.0	49	176	51.0	1
frozen, sweetened	0.70	327	8	0.0	81	188		2
Mulberries								
raw	2.59	271	14	0.0	4	51	4.2	8
Nutmeg, pickled	0.09	3	88	0.0	1	1	3.4	1
Nectarines								
raw	0.20	288	0	0.0	100	7	101.0	8
Oheloberries								
raw	0.13	54	2	0.0	116	8	4.2	7
Olive								
olive	0.31	83	4	0.0	25	1	149.0	56
ripe, canned, large	0.15	0	38	0.0	2	0	0.3	85
Orange								
orange	0.60	29	1	0.0	6	11	35.4	9
Florida, raw	0.16	312	1	0.0	37	83	38.8	4

FRUITS

FOOD	AMOUNT	CALORIES (kcal)	PROTEIN (g)	FAT (g)	CARBOHY-DRATES (g)	FIBER (g)	CALCIUM (mg)
Orange (continued)							
mandarin/tangerine	1 oz	13	0.31	0.09	2.6	0.2	5.1
navels, California, raw	1 cup	76	1.70	0.15	19.2	2.8	66.0
neck	1 oz	9	0.14	0.06	2.0	0.1	4.0
raw, all common varieties, whole	131 g	62	1.23	0.16	15.4	3.1	52.4
raw, sections without membranes	1 cup	85	1.69	0.22	21.2	3.6	72.0
unpeeled, raw	1 cup	68	2.21	0.51	26.4	4.1	119.0
valencias, California, raw	1 cup	88	1.87	0.54	21.4	4.3	72.0
Orange peel, raw	1 tbsp	6	0.09	0.01	1.5	0.2	10.0
Papaya							
papaya	1 oz	10	0.43	0.03	2.0	0.1	3.1
candied	1 oz	100	0.28	0.17	24.3	0.2	7.7
exotica	1 oz	17	0.28	0.03	3.8	0.1	8.8
raw	1 cup	55	0.85	0.20	13.7	1.3	33.6
Papaya nectar, canned	1 cup	143	0.43	0.38	36.3	1.2	25.0
Passion fruit							
purple, raw	18 g	18	0.40	0.13	4.2	2.2	2.2
PEACHES							
peaches	1 oz	10	0.43	0.09	1.8	0.6	1.4
dried, cooked, sugar added	1 cup	278	2.86	0.60	71.8	6.5	22.0
dehydrated, cooked, sulfured	1 cup	322	4.86	1.03	82.6	6.5	38.0
dehydrated, uncooked	1 cup	376	5.67	1.20	96.5		45.0
dried, cooked, sulfured, no sugar	1 cup	199	2.99	0.65	50.8	6.7	23.2
dried, uncooked, sulfured	1 cup	382	5.78	1.22	98.1	14.0	44.8
frozen, sliced, sweetened	1 cup	235	1.56	0.33	59.9	6.0	6.0
halved, canned in water, dietetic	1 oz	7	0.14	0.03	1.8	0.4	0.6
sliced, canned in water, dietetic	1 oz	7	0.14	0.03	1.8	0.4	0.6
spiced, canned-heavy syrup pack	1 cup	182	0.99	0.24	48.6	1.0	14.5
Canned							
extra heavy syrup pack	1 cup	251	1.22	0.08	68.3	2.6	9.0
extra light syrup	1 cup	104	0.99	0.25	27.4	2.5	12.0
halves/slices, light syrup	1 cup	136	1.13	0.08	36.5	2.5	7.5
heavy syrup pack	1 cup	189	1.15	0.26	51.0	1.1	7.7
juice pack	1 cup	109	1.57	0.08	28.7	2.5	15.0
light syrup pack	1 cup	136	1.13	0.08	36.5	2.5	9.0
canned, water pack	1 cup	59	1.07	0.15	14.9	1.1	4.9
Raw	1 cup	94	1.53	0.20	24.3	4.2	10.9
sliced	1 cup	73	1.19	0.15	18.9	2.7	8.5
whole	87 g	37	0.61	0.08	9.7	1.4	4.4
Peach nectar, canned	1 cup	134	0.67	0.05	34.7	0.4	13.0
PEARS							
dried, cooked, sugar added	1 cup	392	2.41	0.81	104.0	16.2	43.0
dried, cooked, no sugar	1 cup	325	2.32	0.78	86.2		41.0
dried, uncooked	1 cup	472	3.37	1.14	125.0	13.8	60.0
green	1 oz	19	0.11	0.00	4.6	0.5	2.3
halved, canned in water, dietetic	1 oz	9	0.06	0.00	2.4	0.4	1.4
yellow-Chinese	1 oz	10	0.14	0.06	2.2	0.5	3.4

FOOD	IRON (mg)	POTAS-SIUM (mg)	SODIUM (mg)	CHOLES-TEROL (mg)	VITAMIN A (mg)	VITAMIN C (mg)	BETA-CAROTENE (ug)	% OF CALORIES FROM FAT
Orange (continued)								
mandarin/tangerine	0.06	23	1	0.0	9	8	56.7	6
navels, California, raw	0.20	294	1	0.0	30	95	34.7	2
neck	0.06	28	1	0.0	1	15	6.2	5
raw, all common varieties, whole	0.13	237	0	0.0	27	70		2
raw, sections without membranes	0.18	326	0	0.0	37	96		2
unpeeled, raw	1.36	333	3	0.0	43	121	35.7	7
valencias, California, raw	0.16	322	0	0.0	41	87	37.8	6
Orange peel, raw	0.05	13	0	0.0	3	8	2.5	2
Papaya								
papaya	0.20	11	1	0.0	55	20	329.0	3
candied	0.45	28	14	0.0	1	1	9.1	2
exotica	0.17	96	1	0.0	115	20	689.0	2
raw	0.14	359	4	0.0	282	87		3
Papaya nectar, canned	0.85	78	13	0.0	28	8	35.2	2
Passion fruit								
purple, raw	0.29	63	5	0.0	13	5	12.6	6
PEACHES								
peaches	0.28	35	1	0.0	37	1	223.0	8
dried, cooked, sugar added	3.24	789	6	0.0	49	9	48.6	2
dehydrated, cooked, sulfured	5.47	1342	10	0.0	96	17	48.4	3
dehydrated, uncooked	6.39	1567	11	0.0	164	12		3
dried, cooked, sulfured, no sugar	3.38	826	5	0.0	51	10		3
dried, uncooked, sulfured	6.50	1594	11	0.0	346	8		3
frozen, sliced, sweetened	0.93	325	16	0.0	71	235		1
halved, canned in water, dietetic	0.11	30	1	0.0	12	1		4
sliced, canned in water, dietetic	0.11	30	1	0.0	12	1		4
spiced, canned-heavy syrup pack	0.68	206	10	0.0	77	13		1
Canned								
extra heavy syrup pack	0.77	217	21	0.0	34	3	86.5	0
extra light syrup	0.74	183	12	0.0	67	7	86.4	2
halves/slices, light syrup	0.90	243	13	0.0	88	18	87.8	1
heavy syrup pack	0.69	235	15	0.0	85	7		1
juice pack	0.66	317	11	0.0	95	9	94.2	1
light syrup pack	0.90	244	13	0.0	89	6	87.8	1
canned, water pack	0.78	242	7	0.0	130	7		2
Raw	0.24	430	0	0.0	118	14	118.0	2
sliced	0.19	335	0	0.0	91	11		2
whole	0.10	171	0	0.0	47	6		2
Peach nectar, canned	0.47	101	17	0.0	64	13	64.7	0
PEARS								
dried, cooked, sugar added	2.72	687	8	0.0	11	11	11.2	2
dried, cooked, no sugar	2.60	659	7	0.0	11	10		2
dried, uncooked	3.78	959	10	0.0	1	13	0.0	2
green	0.14	22	1	0.0	1	2	3.1	0
halved, canned in water, dietetic	0.14	17	1	0.0		1		0
yellow-Chinese	0.03	25	1	0.0	1	2	4.3	5

FRUITS

FOOD	AMOUNT	CALORIES (kcal)	PROTEIN (g)	FAT (g)	CARBOHY-DRATES (g)	FIBER (g)	CALCIUM (mg)
PEARS (continued)							
Canned							
extra heavy syrup pack	1 cup	254	0.51	0.33	65.9	5.2	12.0
extra light syrup pack	1 cup	116	0.74	0.25	30.1	4.2	17.0
halves, light syrup pack	1 cup	143	0.48	0.08	38.1	5.0	12.5
heavy syrup pack	1 cup	189	0.51	0.33	48.9	2.4	12.8
juice pack	1 cup	124	0.84	0.17	32.1	4.7	22.3
light syrup pack	1 cup	144	0.48	0.08	38.1	5.0	13.0
water pack	1 cup	71	0.46	0.07	19.1	4.1	9.8
Raw							
Asian	122 g	51	0.61	0.28	13.0		5.0
bartlett, with skin	166 g	98	0.65	0.66	25.1	4.7	18.3
bosc, with skin	141 g	83	0.55	0.56	21.3	3.7	15.5
d'Anjou, with skin	200 g	118	0.78	0.80	30.1	5.2	22.0
with skin	1 cup	140	0.93	0.95	35.9	7.1	26.2
Pear nectar, canned	1 cup	149	0.27	0.03	39.4		11.0
Persimmons							
persimmon	1 oz	23	0.14	0.03	5.4	0.2	4.3
dried	1 oz	71	0.54	0.14	16.8	0.6	10.5
Japanese, dried	34 g	93	0.47	0.20	25.0	0.6	8.5
Japanese, raw	168 g	118	0.98	0.31	31.2		13.0
native, raw	25 g	32	0.20	0.10	8.4	0.4	6.8
PINEAPPLE							
pineapple	1 oz	13	0.14	0.03	3.0	0.2	6.8
bits, canned in syrup	1 cup	131	0.90	0.29	33.9	1.9	36.0
bits, canned, water pack	1 cup	79	1.06	0.22	20.4	2.0	36.9
candied	1 oz	87	0.26	0.06	21.4	0.3	2.6
frozen, sweetened	1 cup	208	0.98	0.25	54.4	5.4	22.0
sliced, dietetic, canned/water	1 oz	13	0.09	0.03	3.6	0.5	2.6
raw, diced	1 cup	76	0.61	0.67	19.2	1.9	10.9
Canned							
extra heavy syrup, CNF	1 cup	216	0.88	0.29	55.9	2.3	36.4
extra heavy syrup, USDA	1 cup	217	0.89	0.29	55.9		35.0
heavy syrup pack	1 cup	199	0.89	0.28	51.5	2.3	35.7
juice pack, CNF	1 cup	150	1.05	0.20	39.2	1.8	35.0
juice pack, USDA	1 cup	150	1.04	0.21	39.2	1.8	34.0
light syrup pack	1 cup	131	0.91	0.30	33.9	2.2	35.3
syrup	1 oz	21	0.09	0.06	5.0	0.1	1.7
water pack	1 oz	9	0.12	0.03	2.4	0.3	4.3
Pineapple grapefruit drink	1 cup	129	0.51	0.13	32.2	0.0	15.2
Pineapple orange drink	1 cup	134	0.51	0.00	32.4	0.0	12.7
Pitanga							
raw	7 g	2	0.06	0.03	0.5		0.6
Plantains							
cooked	1 cup	179	1.22	0.28	48.0	3.5	3.0
raw	179 g	218	2.33	0.66	57.1	4.1	5.0
PLUMS							
plums	1 oz	10	0.20	0.00	2.3	0.2	4.8

FOOD	IRON (mg)	POTAS-SIUM (mg)	SODIUM (mg)	CHOLES-TEROL (mg)	VITAMIN A (mg)	VITAMIN C (mg)	BETA-CAROTENE (ug)	% OF CALORIES FROM FAT
PEARS (continued)								
Canned								
extra heavy syrup pack	0.57	166	13	0.0	0	3	0.0	1
extra light syrup pack	0.49	110	5	0.0	0	5	0.0	2
halves, light syrup pack	0.70	166	13	0.0	0	3	0.0	0
heavy syrup pack	0.56	166	13	0.0	0	3		2
juice pack	0.72	238	10	0.0	1	4	2.5	1
light syrup pack	0.70	165	13	0.0	0	2	0.0	1
water pack	0.51	129	5	0.0	0	2	0.0	1
Raw								
Asian		148	0	0.0	0	2	0.0	5
bartlett, with skin	0.42	208	0	0.0	3	7		6
bosc, with skin	0.35	176	1	0.0	3	6		6
d'Anjou, with skin	0.50	250	1	0.0	4	8		6
with skin	0.59	297	0	0.0	5	10	4.8	6
Pear nectar, canned	0.65	33	9	0.0	0	3		0
Persimmons								
persimmon	0.11	32	0	0.0	15	5	91.3	1
dried	0.31	131	2		0	30	0.0	2
Japanese, dried	0.25	273	1	0.0	19	0	73.8	2
Japanese, raw	0.26	270	3	0.0	364	13		2
native, raw	0.63	78	78	0.0	54	17	54.2	3
PINEAPPLE								
pineapple	0.40	28	9	0.0	13	4	76.5	2
bits, canned in syrup	0.98	266	3	0.0	4	19		2
bits, canned, water pack	0.98	312	2	0.0	4	19	4.9	3
candied	0.34	23	11	0.0	1	0	4.5	1
frozen, sweetened	0.98	245	5	0.0	7	20	9.8	1
sliced, dietetic, canned/water	0.11	24	1	0.0	1	2		2
raw, diced	0.57	175	2	0.0	4	24		8
Canned								
extra heavy syrup, CNF	0.99	265	3	0.0	3	19	2.6	1
extra heavy syrup, USDA	0.98	265	3	0.0	4	19		1
heavy syrup pack	0.97	265	3	0.0	3	19	2.6	1
juice pack, CNF	0.70	305	3	0.0	10	24	10.0	1
juice pack, USDA	0.70	304	4	0.0	10	24	10.0	1
light syrup pack	0.98	265	3	0.0	3	11	2.5	2
syrup	0.14	5	1	0.0	1	3	5.7	2
water pack	0.11	36	0	0.0	1	2	0.6	3
Pineapple grapefruit drink	0.81	139	56	0.0	0	68	10.1	1
Pineapple orange drink	0.68	121	8	0.0	134	63	134.0	0
Pitanga								
raw	0.01	7	0	0.0	11	2		11
Plantains								
cooked	0.89	716	8	0.0	140	17	140.0	1
raw	1.07	893	7	0.0	202	33	202.0	3
PLUMS								
plums	0.79	15	2	0.0	9	3	54.1	0

FRUITS

FOOD	AMOUNT	CALORIES (kcal)	PROTEIN (g)	FAT (g)	CARBOHY-DRATES (g)	FIBER (g)	CALCIUM (mg)
PLUMS (continued)							
Canned, purple							
extra heavy syrup	1 cup	265	0.93	0.26	68.7	2.6	24.0
light syrup, CNF	1 cup	159	0.93	0.25	41.0	2.5	22.7
light syrup, USDA	1 cup	158	0.93	0.26	41.0	2.5	24.0
heavy syrup pack	1 cup	230	0.93	0.26	60.0	1.1	24.0
juice pack	1 cup	146	1.30	0.06	38.2	1.0	25.0
water pack	1 cup	102	0.96	0.02	27.5	1.2	17.0
Raw							
raw	1 cup	160	2.31	1.81	38.0	3.5	11.7
Japanese & hybrid	66 g	36	0.52	0.41	8.6	1.4	2.6
prune type	28.4 g	20	0.00	0.00	6.0	0.6	3.0
Pomegranates							
raw	154 g	105	1.46	0.46	26.4	1.1	4.6
Pricklypears							
raw	103 g	42	0.75	0.53	9.9	5.6	57.7
Prunes							
prune	1 oz	83	0.65	0.17	19.8	0.4	15.6
canned, heavy syrup pack	1 cup	246	2.04	0.47	65.1	8.6	39.8
dehydrated, cooked	1 cup	317	3.46	0.68	83.2	18.5	68.0
dehydrated, uncooked	1 cup	448	4.89	0.97	118.0	9.5	96.0
Prunes, dried							
cooked, w/sugar	1 cup	295	2.59	0.51	78.3	7.6	51.0
cooked, w/out sugar	1 cup	227	2.47	0.49	59.5	7.5	48.0
uncooked, CNF	1 cup	339	3.71	0.74	89.1	10.4	72.4
uncooked, USDA	1 cup	385	4.20	0.83	101.0	11.0	82.0
Prune whip	1 cup	194	6.04	0.20	45.0	3.6	25.6
Pummelo							
sections, raw	1 cup	72	1.44	0.08	18.3	1.9	7.6
Quince							
raw	92 g	52	0.37	0.09	14.1	1.8	10.1
Raisins							
raisins	1 oz	84	0.65	0.11	20.1	0.2	22.7
seeded	1 cup	488	4.16	0.90	129.0	8.7	46.0
Sun Maid® currant, zantesun	100 g	290	3.40	0.50	74.4	0.9	85.7
Raisins, seedless	1 cup	435	4.67	0.67	115.0	6.1	71.1
golden, seedless	1 cup	498	5.60	0.76	131.0	4.1	87.0
packet	14 g	42	0.45	0.06	11.1	0.7	6.9
sultana	1 cup	511	5.49	0.78	135.0	6.2	83.5
Sun Maid® Golden	100 g	294	3.18	0.26	77.5	0.9	54.0
Sun Maid® Natural	100 g	300	3.30	0.40	77.5	6.8	60.0
Raspberries							
canned, heavy syrup pack	1 cup	234	2.12	0.31	59.8	6.5	27.0
frozen, sweetened	1 cup	258	1.75	0.40	65.4	11.0	37.5
raw	1 cup	60	1.12	0.68	14.2	5.5	27.1
Rhubarb							
cooked from frozen, added sugar	1 cup	278	0.94	0.12	74.9	4.8	348.0
cooked from raw, added sugar	1 cup	380	1.00	0.00	97.0	5.4	211.0
petioles	1 oz	9	0.34	0.37	1.2	0.3	71.7
raw	1 cup	26	1.09	0.24	5.5	2.2	105.0

FOOD	IRON (mg)	POTAS-SIUM (mg)	SODIUM (mg)	CHOLES-TEROL (mg)	VITAMIN A (mg)	VITAMIN C (mg)	BETA-CAROTENE (ug)	% OF CALORIES FROM FAT
PLUMS (continued)								
Canned, purple								
extra heavy syrup	2.15	232	50	0.0	66	1	67.9	1
light syrup, CNF	2.17	234	50	0.0	66	16	65.5	1
light syrup, USDA	2.16	233	50	0.0	67	1	65.5	1
heavy syrup pack	2.17	234	50	0.0	67	1		1
juice pack	0.84	389	3	0.0	254	7	255.0	0
water pack	0.40	314	2	0.0	228	7	227.0	0
Raw								
raw	0.29	502	0	0.0	93	28	93.4	10
Japanese & hybrid	0.07	114	0	0.0	21	6		10
prune type	0.10	48	0	0.0	8	1		0
Pomegranates								
raw	0.46	399	5	0.0	0	9	0.0	4
Pricklypears								
raw	0.31	227	5	0.0	5	14		11
Prunes								
prune	0.57	189	3	0.0	0	0	0.0	2
canned, heavy syrup pack	0.96	529	7	0.0	187	7		2
dehydrated, cooked	3.28	988	5	0.0	146	0	86.8	2
dehydrated, uncooked	4.64	1397	7	0.0	233	0	263.0	2
Prunes, dried								
cooked, w/sugar	2.48	741	4	0.0	68	6		2
cooked, w/out sugar	2.35	708	4	0.0	65	6		2
uncooked, CNF	3.52	1058	6	0.0	283	5	283.0	2
uncooked, USDA	3.99	1200	6	0.0	320	5		2
Prune whip	0.98	333	242	0.0	23	5	22.5	1
Pummelo								
sections, raw	0.21	410	2	0.0	0	116		1
Quince								
raw	0.64	181	4	0.0	4	14	3.7	2
Raisins								
raisins	0.99	179	4	0.0	0	0	0.0	1
seeded	4.27	1362	47	0.0	0	9	1.7	2
Sun Maid® currant, zantesun	2.40	730	10	0.0	8	41	12.0	2
Raisins, seedless								
	3.02	1089	17	0.0	1	5		1
golden, seedless	2.95	1232	20	0.0	7	5	0.6	1
packet	0.29	105	2	0.0	0	0		1
sultana	3.54	1279	20	0.0	2	6		1
Sun Maid® Golden	1.60	715	15	0.0	2	3	1.0	1
Sun Maid® Natural	2.10	751	12		2	3		1
Raspberries								
canned, heavy syrup pack	1.08	241	9	0.0	9	22	7.7	1
frozen, sweetened	1.63	285	3	0.0	15	41		1
raw	0.70	187	0	0.0	16	31		10
Rhubarb								
cooked from frozen, added sugar	0.50	230	2	0.0	17	8		0
cooked from raw, added sugar	1.60	548	5	0.0	22	16		0
petioles	0.14	36	1	0.0	9	4	51.6	35
raw	0.27	351	5	0.0	12	10	12.2	8

FRUITS

FOOD	AMOUNT	CALORIES (kcal)	PROTEIN (g)	FAT (g)	CARBOHY-DRATES (g)	FIBER (g)	CALCIUM (mg)
Rhubarb (continued)							
raw, diced	1 cup	26	1.10	0.24	5.5	2.2	105.0
Roselle							
raw	1 cup	28	0.55	0.37	6.5	2.3	123.0
Salmonberries, Alaska	1 cup	44	1.00	0.10	10.0	1.0	14.0
Sapodilla							
raw	170 g	140	0.74	1.87	33.9	9.0	36.0
Sapotes							
raw	225 g	302	4.77	1.35	76.0		87.8
Soursop							
raw, pulp	1 oz	18	0.37	0.11	4.0	0.5	3.4
	1 cup	149	2.25	0.68	37.9		31.5
Strawberries							
strawberries	1 oz	7	0.20	0.09	1.2	0.5	5.4
canned, heavy syrup pack	1 cup	234	1.42	0.65	59.8	3.1	33.0
raw, whole	1 cup	45	0.91	0.55	10.5	2.7	20.9
sweetened, sliced, California	1 cup	182	2.00	0.00	50.0		0.0
unsweetened, whole, California	1 cup	100	2.00	0.00	26.0	4.0	0.0
Strawberries, frozen							
sweetened, sliced	1 cup	245	1.36	0.33	66.1	19.8	28.0
sweetened, whole	1 cup	199	1.33	0.36	53.5	5.6	28.1
unsweetened, CNF	1 cup	52	0.64	0.16	13.6	2.4	23.8
unsweetened, USDA	1 cup	52	0.64	0.16	13.6	3.9	23.8
Sugar apples							
raw	1 cup	236	5.14	0.73	59.1	11.0	59.0
Tamarinds							
fresh pods	1 oz	89	0.99	0.28	20.6	0.4	48.2
raw	2 g	5	0.06	0.01	1.3	0.1	1.5
Tangerines							
canned, juice pack	1 cup	92	1.54	0.08	23.8	1.5	27.4
canned, light syrup pack	1 cup	154	1.13	0.25	40.8	1.4	17.6
mandarins, canned, juice pack	1 cup	92	1.54	0.08	23.8	0.9	27.4
mandarins, canned, light syrup	1 cup	154	1.13	0.25	40.8	0.9	17.6
raw, peeled	84 g	37	0.53	0.16	9.4	1.5	12.0
Water apple	1 oz	5	0.23	0.03	0.9	0.2	0.6
Watermelon							
raw	1 oz	8	0.17	0.06	1.7	0.1	1.7
	1 cup	51	0.99	0.69	11.5	0.6	12.8

FOOD	IRON (mg)	POTAS-SIUM (mg)	SODIUM (mg)	CHOLES-TEROL (mg)	VITAMIN A (mg)	VITAMIN C (mg)	BETA-CAROTENE (ug)	% OF CALORIES FROM FAT
Rhubarb (continued)								
raw, diced	0.27	351	5	0.0	12	.10	12.2	9
Roselle								
raw	0.84	119	3	0.0	16	7		12
Salmonberries, Alaska	0.60	108	42		155	0		2
Sapodilla								
raw	1.36	328	20	0.0	10	25	10.2	12
Sapotes								
raw	2.25	774	23	0.0	92	45		4
Soursop								
raw, pulp	0.14	83	1	0.0	1	8	4.3	6
	1.35	626	32	0.0	1	46		4
Strawberries								
strawberries	0.28	19	1	0.0	2	15	10.2	12
canned, heavy syrup pack	1.24	218	9	0.0	7	80	7.6	3
raw, whole	0.57	247	1	0.0	4	85		12
sweetened, sliced, California	1.44	93	3	0.0	0	96		0
unsweetened, whole, California	1.44	418	6	0.0	0	84	7.6	0
Strawberries, frozen								
sweetened, sliced	1.49	249	8	0.0	6	106		1
sweetened, whole	1.20	250	3	0.0	7	101		2
unsweetened, CNF	1.12	221	3	0.0	6	61	6.0	3
unsweetened, USDA	1.12	221	3	0.0	7	61	6.0	3
Sugar apples								
raw	1.50	619	24	0.0	2	91	2.5	3
Tamarinds								
fresh pods	3.12	45	3		1	3	5.7	3
raw	0.06	13	1	0.0	0	0	0.1	2
Tangerines								
canned, juice pack	0.67	331	13	0.0	212	85	-	1
canned, light syrup pack	0.93	197	15	0.0	212	50		1
mandarins, canned, juice pack	0.67	331	12	0.0	212	85	212.0	1
mandarins, canned, light syrup	0.93	197	15	0.0	212	43	212.0	1
raw, peeled	0.09	132	1	0.0	77	26		4
Water apple	0.06	14	0	0.0	0	5	2.0	5
Watermelon								
raw	0.06	22	1	0.0	19	2	116.0	6
	0.27	186	3	0.0	59	15		12

NUT & SEED PRODUCTS

FOOD	AMOUNT	CALORIES (kcal)	PROTEIN (g)	FAT (g)	CARBO- HYDRATES (g)	FIBER (g)
NUTS						
Acorns						
raw	1 oz	105	1.75	6.78	11.5	0.73
dried	1 oz	145	2.30	8.92	15.2	0.96
Acorn flour, full-fat	1 oz	142	2.13	8.57	15.5	0.80
Almonds	1 oz					
dried, unblanched	1 oz	167	5.66	14.83	5.7	0.77
dried, blanched	1 oz	166	5.80	14.92	5.2	0.65
dry roasted, unblanched	1 oz	167	4.64	14.65	6.8	1.40
oil roasted, unblanched	1 oz	176	5.79	16.38	4.5	1.40
oil roasted, blanched	1 oz	174	5.41	16.06	5.1	0.89
toasted, unblanched	1 oz	167	5.79	14.42	6.5	1.41
Almond butter						
plain	1 tbsp	101	2.41	9.46	3.3	0.24
honey & cinnamon	1 tbsp	96	2.53	8.35	4.3	0.24
Almond meal, partially defatted	1 oz	116	11.22	5.20	8.2	0.65
Almond paste	1 oz	127	3.37	7.72	12.3	1.70
Almond powder						
full-fat	1 oz	168	5.63	14.67	6.3	0.54
partially defatted	1 oz	112	10.64	4.54	9.0	0.80
Beechnuts, dried	1 oz	164	1.76	14.20	9.5	1.05
Brazilnuts, dried, unblanched	1 oz	186	4.07	18.81	3.6	0.65
Butternuts, dried	1 oz	174	7.07	16.18	3.4	0.53
Cashew nuts						
dry roasted	1 oz	163	4.35	13.16	9.2	0.20
oil roasted	1 oz	163	4.59	13.69	8.1	0.36
Cashew butter, plain	1 oz	167	4.99	14.03	7.8	0.22
Chestnuts, Chinese						
raw	1 oz	64	1.19	0.32	13.9	0.47
dried	1 oz	103	1.94	0.51	22.6	0.76
boiled & steamed	1 oz	44	0.82	0.22	9.5	0.32
roasted	1 oz	68	1.27	0.34	14.8	0.50
Chestnuts, European						
raw, unpeeled	1 oz	60	0.69	0.64	12.9	0.48
raw, peeled	1 oz	56	0.46	0.35	12.5	0.27
dried, unpeeled	1 oz	106	1.81	1.26	21.9	1.55
dried, peeled	1 oz	105	1.42	1.11	22.2	1.42
boiled & steamed	1 oz	37	0.57	0.39	7.8	0.20
roasted	1 oz	70	0.90	0.62	15.0	0.54
Chestnuts, Japanese						
raw	1 oz	44	0.64	0.15	9.9	0.28
dried	1 oz	102	1.49	0.35	23.1	0.64
boiled & steamed	1 oz	16	0.23	0.05	3.5	0.10
roasted	1 oz	57	0.84	0.23	12.8	0.31
Coconut meat						
raw	45 g	159	1.50	15.07	6.8	1.92
dried, creamed	1 oz	194	1.51	19.62	6.1	1.12
dried, unsweetened	1 oz	187	1.95	18.32	6.7	1.51
dried, sweetened, flaked, canned	4 oz	505	3.82	36.13	46.6	2.44

FOOD	CALCIUM (mg)	IRON (mg)	POTAS-SIUM (mg)	SODIUM (mg)	CHOLES-TEROI (mg)	% OF CALORIES FROM FAT
NUTS						
Acorns						
raw	12	0.22	153	0	0	58
dried	15	0.30	201	0	0	55
Acorn flour, full-fat	12	0.34	202		0	54
Almonds						
dried, unblanched	75	1.04	208	3	0	80
dried, blanched	70	1.03	213	3	0	81
dry roasted, unblanched	80	1.08	219	3	0	79
oil roasted, unblanched	66	1.09	194	3	0	84
oil roasted, blanched	55	1.51	197	3	0	83
toasted, unblanched	80	1.40	220	3	0	78
Almond butter						
plain	43	0.59	121	2	0	84
honey & cinnamon	43	0.59	120	2	0	78
Almond meal, partially defatted	120	2.41	398	2	0	40
Almond paste	65	0.90	184	3	0	55
Almond powder						
full-fat	62	0.80	201	2	0	79
partially defatted	67	0.99	204	3	0	36
Beechnuts, dried	0				0	78
Brazilnuts, dried, unblanched	50	0.97	170	0	0	91
Butternuts, dried	15	1.14	119	0	0	84
Cashew nuts						
dry roasted	13	1.70	160	4	0	73
oil roasted	12	1.16	151	5	0	76
Cashew butter, plain	12	1.43	155	4	0	76
Chestnuts, Chinese						
raw	5	0.40	127	1	0	5
dried	8	0.65	206	2	0	4
boiled & steamed	3	0.27	87	1	0	5
roasted	5	0.43	135	1	0	5
Chestnuts, European						
raw, unpeeled	8	0.29	147	1	0	10
raw, peeled	5	0.27	137	1	0	6
dried, unpeeled	19	0.68	280	11	0	11
dried, peeled	18	0.68	281	11	0	10
boiled & steamed	13	0.49	203	8	0	9
roasted	8	0.26	168	1	0	8
Chestnuts, Japanese						
raw	9	0.41	94	4	0	3
dried	20	0.96	218	10	0	3
boiled & steamed	3	0.15	34	1	0	3
roasted	10	0.60			0	4
Coconut meat						
raw	6	1.09	160	9	0	85
dried, creamed	7	0.95	156	11	0	91
dried, unsweetened	7	0.94	154	11	0	88
dried, sweetened, flaked, canned	16	2.10	369	23	0	64

NUT & SEED PRODUCTS

FOOD	AMOUNT	CALORIES (kcal)	PROTEIN (g)	FAT (g)	CARBO-HYDRATES (g)	FIBER (g)
NUTS (continued)						
Coconut meat (continued)						
dried, sweetened, flaked, packaged	7-oz pkg	944	6.52	63.98	94.7	4.17
dried, sweetened, shredded	7-oz pkg	997	5.73	70.62	94.8	4.33
dried, toasted	1 oz	168	1.51	13.35	12.6	0.68
Coconut cream						
raw	1 tbsp	49	0.54	5.20	1.0	
canned, sweetened	1 tbsp	36	0.51	3.37	1.5	
Coconut milk						
raw	1 tbsp	35	0.34	3.58	0.8	
canned	1 tbsp	30	0.30	3.20	0.4	
frozen	1 tbsp	30	0.24	3.12	0.8	
Coconut water	1 tbsp	3	0.11	0.03	0.5	0.00
Filberts or hazelnuts						
dried, unblanched	1 oz	179	3.70	17.79	4.3	1.08
dried, blanched	1 oz	191	3.61	19.11	4.5	0.51
dry roasted, unblanched	1 oz	188	2.84	18.83	5.0	1.12
oil roasted, unblanched	1 oz	187	4.05	18.06	5.4	0.71
Formulated, wheat-based						
unflavored (uncolored, salted)	1 oz	177	3.92	16.39	6.7	0.23
flavored, macadamia flavored	1 oz	176	3.18	16.05	7.9	0.17
flavored, all other flavors	1 oz	184	3.72	17.69	5.9	0.28
Ginkgo nuts						
raw	1 oz	52	1.23	0.48	10.6	0.14
dried	1 oz	99	2.94	0.57	20.5	0.28
canned	1 oz	32	0.65	0.46	6.2	0.46
Hickory nuts, dried	1 oz	187	3.61	18.28	5.1	0.92
Macadamia nuts						
dried	1 oz	199	2.36	20.94	3.9	1.50
oil roasted	1 oz	204	2.06	21.73	3.6	0.49
Mixed nuts						
dry roasted, w/ peanuts	1 oz	169	4.91	14.61	7.2	0.26
oil roasted, w/ peanuts	1 oz	175	4.76	16.00	6.0	0.61
oil roasted w/out peanuts	1 oz	175	4.41	15.95	6.3	0.63
Peanut kernels						
dried	1 oz	161	7.29	13.97	4.6	1.39
oil roasted	1 oz	165	7.60	13.97	5.2	0.68
Peanut butter, smooth type	1 tbsp	95	4.56	8.18	2.5	0.53
Peanut flour, defatted	1 tbsp	13	2.09	0.02	1.3	0.16
Pecans						
dried	1 oz	190	2.20	19.21	5.1	0.45
dry roasted	1 oz	187	2.26	18.35	6.3	0.47
oil roasted	1 oz	195	1.97	20.22	4.5	0.46
Pecan flour	1 oz	93	9.05	0.41	14.4	0.43
Pilinuts-Canarytree, dried	1 oz	204	3.07	22.59	1.1	0.80
Pine nuts						
Pignolia, dried	1 oz	146	6.82	14.40	4.0	0.23
Pinyon, dried	1 oz	161	3.29	17.32	5.4	1.34

FOOD	CALCIUM (mg)	IRON (mg)	POTAS-SIUM (mg)	SODIUM (mg)	CHOLES-TEROI (mg)	% OF CALORIES FROM FAT
NUTS (continued)						
Coconut meat (continued)						
dried, sweetened, flaked, packaged	28	3.58	629	509	0	61
dried, sweetened, shredded	30	3.81	670	522	0	64
dried, toasted	8	0.96	157	11	0	72
Coconut cream						
raw	2	0.34	49	1	0	96
canned, sweetened	0	0.10	19	10	0	84
Coconut milk						
raw	2	0.25	39	2	0	92
canned	3	0.50	33	2	0	96
frozen	1	0.12	35	2	0	94
Coconut water	4	0.04	38	16	0	9
Filberts or hazelnuts						
dried, unblanched	53	0.93	126	1	0	89
dried, blanched	55	0.96	131	1	0	90
dry roasted, unblanched	55	0.96	131	1	0	90
oil roasted, unblanched	56	0.97	132	1	0	87
Formulated, wheat-based						
unflavored (uncolored, salted)	7	0.68	90	143	0	83
flavored, macadamia flavored	6	0.57	74	13	0	82
flavored, all other flavors	6	0.74	91	26	0	87
Ginkgo nuts						
raw	1	0.28	145	2	0	8
dried	6	0.45	283	4	0	5
canned	1	0.08	51	87	0	13
Hickory nuts, dried	17	0.60	124	0	0	88
Macadamia nuts						
dried	20	0.68	104	1	0	95
oil roasted	13	0.51	94	2	0	96
Mixed nuts						
dry roasted, w/ peanuts	20	1.05	169	3	0	78
oil roasted, w/ peanuts	31	0.91	165	3	0	82
oil roasted w/out peanuts	30	0.73	154	3	0	82
Peanut kernels						
dried	17	0.92	204	5	0	78
oil roasted	24	0.54	200	4	0	76
Peanut butter, smooth type	5	0.29	110	3	0	77
Peanut flour, defatted	6	0.08	52	1	0	1
Pecans						
dried	10	0.60	111	0	0	91
dry roasted	10	0.62	105	0	0	88
oil roasted	10	0.60	102	0	0	93
Pecan flour	9	0.56	95	0	0	4
Pilinuts-Canarytree, dried	41	1.00	144	1	0	100
Pine nuts						
Pignolia, dried	7	2.61	170	1	0	89
Pinyon, dried	2	0.87	178	20	0	97

NUT & SEED PRODUCTS

FOOD	AMOUNT	CALORIES (kcal)	PROTEIN (g)	FAT (g)	CARBO-HYDRATES (g)	FIBER (g)
NUTS (continued)						
Pistachio nuts						
dried	1 oz	164	5.84	13.74	7.0	0.53
dry roasted	1 oz	172	4.24	15.00	7.8	0.51
Soybean kernels, roasted & toasted	1 oz	129	10.51	6.80	8.6	1.01
Walnuts						
Black, dried	1 oz	172	6.91	16.07	3.4	1.83
English or Persian, dried	1 oz	182	4.06	17.57	5.2	1.31
SEEDS						
Breadfruit seeds						
raw	1 oz	54	2.10	1.59	8.3	0.48
boiled	1 oz	48	1.51	0.65	9.0	0.51
roasted	1 oz	59	1.76	0.77	11.3	0.62
Breadnut tree seeds						
raw	1 oz	62	1.69	0.28	13.1	0.72
dried	1 oz	104	2.45	0.48	22.5	1.59
Chia seeds, dried	1 oz	134	4.72	7.46	13.6	7.19
Cottonseed kernels, roasted	1 tbsp	51	3.26	3.63	2.1	0.20
Cottonseed flour						
partially defatted	1 tbsp	18	2.05	0.31	2.0	0.10
low-fat	1 oz	94	14.15	0.40	10.2	0.69
Cottonseed meal, partially defatted	1 oz	104	13.94	1.35	10.9	0.69
Lotus seeds						
raw	1 oz	25	1.17	0.15	4.9	0.18
dried	1 oz	94	4.38	0.56	18.3	0.69
Pumpkin & squash seeds						
whole, roasted	1 oz	127	5.27	5.51	15.2	10.20
kernels, dried	1 oz	154	6.97	13.02	5.0	0.63
kernels, roasted	1 oz	148	9.36	11.96	3.8	0.51
Safflower seed kernels, dried	1 oz	147	4.59	10.92	9.7	0.70
Safflower seed meal, partially defatted	1 oz	97	10.11	0.68	13.8	2.16
Sesame seeds, whole						
dried	1 tbsp	52	1.60	4.47	2.1	0.41
roasted & toasted	1 oz	161	4.82	13.63	7.3	2.41
Sesame seed kernels						
dried	1 tbsp	47	2.11	4.38	0.7	0.24
toasted	1 oz	161	4.82	13.63	7.4	1.42
Sesame butter						
paste	1 oz	169	5.14	14.45	7.2	1.55
tahini, from raw & stone ground kernels	1 oz	162	5.06	13.63	7.4	1.42
tahini, from unroasted kernels	1 oz	173	5.10	16.03	5.0	0.86
tahini, from roasted & toasted kernels	1 oz	169	4.83	15.27	6.0	1.42

FOOD	CALCIUM (mg)	IRON (mg)	POTAS-SIUM (mg)	SODIUM (mg)	CHOLES-TEROI (mg)	% OF CALORIES FROM FAT
NUTS (continued)						
Pistachio nuts						
dried	38	1.92	310	2	0	75
dry roasted	20	0.90	275	2	0	78
Soybean kernels, roasted & toasted	39	1.26	417	1	0	47
Walnuts						
Black, dried	16	0.87	149	0	0	84
English or Persian, dried	27	0.69	142	3	0	87
SEEDS						
Breadfruit seeds						
raw	10	1.04			0	27
boiled	17	0.17			0	12
roasted	24	0.26			0	12
Breadnut tree seeds						
raw	28	0.59			0	4
dried	27	1.31			0	4
Chia seeds, dried	150	2.84			0	50
Cottonseed kernels, roasted	10	0.54	135	3	0	64
Cottonseed flour						
partially defatted	24	0.63	89	2	0	16
low-fat	135	3.57	500	10	0	4
Cottonseed meal, partially defatted	143	3.79	531	10	0	12
Lotus seeds						
raw	12	0.27	104	0	0	5
dried	46	1.00	389	1	0	5
Pumpkin & squash seeds						
whole, roasted	16	0.94	261	5	0	39
kernels, dried	12	4.25	229	5	0	76
kernels, roasted	12	4.24	229	5	0	73
Safflower seed kernels, dried	22				0	67
Safflower seed meal, partially defatted	22				0	6
Sesame seeds, whole						
dried	88	1.31	42	1	0	77
roasted & toasted	281	4.19	135	3	0	76
Sesame seed kernels						
dried	10	0.62	33	3	0	84
toasted	37	2.21	115	11	0	76
Sesame butter						
paste	273	5.45	165	3	0	77
tahini, from raw & stone ground kernels	119	0.71	118	21	0	76
tahini, from unroasted kernels	40	1.80	130	0	0	83
tahini, from roasted & toasted kernels	121	2.54	118	33	0	81

NUT & SEED PRODUCTS

FOOD	AMOUNT	CALORIES (kcal)	PROTEIN (g)	FAT (g)	CARBO-HYDRATES (g)	FIBER (g)
NUTS (continued)						
Sesame flour, made from sesame seed kernels						
high-fat	1 oz	149	8.74	10.54	7.5	1.81
partially defatted	1 oz	109	11.45	3.38	9.9	1.71
low-fat	1 oz	95	14.24	0.50	10.0	1.42
Sesame meal, partially defatted	1 oz	161	4.82	13.63	7.4	1.14
Sisymbrium sp. seeds, whole, dried	1 oz	90	3.45	1.31	16.5	8.43
Sunflower seed kernels						
dried	1 oz	162	6.47	14.08	5.3	1.18
dry roasted	1 oz	165	5.49	14.14	6.8	0.51
oil roasted	1 oz	175	6.07	16.32	4.1	0.51
toasted	1 oz	176	4.89	16.13	5.8	0.52
Sunflower seed butter	1 oz	165	5.58	13.56	7.7	0.43
Sunflower seed flour, partially defatted	1 tbsp	16	2.40	0.08	1.7	0.26
Watermelon seed kernels, dried	1 oz	158	8.05	13.45	4.3	0.86

FOOD	CALCIUM (mg)	IRON (mg)	POTAS- SIUM (mg)	SODIUM (mg)	CHOLES- TEROI (mg)	% OF CALORIES FROM FAT
NUTS (continued)						
Sesame flour, made from sesame seed kernels						
high-fat	45	4.31	120	12	0	64
partially defatted	43	4.06	121	12	0	28
low-fat	42	4.04	113	11	0	5
Sesame meal, partially defatted	43	4.13	115	11	0	76
Sisymbrium sp. seeds, whole, dried	464	0.03	605	26	0	13
Sunflower seed kernels						
dried	33	1.92	196	1	0	78
dry roasted	20	1.08	241	1	0	77
oil roasted	16	1.90	137	1	0	84
toasted	16	1.93	139	1	0	82
Sunflower seed butter	35	1.35	20	1	0	74
Sunflower seed flour, partially defatted	6	0.33	3	0	0	5
Watermelon seed kernels, dried	15	2.07	184	28	0	77

SOUPS & SAUCES

FOOD	AMOUNT	CALO-RIES (kcal)	PROTEIN (g)	FAT (g)	MONO-UN-SATURATED FAT (g)	POLY-UN-SATURATED FAT (g)	SATU-RATED FAT (g)
Catsup, tomato	1 tbsp	15	0.00	0.00	0.00	0.00	0.00
Heinz®							
lite	1 tbsp	8	0.20	0.00	0.00	0.00	0.00
low sodium	1 tbsp	8	0.20	0.00	0.00	0.00	0.00
Hunt's®	100 g	115	1.08	0.13	0.03	0.07	0.03
bottle	100 g	114	1.27	0.15	0.03	0.09	0.03
bag in box	100 g	115	1.16	0.14			
Dip							
Fritos® jalapeno bean	1 oz	33	1.50	1.10	0.28	0.67	0.15
Kraft®							
bacon & horseradish	1 tbsp	30	0.50	2.50			
buttermilk	1 tbsp	40	0.50	3.50			
clam	1 tbsp	30	0.50	2.00			
French onion	1 tbsp	30	0.50	2.00			
garlic	1 tbsp	30	0.50	2.00			
green onion	1 tbsp	25	0.50	2.00			
guacamole	1 tbsp	25	0.50	2.00			
jalapeno pepper	1 tbsp	25	0.50	2.00			
nacho cheese	1 tbsp	28	1.00	2.00			1.00
Horseradish	1 tbsp	6	0.20	0.00	0.00	0.00	0.00
Mustard							
yellow	1 tsp	5	0.10	0.10	0.00	0.00	0.00
brown	1 cup	228	14.80	15.80			
Featherweight® low sodium	1 tsp	4	0.20	0.20			
Grey Poupon® Dijon	100 g	126	6.29	6.29			
Relish, corn, Legout®	1 oz	40	0.50	0.00	0.00	0.00	0.00
Relish, hamburger	1 tbsp	19	0.09	0.08	0.04	0.02	0.01
Heinz®	1 oz	30	0.00	0.00	0.00	0.00	0.00
Vlasic®	1 oz	40	0.00	0.00	0.00	0.00	0.00
Relish, hot dog	1 tbsp	14	0.23	0.07	0.04	0.02	0.01
Heinz®	1 oz	35	0.00	0.00	0.00	0.00	0.00
Vlasic®	1 oz	40	0.00	1.00	0.14	0.06	0.02
Relish, pepper, Legout®	1 oz	35	0.00	0.00	0.00	0.00	0.00
Relish, pickle							
Heinz® dill	1 oz	2	0.00	0.00	0.00	0.00	0.00
Vlasic®							
hot piccalilli	1 oz	35	0.00	0.00	0.00	0.00	0.00
India	1 oz	30	0.00	0.00	0.00	0.00	0.00
Relish, pickle, sweet	1 tbsp	19	0.06	0.07	0.03	0.02	0.01
cut or chopped	1 cup	193	0.70	0.84	0.24	0.14	0.20
Vlasic®	1 oz	30	0.00	0.00	0.00	0.00	0.00
Relish, sour, cut or chopped	1 cup	27	0.98	1.26	0.78	0.27	0.08

SOUPS, Canned (condensed, unless otherwise indicated)

FOOD	AMOUNT	CALO-RIES (kcal)	PROTEIN (g)	FAT (g)	MONO-UN-SATURATED FAT (g)	POLY-UN-SATURATED FAT (g)	SATU-RATED FAT (g)
Asparagus, cream of	10¾ oz	210	5.55	9.94	2.30	4.46	2.50
prepared w/milk	10¾ oz	392	15.33	19.87	5.03	5.44	8.08
Campbell's®	1 oz	20	0.50	0.99	0.18	0.24	0.25
Bean w/bacon	11½ oz	420	19.16	14.42	5.29	4.42	3.71
Campbell's®	1 oz	35	1.50	1.00	0.24	0.20	0.17
Healthy Choice	1 serving	140	6.00	4.00			
less salt	1 oz	35	1.50	1.00			

FOOD	CARBO-HYDRATES (mg)	FIBER (mg)	CALCIUM (mg)	IRON (mg)	POTAS-SIUM (mg)	SODIUM (mg)	CHOLES-TEROL (mg)	% OF CALORIES FROM FAT
Catsup, tomato	4.0	0.24	3	0.10	54	156	0	0
Heinz®								
lite	2.0		7	0.10	54	110	0	0
low sodium	2.0		7	0.10	54	90	0	0
Hunt's®	29.4	1.60	20	1.13	363	1139	0	1
bottle	28.7	1.60	20	1.32	363	1197	0	1
bag in box	29.0		25	1.22		1134		1
Dip								
Fritos® jalapeno bean	2.9	1.90	7	0.39	77	163	1	30
Kraft®								
bacon & horseradish	1.5					100	0	75
buttermilk	1.0					135	3	79
clam	1.5					115	5	60
French onion	1.5					120	0	60
garlic	1.5					80	0	60
green onion	1.5					85	0	72
guacamole	1.5					108	0	72
jalapeno pepper	1.5					80	0	72
nacho cheese	1.0		20		30	100	5	65
Horseradish	1.4	0.30	9	0.10	44	165	0	0
Mustard								
yellow	0.1	0.06	4	0.10	7	65	0	18
brown	13.3	2.10	310	4.50	325	3268	0	62
Featherweight® low sodium	0.3		4	0.10	7	1	0	45
Grey Poupon® Dijon	6.2	0.84	20	0.00	157	2516	0	45
Relish, corn, Legout®	9.5		0	0.54	40	115	0	0
Relish, hamburger	5.1		1	0.17	11	164	0	4
Heinz®	7.0		6	0.19		325	0	0
Vlasic®	9.0		0	0.00		255	0	0
Relish, hot dog	3.5		1	0.19	12	164	0	5
Heinz®	8.0		6	0.19		200	0	0
Vlasic®	8.0	0.43	0	0.36	57	255	0	23
Relish, pepper, Legout®	8.0		0	2.70	48	120	0	0
Relish, pickle								
Heinz® dill	1.0	0.54	0	0.00	57	415	0	0
Vlasic®								
hot piccalilli	8.0	0.43	0	0.00	57	165	0	0
India	8.0	0.54	0	0.00	57	205	0	0
Relish, pickle, sweet	5.2		0	0.13	4	122	0	3
cut or chopped	47.6	2.66	28	1.40	280	997	0	4
Vlasic®	8.0	0.54	0	0.00	57	220	0	0
Relish, sour, cut or chopped	3.7	2.66	41	0.42	280	1894	0	43
SOUPS, Canned (condensed, unless otherwise indicated)								
Asparagus, cream of	25.9	1.83	70	1.95	421	2385	12	43
prepared w/milk	39.8	1.81	424	2.10	872	2528	54	46
Campbell's®	2.5	0.07	5	0.09	31	205	2	45
Bean w/bacon	55.3	4.24	196	4.97	978	2311	6	31
Campbell's®	5.2	0.96	15	0.45	45	210	0	26
Healthy Choice	22.0		60	1.80	500	470	5	26
less salt	5.2		15	0.45		118		26

SOUPS & SAUCES

FOOD	AMOUNT	CALO-RIES (kcal)	PROTEIN (g)	FAT (g)	MONO-UN-SATURATED FAT (g)	POLY-UN-SATURATED FAT (g)	SATU-RATED FAT (g)
SOUPS, Canned (continued)							
Bean w/frankfurters	11¼ oz	454	24.24	16.94	6.64	3.99	5.14
Bean w/ham, chunky, ready to serve	19¼ oz	519	28.34	19.11	8.62	2.14	7.49
Campbell's®							
bacon & ham, microwave	1 oz	31	1.07	0.67	0.24	0.20	0.17
ham, chunky	1 oz	26	1.27	0.82	0.19	0.07	0.19
ham'n butter, chunky	1 oz	26	1.12	0.93			
ham, homestyle	1 oz	19	1.30	0.37	0.15	0.12	0.10
homestyle	1 oz	32	1.50	0.25	0.10	0.07	0.08
Beef, Campbell's®	1 oz	20	1.25	0.50			
chunky, ready to serve	1 oz	19	1.40	1.25	0.19	0.04	0.17
country vegetable	1 serving	170	12.00	4.00	0.89	0.13	0.94
vegetable, pasta, homestyle	1 oz	13	1.12	0.19	0.08	0.03	0.08
Beef broth or bouillon	6 g	14	0.96	0.53	0.22	0.02	0.27
ready to serve	14 oz	27	4.53	0.87	0.37	0.04	0.44
Campbell's®	1 oz	4	0.75	0.00	0.00	0.00	0.00
Health Valley® fat free	1 oz	1	0.15	0.15			
Swanson® canned	1 oz	2	0.28	0.14	0.07	0.03	0.04
Beef, chunky, ready to serve	19 oz	383	26.33	11.55	4.81	0.46	5.73
Beef noodle	10¾ oz	204	11.74	7.49	3.01	1.18	2.79
Campbell's®	1 oz	17	1.00	0.75	0.15	0.03	0.15
homestyle	1 oz	20	1.25	1.00	0.15	0.03	0.15
microwave	1 oz	96	4.43	1.48	0.15	0.03	0.15
Bean, black	11 oz	285	15.07	4.12	1.51	1.27	1.06
prepared w/water	11 oz	282	13.69	3.66	1.32	1.14	0.96
Health Valley®							
fat free	1 oz	9	1.20	0.13	0.01	0.06	0.04
natural	1 oz	20	0.93	0.4	0.06	0.05	0.05
Broccoli, cream of, Campbell's®	1 oz	20	0.25	1.25	0.48	0.27	0.49
w/milk	1 oz	17	0.62	0.87			
Cauliflower	1 cup	68	2.89	1.72	0.74	0.65	0.26
Celery, cream of	10¾ oz	219	4.03	13.59	3.14	6.09	3.41
prepared w/milk	10¾ oz	400	13.81	23.51	5.98	6.44	9.60
Campbell's®	1 oz	25	0.50	1.75	0.22	0.30	0.31
Cheddar cheese	11 oz	377	13.17	25.43	7.20	0.72	16.18
prepared w/milk	11 oz	558	22.93	35.33	9.95	1.07	22.13
Campbell's®	1 oz	27	1.00	1.50	0.45	0.05	1.00
Chicken							
& dumplings	10½ oz	236	13.65	13.44	6.15	3.16	3.19
broth	10¾ oz	94	13.48	3.17	1.42	0.66	0.95
broth prepared w/water	10¾ oz	95	11.98	3.37	1.54	0.71	1.01
cream of	10¾ oz	283	8.33	17.89	7.97	3.62	5.05
cream of, prepared w/milk	10¾ oz	464	18.11	27.79	10.81	3.97	11.23
chunky, ready to serve	10¾ oz	216	15.43	8.05	3.61	1.69	2.40
gumbo	10¾ oz	137	6.41	3.48	1.59	0.85	0.79
noodle	10½ oz	182	9.62	5.52	2.46	1.22	1.45
noodle, prepared w/water	10½ oz	182	9.83	5.96	2.70	1.35	1.58
noodle w/meatballs, ready to serve	20 oz	227	18.54	8.16	3.66	1.71	2.44

FOOD	CARBO-HYDRATES (mg)	FIBER (mg)	CALCIUM (mg)	IRON (mg)	POTAS-SIUM (mg)	SODIUM (mg)	CHOLES-TEROL (mg)	% OF CALORIES FROM FAT
SOUPS, Canned (continued)								
Bean w/frankfurters	53.4	4.15	210	5.68	1158	2651	29	34
Bean w/ham, chunky, ready to serve	60.9		177	7.26		2184	49	33
Campbell's®								
bacon & ham, microwave	5.0	0.96	8	0.24	45	111	0	20
ham, chunky	3.4	0.48	9	0.25	36	101	1	28
ham'n butter, chunky	3.1		4	0.17		110		32
ham, homestyle	2.7	0.96	6	0.28	45	93	0	17
homestyle	6.2	0.96	15	0.36	40	175	0	7
Beef, Campbell's®	2.5		0	0.18		208		22
chunky, ready to serve	2.2	0.18	2	0.17	30	102	6	60
country vegetable	21.0	0.54	19	1.24	191	960	5	21
vegetable, pasta, homestyle	1.6	0.07	2	0.17	16	98	1	13
Beef broth or bouillon	1.4	0.01	4		27	1019	1	34
ready to serve	0.0	Trace	25	0.67	214	1294	1	29
Campbell's®	0.2	0.00	0	0.00	15	205	0	0
Health Valley® fat free	0.2	0.00	0	0.00	12	1	0	90
Swanson® canned	0.1	0.00	0	0.00	24	103	0	50
Beef, chunky, ready to serve	43.9	1.62	69	5.20	755	1947	32	27
Beef noodle	21.8	0.31	36	2.67	241	2313	12	33
Campbell's®	1.7	0.17	0	0.20	57	208	5	39
homestyle	1.7	0.17	0	0.18	57	203	5	45
microwave	16.9	0.17	15	1.07	57	939	5	14
Bean, black	48.1		110	4.68	780	3026	0	13
prepared w/water	48.1	3.18	110	5.24	663	2910	0	12
Health Valley®								
fat free	1.2	2.27	8	0.60	112	39	0	13
natural	3.1	2.25	8	0.60	41	3	0	18
Broccoli, cream of, Campbell's®	2.0	0.22	5	0.09	43	198	3	56
w/milk	1.7	0.11	19	0.05	21	106		45
Cauliflower	10.7	0.19				841	Trace	23
Celery, cream of	21.4	0.92	98	1.52	299	2308	34	56
prepared w/milk	35.2	0.92	451	1.67	751	2451	78	53
Campbell's®	2.0	0.09	5	0.00	25	205	3	63
Cheddar cheese	25.5		345	1.81	374	2331	72	61
prepared w/milk	39.3		698	1.95	826	2474	116	57
Campbell's®	2.5	0.11	25	0.09	39	203	5	49
Chicken								
& dumplings	14.6		35	1.52	283	2093	80	51
broth	2.2	Trace	17	1.25	519	1909	3	30
broth prepared w/water	2.2	Trace	21	1.23	510	1886	2	32
cream of	22.5	0.31	83	1.47	212	2397	24	57
cream of, prepared w/milk	36.3	0.31	437	1.62	664	2540	66	54
chunky, ready to serve	20.9	0.31	29	2.10	214	1078	37	34
gumbo	20.3	0.61	59	2.17	183	2321	9	23
noodle	22.7	0.30	32	1.84	134	2257	15	27
noodle, prepared w/water	22.7	0.59	41	1.89	135	2692	18	29
noodle w/meatballs, ready to serve	19.1	1.25	69	3.97		2376	23	32

SOUPS & SAUCES

FOOD	AMOUNT	CALO-RIES (kcal)	PROTEIN (g)	FAT (g)	MONO-UN-SATURATED FAT (g)	POLY-UN-SATURATED FAT (g)	SATU-RATED FAT (g)
SOUPS, Canned (continued)							
Chicken (continued)							
rice	10½ oz	146	8.60	4.65	2.21	1.01	1.11
rice, chunky, ready to serve	19 oz	286	27.54	7.17	3.21	1.50	2.14
vegetable	10½ oz	181	8.77	6.91	3.10	1.45	2.07
Campbell's®							
alphabet	1 oz	20	0.75	0.75	0.13	0.07	0.08
barley	1 oz	17	0.75	0.50	0.03	0.01	0.03
broth	1 oz	7	0.25	0.50	0.07	0.03	0.05
broth, low salt	1 oz	3	0.29	0.10	0.00	0.00	0.00
broth, noodles	1 oz	11	0.25	0.25	0.12	0.06	0.07
chunky	1 oz	17	1.12	0.46	0.13	0.07	0.08
chunky, low sodium	1 cup	173	12.60	5.02			
chunky, ready to eat	1 cup	178	12.70	6.63	2.97	1.39	1.98
chicken chowder, chunky	1 oz	32	1.30	1.95	0.13	0.07	0.08
cream of	1 oz	27	0.50	1.75	0.51	0.19	0.53
cream of, less salt	1 oz	27	0.75	1.75			
country vegetable	1 serving	150	10.00	4.00	1.87	0.87	1.26
curly noodle	1 oz	20	0.75	0.75	0.13	0.07	0.08
dumplings	1 oz	20	1.00	0.75			
gumbo	1 oz	15	0.50	0.04	0.08	0.04	0.04
gumbo, sausage	1 oz	13	1.02	0.37	0.08	0.04	0.04
minestrone	1 oz	17	1.40	0.56			
mushroom, chunky	1 oz	26	1.14	1.81	0.58	0.65	0.58
mushroom, creamy	1 oz	30	0.75	2.00	0.58	0.65	0.58
noodle	1 oz	15	0.75	0.50	0.13	0.07	0.08
noodle, chunky	1 oz	19	1.30	0.65	0.13	0.07	0.08
noodle, Healthy Choice	1 serving	60	3.00	2.00			
noodle, hearty	1 serving	80	9.00	2.00			
noodle, homestyle	1 oz	17	0.75	0.75	0.13	0.07	0.08
noodle, less salt	1 oz	15	0.75	0.50			
noodle, microwave	1 oz	104	5.18	2.22	0.13	0.07	0.08
noodle, mushroom	1 serving	180	12.00	7.00	2.07	2.59	2.34
nuggets, chunky	1 oz	18	1.02	0.56	0.13	0.07	0.08
rice	1 oz	15	0.50	0.75	0.11	0.05	0.05
rice, chunky	1 oz	15	1.05	0.42	0.17	0.08	0.11
rice, Healthy Choice	1 serving	60	2.00	2.00			
rice, homestyle	1 oz	14	1.30	0.09	0.04	0.02	0.03
rice, less salt	1 oz	15	0.50	0.75			
vegetable	1 oz	17	0.75	0.75	0.33	0.16	0.22
vegetable, chunky	1 oz	18	1.05	0.63	0.30	0.14	0.20
& stars	1 oz	15	0.75	0.50	0.13	0.07	0.08
Health Valley®							
broth	1 oz	3	0.58	0.15			
natural broth	1 oz	5	0.58	0.23	0.07	0.03	0.05
Swanson's®							
broth, canned	1 oz	4	0.28	0.28	0.13	0.06	0.08
broth, clear, canned	1 oz	3	0.28	0.14	0.07	0.03	0.04
stew, canned	1 oz	21	1.18	0.92	0.33	0.16	0.22

FOOD	CARBO-HYDRATES (mg)	FIBER (mg)	CALCIUM (mg)	IRON (mg)	POTAS-SIUM (mg)	SODIUM (mg)	CHOLES-TEROL (mg)	% OF CALORIES FROM FAT
SOUPS, Canned (continued)								
Chicken (continued)								
rice	17.4	0.30	42	1.82	244	1980	15	29
rice, chunky, ready to serve	29.1		78	4.20		1994	27	23
vegetable	20.8	0.30	43	2.13	374	2297	21	34
Campbell's®								
alphabet	2.5	0.09	0	0.18	7	200	1	34
barley	2.5	0.22	0	0.09	18	213	0	26
broth	0.5	0.00	0	0.00	24	178	0	60
broth, low salt	0.1		2	0.07		8	0	30
broth, noodles	2.0	0.09	0	0.00	7	215	1	20
chunky	1.9	0.09	4	0.13	7	113	1	25
chunky, low sodium	15.1		28	1.76	264	78		26
chunky, ready to eat	17.3	0.75	24	1.73	176	887	30	34
chicken chowder, chunky	2.1	0.09	2	0.13	7	112	1	56
cream of	2.2	0.03	5	0.00	31	203	3	57
cream of, less salt	2.2		5	0.00		118	1	57
country vegetable	19.0	1.61	27	1.86	188	1080	32	24
curly noodle	2.7	0.09	0	0.18	7	200	1	34
dumplings	2.2		0	0.09		240		34
gumbo	2.0	0.23	5	0.00	9	225	1	2
gumbo, sausage	1.4	0.23	6	0.17	9	101	1	26
minestrone	1.5		6	0.17		88		30
mushroom, chunky	1.2	0.03	2	0.10	48	122	14	63
mushroom, creamy	2.0	0.03	5	0.09	48	230	14	60
noodle	2.0	0.09	0	0.09	7	225	1	30
noodle, chunky	1.8	0.09	2	0.17	7	106	1	32
noodle, Healthy Choice	8.0		0	0.72	270	460	15	30
noodle, hearty	7.0		20	1.08	400	470	25	23
noodle, homestyle	2.0	0.09	0	9.98	7	220	1	39
noodle, less salt	2.0		0	0.09		110	4	30
noodle, microwave	16.2	0.09	0	1.07	7	991	1	19
noodle, mushroom	18.0	2.36	88	2.70	294	1010	97	35
nuggets, chunky	2.2	0.09	4	0.13	7	98	1	28
rice	1.7	0.09	0	0.00	12	198	1	45
rice, chunky	1.6	0.11	4	0.08	13	112	1	26
rice, Healthy Choice	7.0		0	0.36	180	480	10	30
rice, homestyle	0.9	0.09	2	0.10	43	101	6	6
rice, less salt	1.7		0	0.00		120	2	45
vegetable	2.0	0.17	0	0.20	20	213	3	39
vegetable, chunky	2.0	0.17	2	0.11	20	114	3	32
& stars	1.7	0.09	0	0.09	7	218	1	30
Health Valley®								
broth	0.1	0.00	0	0.05	17	42	0	45
natural broth	0.1	0.00	0	0.05	17	0	0	41
Swanson's®								
broth, canned	0.2	0.06	0	0.00	20	124	2	60
broth, clear, canned	0.1	0.17	0	0.00	13	80	1	45
stew, canned	1.9	0.17	3	0.09	20	130	3	39

SOUPS & SAUCES

FOOD	AMOUNT	CALO-RIES (kcal)	PROTEIN (g)	FAT (g)	MONO-UN-SATURATED FAT (g)	POLY-UN-SATURATED FAT (g)	SATU-RATED FAT (g)
SOUPS, Canned (continued)							
Chili beef	11¼ oz	411	16.24	16.04	6.71	0.64	7.99
Campbell's®	1 oz	35	1.25	1.25	0.32	0.03	0.38
chunky	1 oz	26	1.91	0.64	0.31	0.05	0.28
microwave	1 oz	25	0.93	0.53	0.23	0.02	0.28
Clam chowder, Manhattan	10¾ oz	187	5.31	5.37	0.93	3.09	0.99
chunky, ready to serve	19 oz	299	16.28	7.60	2.19	0.28	4.73
prepared w/water	10¾ oz	190	10.16	5.62	1.01	3.20	1.07
Campbell's®	1 oz	17	0.50	0.50	0.08	0.08	0.15
chunky	1 oz	15	0.65	0.37	0.08	0.08	0.15
Clam chowder, New England	10¾ oz	214	13.21	6.10	2.62	2.29	0.91
prepared w/water	10¾ oz	230	11.69	7.00	2.97	2.67	1.01
prepared w/milk	10¾ oz	396	22.97	16.03	5.48	2.62	7.16
Campbell's®	1 serving	250	7.00	15.00	2.45	1.18	3.20
chunky	1 oz	27	0.84	1.58	0.26	0.13	0.34
w/milk	1 oz	37	1.75	1.75	0.26	0.13	0.34
Health Valley® natural	1 oz	13	0.93	0.27	0.09	0.03	0.15
Consomme, with gelatin	10½ oz	71	13.02	0.00	0.00	0.00	0.00
canned, prepared w/water	1 cup	29	5.35	0.00	0.00	0.00	0.00
Campbell's® condensed	1 oz	6	1.00	0.00	0.00	0.00	0.00
Corn							
Campbell's® low sodium	1 serving	191	3.00	5.00			
Health Valley® country corn, fat free	1 oz	9	0.53	0.13			
Crab, ready to serve	13 oz	114	8.30	2.29	1.02	0.60	0.57
Creole style, chunky, Campbell's®	1 oz	22	1.02	0.74			
Escarole, ready to serve	19½ oz	61	3.43	4.04	1.81	0.85	1.21
Gazpacho, ready to serve	13 oz	87	13.14	3.39	0.82	1.99	0.43
Lentil w/ham, ready to serve	20 oz	320	21.18	6.35	2.94	0.73	2.56
Campbell's® hearty, homestyle	1 oz	16	1.02	0.19	0.09	0.04	0.06
Health Valley®							
& carrot	1 oz	9	1.07	0.13			
natural, no salt	1 oz	23	1.07	0.27			
Mediterranean, chunky, Campbell's®	1 oz	18	0.42	0.63	0.19	0.17	0.07
Minestrone	10½ oz	202	10.37	6.11	1.67	2.70	1.32
chunky, ready to serve	19 oz	285	11.46	6.32	2.06	0.58	3.34
Campbell's®	1 oz	20	0.75	0.50			
chunky	1 oz	17	0.63	0.42			
hearty minestrone, Healthy Choice	1 serving	90	4.00	3.00			
homestyle	1 oz	13	0.37	0.28			
Health Valley®							
fat free	1 oz	11	0.80	0.13			
natural, no salt	1 oz	17	0.80	0.40			
Mushroom	16.7 g	74	1.70	3.73	1.72	1.19	0.63
Mushroom, cream of	10¾ oz	313	4.91	23.09	4.40	10.84	6.26
prepared w/water	10¾ oz	314	5.65	21.80	4.15	10.26	5.93
prepared w/milk	10¾ oz	494	14.69	32.99	7.24	11.18	12.44
Mushroom w/beef stock Campbell's®	10¾ oz	208	7.66	9.79	3.42	1.90	3.78

FOOD	CARBO-HYDRATES (mg)	FIBER (mg)	CALCIUM (mg)	IRON (mg)	POTAS-SIUM (mg)	SODIUM (mg)	CHOLES-TEROL (mg)	% OF CALORIES FROM FAT
SOUPS, Canned (continued)								
Chili beef	52.1	3.51	105	5.18	1275	2513	32	35
Campbell's®	4.9	1.08	5	0.36	60	210	1	32
chunky	3.3	0.44	5	0.41	59	102	3	22
microwave	4.2	1.08	5	0.24	60	116	1	19
Clam chowder, Manhattan	29.7	0.92	56	3.97	458	2446	6	26
chunky, ready to serve	42.2	1.08	151	5.93	862	2245	32	23
prepared w/water	29.7	1.19	83	4.60	636	4394	6	27
Campbell's®	2.5	0.26	5	0.09	38	205	1	26
chunky	2.2	0.26	6	0.17	38	103	1	22
Clam chowder, New England	26.5		99	3.45	278	2266	12	26
prepared w/water	30.2	0.65	105	3.61	355	2221	12	27
prepared w/milk	40.3		453	3.59	729	2409	54	36
Campbell's®	22.0	1.61	202	1.61	325	1050	24	54
chunky	2.4	0.17	6	0.17	34	112	3	53
w/milk	4.2	0.17	25	0.18	34	233	3	42
Health Valley® natural	1.8	0.24	8	0.48	79	19	2	18
Consomme, with gelatin	4.2		21	1.28	373	1550	0	0
canned, prepared w/water	1.7		10	0.53	154	636	0	0
Campbell's® condensed	0.5		0	0.09		188	0	0
Corn								
Campbell's® low sodium	31.0		28	0.80	164	33		24
Health Valley® country corn, fat free	1.7	0.40	5	0.10	48	39	0	13
Crab, ready to serve	15.5	0.81	99	1.85	493	1866	10	18
Creole style, chunky, Campbell's®	2.8		6	0.17		85		30
Escarole, ready to serve	3.9	1.66	72	1.66		8618	6	60
Gazpacho, ready to serve	1.1	1.18	37	1.48	338	1790	0	35
Lentil w/ham, ready to serve	46.2	3.20	96	6.04	815	3014	17	18
Campbell's® hearty, homestyle	2.6	0.68	6	0.33	38	86	1	11
Health Valley®								
& carrot	1.3	2.00	8	0.60	85	39	0	13
natural, no salt	3.7	2.27	8	0.60	48	3	0	11
Mediterranean, chunky, Campbell's®	2.5	0.14	6	0.11	47	106	0	32
Minestrone	27.3	1.79	83	2.23	760	2217	3	27
chunky, ready to serve	46.5		136	3.97		1940	11	20
Campbell's®	3.2		5	0.18		225		22
chunky	2.5		8	0.19		91		23
hearty minestrone, Healthy Choice	13.0		40	0.72	540	430	2	30
homestyle	2.0		7	0.10		113		19
Health Valley®								
fat free	1.6	0.53	5	0.19	45	31	0	11
natural, no salt	2.5	1.67	8	0.24	35	15	0	21
Mushroom	8.5	0.06	51		153	782	0	45
Mushroom, cream of	22.5	0.61	78	1.28	203	2469	3	66
prepared w/water	22.5	1.13	111	1.25	244	2507	6	62
prepared w/milk	36.4	0.61	432	1.43	655	2612	48	60
Mushroom w/beef stock Campbell's®	22.6		25	2.04	384	2358	18	42

SOUPS & SAUCES

FOOD	AMOUNT	CALO-RIES (kcal)	PROTEIN (g)	FAT (g)	MONO-UN-SATURATED FAT (g)	POLY-UN-SATURATED FAT (g)	SATU-RATED FAT (g)
SOUPS, Canned (continued)							
Mushroom w/beef stock (continued)							
beefy mushroom	1 oz	15	1.00	0.75	0.34	0.10	0.32
cream of	1 oz	25	0.50	1.75	0.34	0.53	0.59
cream of, Healthy Choice	1 serving	60	1.00	2.00			
cream of, less salt	1 oz	25	0.50	1.75			
cream of, low salt	1 oz	20	0.29	1.33	0.20	0.21	0.28
cream of, low sodium	1 serving	210	3.00	14.00			
golden	1 oz	17	0.50	0.75	0.15	0.38	0.22
Health Valley®							
barley, natural	1 oz	13	0.67	0.27	0.03	0.01	0.03
Nacho cheese, Campbell's®	1 oz	27	1.00	2.00	0.46	0.05	1.03
w/milk	1 oz	45	2.00	3.00	0.46	0.05	1.03
Noodle, Campbell's®							
broth, microwave	1 oz	96	4.43	1.48	0.13	0.07	0.08
w/ground beef	1 oz	22	1.00	1.00	0.15	0.06	0.13
Onion	10½ oz	138	9.12	4.23	1.82	1.59	0.63
Campbell's®							
cream of	1 oz	25	0.50	1.25	0.37	0.18	0.46
cream of, prepared w/milk & water	1 oz	35	1.00	1.75	0.37	0.18	0.46
French onion	1 oz	15	0.50	0.50	0.09	0.08	0.03
Oyster stew	10½ oz	144	5.13	9.32	2.20	0.39	6.09
prepared w/milk	10½ oz	325	14.90	19.25	5.05	0.74	12.27
Campbell's®	1 oz	17	0.50	1.25	0.36	0.10	0.79
w/milk	1 oz	35	1.50	2.25	0.47	0.13	1.02
Pasta e Fagioli, home recipe	1 cup	194	8.69	4.98	3.06	0.61	0.92
Pea, green (including cream of pea)	11¼ oz	398	20.86	7.13	2.42	0.92	3.42
prepared w/milk	11¼ oz	579	30.62	17.05	5.30	1.26	9.71
split w/ham (including split pea)	11½ oz	459	25.03	10.69	4.37	1.54	4.28
chunky, ready to serve	19 oz	413	24.90	8.95	3.66	1.29	3.58
Campbell's®							
green pea	1 oz	40	2.00	0.75	0.11	0.04	0.16
split, ham, chunky	1 serving	21	1.12	0.56	0.19	0.07	0.19
split, ham, homestyle	1 oz	21	1.49	0.09	0.00	0.00	0.00
split, ham, bacon	1 oz	40	2.25	1.00	0.19	0.07	0.19
split, ham, bacon, low salt	1 oz	21	1.12	0.37	0.11	0.04	0.16
Health Valley®							
split pea, carrot, fat free	1 oz	7	0.67	0.13	0.01	0.06	0.02
split pea, natural	1 oz	12	1.20	0.13	0.05	0.02	0.07
Pepperpot	10½ oz	251	15.47	11.26	4.89	0.86	5.01
Campbell's®	1 oz	22	1.25	1.00	0.24	0.04	0.24
Pepper steak, chunky, Campbell's®	1 oz	17	1.30	0.28			
Potato, cream of	10¾ oz	178	4.24	5.73	1.34	1.01	2.96
prepared w/milk	10¾ oz	360	14.02	15.66	4.20	1.36	9.14
Campbell's®							
cream of	1 oz	20	0.25	0.75	0.07	0.05	0.14
cream of, w/milk & water	1 oz	30	0.75	1.00			
Health Valley® leek, natural	1 oz	17	0.53	0.27	0.07	0.05	0.14

FOOD	CARBO-HYDRATES (mg)	FIBER (mg)	CALCIUM (mg)	IRON (mg)	POTAS-SIUM (mg)	SODIUM (mg)	CHOLES-TEROL (mg)	% OF CALORIES FROM FAT
SOUPS, Canned (continued)								
Mushroom w/beef stock (continued)								
beefy mushroom	1.2	0.03	0	0.09	67	240	19	45
cream of	2.0	0.06	0	0.00	31	205	2	63
cream of, Healthy Choice	9.0		0	0.36	440	460	5	30
cream of, less salt	2.0		5	0.00		120	1	63
cream of, low salt	1.7	0.06	6	0.10	12	5	0	60
cream of, low sodium	18.0		60	1.08		55		60
golden	2.2	0.06	0	0.09	12	218	0	39
Health Valley®								
barley, natural	2.1	1.13	3	1.20	31	3	0	18
Nacho cheese, Campbell's®	2.0	0.11	10	0.00	39	185	5	65
w/milk	3.2	0.11	50	0.09	39	200	5	60
Noodle, Campbell's®								
broth, microwave	16.9	0.09	0	1.07	7	1005	1	14
w/ground beef	2.5	0.09	0	0.18	12	205	1	40
Onion	19.8	1.19	64	1.64	167	2563	0	28
Campbell's®								
cream of	3.0	0.09	5	0.00	35	208	4	45
cream of, prepared w/milk & water	3.7	0.09	20	0.09	35	215	4	45
French onion	2.2	0.11	5	0.09	8	225	0	30
Oyster stew	9.8		52	2.38	119	2384	33	58
prepared w/milk	23.7		406	2.53	571	2526	77	53
Campbell's®	1.2	0.00	0	0.36	52	210	10	64
w/milk	2.5	0.00	25	0.36	52	223	10	58
Pasta e Fagioli, home recipe	29.6		62	2.72	522	790	3	23
Pea, green (including cream of pea)	64.3	1.60	66	4.73	463	2397	0	16
prepared w/milk	78.1	1.60	420	4.88	914	2541	43	27
split w/ham (including split pea)	67.8	1.63	53	5.53	969	2446	20	21
chunky, ready to serve	60.1		74	4.80		2167	16	20
Campbell's®								
green pea	6.2	0.31	0	0.36	22	205	0	17
split, ham, chunky	3.0	0.48	2	0.17	36	100	1	23
split, ham, homestyle	3.5		4	0.25		122	0	4
split, ham, bacon	5.9	0.48	0	0.45	36	195	1	22
split, ham, bacon, low salt	3.4	0.09	4	0.17	22	3	0	16
Health Valley®								
split pea, carrot, fat free	1.0	0.40	8	0.24	79	39	0	18
split pea, natural	1.4	1.67	8	0.24	51	3	0	10
Pepperpot	22.8	1.19	57	2.18	370	2360	24	40
Campbell's®	2.2	0.06	5	0.18	18	243	1	40
Pepper steak, chunky, Campbell's®	2.2		2	0.17		98		15
Potato, cream of	27.8		48	1.16	332	2431	15	29
prepared w/milk	41.6		402	1.31	784	2574	54	39
Campbell's®								
cream of	3.0	0.06	0	0.00	16	218	1	34
cream of, w/milk & water	3.7		20	0.09		225		30
Health Valley® leek, natural	3.0	0.99	5	0.36	37	3	0	14

SOUPS & SAUCES

FOOD	AMOUNT	CALO-RIES (kcal)	PROTEIN (g)	FAT (g)	MONO-UN-SATURATED FAT (g)	POLY-UN-SATURATED FAT (g)	SATU-RATED FAT (g)
SOUPS, Canned (continued)							
Ramen, Campbell's®							
beef flavor	1 oz	127	3.32	5.32			
beef, low fat	1 oz	110	3.49	1.00			
beef, low fat, block	1 oz	107	3.32	0.67			
beef, vegetable	1 oz	123	2.73	4.54	.094	0.01	0.10
chicken flavor	1 oz	127	3.32	5.32	0.07	0.05	0.04
chicken, low fat	1 oz	102	3.25	0.93			
chicken, vegetable	1 oz	123	2.73	4.54	0.15	0.08	0.10
oriental flavor	1 oz	127	3.32	5.32	0.05	0.03	0.03
oriental flavor, low fat	1 oz	110	3.49	1.00	0.06	0.05	0.05
oriental flavor, vegetable	1 oz	123	2.73	4.54	0.10	0.09	0.03
pork flavor	1 oz	133	3.32	5.32	0.21	0.06	0.16
pork flavor, low fat, block	1 oz	100	2.67	0.67			
shrimp, low fat	1 oz	105	3.17	0.91			
shrimp, vegetable	1 oz	127	2.73	4.54	0.21	0.10	0.16
Ratatouille, home recipe	1 cup	266	2.41	24.60	17.90	2.22	3.34
Scotch broth	10½ oz	195	12.07	6.38	1.89	1.33	2.71
Campbell's®	1 oz	20	1.00	0.75	0.09	0.07	0.13
Shrimp, cream of	10¾ oz	219	6.77	12.63	3.64	0.47	7.86
prepared w/milk	10¾ oz	400	16.55	22.54	6.51	0.84	14.04
Campbell's®	1 oz	22	0.50	1.50	0.24	0.03	0.52
w/cream, milk	1 oz	40	1.25	2.50	0.68	0.41	0.68
Sirloin burger, Campbell's®							
chunky	1 oz	20	1.12	0.84			
country vegetable	1 serving	200	10.00	8.00	1.78	1.56	0.62
Steak & potato, chunky, Campbell's®	1 oz	19	1.30	0.46			
Stock pot	11 oz	242	11.82	9.48	2.47	4.27	2.10
Teddy Bear, Campbell's®	1 oz	17	0.75	0.50	0.13	0.07	0.08
Tomato	10¾ oz	208	5.00	4.67	1.04	2.33	0.88
beef w/noodle	10¾ oz	341	10.83	10.43	4.20	1.65	3.86
prepared w/milk	10¾ oz	389	14.78	14.59	3.89	2.68	7.07
rice	11 oz	291	5.13	6.61	1.47	3.29	1.25
Tomato bisque	11 oz	300	5.49	6.10	1.66	2.70	1.31
prepared w/milk	11 oz	481	15.27	16.02	4.54	3.00	7.61
Campbell's®	1 oz	22	0.25	0.50	0.08	0.12	0.12
bisque	1 oz	30	0.50	0.75	0.08	0.12	0.12
cream of, homestyle	1 oz	27	0.25	0.75	0.19	0.13	0.33
cream of, milk	1 oz	45	1.25	1.75	0.19	0.13	0.33
garden	1 oz	14	0.19	0.28	0.08	0.10	0.10
Healthy Choice	1 serving	90	1.00	2.00			
less salt	1 oz	22	0.25	0.50	0.05	0.11	0.04
less salt, milk	1 oz	37	1.25	1.00	0.05	0.11	0.04
low salt	1 oz	18	0.38	0.57	0.05	0.11	0.04
w/milk	1 oz	37	1.25	1.00	0.19	0.13	0.33
med/skim milk	1 serving	130	5.00	2.00			
rice, old fashioned	1 oz	27	0.25	0.50	0.12	0.27	0.11

FOOD	CARBO-HYDRATES (mg)	FIBER (mg)	CALCIUM (mg)	IRON (mg)	POTAS-SIUM (mg)	SODIUM (mg)	CHOLES-TEROL (mg)	% OF CALORIES FROM FAT
SOUPS, Canned (continued)								
Ramen, Campbell's®								
beef flavor	17.2		13	0.96		672		38
beef, low fat	21.9		10	0.90		799		8
beef, low fat, block	21.2		0	1.20		592		6
beef, vegetable	17.2	0.06	9	0.82	20	694	1	33
chicken flavor	17.2	0.09	13	1.20	1	646	0	38
chicken, low fat	20.4		9	0.84		697		8
chicken, vegetable	17.2	0.09	9	0.82	19	667	1	33
oriental flavor	17.2	0.09	13	1.20	6	619	0	38
oriental flavor, low fat	21.9	0.35	10	0.90	9	699	4	8
oriental flavor, vegetable	17.2	0.06	9	1.23	25	549	0	33
pork flavor	17.2	0.10	0	0.96	25	572	4	36
pork flavor, low fat, block	20.6		0	1.80		759		6
shrimp, low fat	20.4		9	1.23		585		8
shrimp, vegetable	18.1	0.24	9	0.82	28	540	13	32
Ratatouille, home recipe	11.8		56	1.27	485	329	0	83
Scotch broth	23.0		37	2.03	387	2461	12	29
Campbell's®	2.2	0.14	0	0.09	19	218	1	34
Shrimp, cream of	19.9		43	1.28		2373	40	52
prepared w/milk	33.7		397	1.43		2516	84	51
Campbell's®	2.0	0.03	0	0.00	18	203	3	60
w/cream, milk	3.2	0.02	37	0.09	51	215	16	56
Sirloin burger, Campbell's®								
chunky	2.1		4	0.25		115		37
country vegetable	21.0	1.35	62	1.83	444	1100	0	36
Steak & potato, chunky, Campbell's®	2.2		2	0.17		106		22
Stock pot	27.9	1.25	53	2.11	577	2546	9	35
Teddy Bear, Campbell's®	2.7	0.09	0	0.18	7	198	1	26
Tomato	40.3	1.22	32	4.27	641	2120	0	20
beef w/noodle	51.4		43	2.71	537	2230	9	28
prepared w/milk	54.1	1.20	386	4.41	1092	2263	42	34
rice	53.2	1.56	56	1.93	803	1981	3	20
Tomato bisque	57.6		98	1.99	1014	2546	11	18
prepared w/milk	71.4		452	2.13	1465	2689	53	30
Campbell's®	4.2	0.06	0	0.09	36	170	0	20
bisque	5.4	0.06	10	0.09	36	205	0	23
cream of, homestyle	4.9	0.06	0	0.09	51	203	2	25
cream of, milk	6.2	0.06	25	0.09	51	215	2	35
garden	2.7	0.06	7	0.17	36	86	0	18
Healthy Choice	17.0		0	0.36	220	430	0	20
less salt	4.2	0.06	0	0.09	31	108	0	20
less salt, milk	5.4	0.06	37	0.18	31	123	0	24
low salt	2.8	0.06	4	0.14	31	4	0	28
w/milk	5.4	0.06	37	0.18	51	185	2	24
med/skim milk	22.0		150	0.72	400	490	5	14
rice, old fashioned	5.4	0.37	0	0.09	73	183	0	16

SOUPS & SAUCES

FOOD	AMOUNT	CALO-RIES (kcal)	PROTEIN (g)	FAT (g)	MONO-UN-SATURATED FAT (g)	POLY-UN-SATURATED FAT (g)	SATU-RATED FAT (g)
SOUPS, Canned (continued)							
zesty	1 oz	25	0.25	0.50	0.08	0.12	0.12
Health Valley®							
natural	1 oz	17	0.40	0.40	0.08	0.12	0.12
vegetable, fat free	1 oz	7	0.67	0.13	0.03	0.01	0.04
Turkey							
chunky, ready to serve	18¾ oz	306	23.04	9.95	4.01	2.44	2.75
noodle	10¾ oz	168	9.49	4.83	1.96	1.19	1.35
vegetable	10½ oz	179	7.51	7.36	3.23	1.62	2.18
Campbell's®							
noodle	1 oz	17	0.75	0.50	0.09	0.06	0.07
vegetable	1 oz	17	0.50	0.75	0.30	0.15	0.20
vegetable, chunky	1 oz	16	0.96	0.64	0.30	0.15	0.20
Vegetable							
chunky, ready to serve	19 oz	274	7.87	8.30	3.57	3.12	1.23
vegetarian	10½ oz	176	5.12	4.70	2.02	1.77	0.70
w/beef	10¾ oz	192	13.57	4.61	1.94	0.28	2.06
w/beef broth	10½ oz	197	7.21	4.64	1.34	1.91	1.08
Campbell's®	1 oz	22	0.75	0.50	0.23	0.07	0.20
beef	1 oz	17	1.00	0.50	0.12	0.04	0.12
beef, less salt	1 oz	17	1.00	0.50			
beef, low salt	1 oz	17	1.30	0.46	0.13	0.11	0.04
beef, microwave	1 oz	13	0.67	0.27	0.09	0.01	0.10
beef, chunky	1 oz	18	1.21	0.56	0.19	0.17	0.07
beef, Healthy Choice	1 serving	70	5.00	2.00			
chunky	1 oz	15	0.37	0.37	0.15	0.17	0.06
country vegetable, homestyle	1 oz	11	0.37	0.19	0.06	0.08	0.05
healthy	1 serving	90	3.00	2.00			
hearty, Healthy Choice	1 serving	110	3.00	3.00			
hearty beef, Healthy Choice	1 serving	120	9.00	3.00			
homestyle	1 oz	15	0.50	0.50	0.07	0.09	0.05
less salt	1 oz	22	0.75	0.50			
microwave	1 oz	106	4.11	1.18	0.07	0.09	0.05
old fashioned	1 oz	15	0.50	0.50	0.07	0.09	0.05
vegetarian	1 oz	20	0.50	0.50	0.10	0.09	0.03
Health Valley®							
barley, fat free	1 oz	8	0.53	0.13			
w/chicken	1 oz	17	2.67	0.27	0.13	0.06	0.08
14 vegetable, fat free	1 oz	1	0.53	0.13			
5 bean	1 oz	15	0.53	0.27	0.08	0.13	0.06
5 bean, fat free	1 oz	13	1.07	0.13			
natural	1 oz	15	0.53	0.13	0.04	0.06	0.03
Wonton, Campbell's®	1 oz	10	0.50	0.25	0.12	0.04	0.09
SOUPS, Dehydrated							
Asparagus, cream of	63.8 g	234	8.77	6.89	2.96	2.59	1.03
prepared w/water	1128.5 g	265	9.94	7.81	3.35	2.92	1.16
Bean w/bacon	1 cup	105	5.50	2.16	0.94	0.16	0.96
Beef broth, cubed	3.6 g	6	0.62	0.14	0.06	0.01	0.07
Chicken broth or bouillon	6 g	16	1.00	0.83	0.32	0.27	0.21

FOOD	CARBO-HYDRATES (mg)	FIBER (mg)	CALCIUM (mg)	IRON (mg)	POTAS-SIUM (mg)	SODIUM (mg)	CHOLES-TEROL (mg)	% OF CALORIES FROM FAT
SOUPS, Canned (continued)								
zesty	4.9	0.06	5	0.18	36	190	0	18
Health Valley®								
natural	2.8	0.16	3	0.36	88	5	0	21
vegetable, fat free	1.0	0.40	5	0.14	79	39	0	18
Turkey								
chunky, ready to serve	31.7	2.13	112	4.31	814	2082	21	29
noodle	20.9	0.31	28	2.29	183	1983	12	26
vegetable	21.0		40	1.85	426	2202	3	37
Campbell's®								
noodle	2.2	0.09	0	0.09	9	220	1	26
vegetable	2.0	0.17	0	0.09	38	178	1	39
vegetable, chunky	1.7	0.17	4	0.12	38	113	1	36
Vegetable								
chunky, ready to serve	42.7	2.70	126	3.67	889	2269	0	27
vegetarian	29.1	1.19	52	2.62	509	2001	0	24
w/beef	24.7	0.76	41	2.70	420	2326	12	22
w/beef broth	31.8	1.49	43	2.35	467	1969	6	21
Campbell's®	3.4	0.50	5	0.09	71	208	4	20
beef	2.5	0.07	0	0.18	16	195	1	26
beef, less salt	2.5		0	0.18		118	2	26
beef, low salt	1.7	0.10	4	0.17	31	8	0	25
beef, microwave	2.1	0.06	3	0.14	20	111	1	18
beef, chunky	1.8	0.14	4	0.17	47	102	0	28
beef, Healthy Choice	9.0		20	1.08	360	490	5	26
chunky	2.6	0.14	6	0.17	47	102	0	22
country vegetable, homestyle	1.8	0.06	6	0.13	23	99	0	15
healthy	14.0		20	0.72	410	500	5	20
hearty, Healthy Choice	17.0		40	0.72	550	480	0	25
hearty beef, Healthy Choice	15.0		20	1.08	620	490	15	23
homestyle	2.2	0.06	5	0.09	23	220	0	30
less salt	3.4		0	0.09		125	1	20
microwave	18.7	0.06	12	1.06	23	775	0	10
old fashioned	2.2	0.06	0	0.09	23	220	0	30
vegetarian	3.2	0.51	0	0.18	25	198	0	22
Health Valley®								
barley, fat free	1.4	0.53	5	0.14	48	36	0	15
w/chicken	0.9	0.53	3	0.20	51	8	2	14
14 vegetable, fat free	1.2	0.40	5	0.14	68	35	0	
5 bean	2.8	1.41	5	0.24	40	8	0	16
5 bean, fat free	1.8	0.40	5	0.19	96	35	0	9
natural	2.6	1.12	5	0.24	40	5	0	8
Wonton, Campbell's®	1.2	0.11	0	0.09	33	213	7	23
SOUPS, Dehydrated								
Asparagus, cream of	35.5	0.51				3177	1	27
prepared w/water	40.3	0.58				3602	1	27
Bean w/bacon	16.3	1.53			327	930	3	19
Beef broth, cubed	0.5			0.08	15	864	Trace	21
Chicken broth or bouillon	1.0	0.01	11	0.06	19	1115	1	47

SOUPS & SAUCES

FOOD	AMOUNT	CALORIES (kcal)	PROTEIN (g)	FAT (g)	MONO-UN-SATURATED FAT (g)	POLY-UN-SATURATED FAT (g)	SATURATED FAT (g)
SOUPS, Dehydrated (continued)							
Chicken broth, cubed	4.8 g	9	0.70	0.23	0.09	0.08	0.06
Chicken, cream of	18.3 g	80	1.33	3.97	0.87	0.30	2.52
Chicken noodle	11.1 g	38	2.13	0.85	0.37	0.25	0.19
Campbell's®							
recipe mix	1 oz	12	0.62	0.25	0.12	0.06	0.07
recipe mix, hearty noodle	1 oz	11	0.50	0.13	0.03	0.05	0.04
meat, creamy, dry	1 oz	15	0.50				
meat, dry	1 oz	15	1.00	0.33	0.15	0.07	0.12
Chicken rice	1 cup	60	2.44	1.44	0.63	0.42	0.32
Campbell's® microwave	1 oz	13	0.40	0.53	0.11	0.05	0.05
Chicken vegetable	10.6 g	37	2.01	0.59	0.23	0.11	0.14
Clam chowder, Manhattan	1 cup	65	2.07	1.55	0.72	0.50	0.26
Clam chowder, New England	1 cup	95	2.79	3.67	1.70	1.17	0.62
Consomme, w/gelatin added	56.7 g	77	9.75	0.06	0.03	0.02	0.01
Leek	78 g	294	8.78	8.50	3.55	0.34	4.23
prepared w/water	1 pkt	319	9.51	9.21	3.87	0.37	4.60
Minestrone	78 g	279	15.60	6.08	2.59	0.35	2.87
prepared w/water	1 pkt	358	19.99	7.79	3.31	0.45	3.67
Mushroom	serving	441	10.20	22.30	10.30	7.15	3.78
Noodle, Campbell's®							
chicken broth, dry	1 oz	15	0.67	0.33			
recipe mix	1 oz	14	0.62	0.25	0.07	0.10	0.08
Onion, Campbell's®	7.1 g	21	0.82	0.42	0.25	0.05	0.10
recipe mix	1 oz	4	0.13	0.00	0.00	0.00	0.00
Oxtail	74.4 g	280	11.16	10.12	4.23	0.40	5.04
prepared w/water	1 pkt	318	12.64	11.46	4.81	0.46	5.73
Pea, green or split	28 g	100	5.74	1.18	0.72	0.29	0.43
prepared w/water	1 pkt	101	5.83	1.20	0.56	0.23	0.33
Tomato	21.3 g	77	1.84	1.78	0.29	0.17	0.81
Tomato vegetable	38.5 g	125	4.52	1.96	0.73	0.19	0.89
prepared w/water	6 fl oz	41	1.49	0.65	0.25	0.06	0.30
Vegetable beef	74.4 g	256	14.07	5.36	2.24	0.21	2.67
prepared w/water	1 pkt	240	13.21	5.03	2.10	0.20	2.49
Vegetable, cream of	17.7 g	79	1.42	4.27	1.90	1.11	1.07
Campbell's® recipe mix	1 oz	5	0.13	0.00	0.00	0.00	0.00
SAUCES, Dehydrated							
Béarnaise	1 cup	60	2.32	1.49	0.64	0.56	0.22
prepared w/milk & butter	1 cup	701	8.32	68.24	19.92	3.03	41.77
Cheese	35.2 g	158	7.99	8.95	2.97	1.29	4.24
prepared w/milk	1 cup	307	16.01	17.10	5.31	1.58	9.32
Curry	1 cup	121	2.65	6.54	2.81	2.46	0.97
prepared w/milk	1 cup	270	10.69	14.70	5.16	2.76	6.05
Hollandaise, w/butterfat, prepared w/water	1 cup	237	4.72	19.74	5.94	0.93	11.60
Hollandaise, w/vegetable oil	1 cup	62	2.27	1.53	0.67	0.45	0.32
prepared w/milk & butter	1 cup	703	8.27	68.29	19.95	2.93	41.87

FOOD	CARBO-HYDRATES (mg)	FIBER (mg)	CALCIUM (mg)	IRON (mg)	POTAS-SIUM (mg)	SODIUM (mg)	CHOLES-TEROL (mg)	% OF CALORIES FROM FAT
SOUPS, Dehydrated (continued)								
Chicken broth, cubed	1.1			0.09	18	1152	1	23
Chicken, cream of	9.9	0.87	57		160	882	2	45
Chicken noodle	5.3	0.05	23	0.36	23	931	2	20
Campbell's®								
recipe mix	2.0	0.09	2	0.14	7	89	1	18
recipe mix, hearty noodle	1.8	0.23	2	0.09	35	105	4	10
meat, creamy, dry	2.0		3	0.00		170		0
meat, dry	2.0	0.24	0	0.12	28	128	13	20
Chicken rice	9.2	0.03	7	0.10	12	980	3	22
Campbell's® microwave	1.8	0.09	0	0.48	12	109	1	36
Chicken vegetable	5.8			0.44	51	604	2	14
Clam chowder, Manhattan	10.8	0.57				1336		21
Clam chowder, New England	12.8	0.20	76		205	745	1	35
Consomme, w/gelatin added	9.2	0.06				14855	0	1
Leek	47.4	1.09				4009	9	26
prepared w/water	51.3	1.19				4345	11	26
Minestrone	41.8	1.48				3604	6	20
prepared w/water	53.5	1.90	14			4618	11	20
Mushroom	51.2	0.30	306	0.20	915	4681	2	46
Noodle, Campbell's®								
chicken broth, dry	2.5		3	0.18		152		20
recipe mix	2.3	0.23	2	0.18	35	87	4	16
Onion, Campbell's®	3.8	0.17	10	0.11	47	636	0	18
recipe mix	0.8	0.11	0	0.00	7	87	0	0
Oxtail	35.6	0.52				4806	11	33
prepared w/water	40.3	0.59				5443	11	32
Pea, green or split	16.9	0.52	17	0.75	178	914	0	11
prepared w/water	17.2	0.52	16	0.76	181	927	2	11
Tomato	14.5	0.32	40	0.32	221	707	1	21
Tomato vegetable	23.0	1.19	18	1.43	233	2588	1	14
prepared w/water	7.6	0.40	6	0.47	77	856	Trace	14
Vegetable beef	28.4	0.74		4.10		4806	6	19
prepared w/water	36.1	0.69		3.85		4513	5	19
Vegetable, cream of	9.2	0.11			72	877	0	49
Campbell's® recipe mix	1.0	0.06	2	0.00	9	89	0	0
SAUCES, Dehydrated								
Béarnaise	9.8	0.03				559	Trace	22
prepared w/milk & butter	17.5	0.03				1265	189	88
Cheese	11.8	0.04	280	0.15	183	1447	18	51
prepared w/milk	23.2	0.04	570	0.27	554	1566	53	50
Curry	14.3	0.37				1155	Trace	49
prepared w/milk	25.7	0.37	485			1276	35	49
Hollandaise, w/butterfat, prepared w/water	13.7	0.04	124	0.90	124	1565	51	75
Hollandaise, w/vegetable oil	10.3	0.03				429	Trace	22
prepared w/milk & butter	17.9	0.03				1134	189	87

193

SOUPS & SAUCES

FOOD	AMOUNT	CALO-RIES (kcal)	PROTEIN (g)	FAT (g)	MONO-UN-SATURATED FAT (g)	POLY-UN-SATURATED FAT (g)	SATU-RATED FAT (g)
SAUCES, Dehydrated (continued)							
Mushroom	1 cup	79	3.26	2.16	0.93	0.81	0.32
prepared w/milk	1 cup	228	11.29	10.31	3.27	1.10	5.40
Sour cream	1 cup	360	11.05	22.11	7.54	2.47	11.02
prepared w/milk	1 cup	509	19.08	30.26	3.55	2.76	16.10
Spaghetti	42 g	118	2.52	0.42	0.12	0.01	0.27
w/mushrooms	39 g	118	3.90	3.51	0.99	0.10	2.23
Stroganoff	1 cup	195	6.73	5.30	1.43	0.15	3.44
prepared w/milk & water	1 cup	271	11.70	10.70	3.01	0.35	6.77
Sweet & sour	1 cup	294	0.76	0.08	0.02	0.04	0.01
Teriyaki	46 g	130	4.14	0.92	0.22	0.53	0.13
White	1 cup	92	2.17	5.29	2.35	1.38	1.32
prepared w/milk	1 cup	241	10.20	13.45	4.70	1.68	6.40
SAUCES, Ready to serve							
Alfredo							
Kraft® all natural	1 tbsp	50	2.00	4.00			
Legout® frozen	1 oz	95	1.00	9.50			
Barbecue	1 cup	188	4.50	4.50	1.94	1.71	0.67
Cripple Creek®							
VPP 915-5	1 oz	50	4.00	4.00		0.00	1.00
VPP 920-9	1 oz	60	4.00	4.00		0.00	2.00
pork barbecue	1 oz	40	5.00	2.00		0.00	0.00
Legout®	1 oz	30	0.00	0.00	0.00	0.00	0.00
Kraft®	1 tbsp	23	0.00	0.50			
garlic	1 tbsp	20	0.00	0.00			
hickory smoke	1 tbsp	23	0.00	0.50			
hickory smoke, onion	1 tbsp	25	0.00	0.50			
hot	1 tbsp	23	0.00	0.50			
hot, hickory smoke	1 tbsp	23	0.00	0.50			
Italian season	1 tbsp	25	0.00	0.50			
Kansas City style	1 tbsp	25	0.00	0.50			
mesquite smoke	1 tbsp	23	0.00	0.50			
onion bits	1 tbsp	25	0.00	0.50			
thick n spicy	1 tbsp	30	0.00	0.50			
thick n spicy, hickory smoke	1 tbsp	25	0.00	0.50			
thick n spicy, honey	1 tbsp	30	0.00	0.50			
thick n spicy, Kansas City style	1 tbsp	30	0.00	0.50			
thick n spicy, mesquite smoke	1 tbsp	25	0.00	0.50			
thick n spicy, original	1 tbsp	25	0.00	0.50			
Béarnaise							
Kraft® w/herb butter, all natural	1 tbsp	70	0.00	7.00	1.68	0.31	3.10
Legout® frozen	1 oz	55	0.50	5.00			
Bordelaise, Legout® frozen	1 oz	23	0.50	1.50			
Cacciatore, Legout® frozen	1 oz	13	0.50	0.50			
Carbonara, Legout® frozen	1 oz	50	6.00	3.50			
Cheese, Kraft®							
cheddar, all natural	1 tbsp	60	2.00	4.00	1.19	0.12	2.69
nacho, all natural	1 tbsp	60	2.00	4.00			
triple, all natural	1 tbsp	60	2.00	4.00			

FOOD	CARBO-HYDRATES (mg)	FIBER (mg)	CALCIUM (mg)	IRON (mg)	POTAS-SIUM (mg)	SODIUM (mg)	CHOLES-TEROL (mg)	% OF CALORIES FROM FAT
SAUCES, Dehydrated (continued)								
Mushroom	12.4	0.23				1414	0	25
prepared w/milk	23.7	0.23				1533	34	41
Sour cream	34.0		256	0.49	363	887	56	55
prepared w/milk	45.4		546	0.61	733	1007	91	54
Spaghetti	26.9		72	1.12	353	3562	0	3
w/mushrooms	19.1		156	0.71	160	3674	11	27
Stroganoff	32.0	0.72	371	1.61	481	2252	14	24
prepared w/milk & water	33.9	0.56	521	1.33	672	1829	38	36
Sweet & sour	72.6		41	1.62	66	779	0	0
Teriyaki	27.6		112	2.79	215	4784	0	6
White	10.0	0.04	133		73	675	Trace	52
prepared w/milk	21.4	0.04	424	0.26	443	796	34	50
SAUCES, Ready to serve								
Alfredo								
Kraft® all natural	2.0					170	15	72
Legout® frozen	2.0		40	0.00	43	165		90
Barbecue	32.0	1.50	48	2.25	435	2038	0	22
Cripple Creek®								
VPP 915-5	3.0		0	0.72	110	180	10	72
VPP 920-9	2.0		0	0.72	95	140	10	60
pork barbecue	3.0		0	0.72	110	115	10	45
Legout®	7.0						0	0
Kraft®	5.0				33	230		20
garlic	4.5				30	210		0
hickory smoke	5.0				30	220		20
hickory smoke, onion	5.5				28	170		18
hot	4.5				30	260		20
hot, hickory smoke	4.5				30	180		20
Italian season	5.0				30	140		18
Kansas City style	5.5		10	0.36	60	135		18
mesquite smoke	5.0				33	205		20
onion bits	5.5				28	170		18
thick n spicy	6.5			0.18	43	210		15
thick n spicy, hickory smoke	6.0			0.18	38	215		18
thick n spicy, honey	6.5		10	0.18	50	170		15
thick n spicy, Kansas City style	6.5		10	0.18	65	135		15
thick n spicy, mesquite smoke	6.0			0.18	35	215		18
thick n spicy, original	6.0			0.18	38	215		18
Béarnaise								
Kraft® w/herb butter, all natural	2.0	0.02	7	0.11	0	95	20	90
Legout® frozen	1.5		10	0.00	18	105		82
Bordelaise, Legout® frozen	1.0		0	0.00	28	170		60
Cacciatore, Legout® frozen	1.5		0	0.00	38	160		36
Carbonara, Legout® frozen	1.5		30	0.00	50	140		63
Cheese, Kraft®								
cheddar, all natural	3.0	0.00	102	0.10	14	220	15	60
nacho, all natural	3.0					220	15	60
triple, all natural	2.0					190	15	60

SOUPS & SAUCES

FOOD	AMOUNT	CALO-RIES (kcal)	PROTEIN (g)	FAT (g)	MONO-UN-SATURATED FAT (g)	POLY-UN-SATURATED FAT (g)	SATU-RATED FAT (g)
SAUCES, Ready to serve (continued)							
Chez instant, Legout®							
prepared	1 oz	35	1.00	1.50			
chef style, light	1 oz	55	1.50	4.00			
Chili	1 tbsp	16	0.40	0.00	0.00	0.00	0.00
low sodium	1 tbsp	8	0.00	0.00	0.00	0.00	0.00
Hunt's®	100 g	117	1.33	0.16	0.04	0.01	0.11
hot dog/beef	1 fl oz	27	2.00	1.00	0.49	0.09	0.41
Gebhardt® hot dog/beef	1 fl oz	27	2.00	1.00	0.49	0.09	0.41
Chili Bowl® hot dog	1 oz	40	2.00	3.00		0.00	1.00
Clam, Legout® frozen	1 oz	28	1.50	1.50			
Creole, Legout® prepared	1 oz	15	0.00	0.00	0.00	0.00	0.00
Enchilada, Rosarita®	1 fl oz	6	0.00	0.00	0.00	0.00	0.00
Guava, cooked	1 cup	86	0.76	0.33	0.03	0.14	0.10
Hollandaise							
Kraft® all natural	1 tbsp	80	1.00	7.00	1.97	0.36	3.64
Legout®	100 g	370	11.00	10.00			
frozen	1 oz	55	0.50	5.00			
Marinara	1 cup	170	4.00	8.38	4.28	2.30	1.20
Legout® frozen	1 oz	15	0.50	0.00	0.00	0.00	0.00
Morney, Legout® frozen	1 oz	40	1.50	2.50			
Murtabak	1 oz	22	1.13	0.96			
Mushroom, Legout® frozen	1 oz	140	4.00	8.00			
Picante	1 fl oz	9	0.30	0.50	0.00	0.00	0.00
Pineapple, S&S® prepared, light	1 oz	35	0.00	0.50			
Pizza, Hunt's® Angela Mia	100 g	56	2.08	0.25			
Plum, La Choy®	1 tbsp	20	0.05	0.01	0.00	0.00	0.00
Salsa							
with green chiles	1 fl oz	10	0.40	0.70	0.00	0.00	0.00
Rosarita®							
mild green chile	1 fl oz	5	0.20	0.00	0.00	0.00	0.00
picante	1 fl oz	5	0.20	0.00	0.00	0.00	0.00
Satay	1 oz	43	4.22	0.37			
Spaghetti, tomato based	1 cup	271	4.53	11.90	6.07	3.25	1.70
Prego® regular	1 oz	33	0.50	1.25	0.47	0.40	0.39
chunky garden	1 oz	20	0.50	0.50			
marinara	1 oz	25	0.50	1.50	0.24	0.60	0.15
meat flavored	1 oz	35	0.50	1.50	0.80	0.36	0.31
mushroom	1 oz	33	0.50	1.25	0.28	0.14	0.25
mushroom & onion	1 oz	25	0.50	1.00			
mushroom & pepper	1 oz	25	0.50	1.00	0.28	0.14	0.25
mushroom & spice	1 oz	25	0.50	0.75			
mushroom & tomato	1 oz	28	0.25	1.25			
no salt added	1 oz	28	0.50	1.50	0.69	0.37	0.19
onion & garlic	1 oz	28	0.25	1.00			
sausage & pepper	1 oz	40	0.75	2.00			
three cheese	1 oz	25	0.75	0.50	0.12	0.30	0.08
tomato & basil	1 oz	25	0.50	0.50			
tomato & onion	1 oz	28	0.50	1.25			
Legout®							
frozen	1 oz	25	1.50	1.00			

FOOD	CARBO-HYDRATES (mg)	FIBER (mg)	CALCIUM (mg)	IRON (mg)	POTAS-SIUM (mg)	SODIUM (mg)	CHOLES-TEROL (mg)	% OF CALORIES FROM FAT
SAUCES, Ready to serve (continued)								
Chez instant, Legout®								
prepared	4.0		30	0.00	75	260		39
chef style, light	3.0		50	0.18	35	245		65
Chili	3.7		3	0.10	56	201	0	0
low sodium	2.0					10	0	0
Hunt's®	29.1	5.90	20	1.34	370	23	0	1
hot dog/beef	3.0	0.74	10	0.60	66	140	9	33
Gebhardt® hot dog/beef	3.0	0.74	10	0.50	66	140	9	33
Chili Bowl® hot dog	2.0		0	0.36	85	110	5	68
Clam, Legout® frozen	2.0		10	0.36	28	85		49
Creole, Legout® prepared	3.0		0	0.00	50	130	0	0
Enchilada, Rosarita®	1.0	0.31	3	0.10	9	146	10	0
Guava, cooked	22.6	6.78	17	0.43	536	10	0	3
Hollandaise								
Kraft® all natural	3.0	0.00	7	0.15	7	180	20	79
Legout®	60.0		106	0.00	820	590		24
frozen	1.5		10	0.00	18	105		82
Marinara	25.5		45	2.00	1060	1573	0	44
Legout® frozen	3.5	0.00	0	0.36	105	270	0	0
Morney, Legout® frozen	2.0		40	0.00	38	150		56
Murtabak	2.1	0.00	4	0.45	79	91		40
Mushroom, Legout® frozen	12.0		0	1.44	340	1160		51
Picante	1.9		4	0.25	77	218	0	50
Pineapple, S&S® prepared, light	6.5		0	0.00	30	45		13
Pizza, Hunt's® Angela Mia	11.3		19	2.14		280		4
Plum, La Choy®	5.1	0.09	1			4	0	0
Salsa								
with green chiles	2.0		4	0.28	87	111	0	63
Rosarita®								
mild green chile	1.0	0.37	4	0.10	31	251	0	0
picante	1.0	0.47	4	0.10	37	224	1	0
Satay	5.6	1.39	7	0.48	28	36		8
Spaghetti, tomato based	39.7		70	1.62	956	1235	0	40
Prego® regular	5.0	0.48	10	0.27	124	158	5	35
chunky garden	3.5		10	0.27		105		23
marinara	2.5	0.58	5	0.18	128	155	0	54
meat flavored	5.0	0.91	10	0.27	108	165	2	39
mushroom	5.0	0.38	10	0.18	64	158	3	35
mushroom & onion	3.2		5	0.27		123		36
mushroom & pepper	3.5	0.38	5	0.27	64	103	3	36
mushroom & spice	4.2		10	0.27		113		27
mushroom & tomato	3.5		5	0.27		125		41
no salt added	2.7	0.85	10	0.27	109	6	0	49
onion & garlic	4.0		5	0.27		128		33
sausage & pepper	4.7		10	0.27		125		45
three cheese	4.2	0.58	10	0.36	128	103	0	18
tomato & basil	4.5		10	0.27		93		18
tomato & onion	3.5		5	0.27		123		41
Legout®								
frozen	2.0		0	0.36	90	195		36

SOUPS & SAUCES

FOOD	AMOUNT	CALO-RIES (kcal)	PROTEIN (g)	FAT (g)	MONO-UN-SATURATED FAT (g)	POLY-UN-SATURATED FAT (g)	SATU-RATED FAT (g)
SAUCES, Ready to serve (continued)							
Spaghetti, tomato basedf (continued)							
chef style, prepared	1 oz	25	0.50	1.00			
Hunt's® w/tomato bits	100 g	101	2.21	2.65			
Soy	1 tbsp	11	1.56	0.00	0.00	0.00	0.00
La Choy®	1 tbsp	8	0.65	0.15	0.00	0.01	0.00
lite	1 tbsp	0	0.60	0.00	0.00	0.00	0.00
Tamari®	1 tbsp	11	1.89	0.02	0.00	0.01	0.00
Kikkoman® preservative free	1 tbsp	10	1.43	0.00	0.00	0.00	0.00
Shoyu®	1 tbsp	9	0.93	0.01	0.00	0.01	0.00
low sodium	1 tbsp	9	0.93	0.01	0.00	0.01	0.00
Steak, Heinz 57®	1 tbsp	15	0.40	0.20	0.00	0.00	0.00
Sweet & sour							
La Choy®	1 tbsp	23	0.05	0.00	0.00	0.00	0.00
Legout® frozen	1 oz	20	0.00	0.50			
Tabasco	1 tsp	0	0.10	0.00	0.00	0.00	0.00
Taco	1 fl oz	11	0.40	0.70			
Rosarita®	1 fl oz	10	0.30	0.00	0.00	0.00	0.00
Tartar	1 tbsp	75	0.00	8.00	1.80	4.10	1.50
low calorie	1 cup	501	1.34	50.10	11.20	24.60	8.95
Bright Day®	1 tbsp	50	0.00	5.00	1.46	2.83	0.71
Teriyaki	1 tbsp	15	1.07	0.00	0.00	0.00	0.00
La Choy®	1 tbsp	10	0.40	0.00	0.00	0.00	0.00
Kikkoman® CD01400	1 tbsp	14	1.00	0.00	0.00	0.00	0.00
Tomato, canned							
salt added	1 cup	74	3.26	0.42	0.06	0.16	0.06
Spanish	1 cup	81	3.51	0.66	0.10	0.26	0.09
w/herbs & cheese	1 cup	144	5.18	4.72	0.93	2.01	1.53
w/mushrooms	1 cup	86	3.55	0.32	0.03	0.12	0.04
w/onions	1 cup	103	3.82	0.47	0.07	0.19	0.07
Health Valley®	1 oz	9	0.30	0.06	0.01	0.02	0.01
Hunt's®	100 g	28	1.04	0.13	0.03	0.07	0.02
S&W® low sodium	1 cup	90	4.00	0.00	0.00	0.00	0.00
Worcestershire	1 tbsp	12	0.30	0.00	0.00	0.00	0.00
GRAVIES, Canned							
Au jus	1 cup	38	2.86	0.48	0.20	0.02	0.24
Franco®	1 cup	40	0.00	0.00	0.00	0.00	0.00
Beef	1 cup	124	8.73	5.49	2.30	0.21	2.75
Franco®	1 cup	100	0.00	4.00	1.78	0.18	2.04
Legout®	1 cup	80	12.00	0.00	0.00	0.00	0.00
Brown, Legout®	1 cup	100	4.00	0.00	0.00	0.00	0.00
Chicken	1 cup	189	4.59	13.62	6.08	3.58	3.36
Franco®	1 cup	180	0.00	16.00	5.92	3.06	3.90
chicken giblet	1 cup	120	4.00	8.00	3.67	1.90	2.42
Legout®	1 cup	160	4.00	8.00			
Cream, Franco®	1 cup	140	0.00	8.00			
Mushroom	1 cup	120	3.01	6.46	2.78	2.43	0.96
Franco®	1 cup	100	0.00	4.00	0.25	0.02	0.46
Legout®	1 cup	140	4.00	4.00			

FOOD	CARBO-HYDRATES (mg)	FIBER (mg)	CALCIUM (mg)	IRON (mg)	POTAS-SIUM (mg)	SODIUM (mg)	CHOLES-TEROL (mg)	% OF CALORIES FROM FAT
SAUCES, Ready to serve (continued)								
Spaghetti, tomato based (continued)								
chef style, prepared	3.5		0	0.18	80	240		36
Hunt's® w/tomato bits	18.1		24	1.33		1037		24
Soy	1.5	0.00	3	0.49	64	1029	0	0
La Choy®	1.2	0.00	11	0.29	26	1283	0	17
lite	0.8	0.00	8	0.29	26	623	0	0
Tamari®	1.0	0.00	4	0.43	38	1005	0	2
Kikkoman® preservative free	1.0	0.00	3	0.34	39	528	0	0
Shoyu®	1.5	0.00	3	0.36	32	1029	0	1
low sodium	1.5	0.00	3	0.36	32	600	0	1
Steak, Heinz 57®	2.7					265	0	12
Sweet & sour								
La Choy®	5.8	0.01	1	0.05	5	50	0	0
Legout® frozen	3.5		0	0.00	28	135		23
Tabasco	0.1	0.00	0	0.03	3	22	0	
Taco	2.2		6	0.30	88	128	0	57
Rosarita®	2.0	0.47	4	0.30	63	240	1	0
Tartar	1.0		3	0.10	11	98	9	96
low calorie	15.0	0.46	40	2.01	175	1582	114	90
Bright Day®	2.0	0.02	3	0.13	2	40	0	90
Teriyaki	2.8		4	0.31	41	690	0	0
La Choy®	2.6	0.01	6	0.24	32	336	0	0
Kikkoman® CD01400	2.7	0.02	4	0.29	39	602	0	0
Tomato, canned								
salt added	17.6	3.68	34	1.89	908	1482	0	5
Spanish	17.7	3.66	42	8.49	900	1152	0	7
w/herbs & cheese	25.0	3.66	90	2.12	869	1325		30
w/mushrooms	20.7	3.68	32	2.18	931	1107	0	3
w/onions	24.4	3.68	42	2.28	1012	1350	0	4
Health Valley®	1.6	0.04	4	0.22	74	4	0	6
Hunt's®	5.6	1.50	12	1.06	371	625	0	4
S&W® low sodium	18.0	3.39	32	1.74	838	65	0	0
Worcestershire	2.7	0.00	15	0.90	120	147	0	0
GRAVIES, Canned								
Au jus	5.9		10	1.43			1	11
Franco®	8.0	0.91	0	0.00	216	1320	6	0
Beef	11.2		14	1.63	189	117	7	40
Franco®	16.0	0.88	0	0.00	149	1360	24	36
Legout®	4.0		0	0.00	80	1320	0	0
Brown, Legout®	16.0		0	0.48	40	1560	0	0
Chicken	12.9		48	1.12	260	1375	5	65
Franco®	12.0	0.46	0	0.00	396	960	101	80
chicken giblet	12.0	0.46	0	0.00	396	1240	101	60
Legout®	16.0		1	80.00	140	1200		45
Cream, Franco®	16.0		0	0.00		880		51
Mushroom	13.0		17	1.57	253	1359	0	48
Franco®	12.0	0.91	0	0.00	50	1160	0	36
Legout®	20.0		0	7.20	240	1800		26

SOUPS & SAUCES

FOOD	AMOUNT	CALO-RIES (kcal)	PROTEIN (g)	FAT (g)	MONO-UN-SATURATED FAT (g)	POLY-UN-SATURATED FAT (g)	SATU-RATED FAT (g)
GRAVIES, Canned (continued)							
Pork, Franco®	1 cup	160	0.00	12.00	5.89	1.58	4.54
Turkey	1 cup	122	6.20	5.01	2.15	1.17	1.48
Franco®	1 cup	120	0.00	8.00	2.18	2.15	2.54
Legout®	1 cup	160	4.00	8.00			
GRAVIES, Dehydrated							
Au jus	1 cup	32	1.18	1.33	0.56	0.05	0.66
prepared w/water	1 cup	19	0.72	0.81	0.34	0.03	0.40
Beef, Legout®	100 g	350	12.00	4.00			
Brown	1 cup	80	2.57	1.85	0.77	0.07	0.92
prepared w/water	1 cup	9	0.28	0.20	0.08	0.01	0.10
Pillsbury®	4.4 g	16	0.00	0.00	0.00	0.00	0.00
Chicken	1 cup	83	2.61	1.92	0.86	0.45	0.53
Legout®	100 g	350	10.00	4.00			
1 step	100 g	410	10.00	15.00			
Pillsbury®	4.4 g	18	0.00	0.00	0.00	0.00	0.00
Mushroom	1 cup	70	2.13	0.85	0.28	0.03	0.50
Onion	1 cup	77	2.16	0.72	0.22	0.03	0.45
prepared w/water	1 cup	80	2.23	0.74	0.22	0.03	0.46
Pork	1 cup	76	1.92	1.92	0.86	0.22	0.75
Turkey	1 cup	87	2.93	1.87	0.80	0.43	0.55
Legout® 1 step	100 g	400	9.00	13.00			
instant	100 g	350	10.00	3.00			
Unspecified	1 cup	85	3.22	1.98	0.78	0.40	0.71
Pillsbury® homestyle	4.4 g	16	0.00	0.00	0.00	0.00	0.00
Legout® country	100 g	340	10.00	5.00			
SHAKE N BAKE®							
coating, extra crisp, chicken	29.8 g	115	3.00	2.00			
coating, homestyle, chicken	22.7 g	85	1.00	2.00			
Italian herb	20.4 g	77	2.00	1.00			
original barbecue, chicken	24.8 g	93	1.00	2.00			
original barbecue, pork	10.2 g	38	0.00	1.00			
original country	16.8 g	76	1.00	4.00			
original for chicken	19.5 g	77	2.00	2.00			
pork coating, oven	29.8 g	120	3.00	3.00			
seasoning/coating mix	18.6 g	73	1.00	1.00			

FOOD	CARBO-HYDRATES (mg)	FIBER (mg)	CALCIUM (mg)	IRON (mg)	POTAS-SIUM (mg)	SODIUM (mg)	CHOLES-TEROL (mg)	% OF CALORIES FROM FAT
GRAVIES, Canned (continued)								
Pork, Franco®	12.0	0.45	0	0.00	457	1320	110	68
Turkey	12.1		10	1.67			5	37
Franco®	12.0	0.46	0	0.00	457	1160	86	60
Legout®	12.0		0	32.40	120	1480		45
GRAVIES, Dehydrated								
Au jus	3.9	0.02	18			955	1	37
prepared w/water	2.3	0.01	11			579	1	38
Beef, Legout®	66.0		0	0.00	490	4810		10
Brown	13.9	0.11	66	0.23	61	1145	2	21
prepared w/water	1.5	0.01	7	0.03	7	125	Trace	20
Pillsbury®	3.0		0	0.00	0	180	0	0
Chicken	14.3	0.06	39			1133	2	21
Legout®	70.0		0	0.00	830	4660		10
1 step	60.0		0		550	4210		33
Pillsbury®	3.0		0	0.00	5	170	0	0
Mushroom	13.7		49			1402	1	11
Onion	16.2		67			1005	Trace	8
prepared w/water	16.7		69			1036	1	8
Pork	13.4		32			1235	2	23
Turkey	15.0	0.10	50			1500	2	19
Legout® 1 step	62.0		0		490	3610		29
instant	71.0		0	0.00	830	3190		8
Unspecified	14.3		37			1421	1	21
Pillsbury® homestyle	3.0		0	0.00	5	240	0	0
Legout® country	65.0		106	0.00	1160	3390		13
SHAKE N BAKE®								
coating, extra crisp, chicken	21.0		32	1.10	51	825	0	16
coating, homestyle, chicken	15.0		14	0.40	28	971	0	21
Italian herb	14.0		32	0.70	46	618	1	12
original barbecue, chicken	18.0		17	0.40	87	841	0	19
original barbecue, pork	7.0		7	0.20	38	351	0	24
original country	10.0		5	0.30	26	501	0	47
original for chicken	14.0		6	0.30	39	451	0	23
pork coating, oven	21.0		5	0.40	43	688	0	23
seasoning/coating mix	14.0		4	0.40	24	406	0	12

EGGS

FOOD	AMOUNT	CALORIES (kcal)	PROTEIN (g)	FAT (g)	SATU-RATED FAT (g)	CARBO-HYDRATES (g)	FIBER (g)
Egg beaters, no cholesterol, Fleischmann's®	55 g	25	5.00	0.00	0.00	1.0	0.00
Egg, chicken							
scrambled/milk/butter	61 g	101	6.77	7.45	2.24	1.3	0.00
white	1 oz	15	3.01	0.00	0.00	0.6	0.00
whole	1 oz	44	3.66	3.15	0.88	0.2	0.00
whole, scrambled	1 lb	693	46.30	51.00	15.40	9.1	0.00
yolk	1 oz	97	4.25	8.76	1.47	0.3	0.00
Egg, chicken, whole							
hard boiled	1 cup	211	17.10	14.40	4.44	1.5	0.00
hard cooked, no shell	1 egg	77	6.29	5.30	1.63	0.5	0.00
fresh or frozen, raw	1 cup	362	30.30	24.30	7.53	2.9	0.00
fried in butter	1 egg	92	6.23	6.90	1.92	0.6	0.00
fried, margarine & salt	1 cup	366	24.90	27.60	7.67	2.5	0.00
fried in margarine w/salt, large	1 egg	91	6.23	6.90	1.92	0.6	
frozen, salted 10%	1 oz	40	3.10	2.93	0.86	0.3	0.00
frozen, salted 5%	1 oz	43	3.27	3.00	0.90	0.3	0.00
frozen, sugared 10%	1 oz	50	3.10	2.93	0.86	3.1	0.00
frozen, sugared 5%	1 oz	48	3.27	3.00	0.90	1.7	0.00
omelet, margarine/salt	1 cup	334	22.70	25.20	7.00	2.2	0.00
poached	1 oz	42	3.53	2.83	0.88	0.3	0.00
poached, large	1 egg	74	6.22	4.99	1.54	0.6	0.00
scrambled, milk/margarine	1 cup	365	24.40	26.90	8.09	4.8	0.00
Egg, chicken, yolk							
fresh, raw, part white	1 cup	870	40.70	75.00	23.20	4.3	0.00
frozen, raw, 17% white	1 cup	751	38.30	63.20	19.60	4.0	0.00
Egg, chicken, yolk, frozen							
salted, raw	100 g	278	14.20	23.40	7.24	1.4	
sugared, raw	100 g	317	14.20	23.40	7.24	11.5	
whites, raw, cooked	1 lb	208	43.00	0.00	0.00	4.1	0.00
Egg, combination foods							
omelet, two eggs, ham & cheese Swanson's®	1 item	266	18.50	20.00	7.30	1.8	0.00
egg, bacon & cheese biscuit	1 oz	81	3.08	4.23	1.54	7.1	0.14
egg, bacon & cheese muffin	1 oz	71	3.66	3.66	1.52	6.1	0.34
egg, beefsteak & cheese muffin	1 oz	74	3.47	4.08	1.69	0.2	0.34
egg, sausage & cheese biscuit	1 oz	84	3.27	5.09	1.98	6.3	0.12
eggs/mini muffin, low cholesterol	1 oz	53	2.11	2.53	1.05	5.6	0.34
omelets/cheese sauce & ham	1 oz	56	2.71	4.14	1.05	2.1	0.00
scrambled eggs/bacon/home fries	1 oz	61	1.96	4.64		2.8	
scrambled eggs/cheese & pancakes	1 oz	85	2.06	6.76	4.12		
scrambled eggs, home fries	1 oz	57	1.52	4.13		3.0	
scrambled eggs & sausage/hash browns	1 oz	66	2.00	5.23	1.48	2.9	0.17
Egg, large chicken, raw							
white	1 egg	17	3.52	0.00	0.00	0.3	0.00
whole	1 egg	75	6.25	5.01	1.55	0.6	0.00

FOOD	CALCIUM (mg)	IRON (mg)	POTAS-SIUM (mg)	SODIUM (mg)	CHOLES-TEROL (mg)	% OF CALORIES FROM FAT
Egg beaters, no cholesterol, Fleischmann's®	20	1.08	133	80	0	0
Egg, chicken						
scrambled/milk/butter	44	0.73	84	171	215	66
white	2	0.03	42	50	0	0
whole	16	0.68	39	35	120	65
whole, scrambled	296	5.01	576	1168	1469	66
yolk	42	2.24	31	22	208	81
Egg, chicken, whole						
hard boiled	68	1.62	171	169	586	61
hard cooked, no shell	25	0.60	63	62	213	62
fresh or frozen, raw	119	3.50	294	306	1047	60
fried in butter	25	0.72	61	162	211	68
fried, margarine & salt	101	2.87	243	649	856	68
fried in margarine w/salt, large	25	0.72	61	162	211	68
frozen, salted 10%	14	0.53	33	1145	140	65
frozen, salted 5%	15	0.56	35	592	148	64
frozen, sugared 10%	14	0.53	33	35	140	53
frozen, sugared 5%	15	0.56	35	37	148	57
omelet, margarine/salt	92	2.62	222	594	783	68
poached	14	0.41	34	79	122	60
poached, large	25	0.72	60	140	212	61
scrambled, milk/margarine	156	2.64	304	616	788	66
Egg, chicken, yolk						
fresh, raw, part white	333	8.58	228	104	3154	78
frozen, raw, 17% white	282	7.39	243	151	2663	76
Egg, chicken, yolk, frozen						
salted, raw	109	2.75	91	3932	973	76
sugared, raw	105	2.74	90	56	973	66
whites, raw, cooked	24	0.12	587	672	0	0
Egg, combination foods						
omelet, two eggs, ham & cheese Swanson's®	153	1.67	182	598	445	68
egg, bacon & cheese biscuit	48	0.87	43	355	31	47
egg, bacon & cheese muffin	37	0.66	52	188	37	47
egg, beefsteak & cheese muffin	20	0.55	52	149	37	50
egg, sausage & cheese biscuit	36	0.33	53	238	27	55
eggs/mini muffin, low cholesterol	13	0.30	52	84	37	43
omelets/cheese sauce & ham	43	0.26	36	174	84	67
scrambled eggs/bacon/home fries	11	0.32		123		69
scrambled eggs/cheese & pancakes	18	0.53		112		71
scrambled eggs, home fries	13	0.31		83		66
scrambled eggs & sausage/hash browns	9	0.28	74	117	41	71
Egg, large chicken, raw						
white	2	0.01	48	55	0	0
whole	25	0.72	60	63	213	60

EGGS

FOOD	AMOUNT	CALORIES (kcal)	PROTEIN (g)	FAT (g)	SATU-RATED FAT (g)	CARBO-HYDRATES (g)	FIBER (g)
Egg, large chicken, raw (continued)							
whole, raw, Alaska	1 egg	149	12.50	10.00	3.10	1.2	
yolk	1 yolk	59	2.78	5.12	1.59	0.3	0.00
Egg, duck							
whole	1 oz	52	3.88	3.86	1.04	0.4	0.00
whole, fresh, raw	1 egg	130	8.97	9.64	2.58	1.0	0.00
whole, salted	1 oz	56	4.08	4.14	1.04	0.6	0.00
yolk	1 oz	104	3.69	9.87	2.70	0.2	0.00
yolk, salted	1 oz	161	6.46	15.00	1.04	0.0	0.00
Egg, quail, whole	1 oz	48	3.49	3.60	1.00	0.3	0.00
Egg substitute							
frozen	1 cup	384	27.10	26.70	4.63	7.6	0.00
frozen, yolk replaced	1 cup	384	27.10	26.70	4.63	7.6	0.00
liquid	1 cup	211	30.10	8.31	1.65	1.6	0.00
powder	28.4 g	126	15.70	3.69	1.07	6.1	0.00
Healthy Choice® no cholesterol	1 cup	120	20.00	4.00		4.0	
Egg, turtle							
whole	1 oz	35	3.40	2.32		0.0	0.00
white	1 oz	1	0.31	0.00	0.00	0.0	0.00
yolk	1 oz	79	7.43	5.27		0.4	0.00

FOOD	CALCIUM (mg)	IRON (mg)	POTAS- SIUM (mg)	SODIUM (mg)	CHOLES- TEROL (mg)	% OF CALORIES FROM FAT
Egg, large chicken, raw (continued)						
whole, raw, Alaska	49	1.44	121	126	425	60
yolk	23	0.59	16	7	213	78
Egg, duck						
whole	19	1.05	28	30	249	67
whole, fresh, raw	45	2.70	156	102	619	67
whole, salted	21	0.77	43	149	249	67
yolk	47	1.08	22	17	363	85
yolk, salted	52	2.47	22	87	249	84
Egg, quail, whole	16	0.88	38	32	236	68
Egg substitute						
frozen	175	4.75	512	479	5	63
frozen, yolk replaced	175	4.75	512	479	5	63
liquid	133	5.27	828	444	3	35
powder	92	0.90	211	227	162	26
Healthy Choice® no cholesterol	80	2.88	320	360		30
Egg, turtle						
whole	13	0.40	43	34		60
white	4	0.09	35	44	0	0
yolk	44	0.77	37	29		60

DAIRY PRODUCTS

FOOD	AMOUNT	CALORIES (kcal)	PROTEIN (g)	FAT (g)	MONO-UN-SATURATED FAT (g)	POLY-UN-SATURATED FAT (g)	SATURATED fat (g)
CHEESE							
American							
pasteurized process	1 oz	106	6.3	8.86	2.54	0.28	5.58
Golden Image®	1 oz	90	7.0	6.00		2.00	2.00
Kraft® light	1 oz	70	6.0	4.00			3.00
Kraft Light & Lively®	1 oz	70	6.0	4.00			3.00
Kraft® pasteurized loaf	1 oz	110	6.0	9.00			5.00
Kraft® pasteurized slices	1 oz	110	6.0	9.00			5.00
Smart Beat® fat free	1 oz	30	4.0	0.00			
Blue	1 oz	100	6.1	8.15	2.21	0.23	5.30
crumbled, unpacked	1 cup	477	28.9	38.80	10.50	1.08	25.20
Sargento®	1 oz	100	6.1	8.15	0.00	0.00	0.00
Brick	1 oz	105	6.6	8.41	2.44	0.22	5.32
Brie	1 oz	95	5.9	7.85	2.27	0.23	4.94
Sargento®	1 oz	95	5.9	7.35	0.00	0.00	0.00
Burger, Sargento®	1 oz	106	6.3	8.36	0.00	0.00	0.00
Cajun, Sargento®	1 oz	110	7.0	8.99	0.00	0.00	0.00
Camabert							
wedge	38 g	114	7.5	9.22	2.67	0.28	5.80
caraway	1 oz	107	7.1	8.28	2.35	0.24	5.27
Sargento®	1 oz	85	5.6	6.88	0.00	0.00	0.00
Cheddar							
canned	1 oz	85	6.2	5.02	0.00	0.00	0.00
cut pieces	1 oz	114	7.1	9.40	2.66	0.27	5.98
inch cubes	17.2 g	69	4.8	5.70	1.62	0.16	3.63
mild-shredded	1 oz	90	7.0	5.00	0.00	0.00	0.00
past process, spreadery	1 oz	70	5.0	4.00			2.00
process with skim milk	1 cup	483	60.4	15.90			
process spread with milk	1 cup	484	59.4	15.80			
sharp nut log	1 oz	97	5.5	7.48	0.00	0.00	0.00
shredded	1 cup	455	28.1	37.50	10.60	1.06	23.80
Cracker Barrel®							
cheddar/wine	1 oz	100	4.0	7.00			4.00
extra sharp	1 oz	90	5.0	7.00			4.00
sharp	1 oz	100	4.0	7.00			4.00
sharp, lowfat	1 oz	80	9.0	5.00			3.00
Dormans Cheda Jack® low sodium	1 oz	80	8.0	5.00	0.57	0.00	3.00
Dormans® low sodium, lowfat	1 oz	80	8.0	5.00	0.57	0.00	3.00
Healthy Choice® fat free	1 oz	40	9.0	0.00			
Kraft®							
light & lively	1 oz	70	6.0	4.00			2.00
mild light naturals	1 oz	80	9.0	5.00			3.00
pasteurized pimento slices	1 oz	100	6.0	8.00			5.00
past process light	1 oz	70	6.0	4.00			2.00
sharp light naturals	1 oz	80	9.0	5.00			3.00
Pauly® lowfat, low sodium	1 oz	83	9.0	5.00	0.57	0.06	1.20
Pauly® low sodium, lowfat	1 oz	70	10.0	3.00	0.57	0.06	1.20
Savoldi®	100 g	330	23.0	21.00	15.30	1.47	4.20
Savoldi® mild, imitation	1 oz	90	6.0	6.00	0.00	0.00	0.00

FOOD	CARBO-HYDRATES (g)	CALCIUM (mg)	POTAS-SIUM (mg)	SODIUM (mg)	CHOLES-TEROL (mg)	LACTOSE (g)	% OF CALORIES FROM FAT
CHEESE							
American							
pasteurized process	0.4	174	46	406	27	0.45	75
Golden Image®	2.00	200	55	360	5		60
Kraft® light	2.00	200	70	420	15		51
Kraft Light & Lively®	2.00	200	70	420	15		51
Kraft® pasteurized loaf	1.00	150	25	430	25		74
Kraft® pasteurized slices	1.00	150	25	450	25		74
Smart Beat® fat free	2.00	150	90	180			0
Blue	0.6	150	73	396	21	0.28	73
crumbled, unpacked	3.1	712	346	1884	102		73
Sargento®	0.6	150		396	21		73
Brick	0.7	191	38	159	27		72
Brie	0.1	52	43	178	28	0.00	74
Sargento®	0.1	52		178	28		70
Burger, Sargento®	0.4	174		405	27		71
Cajun, Sargento®	0.2	4		164	28		74
Camabert							
wedge	0.1	147	71	320	27	0.00	73
caraway	0.8	191	26	196	26		70
Sargento®	0.1	110		239	20		73
Cheddar							
canned	3.60	77	21	350	0		53
cut pieces	0.3	204	28	176	30	0.20	74
inch cubes	0.2	124	17	107	18	0.12	74
mild-shredded	3.00			180	15	2.70	50
past process, spreadery	3.00	150	150	250	15		51
process with skim milk	25.00	1420	745	3890	239	21.60	30
process spread with milk	26.50	1422	1031	4983	140	21.60	29
sharp nut log	2.5	175		252	18		69
shredded	1.00	815	111	701	119	0.79	74
Cracker Barrel®							
cheddar/wine	3.00	150	100	230	20		63
extra sharp	3.00	150	110	240	20		70
sharp	4.00	150	120	230	20		63
sharp, lowfat	1.00	250	20	220	20		56
Dormans Cheda Jack® low sodium	1.00	200	30	140	19		56
Dormans® low sodium, lowfat	1.00	200	30	140	20	0.20	56
Healthy Choice® fat free	1.00	250	30	200	5		0
Kraft®							
light & lively	2.00	200	80	380	15		51
mild light naturals	0.00	250	20	220	20	0.00	56
pasteurized pimento slices	1.00	150	20	440	25		72
past process light	2.00	200	80	380	15		51
sharp light naturals	1.00	250	20	220	20		56
Pauly® lowfat, low sodium	1.00	200	32	68	14	0.20	54
Pauly® low sodium, lowfat	1.00	300	90	50	10	0.20	39
Savoldi®	8.00	800			0		57
Savoldi® mild, imitation	2.00	150	20	300	0		60

DAIRY PRODUCTS

FOOD	AMOUNT	CALORIES (kcal)	PROTEIN (g)	FAT (g)	MONO-UN-SATURATED FAT (g)	POLY-UN-SATURATED FAT (g)	SATURATED fat (g)
CHEESE (continued)							
Cheddar (continued)							
Sargento®	1 oz	114	7.1	9.40	2.66	0.27	5.98
Sargento® imitation cheddar	1 oz	85	7.0	6.00	0.00	0.00	0.00
Sargento® New York	1 oz	114	7.1	9.40	2.66	0.27	5.90
Smart Beat® sharp, fat free	1 oz	30	4.0	0.00			
Cheshire	1 oz	110	6.6	8.68	2.46	0.25	5.52
Colby	1 oz	112	6.7	9.10	2.63	0.27	5.73
lowfat, lorraine, lites	1 oz	90	8.0	6.00	0.60	0.06	4.00
Kraft® Light Naturals	1 oz	80	9.0	5.00			3.00
Pauly® low sodium, lowfat	1 oz	70	10.0	3.00	0.57	0.06	1.26
Sargento®	1 oz	112	6.7	9.10	0.00	0.00	0.00
Sargento® Jack	1 oz	109	6.8	8.84	0.00	0.00	0.00
Edam	1 oz	101	7.1	7.88	2.30	0.19	4.98
Sargento®	1 oz	101	7.1	7.88	0.00	0.00	0.00
Farmer's Cheese, Sargento®	1 oz	102	6.8	8.00	0.00	0.00	0.00
Feta	1 cup	670	36.1	54.10	11.80	1.50	38.00
	1 oz	75	4.0	6.03	1.31	0.17	4.24
Sargento®	1 oz	75	4.0	6.03	0.00	0.00	0.00
Fontina	1 oz	110	7.3	8.83	2.46	0.47	5.44
Pauly® garlic, lowfat, low sodium	1 oz	80	8.0	6.00	0.00	2.50	3.00
Sargento®	1 oz	110	7.3	8.63	0.00	0.00	0.00
Gjetost	1 oz	132	2.7	8.37	2.23	0.27	5.43
Sargento®	1 oz	132	2.7	8.37	0.00	0.00	0.00
Goat							
fresh-60% to 80% water-17% B.F.	1 cup	506	27.2	42.90			
hard	1 oz	128	8.7	10.10	2.30	0.24	6.98
semi-soft	1 oz	103	6.1	8.46	1.93	0.20	5.85
soft	1 oz	76	5.3	5.98	1.36	0.14	4.13
soft-35% to 60% water-28% B.F.	1 cup	802	44.9	69.20	11.30	1.45	36.60
Gouda	1 cup	892	62.5	68.70	19.40	1.65	44.10
	1 oz	101	7.1	7.78	2.20	0.19	4.99
Sargento®	1 oz	101	7.1	7.78	0.00	0.00	0.00
Gruyere	1 oz	117	8.5	9.17	2.85	0.49	5.36
Havarti, Sargento®	1 oz	118	5.1	10.60	0.00	0.00	0.00
Heart beat® Nucoa	1 oz	50	7.0	2.00	1.43	0.00	0.58
Hot pepper processed	1 oz	106	6.3	8.86	0.00	0.00	0.00
Italian style, grated	1 oz	108	8.2	7.75	0.00	0.00	0.00
Jarlsberg, Sargento®	1 oz	100	7.0	7.00	0.00	0.00	0.00
Limburger	1 oz	93	5.7	7.72	2.44	0.14	4.75
Sargento®	1 oz	93	5.7	7.72	0.00	0.00	0.00
Low Calorie							
0.5% B.F.	1 oz	15	2.00	0.14	0.00	0.00	0.00
3% B.F.	1 oz	17	1.8	0.91	0.00	0.00	0.00
6% B.F.	1 oz	57	6.5	1.70	0.00	0.00	0.00
Monterey Jack	1 oz	106	6.9	8.58	2.48	0.26	5.41
low sodium, lowfat	1 oz	70	10.0	3.00	0.57	0.06	1.26
lowfat, low sodium	1 oz	80	8.0	6.00	0.00	2.50	3.00
Dormans® Monterey low sodium Kraft®	1 oz	80	8.0	5.00	2.35	0.00	2.65

FOOD	CARBO-HYDRATES (g)	CALCIUM (mg)	POTAS-SIUM (mg)	SODIUM (mg)	CHOLES-TEROL (mg)	LACTOSE (g)	% OF CALORIES FROM FAT
CHEESE (continued)							
Cheddar (continued)							
Sargento®	0.3	204	28	176	30	0.20	74
Sargento® imitation cheddar	0.00	200		350	2	0.00	64
Sargento® New York	0.3	204	128	176	30	0.20	74
Smart Beat® sharp, fat free	2.00	150		230			0
Cheshire	1.3	182	27	198	29		71
Colby	0.7	194	36	171	27		73
lowfat, lorraine, lites	1.00	200	32	140	20		60
Kraft® Light Naturals	0.00	250	15	220	20	0.00	56
Pauly® low sodium, lowfat	1.00	300	90	50	10		39
Sargento®	0.7	194		171	27		73
Sargento® Jack	0.4	203		162	27		73
Edam	0.40	207	53	274	25		70
Sargento®	0.40	207		274	25		70
Farmer's Cheese, Sargento®	0.7	219		129	26		71
Feta	10.40	1253	157	2838	226		73
	1.1	140	18	316	25		72
Sargento®	1.1	140		316	25		72
Fontina	0.4	156	18	227	33		72
Pauly® garlic, lowfat, low sodium	0.00			95	20	0.00	68
Sargento®	0.4	156			33		71
Gjetost	12.10	113		170			57
Sargento®	12.10	113		170	0		57
Goat							
fresh-60% to 80% water-17% B.F.	2.9	250	151	800	218		76
hard	0.6	254	14	98	30		71
semi-soft	0.7	84	45	146	22		74
soft	0.2	40	7	104	13		71
soft-35% to 60% water-28% B.F.	0.2	253	151	1426	218		78
Gouda	5.5	1752	302	2052	285		69
	0.6	198	34	232	32		69
Sargento®	0.6	198		232	32		69
Gruyere	0.10	287	23	95	31	0.00	71
Havarti, Sargento®	0.2	228		200	31		81
Heart beat® Nucoa	2.00	199	140	280	0		36
Hot pepper processed	0.4	174		406	27		75
Italian style, grated	0.9	277		106	25		65
Jarlsberg, Sargento®	1.00	200		130	16		63
Limburger	0.1	141	36	227	26	0.00	75
Sargento®	0.1	141		227	26		75
Low Calorie							
0.5% B.F.	1.3	47	46	21	8		8
3% B.F.	0.7	34		28	0		47
6% B.F.	1.1	198			0		27
Monterey Jack	0.1	212	23	152	25	0.00	73
low sodium, lowfat	1.00	300	45	50	10		39
lowfat, low sodium	0.00			95	20	0.00	68
Dormans® Monterey low sodium Kraft®	1.00	200	25	140	18		5

DAIRY PRODUCTS

FOOD	AMOUNT	CALORIES (kcal)	PROTEIN (g)	FAT (g)	MONO-UN-SATURATED FAT (g)	POLY-UN-SATURATED FAT (g)	SATURATED fat (g)
CHEESE (continued)							
Monterey Jack (continued)							
caraway seeds	1 oz	100	7.0	8.00			5.00
jalepeno pepper	1 oz	110	7.0	9.00			5.00
light naturals	1 oz	80	9.0	5.00			3.00
Sargento®	1 oz	106	6.9	8.58	0.00	0.00	0.00
Mozzarella							
52% Water-22.5% B.F.	1 cup	740	51.1	56.80	17.30	2.01	34.60
Skim-52%water-16.5% B.F.	1 cup	664	63.4	41.60	11.80	1.23	26.40
imitation mozzarella, processed	1 oz	80	7.0	6.00	0.00	0.00	0.00
low sodium, lowfat	1 oz	60	10.0	2.00	0.60	0.06	1.34
made from skim milk	1 oz	72	6.9	4.51	1.28	0.13	2.87
made from whole milk	1 oz	80	5.5	6.12	1.86	0.22	3.73
shredded, light	1 oz	60	8.0	3.00	0.00	0.00	0.00
sliced, light	1 oz	60	8.0	3.00	0.00	0.00	0.00
substitute	1 oz	70	3.3	3.47	1.77	0.49	1.05
whole milk	1 oz	90	6.1	6.98	1.86	0.22	3.73
Dormans® low sodium	1 oz	80	9.0	4.00	1.26	0.00	2.74
Healthy Choice® fat free	1 oz	40	9.0	0.00			
Kraft® light naturals	1 oz	80	8.0	4.00			3.00
Kraft® string part skim	1 oz	80	8.0	5.00			3.00
Savoldi®	100 g	300	23.0	21.00	15.30	1.47	4.20
Savoldi® Imitation	1 oz	80	6.0	6.00	0.00	0.00	0.00
Muenster	1 oz	104	6.6	8.52	2.47	0.19	5.42
Dormans® low sodium	1 oz	80	8.0	5.00	2.26	0.00	2.74
Sargento® red rind	1 oz	104	6.6	8.52	0.00	0.00	0.00
Neufchatel	1 oz	74	2.8	6.64	1.92	0.18	4.20
Light	1 oz	80	3.0	7.00			4.00
Packaged Bacon							
Cracker Barrel®	1 oz	90	5.0	7.00			4.00
Kraft® nonfat pasteurized process	1 oz	45	7.0	0.00			
Parmesan							
grated	1 oz	456	41.6	30.00	8.73	0.66	19.10
& Romano grated	1 oz	111	9.6	7.48	0.00	0.00	0.00
Sargento® fresh	1 oz	111	10.1	7.32	0.00	0.00	0.00
Sargento® grated	1 oz	129	11.8	8.51	0.00	0.00	0.00
Pasteurized & Processed							
cheddar, fat free	1 oz	40	8.0	0.00			
mozzarella	1 oz	40	9.0	0.00			
pimento	1 oz	106	6.3	8.84	0.00	0.00	0.00
sharp	1 oz	106	6.3	8.86	0.00	0.00	0.00
Swiss	1 oz	95	7.0	7.09	0.00	0.00	0.00
Healthy Choice® fat free	1 oz	40	6.0	0.00			
Sargento®	1 oz	95	5.7	8.56	0.00	0.00	0.00
Pizza double shredded light	1 oz	70	8.0	4.00	0.00	0.00	0.00
Port du Salut	1 oz	100	6.7	8.00	2.65	0.21	4.73
Port wine-nut log, Sargento®	1 oz	97	5.5	7.48	0.00	0.00	0.00
Pot, Sargento®	1 oz	26	5.0	0.20	0.00	0.00	0.00
Processed							
cheddar	1 oz	92	6.2	6.44	1.94	0.22	4.28

FOOD	CARBO-HYDRATES (g)	CALCIUM (mg)	POTAS-SIUM (mg)	SODIUM (mg)	CHOLES-TEROL (mg)	LACTOSE (g)	% OF CALORIES FROM FAT
CHEESE (continued)							
Monterey Jack (continued)							
caraway seeds	1.00	150	15	180	30		72
jalepeno pepper	1.00	200	15	190	30		74
light naturals	0.00	250	15	220	20	0.00	56
Sargento®	0.1	212		152	25		73
Mozzarella							
52% Water-22.5% B.F.	5.8	1360	176	981	206		69
Skim-52%water-16.5% B.F.	7.2	1712	219	1217	151	0.10	56
imitation mozzarella, processed	0.00	250		310	2	0.00	68
low sodium, lowfat	1.00	208	65	70	8	0.10	30
made from skim milk	0.7	183	24	132	16	0.10	56
made from whole milk	0.6	147	19	106	22	0.10	69
shredded, light	1.00			150	10	0.10	45
sliced, light	1.00			150	10	0.10	45
substitute	6.7	173	129	194	0		45
whole milk	0.70	163	19	118	25	0.20	70
Dormans® low sodium	1.00	208	30	140	15	0.10	45
Healthy Choice® fat free	1.00	250	30	200	5	1.00	0
Kraft® light naturals	1.00	250	25	200	15		45
Kraft® string part skim	1.00	200	25	230	20		56
Savoldi®	8.00	1000			0		63
Savoldi® Imitation	2.00	150	20	330	0		68
Muenster	0.3	203	38	178	27		74
Dormans® low sodium	0.00	204	40	140	18	0.00	56
Sargento® red rind	0.3	203		178	27		74
Neufchatel	0.8	21	32	113	22	0.28	81
Light	1.00	20	30	115	25		79
Packaged Bacon							
Cracker Barrel®	3.00	150	85	280	20		70
Kraft® nonfat pasteurized process	4.00	200	80	420	5		0
Parmesan							
grated	3.7	1376	107	1862	79		59
& Romano grated	0.9	319		397	24		61
Sargento® fresh	0.9	336		454	19		59
Sargento® grated	1.0	390		528	22		59
Pasteurized & Processed							
cheddar, fat free	1.00	200		290	5		0
mozzarella	0.00	200 -	290	5	0.00	0	
pimento	0.4	174		405	27		75
sharp	0.4	174		406	27	0.40	75
Swiss	0.60	219		388	24		67
Healthy Choice® fat free	3.00	200	15	390	5		0
Sargento®	0.8	149		431	25	0.80	81
Pizza double shredded light	1.00			160	10		51
Port du Salut	0.1	184	39	151	35	0.00	72
Port wine-nut log, Sargento®	2.5	169		252	18		69
Pot, Sargento®	0.80	77		1	0		7
Processed							
cheddar	2.3	139	23	412	27	2.10	63

211

DAIRY PRODUCTS

FOOD	AMOUNT	CALORIES (kcal)	PROTEIN (g)	FAT (g)	MONO-UN-SATURATED FAT (g)	POLY-UN-SATURATED FAT (g)	SATURATED fat (g)
CHEESE (continued)							
Processed (continued)							
Pauly® low sodium, lowfat	1 oz	70	6.0	4.00	0.57	0.06	1.25
Provolone	1 oz	100	7.3	7.55	2.10	0.22	4.84
Dormans® low sodium	1 oz	80	9.0	4.00	0.57	0.00	3.00
Sargento®	1 oz	100	7.3	7.55	0.00	0.00	0.00
Quark	1 oz	20	4.0	0.07	0.00	0.00	0.00
Queso Blanco, Sargento®	1 oz	104	6.6	8.52	0.00	0.00	0.00
Queso de Papa, Sargento®	1 oz	114	7.1	9.40	0.00	0.00	0.00
Ricotta							
made with part skim milk	1 cup	340	28.0	19.50	5.69	0.64	12.10
made with whole milk	1 cup	428	27.7	31.90	8.92	0.95	20.40
Frigo® fat free	1 oz	20	4.0	0.00			
Frigo® lowfat, low salt	1 oz	30	3.0	1.00			
Gardenia® lowfat	1 oz	30	3.0	1.00			
Sargento® lite	1 oz	24	2.6	0.80	0.00	0.00	0.00
Sargento® part skim	1 oz	32	2.6	1.90	0.59	0.07	1.25
Roquefort	1 oz	105	6.1	8.69	2.40	0.37	5.46
Romano	1 oz	110	9.0	7.64	2.22	0.17	4.85
Sargento®	1 oz	110	9.0	7.64	0.00	0.00	0.00
Shredded Taco, Light, Sargento®	1 oz	80	8.0	4.00	0.00	0.00	0.00
Smokestick, Sargento®	1 oz	103	7.0	7.09	0.00	0.00	0.00
String							
Sargento®	1 oz	79	7.8	4.85	0.00	0.00	0.00
Sargento® smoked	1 oz	79	7.8	4.85	0.00	0.00	0.00
Swiss	1 oz	107	8.1	7.78	2.06	0.28	5.04
almond nut log	1 oz	94	6.1	7.38	0.00	0.00	0.00
no salt, deli, light	1 oz	100	8.0	8.00	2.06	0.28	5.05
pasteurized process	1 oz	95	7.0	7.09	2.00	0.18	4.55
shredded, light, fancy	1 oz	80	8.0	5.00	0.00	0.00	0.00
Dormans® low sodium, lowfat	1 oz	90	10.0	5.00	2.04	0.00	2.96
Kraft®							
light & lively	1 oz	70	6.0	3.00			2.00
light naturals	1 oz	90	10.0	5.00			3.00
low sodium	1 oz	110	8.0	8.00			5.00
pasteurized	1 oz	90	7.0	7.00			4.00
pasteurized processed	1 oz	70	6.0	3.00			2.00
Pauly® low sodium, lowfat	1 oz	80	9.0	3.00	0.84	0.11	2.05
Pauly® lowfat, low sodium	1 oz	97	9.0	7.00	1.95	0.26	4.79
Sargento®	1 oz	107	8.1	7.78	2.06	0.28	5.04
Sargento® Finland swiss	1 oz	107	8.1	7.78	0.00	0.00	0.00
Sargento® sliced, light	1 oz	80	10.0	5.00	0.00	0.00	0.00
Taco, Sargento®	1 oz	109	6.8	8.84	0.00	0.00	0.00
Tilsit	1 oz	96	6.9	7.36	2.02	0.20	4.76
Tilsiter, Sargento®	1 oz	96	6.9	7.36	0.00	0.00	0.00
Tybo Red Wax, Sargento®	1 oz	98	7.1	7.42	0.00	0.00	0.00
CHEESE FOOD							
American							
pasteurized process	1 oz	93	5.6	6.97	2.04	0.20	4.38
Kraft®	1 oz	90	5.0	7.00			4.00

FOOD	CARBO-HYDRATES (g)	CALCIUM (mg)	POTAS-SIUM (mg)	SODIUM (mg)	CHOLES-TEROL (mg)	LACTOSE (g)	% OF CALORIES FROM FAT
CHEESE (continued)							
Processed (continued)							
Pauly® low sodium, lowfat	2.00	250	40	150	10	1.80	51
Provolone	0.6	214	39	248	20		68
Dormans® low sodium	1.00	200	40	140	17		45
Sargento®	0.6	214		248	20		68
Quark	0.7	9		4	0		3
Queso Blanco, Sargento®	0.3	203		178	27		73
Queso de Papa, Sargento®	0.3	204		176	30		74
Ricotta							
made with part skim milk	12.60	669	308	307	76	3.44	52
made with whole milk	7.4	509	257	207	124	3.69	67
Frigo® fat free	2.00	60		15	3		0
Frigo® lowfat, low salt	1.00	60		10			30
Gardenia® lowfat	2.00	40		130			30
Sargento® lite	1.5	37		23	4	0.43	31
Sargento® part skim	1.10	51	39	27	10	0.43	53
Roquefort	0.5	188	26	513	26		75
Romano	1.0	302	25	340	29		63
Sargento®	1.0	302		340	29		63
Shredded Taco, Light, Sargento®	1.00			220	15		45
Smokestick, Sargento®	0.60	219		388	24		62
String							
Sargento®	0.8	207		150	15 -	55	
Sargento® smoked	0.8	207		150	15		55
Swiss	0.9	272	31	74	26		65
almond nut log	1.5	219		349	21		71
no salt, deli, light	0.00	273	30	8	26	0.00	72
pasteurized process	0.60	219	61	388	24		67
shredded, light, fancy	1.00			120	15		56
Dormans® low sodium, lowfat	0.00	273	30	60	17	0.00	50
Kraft®							
light & lively	2.00	200	80	350	15		3
light naturals	1.00	350	25	70	20		50
low sodium	1.00	250	25	10	25		65
pasteurized	1.00	200	25	420	25		70
pasteurized processed	2.00	200	80	350	15		39
Pauly® low sodium, lowfat	1.00	300	80	35	10		34
Pauly® lowfat, low sodium	1.00	273	32	32	19		65
Sargento®	0.9	272	31	74	26		65
Sargento® Finland swiss	0.9	272		74	26		65
Sargento® sliced, light	1.00			55	15		56
Taco, Sargento®	0.4	203		162	27		73
Tilsit	0.5	198	18	213	29		69
Tilsiter, Sargento®	0.5	198		213	29		69
Tybo Red Wax, Sargento®	0.2	228		200	23		68
CHEESE FOOD							
American							
pasteurized process	2.0	163	79	337	18	2.72	67
Kraft®	2.00	150	65	390	25		70

DAIRY PRODUCTS

FOOD	AMOUNT	CALORIES (kcal)	PROTEIN (g)	FAT (g)	MONO-UN-SATURATED FAT (g)	POLY-UN-SATURATED FAT (g)	SATURATED fat (g)
CHEESE (continued)							
American (continued)							
white	1 oz	90	5.0	7.00			4.00
cheez'n bacon	1 oz	90	6.0	7.00			4.00
garlic	1 oz	90	5.0	7.00			4.00
jalapeno, singles	1 oz	90	5.0	7.00			4.00
jalapeno, tub	1 oz	90	5.0	7.00			4.00
monterey jack	1 oz	90	5.0	7.00			4.00
pimento	1 oz	90	5.0	7.00			4.00
sharp	1 oz	100	6.0	8.00			5.00
swiss	1 oz	90	6.0	7.00			4.00
Velveeta®							
hot mexican	1 oz	100	6.0	7.00			4.00
mild mexican	1 oz	100	6.0	7.00			4.00
shredded	1 oz	100	6.0	7.00			4.00
CHEESE SPREAD							
American, processed	1 oz	82	4.7	6.02	1.76	0.18	3.78
Bacon squeez a snak	1 oz	80	5.0	7.00			4.00
Cheese Whiz® Kraft	1 oz	80	4.0	6.00			3.00
mild mexican	1 oz	80	4.0	6.00			4.00
jalepeno	1 oz	80	4.0	6.00			4.00
Cheese Sticks, Sargento®	1 oz	110	3.0	6.00	0.00	0.00	0.00
Garlic squeez a snak	1 oz	80	5.0	7.00			4.00
Hickory smoke squeez a snak	1 oz	80	5.0	7.00			4.00
Jalapeno squeez a snak	1 oz	80	5.0	6.00			4.00
Sharp-squeez a snak	1 oz	80	5.0	7.00			4.00
Kraft®							
american	1 oz	80	4.0	6.00			3.00
bacon	1 oz	80	5.0	7.00			4.00
jalapeno	1 oz	80	5.0	6.00			4.00
Mohawk Valley® Limburger	1 oz	70	4.0	6.00			3.00
Velveeta Hot Mexican®	1 oz	80	5.0	6.00			3.00
COTTAGE CHEESE							
dry curd, uncreamed	1 cup	123	25.0	0.61	0.16	0.02	0.40
0.1% B.F.	1 oz	26	5.2	0.02	0.01	0.00	0.01
1% B.F.	1 cup	183	31.3	2.58	0.74	0.08	1.63
1% Lowfat, unpacked	1 cup	164	28.0	2.30	0.66	0.07	1.46
2% Lowfat, unpacked	1 cup	203	31.1	4.36	1.24	0.13	2.76
4% Fat, large curd, unpack	1 cup	232	28.1	10.10	2.88	0.32	6.41
4% Fat, small curd, unpack	1 cup	217	26.2	9.47	2.70	0.29	5.99
with fruit, unpacked	1 cup	279	22.4	7.68	2.19	0.24	4.86
Knudsen® fat free	1 cup	140	30.0	0.00			
Lucerne® fat free	1 cup	140	26.0	0.00			
Lucerne® 1% no salt added	1 cup	180	28.0	2.00			
CREAM							
Coffee-table							
15% B.F.	1 cup	383	6.8	36.00	10.40	1.34	22.40
18% B.F.	1 cup	443	6.6	43.20	12.50	1.61	26.90

FOOD	CARBO-HYDRATES (g)	CALCIUM (mg)	POTAS-SIUM (mg)	SODIUM (mg)	CHOLES-TEROL (mg)	LACTOSE (g)	% OF CALORIES FROM FAT
CHEESE (continued)							
American (continued)							
white	2.00	150	70	400	20		70
cheez'n bacon	2.00	150	75	400	25		70
garlic	2.00	150	80	370	20		70
jalapeno, singles	2.00	150	75	450	25		70
jalapeno, tub	2.00	150	80	390	20		70
monterey jack	2.00	150	70	390	25		70
pimento	2.00	150	75	390	25		70
sharp	1.00	150	35	400	25		72
swiss	2.00	200	70	440	25		70
Velveeta®							
hot mexican	3.00	200	75	430	25		63
mild mexican	3.00	150	70	420	25		63
shredded	3.00	150	75	410	20		63
CHEESE SPREAD							
American, processed	2.4	159	69	381	16	2.48	66
Bacon squeez a snak	1.00	150	20	500	20		79
Cheese Whiz® Kraft	2.00	100	65	470	20		68
mild mexican	2.00	100	50	430	20		68
jalepeno	2.00	100	50	430	20		68
Cheese Sticks, Sargento®	10.00			268	9		49
Garlic squeez a snak	1.00	150	20	430	20		79
Hickory smoke squeez a snak	1.00	150	20	440	20		79
Jalapeno squeez a snak	1.00	150	25	510	20		68
Sharp-squeez a snak	1.00	150	20	440	20		79
Kraft®							
american	2.00	150	55	470	15		68
bacon	1.00	150	25	560	20		79
jalapeno	2.00	150	95	470	20		68
Mohawk Valley® Limburger	0.00	100	15	420	20	0.00	77
Velveeta Hot Mexican®	3.00	150	95	520	20		68
COTTAGE CHEESE							
dry curd, uncreamed	2.6	46	47	19	10		4
0.1% B.F.	0.9	9	24	53	3	0.58	1
1% B.F.	6.8	154	216	1026	11		13
1% Lowfat, unpacked	6.1	138	193	918	10	6.15	13
2% Lowfat, unpacked	8.20	155	217	918	19	7.23	19
4% Fat, large curd, unpack	6.0	135	189	911	34	1.35	39
4% Fat, small curd, unpack	5.6	126	177	850	31	1.26	39
with fruit, unpacked	30.10	108	151	915	25		25
Knudsen® fat free	6.00	120		600	10		0
Lucerne® fat free	8.00	80		840	10		0
Lucerne® 1% no salt added	8.00	120		80			10
CREAM							
Coffee-table							
15% B.F.	9.6	242	303	97	12		85
18% B.F.	9.0	234	296	96	147		88

DAIRY PRODUCTS

FOOD	AMOUNT	CALORIES (kcal)	PROTEIN (g)	FAT (g)	MONO-UN-SATURATED FAT (g)	POLY-UN-SATURATED FAT (g)	SATURATED fat (g)
CREAM (continued)							
20% B.F.	1 cup	483	6.4	48.00	13.90	1.79	29.90
Light-fluid	1 cup	469	6.5	46.30	13.40	1.72	28.90
Cream							
Half & Half® 10% B.F.	1 cup	285	7.2	24.20	6.98	0.91	15.10
Half & Half® 12% B.F.	1 cup	326	7.1	29.00	8.38	1.09	18.10
Half & Half® milk and cream fluid	1 cup	315	7.2	27.80	8.04	1.03	17.30
imitation liquid, non dairy, frozen	1 cup	333	2.5	24.40	18.50	0.07	4.75
imitation, non dairy, powdered	1 cup	514	4.5	33.40	0.91	0.01	30.60
26% Fat	1 oz	71	0.7	7.12			
Whipped							
imitation, non dairy, frozen	1 cup	239	0.9	19.00	1.21	0.39	16.30
imitation, non dairy, powder	1 cup	151	2.9	9.93	0.68	0.16	8.55
imitation, pressurized	1 cup	154	1.9	13.30	3.85	0.50	8.30
imitation, pressurized	1 cup	184	0.7	15.60	1.35	0.17	13.20
Whipping							
32% B.F.	1 cup	722	5.0	76.50	22.40	2.31	47.80
35% B.F.	1 cup	780	5.0	83.30	24.20	2.88	51.90
heavy, unwhipped, fluid	1 cup	821	4.9	88.10	25.40	3.27	54.80
light, unwhipped, fluid	1 cup	699	5.2	73.90	21.70	2.11	46.20
Cream Cheese	1 oz	100	2.2	10.00	2.82	0.37	6.31
Low calorie, 20% B.F.	1 oz	64	2.6	5.06	0.62	0.06	1.01
Healthy Choice® fat Free herb/garlic	1 oz	30	6.0	0.00			
Healthy Choice® fat Free strawberry	1 oz	30	5.0	0.00			
Philadelphia® Cream Cheese	1 oz	100	2.0	10.00			6.00
Chives	1 oz	90	2.0	9.00			5.00
Chives/onion	1 oz	100	2.0	9.00			5.00
Herb/garlic	1 oz	100	1.0	9.00			5.00
Olives/pimento	1 oz	90	2.0	8.00			5.00
Olive/pimento	1 oz	90	2.0	8.00	2.38	0.31	5.32
Pasteurized	1 oz	60	3.0	5.00			3.00
Pimento	1 oz	90	2.0	9.00			5.00
Pineapple	1 oz	90	1.0	8.00			5.00
Smoked salmon	1 oz	90	2.0	9.00			5.00
Soft	1 oz	100	1.0	10.00			5.00
Strawberries	1 oz	90	1.0	8.00			5.00
Whipped	1 oz	100	2.0	10.00			6.00
Whipped/chives	1 oz	90	2.0	8.00			5.00
Whipped/onions	1 oz	90	2.0	8.00			5.00
Whipped/salmon	1 oz	90	2.0	8.00			5.00
Philadelphia light processed	1 oz	60	3.0	5.00	1.85	0.15	3.00
Creamer							
non dairy	1 oz	107	1.0	0.40	0.03	0.01	0.36
Coffeemate® non dairy liquid	1 tbsp	16	0.0	1.00		0.00	0.00
Coffeemate® non dairy lite liquid	1 tsp	8	0.0	0.00	0.00	0.00	0.00
Non dairy, Cremora Lite® liquid	1 tsp	21	1.0	1.00	1.00	0.00	0.00
Dairifree milk substitute, Canopro®	1 cup	71	6.4	1.10		0.13	0.22

FOOD	CARBO-HYDRATES (g)	CALCIUM (mg)	POTAS-SIUM (mg)	SODIUM (mg)	CHOLES-TEROL (mg)	LACTOSE (g)	% OF CALORIES FROM FAT
CREAM (continued)							
20% B.F.	8.6	228	291	96	165		89
Light-fluid	8.7	231	292	95	159		89
Cream							
Half & Half® 10% B.F.	10.70	258	318	100	76		76
Half & Half® 12% B.F.	10.30	253	313	99	94		80
Half & Half® milk and cream fluid	10.40	254	314	98	89		79
imitation liquid, non dairy, frozen	27.90	22	466	194	0		66
imitation, non dairy, powdered	51.60	21	763	170	0		58
26% Fat	1.1	19	21	16			90
Whipped							
imitation, non dairy, frozen	17.30	5	14	19	0		72
imitation, non dairy, powder	13.20	72	121	53	8		59
imitation, pressurized	7.4	61	88	78	46		78
imitation, pressurized	11.30	4	13	43	0		76
Whipping							
32% B.F.	7.4	163	222	86	276	6.70	95
35% B.F.	6.7	158	196	86	306	6.70	96
heavy, unwhipped, fluid	6.6	154	179	89	326	6.66	97
light, unwhipped, fluid	7.0	166	231	82	265	6.69	95
Cream Cheese	0.7	23	34	85	31	0.48	90
Low calorie, 20% B.F.	1.0	26	40	198	18	0.50	71
Healthy Choice® fat Free herb/garlic	2.00	200	30	200	5		0
Healthy Choice® fat Free strawberry	2.00	200	30	200	3		0
Philadelphia® Cream Cheese	1.00	20	25	90	30		90
Chives	1.00	20	30	125	30		90
Chives/onion	2.00	20	45	100	30		81
Herb/garlic	2.00	40	70	160	25		81
Olives/pimento	2.00	20	40	160	25		80
Olive/pimento	2.00	20	34	180	31		80
Pasteurized	2.00	40	60	160	10		75
Pimento	1.00	20	30	150	30		90
Pineapple	4.00	20	40	90	25		80
Smoked salmon	1.00	20	40	180	25		90
Soft	2.00	40	55	100	30		90
Strawberries	4.00	20	65	75	20		80
Whipped	1.00	20	30	85	30		90
Whipped/chives	1.00	20	40	150	30		80
Whipped/onions	2.00	20	45	170	25		80
Whipped/salmon	2.00	20	45	170	30		80
Philadelphia light processed	2.00	40	34	160	10		75
Creamer							
non dairy	24.90	3	223	30	0		3
Coffeemate® non dairy liquid	2.00		20	5	0		56
Coffeemate® non dairy lite liquid	2.00		15	0	0		0
Non dairy, Cremora Lite® liquid	2.00	0	5	5	0		43
Dairifree milk substitute, Canopro®	8.90	338	7	105	0		14

DAIRY PRODUCTS

FOOD	AMOUNT	CALORIES (kcal)	PROTEIN (g)	FAT (g)	MONO-UN-SATURATED FAT (g)	POLY-UN-SATURATED FAT (g)	SATURATED fat (g)
MILK							
Buttermilk							
cultured, fluid	1 cup	99	8.1	2.16	0.62	0.08	1.34
dried, sweet cream	1 cup	464	41.2	6.94	2.00	0.26	4.32
Chocolate							
cocoa, whole, homemade	1 cup	218	9.1	9.05	2.65	0.33	5.61
1% fat, fluid	1 cup	158	8.1	2.50	0.75	0.09	1.54
2% fat, fluid	1 cup	179	8.0	5.00	1.47	0.18	3.10
pasteurized	1 oz	19	1.0	0.57	0.17	0.02	0.37
whole, vitamin D	1 cup	208	7.9	8.48	2.48	0.31	5.26
Condensed							
sweet	1 oz	95	2.5	2.52	0.69	0.10	1.55
sweetened, canned	1 cup	982	24.2	26.60	7.43	1.03	16.80
Cow, fresh	1 oz	18	0.9	1.22	0.27	0.04	0.59
Dry, skim, powder, instantized	1 cup	244	23.9	0.49	0.13	0.02	0.32
Eggnog, commercial	1 cup	342	9.7	19.00	5.67	0.86	11.30
Evaporated	1 oz	42	2.2	2.41	0.34	0.04	0.67
part skim, canned, 2% fat	1 cup	233	18.7	5.08	1.57	0.17	3.08
skim, canned	1 fl oz	25	2.4	0.06	0.02	0.00	0.04
skim, canned, 0.2% B.F.	1 cup	199	19.3	0.51	0.16	0.02	0.31
whole, canned	1 cup	338	17.2	19.10	5.90	0.61	11.60
whole, canned, 7.8% B.F.	1 cup	344	17.2	19.70	6.07	0.64	11.90
Filled							
filled	1 oz	96	2.5	2.66	0.03	0.00	0.88
Filled, condensed	1 oz	97	2.4	3.37	0.69	0.10	1.55
Fluid							
fluid, skim	1 cup	86	8.4	0.44	0.12	0.02	0.29
fluid, whole, pasturized, 3.3% B.F.	1 cup	150	8.0	8.15	2.35	0.30	5.07
Full cream, pasteurized	1 oz	21	1.0	0.96			
Goat, whole, fluid	1 cup	168	8.7	10.10	2.71	0.36	6.51
Human, whole, mature	1 cup	171	2.5	10.80	4.08	1.22	4.94
Imitation							
imitation	1 cup	150	4.3	8.32	4.88	1.19	1.87
Health Valley Soy Moo®	1 cup	160	8.0	0.00	0.00	0.00	0.00
Indian buffalo, whole	1 cup	236	9.2	16.80	4.36	0.36	11.20
Lowfat, pasteurized	1 oz	15	1.2	0.48	0.01	0.00	0.03
Malted							
beverage	1 cup	237	10.4	9.80	2.78	0.56	5.96
chocolate, beverage	1 cup	229	9.1	8.90	2.57	0.38	5.52
chocolate, powdered	1 tsp	26	0.4	0.27	0.07	0.03	0.15
chocolate flavor	1 cup	228	9.0	9.01	2.57	0.38	5.53
chocolate flavor, prepared	1 cup	229	9.1	8.90	2.57	0.38	5.53
natural flavor	1 cup	236	10.3	9.80	2.78	0.56	5.95
natural flavor, prepared	1 cup	237	10.4	9.80	2.78	0.56	5.96
powdered	1 tsp	29	0.8	0.57	0.14	0.08	0.29
Non dairy							
Tofu Magic®	1 cup	90	2.0	5.00			
Sovex® Tofu	1 cup	90	2.0	5.00			

FOOD	CARBO-HYDRATES (g)	CALCIUM (mg)	POTAS-SIUM (mg)	SODIUM (mg)	CHOLES-TEROL (mg)	LACTOSE (g)	% OF CALORIES FROM FAT
MILK							
Buttermilk							
cultured, fluid	11.70	285	371	257	9	9.07	20
dried, sweet cream	58.80	1421	1910	621	83		13
Chocolate							
cocoa, whole, homemade	25.80	298	480	123	33		37
1% fat, fluid	26.10	287	426	152	7		14
2% fat, fluid	26.00	284	422	150	17		25
pasteurized	2.5	31	34	14	3		26
whole, vitamin D	25.80	280	417	149	30		37
Condensed							
sweet	15.60	94	2	35	10		24
sweetened, canned	166.00	868	1136	389	104		24
Cow, fresh	0.9	30	19	3	4		60
Dry, skim, powder, instantized	35.50	837	1160	373	12		2
Eggnog, commercial	34.40	330	420	138	149		50
Evaporated	2.9	76	1	39	4		51
part skim, canned, 2% fat	28.00	700	806	281	20		20
skim, canned	3.6	92	106	37	1		2
skim, canned, 0.2% B.F.	29.10	741	849	294	9		2
whole, canned	25.30	658	764	267	73		51
whole, canned, 7.8% B.F.	25.30	657	764	267	74		52
Filled							
filled	15.50	92	2	38	1		25
Filled, condensed	14.30	78	74	30	10		31
Fluid							
fluid, skim	11.90	302	406	126	4	10.80	5
fluid, whole, pasturized, 3.3% B.F.	11.40	291	370	120	33	11.40	49
Full cream, pasteurized	2.0	31	28	10			42
Goat, whole, fluid	10.90	326	499	122	28		54
Human, whole, mature	17.00	79	126	42	34		57
Imitation							
imitation	15.00	79	279	191	0		50
Health Valley Soy Moo®	34.00	74	420	210	0		0
Indian buffalo, whole	12.60	412	434	127	46		65
Lowfat, pasteurized	1.3	37	23	10	1		30
Malted							
beverage	27.30	354	529	223	37		37
chocolate, beverage	29.80	304	499	172	34		35
chocolate, powdered	6.1	4	43	18	0		9
chocolate flavor	29.90	305	498	172	34	10.90	36
chocolate flavor, prepared	29.80	304	499	172	34	10.90	35
natural flavor	27.30	355	530	223	37		37
natural flavor, prepared	27.30	354	529	223	37		37
powdered	5.30	21	53	34	1		18
Non dairy							
Tofu Magic®	10.00	500	10	120			50
Sovex® Tofu	10.00	500		120	0		50

DAIRY PRODUCTS

FOOD	AMOUNT	CALORIES (kcal)	PROTEIN (g)	FAT (g)	MONO-UN-SATURATED FAT (g)	POLY-UN-SATURATED FAT (g)	SATURATED fat (g)
MILK (continued)							
Nonfat							
skim, fluid	1 cup	86	8.4	0.44	0.12	0.02	0.29
skim, instantized, envelope	91 g	326	31.9	0.66	0.17	0.03	0.42
skim, instantized, dried	1 cup	244	23.9	0.49	0.13	0.02	0.32
skim, milk solids added	1 cup	90	8.8	0.61	0.16	0.02	0.40
skim, protein fortified	1 cup	100	9.7	0.62	0.16	0.02	0.40
1% fat							
lowfat, fluid	1 cup	102	8.0	2.59	0.75	0.10	1.61
nonfat milk solids added	1 cup	104	8.5	2.38	0.69	0.09	1.48
protein fortified	1 cup	119	9.7	2.88	0.83	0.11	1.79
Powder							
instant, full cream	1 oz	140	7.7	7.54	0.25	0.03	0.55
skim	1 oz	100	7.1	0.74	0.03	0.00	0.07
Sheep, whole, fluid	1 cup	264	14.7	17.20	4.22	0.76	11.30
Soy, fluid	1 cup	79	6.6	4.58	0.78	2.00	0.51
Soybean							
no sugar	1 oz	17	1.1	0.34			
packet	1 oz	18	0.4	0.62			
Sterilized	1 oz	18	0.9	0.96	0.27	0.04	0.59
2% fat							
lowfat, fluid	1 cup	121	8.1	4.68	1.35	0.17	2.92
nonfat milk solids added	1 cup	125	8.5	4.70	1.36	0.18	2.93
fluid, protein fortified	1 cup	137	9.7	4.87	1.41	0.18	3.03
Whole							
dry	1 cup	635	33.7	34.20	10.10	0.85	21.40
low sodium	1 cup	149	7.6	8.44	2.44	0.31	5.26
regular, 3.3% fat fluid	1 cup	150	8.0	8.15	2.35	0.30	5.07
Milkshake							
chocolate, thick	300 g	356	9.2	8.10	2.34	0.30	5.04
vanilla, thick	313 g	350	12.1	9.48	2.74	0.35	5.90
Mocha mix non dairy	1 tbsp	20	1.0	2.40	0.80	0.80	0.80
SOUR CREAM							
cultured	1 cup	493	7.3	48.20	13.90	1.79	30.00
imitation	1 oz	59	0.7	5.53	0.17	0.02	5.04
imitation, non fat, dry milk added	235 g	415	8.0	39.00	4.96	1.19	31.20
14% B.F.	1 cup	350	6.9	32.20	9.31	1.20	20.00
18% B.F.	1 cup	432	7.1	41.40	12.00	1.54	25.80
substitute	1 tbsp	30	0.0	3.00	0.09	0.01	2.56
Half & Half®	1 tbsp	20	0.4	1.80	0.52	0.07	1.12
Knudsen® fat free	15 g	9	1.0	0.00			
Knudsen® light	15 g	18	0.5	1.00			
Land O Lakes® fat free	14 g	8	1.5	0.00			
Molly McButter®	1 tsp	8	0.0	0.00	0.00	0.00	0.00
Whey							
acid, dry	1 tbsp	10	0.3	0.02	0.00	0.00	0.01
acid, fluid	1 cup	59	1.9	0.22	0.06	0.01	0.14
sweet, dry	1 tbsp	26	1.0	0.08	0.02	0.00	0.05
sweet, fluid	1 cup	66	2.1	0.89	0.25	0.03	0.57

FOOD	CARBO-HYDRATES (g)	CALCIUM (mg)	POTAS-SIUM (mg)	SODIUM (mg)	CHOLES-TEROL (mg)	LACTOSE (g)	% OF CALORIES FROM FAT
MILK (continued)							
Nonfat							
skim, fluid	11.90	302	406	126	4	10.80	5
skim, instantized, envelope	47.50	1120	1552	499	17	45.90	2
skim, instantized, dried	35.50	837	1160	373	12	34.30	2
skim, milk solids added	12.30	316	418	130	5	10.80	6
skim, protein fortified	13.70	352	446	144	5	10.80	6
1% fat							
lowfat, fluid	11.70	300	381	123	10	11.20	23
nonfat milk solids added	12.20	313	397	128	10	11.30	21
protein fortified	13.60	349	444	143	10	11.30	22
Powder							
instant, full cream	10.30	179	211	85	4	10.30	48
skim	16.20	331	325	135	1	15.10	7
Sheep, whole, fluid	13.10	474	334	108	66		59
Soy, fluid	4.3	10	338	29	0		52
Soybean							
no sugar	2.3	6	18	1			18
packet	2.7	2	12	1			31
Sterilized	1.30	26	32	19	4		49
2% fat							
lowfat, fluid	11.70	297	377	122	18	11.20	35
nonfat milk solids added	12.20	313	397	128	18	11.30	34
fluid, protein fortified	13.50	352	447	145	19	11.30	32
Whole							
dry	49.20	1168	1702	475	124	46.00	48
low sodium	10.90	246	617	6	33	10.90	51
regular, 3.3% fat fluid	11.40	291	370	120	33	12.00	49
Milkshake							
chocolate, thick	63.50	396	672	333	32	14.40	20
vanilla, thick	55.60	457	572	299	37	15.70	24
Mocha mix non dairy	1.00		20	5	0		100
SOUR CREAM							
cultured	9.8	268	331	123	102		88
imitation	1.8	1	46	29	0		84
imitation, non fat, dry milk added	11.00	266	380	240	0		85
14% B.F.	9.80	245	304	99	91		83
18% B.F.	9.8	258	320	112	97		86
substitute	0.00	0	30	15	0	0.00	90
Half & Half®	0.6	16	19	6	6		81
Knudsen® fat free	1.50	20		10			0
Knudsen® light	1.00	20		10	5		51
Land O Lakes® fat free	0.50	10		8			0
Molly McButter®	2.00		16	130	0		0
Whey							
acid, dry	2.1	59	66	28	0		2
acid, fluid	12.60	253	352	118	1	11.10	3
sweet, dry	5.5	59	155	80	0		3
sweet, fluid	12.60	115	396	132	5	11.10	12

DAIRY PRODUCTS

FOOD	AMOUNT	CALORIES (kcal)	PROTEIN (g)	FAT (g)	MONO-UN-SATURATED FAT (g)	POLY-UN-SATURATED FAT (g)	SATURATED fat (g)
YOGURT							
apricot	1 oz	76	0.9	5.67	0.00	0.00	0.00
beverage	1 cup	170	6.3	2.16	0.59	0.06	1.39
coffee & vanilla flavor, 1.9% B.F	1 cup	225	10.0	4.65	1.28	0.13	3.00
cherry/mixed berry, custard style	170 g	190	7.0	4.00	0.00	0.00	0.00
Yogurt, fruit at bottom							
<1% B.F.	1 cup	152	10.5	0.47	0.13	0.01	0.30
>4% B.F.	1 cup	352	7.6	14.70	4.07	0.42	9.49
1% To 2% B.F.	1 cup	247	9.7	3.77	1.05	0.10	2.43
2% To 4% B.F.	1 cup	21	9.5	7.35	2.02	0.21	4.74
Yogurt, fruit flavors							
custard style	170 g	150	6.0	3.00	0.51	0.05	1.18
lowfat, added solids	1 cup	231	9.9	2.45	0.67	0.07	1.58
Dannon® original coffee lowfat	227 g	200	10.0	3.00	0.78	0.08	1.83
Dannon® peach/strawberry lowfat	125 g	60	6.0	0.00	0.00	0.00	0.00
Light n Lively® strawberry	125 g	50	4.0	0.00	0.00	0.00	0.00
Yoplait® fat free	170 g	150	7.0	0.00	0.00	0.00	0.00
Yoplait® light	170 g	80	7.0	0.00	0.00	0.00	0.00
Yoplait® original	170 g	190	8.0	3.00	0.00	0.00	0.00
Fruit, stirred or Swiss style	1 cup	249	11.0	4.12	1.14	0.12	2.66
Yogurt, plain							
lowfat, milk solids added	1 cup	144	11.9	3.52	0.97	0.10	2.27
nonfat, milk solids added	1 cup	127	13.0	0.41	0.11	0.01	0.26
nonfat	227 g	120	13.0	0.00	0.00	0.00	0.00
stirred or Swiss style	1 cup	168	12.5	5.07	1.41	0.13	3.27
whole milk, no solids	1 cup	139	7.9	7.38	2.03	0.21	4.76
<1% B.F.	1 cup	124	12.3	0.25	0.07	0.01	0.16
2%->4% B.F.	1 cup	182	11.6	6.84	1.88	0.19	4.41
>4% B.F.	1 cup	255	9.8	14.40	3.93	0.40	9.28
Yoplait® original	170 g	130	10.0	3.00	0.72	0.08	1.70
Yogurt, vanilla							
custard style	227 g	180	7.0	4.00	0.78	0.08	1.83
Yoplait® nonfat	227 g	180	11.0	0.00	0.00	0.00	0.00
Yoplait® original	170 g	180	9.0	3.00	0.58	0.06	1.37

FOOD	CARBO-HYDRATES (g)	CALCIUM (mg)	POTAS-SIUM (mg)	SODIUM (mg)	CHOLES-TEROL (mg)	LACTOSE (g)	% OF CALORIES FROM FAT
YOGURT							
apricot	5.2	36	43	23	0		67
beverage	32.80	260	399	98	13		11
coffee & vanilla flavor, 1.9% B.F	38.00	322	356	141	13		19
cherry/mixed berry, custard style	32.00	200	290	95	20	5.62	19
Yogurt, fruit at bottom							
<1% B.F.	26.40	393	483	172	7	5.00	3
>4% B.F.	41.00	263	452	104	15	8.09	38
1% To 2% B.F.	43.10	299	440	122	15	8.09	14
2% To 4% B.F.	43.50	350	459	147	25	8.09	24
Yogurt, fruit flavors							
custard style	25.00	150	260	100	10	5.62	18
lowfat, added solids	43.20	345	442	133	10	7.49	10
Dannon® original coffee lowfat	34.00	389	498	140	11		14
Dannon® peach/strawberry lowfat	8.00	300	179	70	5	1.88	0
Light n Lively® strawberry	8.00	58	10	55	0	1.88	0
Yoplait® fat free	31.00	250	390	95	5	5.62	0
Yoplait® light	13.00	150	270	80	5	2.50	0
Yoplait® original	32.00	250	350	110	10	5.62	14
Fruit, stirred or Swiss style	42.30	338	449	136	15	8.09	15
Yogurt, plain							
lowfat, milk solids added	16.00	415	531	159	14	8.40	22
nonfat, milk solids added	17.40	452	579	174	4	8.40	3
nonfat	18.00	450	590	160	5	8.40	0
stirred or Swiss style	16.90	447	578	155	22	9.07	27
whole milk, no solids	10.60	274	351	105	29	8.40	48
<1% B.F.	17.80	412	582	175	5	9.07	2
2%->4% B.F.	16.40	394	557	150	24	9.07	34
>4% B.F.	18.10	370	511	139	44	9.07	51
Yoplait® original	15.00	300	370	140	15	6.29	21
Yogurt, vanilla							
custard style	30.00	250	300	110	20		20
Yoplait® nonfat	35.00	400	500	140	5		0
Yoplait® original	29.00	250	390	120	10		15

THE GOOD-SENSE FOOD GUIDE PYRAMID
Your guide to daily food choices

Fats, Oils & Sweets
USE SPARINGLY

Milk, Yogurt,
Cheese Group
2-3 SERVINGS

Vegetable
Group
3-5 SERVINGS

Meat, Poultry, Fish,
Dry Beans, Eggs &
Nuts Group
2-3 SERVINGS

Fruit Group
2-4 SERVINGS

Bread, Cereal, Rice
& Pasta Group
6-11 SERVINGS

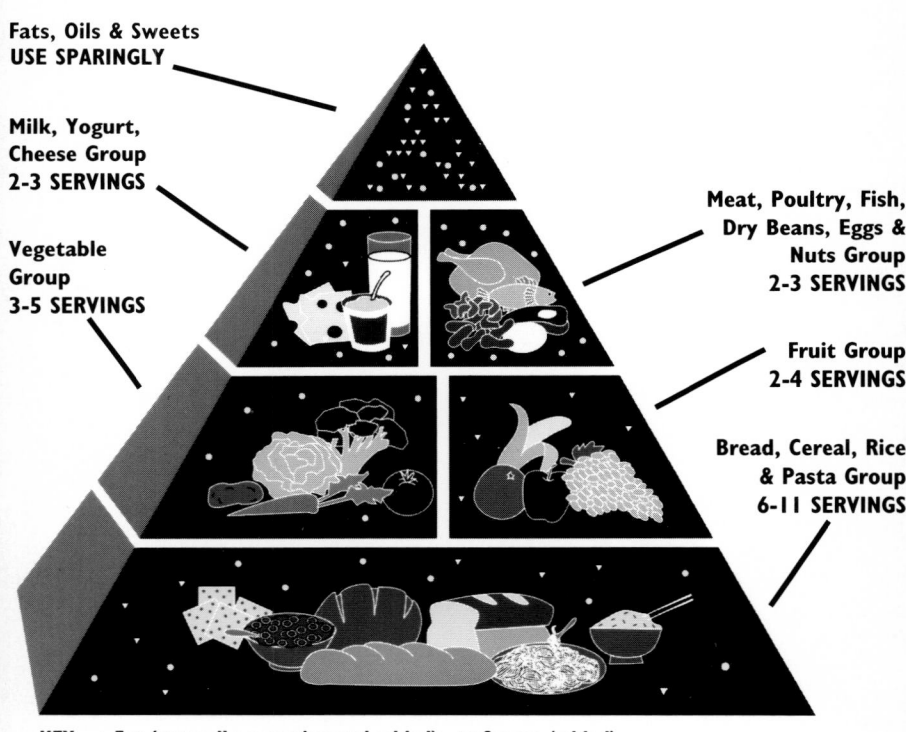

KEY • Fat (naturally occurring and added) ▼ Sugars (added)

FISH, POULTRY, BEEF, LAMB, VEAL, PORK, SAUSAGES, AND LUNCHEON MEAT

This section contains foods from the third level of the Food Guide Pyramid. As the levels progress up the Pyramid, the recommended number of servings per day for each level is lower than for the previous level. Therefore, two to three servings are suggested here. These foods all come from animals. They are important sources of protein, B vitamins, calcium, iron, and zinc. The Fish charts have columns for DHA3 and EPA3, which are omega-3 fatty acids. The omega-3 fats in fish may be of preventive importance in relation to coronary heart disease.

The foods in this section contain important nutrients and vitamins. However, certain cuts of meat as well as poultry skin, are high in fat.

The changes that occur in cooking meat are complex and some of the varying nutritive values for one type of meat is confusing. Solids and moisture are lost from both lean and fat tissue. High retention of fat in the lean could be caused by migration of lipid from the separable fat during cooking. Low retention of nutrients may be attributed to loss into cooking juices, drippings or breakdown by heat.

FISH

FOOD	AMOUNT	CALORIES (kcal)	PROTEIN (g)	FAT (g)	CARBO-HYDRATES (g)	FIBER (g)	CALCIUM (mg)
Abalone							
cooked, fried	85.0 g	161	16.7	5.8	9.4	0.3	32.0
raw	1 oz	29	4.9	0.2	1.7		9.0
Agutuk							
fish with shortening, Alaska	1 cup	473	9.0	44.4	10.5		
fish/berry with seal oil, Alaska	1 cup	350	3.4	32.2	13.2	0.5	7.5
Alewife, with bone, baked or broiled	1 cup	626	61.3	41.8	1.0		72.8
Anchovy							
dried, cleaned	1 oz	75	17.2	0.6	0.1	0.0	142.0
dried, whole	1 oz	73	16.1	0.9	0.3	0.0	447.0
European, raw	85.0 g	111	17.3	4.1	0.0	0.0	125.0
fillet, canned	4.0 g	8	1.2	0.4	0.0	0.0	9.2
whole	1 oz	22	4.7	0.3	0.2	0.0	38.0
Arctic char, raw	1 cup	414	52.5	21.0	0.0	4.1	18.7
Bass							
black, baked	1 oz	32	5.3	1.4	0.0	0.0	22.7
freshwater, broiled	62.0 g	90	15.0	2.9	0.0		64.0
freshwater, raw fillet	79.0 g	90	14.9	2.9	0.0		63.0
sharptooth bass	1 oz	26	5.7	0.4	0.0	0.0	12.8
striped, broiled	124.0 g	154	28.2	3.7	0.0		
striped, oven fried	200.0 g	392	43.0	17.0	13.4	0.3	
striped, raw	159.0 g	154	28.2	3.7	0.0		
Blackfish, whole, Alaska	1 oz	86	15.5	1.8	1.0		236.0
Bladder, dried	1 oz	97	23.0	0.5	0.0	0.0	5.4
Bluefish							
baked with butter	155.0 g	246	40.6	8.1	0.0	0.0	44.6
bluefish, broiled	117.0 g	186	30.1	6.4	0.0		10.0
raw	150.0 g	186	30.1	6.4	0.0		10.0
Bream							
African	1 oz	27	4.7	0.8	0.3	0.0	7.9
threadfin, Japanese	1 oz	28	5.2	0.6	0.3	0.0	15.0
Burbot							
broiled	90.0 g	104	22.3	0.9	0.0		58.0
raw	116.0 g	104	22.4	0.9	0.0		58.0
Butterfish							
broiled	25.0 g	47	5.5	2.6	0.0		
raw	32.0 g	47	5.5	2.6	0.0		
Carp							
big head	1 oz	36	4.6	1.9	0.6	0.0	9.4
common	1 oz	20	4.4	0.6	0.5	0.0	7.1
cooked, dry heat	170.0 g	276	38.9	12.2	0.0		89.0
grass	1 oz	28	4.8	1.0	0.0	0.0	7.9
Japanese	1 oz	41	4.6	2.6	0.0	0.0	9.9
raw	218.0 g	276	38.9	12.2	0.0		89.0
	1 oz	38	4.9	1.9	0.3	0.0	7.1
Catfish							
breaded, fried	85.0 g	195	15.4	11.3	6.8	0.8	37.4
catfish eel	1 oz	34	5.0	1.4	0.3	0.0	4.0

FOOD	IRON (mg)	POTAS-SIUM (mg)	SODIUM (mg)	CHOLES-TEROL (mg)	MAGNE-SIUM (mg)	DHA3 (gm)	EPA3 (gm)	% OF CALORIES FROM FAT
Abalone								
cooked, fried	3.23	241	502	80	47.0		0.05	32
raw	0.90		85	24	13.7		0.01	6
Agutuk								
fish with shortening, Alaska	0.20	143	25					84
fish/berry with seal oil, Alaska	0.30	67	21	6	2.0			83
Alewife, with bone, baked or broiled	3.90			109	88.3			60
Anchovy								
dried, cleaned	0.85	256	1125					8
dried, whole	1.50	192	103					11
European, raw	2.76	325	88		35.0			33
fillet, canned	0.19	22	147	3	2.8	0.05	0.03	42
whole	0.17	37	162					13
Arctic char, raw	0.60	1432	133	0	211.0			46
Bass								
black, baked	0.42	101	20	19	8.7	0.10	0.27	39
freshwater, broiled	1.18	283	56	54	24.0	0.28	0.19	29
freshwater, raw fillet	1.18	281	55	54	24.0	0.28	0.19	29
sharptooth bass	0.09	62	15	14	14.1			13
striped, broiled	1.34		110	127		0.93	0.27	22
striped, oven fried								39
striped, raw	1.33		110	127		0.93	0.27	22
Blackfish, whole, Alaska	4.60							18
Bladder, dried	0.54	4	4					5
Bluefish								
baked with butter	1.10		161	108	43.3			30
bluefish, broiled	0.72	558	90	88	49.0	0.78	0.38	31
raw	0.72	558	90	88	50.0	0.79	0.38	31
Bream								
African	0.31	72	14					26
threadfin, Japanese	0.23	79	70					19
Burbot								
broiled	1.04	466	112	69	37.0	0.11	0.08	8
raw	1.04	469	112	69	37.0	0.11	0.08	8
Butterfish								
broiled	0.16	120	29	21				49
raw	0.16	120	28	21				49
Carp								
big head	0.45	60	14					48
common	0.45	81	19	28	10.1			27
cooked, dry heat	2.69	726	107	143	64.0	0.25	0.52	40
grass	0.40	51	14					32
Japanese	0.28	86	12	28	10.1			55
raw	2.69	726	107	143	64.0	0.25	0.52	40
	0.54	79	7	28	10.1			45
Catfish								
breaded, fried	1.22	289	238	69	23.0			52
catfish eel	0.23	78	22					38

FISH

FOOD	AMOUNT	CALORIES (kcal)	PROTEIN (g)	FAT (g)	CARBO-HYDRATES (g)	FIBER (g)	CALCIUM (mg)
Catfish-channel							
cooked, dry heat	143.0 g	218	26.8	11.5	0.0		13.0
raw	159.0 g	214	24.7	12.1	0.0		14.0
wild, breaded/fried	87.0 g	199	15.7	11.6	7.0		38.0
wild, cooked, dry	143.0 g	150	26.4	4.1	0.0		16.0
wild, raw	159.0 g	152	26.0	4.5	0.0		23.0
giant sea	1 oz	22	5.2	0.1	0.2	0.0	4.5
Malaysia river	1 oz	34	4.7	1.6	0.2	0.0	3.1
river	1 oz	24	5.1	0.3	0.3	0.0	4.5
Chiton, leathery, gumboots, Alaska	1 oz	83	17.1	1.6	0.0		121.0
Cisco							
raw	85.0 g	84	16.1	1.6	0.0	0.0	15.3
smoked	85.0 g	151	13.9	10.1	0.0	0.0	22.0
Clams							
breaded, fried	85.0 g	172	12.1	8.8	8.9	0.3	53.6
cooked, moist heat	85.0 g	126	21.7	1.7	4.4	0.0	78.0
raw, meat only	85.0 g	63	10.9	0.8	2.2	0.0	39.1
Mrs. Paul's® fried	1 oz	80	4.0	3.6	8.4	0.1	0.0
Clams, canned							
liquid, all varieties	1 cup	6	1.0	0.1	0.2	0.0	31.0
mixed species	1 cup	236	40.9	3.1	8.2	0.0	148.0
solids and liquids	1 oz	13	2.3	0.3	0.7	0.0	15.7
Cockles							
Alaska	1 oz	79	13.5	0.7	4.7		30.0
boiled	1 oz	17	2.4	0.1	1.4	0.0	13.9
fresh	1 oz	21	3.4	0.3	1.1	0.0	67.5
Cod							
canned, solids & liquids	85.0 g	89	19.4	0.7	0.0	0.0	18.0
coral	1 oz	23	5.2	0.1	0.1	0.0	13.6
gray, Pacific, raw	1 oz	23	5.1	0.2	0.0	0.0	2.0
Pacific, broiled	90.0 g	95	20.6	0.7	0.0		8.0
Pacific, raw	116.0 g	95	20.8	0.7	0.0		8.0
scrod, Atlantic, baked or broiled	1 cup	273	59.3	2.2	0.0	0.0	36.4
scrod, Atlantic, raw	1 oz	23	5.1	0.2	0.0	0.0	4.5
scrod, Atlantic, smoked	1 cup	233	49.4	2.5	0.0	0.0	16.5
tongues/cheeks, Atlantic, raw	1 oz	21	4.1	0.3	0.0	0.0	4.8
Cod, Atlantic							
cooked, dry heat	180.0 g	189	41.1	1.6	0.0	0.0	25.0
dry, salted	85.0 g	246	53.4	2.0	0.0	0.0	136.0
raw	85.0 g	70	15.1	0.6	0.0	0.0	13.0
Crab							
Alaska king, raw	85.0 g	71	15.6	0.5	0.0	0.0	39.1
baked with flour/egg	109.0 g	160	28.5	2.3	4.2		415.0
deviled	1 cup	451	27.4	22.6	31.9	2.3	113.0
dungeness, cooked/moist	127.0 g	140	28.4	1.6	1.2		75.0
dungeness, raw	85.0 g	73	14.8	0.8	0.6	0.0	39.1
imperial	1 cup	323	32.1	16.7	8.6	0.0	132.0
jonah, steamed	1 oz	28	4.6	0.5	0.9	0.0	27.2
meat, king, canned, unpacked	1 cup	135	24.0	3.2	1.0	0.0	61.0
queen, cooked/moist	1 oz	33	6.7	0.4	0.0		9.3

FOOD	IRON (mg)	POTAS- SIUM (mg)	SODIUM (mg)	CHOLES- TEROL (mg)	MAGNE- SIUM (mg)	DHA3 (gm)	EPA3 (gm)	% OF CALORIES FROM FAT
Catfish-channel								
cooked, dry heat	1.17	459	115	91	37.0	0.18	0.07	47
raw	0.79	476	84	74	36.0	0.33	0.11	51
wild, breaded/fried	1.24	296	244	70	24.0	0.19	0.10	52
wild, cooked, dry	0.50	599	71	103	40.0	0.20	0.14	24
wild, raw	0.47	569	69	92	37.0	0.37	0.21	27
giant sea	0.14	123	24	26	9.1	0.00	0.00	2
Malaysia river	0.14	72	10	26	9.1			42
river	0.28	84	4	26	9.1			10
Chiton, leathery, gumboots, Alaska	16.00							17
Cisco								
raw	0.31	301	47	41	26.4			18
smoked	0.41	249	409	27	14.0			60
Clams								
breaded, fried	11.80	277	309	52	11.9			46
cooked, moist heat	23.80	534	95	57	16.0	0.12	0.12	12
raw, meat only	11.90	267	48	29	7.7			12
Mrs. Paul's®fried	0.43	94	180	6	4.1			41
Clams, canned								
liquid, all varieties	37.70	848	516	0	26.0	0.00	0.00	8
mixed species	44.70	1005	179	107	30.0			12
solids and liquids	1.17	40	15	18				23
Cockles								
Alaska	16.20							8
boiled	2.24	37	99					8
fresh	3.74	79	75					15
Cod								
canned, solids & liquids	0.41	449	185	47	35.0			8
coral	0.11	74	31	14	12.0			6
gray, Pacific, raw	0.07	114	20	11	6.8			7
Pacific, broiled	0.30	465	82	43	28.0	0.16	0.09	7
Pacific, raw	0.31	467	82	43	28.0	0.16	0.01	7
scrod, Atlantic, baked or broiled	1.27	634	203	143	109.0			7
scrod, Atlantic, raw	0.11	117	15	12	9.1			7
scrod, Atlantic, smoked	3.84	946	2315	211	148.0			10
tongues/cheeks, Atlantic, raw	0.09	53	54	14	8.8			14
Cod, Atlantic								
cooked, dry heat	0.88	440	141	99	76.0	0.27	0.01	7
dry, salted	2.13	1239	5973	129	113.0			7
raw	0.32	351	46	37	27.0			7
Crab								
Alaska king, raw	0.50	173	711	36	41.7			6
baked with flour/egg	1.38	598	550	184	82.0			13
deviled	2.90	398	2081	223	63.7			45
dungeness, cooked/moist	0.54	519	480	96	73.0	0.02	0.36	10
dungeness, raw	0.32	301	251	50	38.3			10
imperial	2.00	288	1602	275	57.3			47
jonah, steamed	9.32	79	78	0	9.3			17
meat, king, canned, unpacked	1.10	149	675	135	29.0			21
queen, cooked/moist		57	196	20		0.04	0.09	12

FISH

FOOD	AMOUNT	CALORIES (kcal)	PROTEIN (g)	FAT (g)	CARBO-HYDRATES (g)	FIBER (g)	CALCIUM (mg)
Crab (continued)							
queen, raw	1 oz	25	5.2	0.3	0.0		7.3
red, steamed	1 oz	22	4.3	0.3	0.4	0.0	11.6
snow, spider, Atlantic, canned	1 oz	20	4.1	0.2	0.1	0.0	11.6
soft shell, fried	125.0 g	334	11.0	17.9	31.2		55.0
steamed, pieces	1 cup	150	30.0	2.4	0.0	0.0	91.5
swimming, boiled	1 oz	30	5.4	0.7	0.7	0.0	64.1
Mrs. Paul's® deviled miniatures	1 oz	69	2.6	3.4	7.1	0.2	17.1
Surimi® imitation	85.0 g	87	10.2	1.1	8.7	0.0	11.1
Crab, blue							
canned	1 cup	134	27.7	1.7	0.0	0.0	136.0
cooked, moist heat	1 cup	138	27.3	2.4	0.0	0.0	140.0
raw	21.0 g	18	3.8	0.2	0.0	0.0	19.0
sea, boiled	1 oz	24	5.1	0.3	0.1	0.0	47.6
Crab cake	60.0 g	160	11.2	10.4	5.1		202.0
Crab salad	100.0 g	145	11.8	8.5	4.9	0.3	38.0
Crayfish							
cooked, moist heat	1 oz	25	5.0	0.4	0.0		14.3
raw	1 oz	20	4.2	0.3	0.0		7.0
wild, cooked, moist heat	1 oz	25	4.7	0.3	0.0		17.0
wild, raw	1 oz	22	4.5	0.3	0.0		7.7
Croaker							
Atlantic, raw	79.0 g	83	14.0	2.5	0.0		12.0
breaded, fried	85.0 g	188	15.5	10.8	6.4	0.3	27.0
Cusk							
broiled	95.0 g	106	23.1	0.8	0.0		12.0
raw	1 oz	25	5.4	0.2	0.0	0.0	2.8
raw	85.0 g	74	16.1	0.6	0.0	0.0	9.0
Cuttlefish							
cooked/moist	1 oz	45	9.2	0.4	0.5		51.0
dried	1 oz	85	17.2	0.8	2.3	0.0	27.2
fresh	1 oz	25	4.5	0.4	0.0	0.0	6.5
raw	1 oz	22	4.6	0.2	0.2		25.7
Devilfish, myoxocephalus, Alaska	1 oz	101	11.7	5.3	0.7		12.0
Dolphinfish							
broiled	159.0 g	174	37.7	1.4	0.0		
raw	204.0 g	174	37.7	1.4	0.0		
Drum							
freshwater, broiled	154.0 g	236	34.6	9.7	0.0		118.0
freshwater, raw	198.0 g	236	34.7	9.8	0.0		119.0
Eel							
cooked, dry heat	85.0 g	201	20.1	12.7	0.0	0.0	22.1
raw, all varieties	85.0 g	156	15.7	9.9	0.0	0.0	17.0
Eulachon							
smoked, Alaska	1 oz	308	20.5	24.8	0.8		30.0
whole, Alaska	63.0 g			11.8			
Featherback	1 oz	30	5.7	0.7	0.1	0.0	24.7
Fillet of fish divan							
Lean Cuisine Dinner®	351.0 g	270	31.0	10.0	16.0		

FOOD	IRON (mg)	POTAS-SIUM (mg)	SODIUM (mg)	CHOLES-TEROL (mg)	MAGNE-SIUM (mg)	DHA3 (gm)	EPA3 (gm)	% OF CALORIES FROM FAT
Crab (continued)								
queen, raw		49	153	16		0.03	0.07	12
red, steamed	0.26	73	102	28	7.8			11
snow, spider, Atlantic, canned	0.24	37	200	25	7.0			10
soft shell, fried	1.81	163	1118	45	25.0			48
steamed, pieces	1.18	406	1662	82	52.7	0.18	0.46	14
swimming, boiled	0.28	47	76					19
Mrs. Paul's® deviled miniatures	0.31	76	154	6	7.5			45
Surimi® imitation	0.33	77	715	17	36.6			12
Crab, blue								
canned	1.13	505	450	120	52.7			11
cooked, moist heat	1.22	437	376	135	45.0	0.31	0.33	16
raw	0.15	69	62	16	7.0			12
sea, boiled	0.17	58	91					13
Crab cake	1.12	162	492	82	25.0			59
Crab salad	0.60	260	487	69	26.0			53
Crayfish								
cooked, moist heat	0.31	67	28	39	9.3	0.01	0.04	13
raw	0.15	74	18	30	8.7	0.01	0.03	12
wild, cooked, moist heat	0.23	84	27	38	9.3	0.01	0.03	12
wild, raw	0.24	86	16	32	7.7	0.01	0.03	11
Croaker								
Atlantic, raw	0.29	273	44	48	31.0	0.08	0.10	27
breaded, fried	0.73	289	296	71	35.0	0.08	0.10	52
Cusk								
broiled	1.01	477	38	50	38.0			7
raw	0.24	111	9	12	8.8			7
raw	0.71	333	27	35	27.0			7
Cuttlefish								
cooked/moist	3.07	181	211	63		0.04	0.02	8
dried	0.77	172	294					8
fresh	0.51	17	27					15
raw	1.70	100	105	32		0.02	0.01	8
Devilfish, myoxocephalus, Alaska	0.40							47
Dolphinfish								
broiled	2.30	848	179	149		0.18	0.04	7
raw	2.31	849	179	149		0.18	0.04	7
Drum								
freshwater, broiled	1.78	543	148	126	59.0	0.57	0.45	37
freshwater, raw	1.78	544	149	127	59.0	0.57	0.46	37
Eel								
cooked, dry heat	0.54	297	55	137	22.1			57
raw, all varieties	0.43	232	43	107	26.4			57
Eulachon								
smoked, Alaska	12.20							72
whole, Alaska				27				
Featherback	0.06	74	6					21
Fillet of fish divan								
Lean Cuisine Dinner®		850	780	85		0.00	0.00	33

FISH

FOOD	AMOUNT	CALORIES (kcal)	PROTEIN (g)	FAT (g)	CARBO-HYDRATES (g)	FIBER (g)	CALCIUM (mg)
Fillet of fish florentine							
Lean Cuisine Dinner®	255.0 g	240	26.0	9.0	13.0		
Fish ball	1 oz	30	1.5	0.4	5.3	0.0	109.0
Fish cakes							
fried	1 cup	361	30.9	16.8	19.5	2.3	23.1
frozen, fried, reheated	1 cup	567	19.3	37.6	36.1	0.0	23.1
Fish curry, canned	1 oz	27	3.4	0.5	2.2	0.0	77.7
Fish and chips							
Swanson® dinner	1 oz	50	2.0	2.1	6.0	0.6	6.0
Van de Kamps® dinner	224.0 g	500	16.0	30.0	45.0	4.7	34.8
Fish dijon, light, Mrs.Paul's®	1 oz	23	2.4	0.6	1.9		22.9
Fish eggs							
caviar, sturgeon, granular	1 tbsp	40	3.9	2.9	0.6	0.0	44.0
carp/cod/pike/shad, roe, raw	1 oz	39	6.3	1.8	0.4	0.0	6.3
Fish fillets, breaded, frozen, Healthy Choice®	49.6 g	80	6.0	2.5	8.0		10.0
Fish fillet jardiniere, Lean Cuisine®	319.0 g	290	31.0	10.0	18.0		150.0
Fish flakes, canned	1 cup	183	40.8	1	0.0	0.0	80.8
Fish florentine, light, Mrs.Paul's®	1 oz	28	3.13	1.0	1.3		50.0
Fish flour							
from fillets	1 oz	113	26.4	0.0	0.0	0.0	261.0
from fillet waste	1 oz	87	20.1	0.1	0.0	0.0	1712
Fish flour, from whole fish	1 oz	95	22.1	0.1	0.0	0.0	1307
Fish loaf, cooked	1 cup	260	29.6	7.8	15.3	1.5	23.1
Fish mornay, light, Mrs.Paul's®	1 oz	26	2.67	1.1	1.33		33.3
Fish roe, fresh	1 oz	41	6.4	1.6	0.2	0.0	3.7
Fish satay snack	1 oz	108	3.9	3.5	15.2	0.2	23.0
Fish sticks							
breaded, frozen, cooked	1 oz	77	4.4	3.5	6.8	0.7	5.7
breaded, frozen, Healthy Choice®	68.0 g	120	8.0	4.0	14.0		20.0
Flatfish							
battered, fried	91.0 g	211	13.3	11.2	15.4		17.0
cooked, dry heat	85.0 g	100	20.5	1.3	0.0	0.0	15.3
raw	85.0 g	78	16.0	1.0	0.0	0.0	15.0
Flounder							
flesh, air dried, Alaska	1 cup	429	70.4	14.2	0.0		
Gefiltefish							
commercial, with broth	42.0 g	35	3.8	0.7	3.1	0.0	9.7
Goby	1 oz	21	4.9	0.1	0.2	0.0	8.2
Goldeye							
raw	1 oz	37	4.6	1.9	0.0	0.0	26.2
Gouramy							
giant	1 oz	29	5.0	0.9	0.2	0.0	6.8
snakeskin	1 oz	25	5.1	0.5	0.1	0.0	13.3
Grayling, Arctic, Alaska	1 oz	93	20.5	1.5	0.2	1.0	0.4
Grouper							
cooked, dry heat	85.0 g	100	21.1	1.1	0.0	0.0	18.0
greasy	1 oz	23	5.5	0.1	0.0	0.0	18.1
raw, all varieties	85.0 g	78	16.5	0.9	0.0	0.0	23.0
Grunter, silver	1 oz	24	5.5	0.1	0.1	0.0	6.5

FOOD	IRON (mg)	POTAS-SIUM (mg)	SODIUM (mg)	CHOLES-TEROL (mg)	MAGNE-SIUM (mg)	DHA3 (gm)	EPA3 (gm)	% OF CALORIES FROM FAT
Fillet of fish florentine								
Lean Cuisine Dinner®		540	700	100		0.00	0.00	34
Fish ball	0.91	5	1794					12
Fish cakes								
fried	0.84	731	372	88	37.8			42
frozen, fried, reheated	0.84	731	372	55	61.7			60
Fish curry, canned	1.05	49	183	5	8.7			15
Fish and chips								
Swanson® dinner	0.18	100	96	4	6.6			38
Van de Kamps® dinner	2.22	785	551	33	52.6	0.00	0.00	54
Fish dijon, light, Mrs.Paul's®	0.08		74	7				22
Fish eggs								
caviar, sturgeon, granular	1.90	29	240	94	48.0			64
carp/cod/pike/shad, roe, raw	0.17	63	26	106	5.6			42
Fish fillets, breaded, frozen, Healthy Choice®	0.90	115	175	15				28
Fish fillet jardiniere, Lean Cuisine®	0.36	900	840	110				31
Fish flakes, canned	1.32	460	68	115	51.2			5
Fish florentine, light, Mrs.Paul's®	0.14		103	12				33
Fish flour								
from fillets	2.27	23	11	75		0.00	0.00	0
from fillet waste	15.30	153	62	57		0.00	0.00	1
Fish flour, from whole fish	11.60	122	48	63		0.00	0.00	1
Fish loaf, cooked	0.84	731	372	84	37.8			27
Fish mornay, light, Mrs.Paul's®	0.08	74	9					39
Fish roe, fresh	0.51	43	41	121	6.5			36
Fish satay snack	1.16	101	238					29
Fish sticks								
breaded, frozen, cooked	0.21	74	165	32	7.1			40
breaded, frozen, Healthy Choice®		160	250	20				30
Flatfish								
battered, fried	1.92	292	484	31	22.0			48
cooked, dry heat	0.29	292	89	58	49.3			12
raw	0.30	307	69	41	27.0			12
Flounder								
flesh, air dried, Alaska								30
Gefiltefish								
commercial, with broth	1.04	38	220	13	3.7			19
Goby	0.23	76	9	0		0.00	0.00	4
Goldeye								
raw	0.22	79	20	10	8.8			47
Gouramy								
giant	0.14	93	6					28
snakeskin	0.37	80	3					17
Grayling, Arctic, Alaska	1.00	339	81	58				15
Grouper								
cooked, dry heat	0.96	403	45	40	32.0	0.18	0.03	10
greasy	0.14	98	22					4
raw, all varieties	0.75	410	45	31	26.0			10
Grunter, silver	0.20	130	16					10

FISH

FOOD	AMOUNT	CALORIES (kcal)	PROTEIN (g)	FAT (g)	CARBO-HYDRATES (g)	FIBER (g)	CALCIUM (mg)
Haddock							
baked or broiled	1 cup	291	63.0	2.4	0.0	0.1	109.0
breaded, fried	85.0 g	140	17.0	5.0	5.0	0.3	34.0
broiled	85.0 g	95	20.6	0.8	0.0	0.0	35.7
raw	1 oz	25	5.4	0.2	0.0	0.0	9.4
raw	85.0 g	74	16.1	0.6	0.0	0.0	28.0
smoked	85.0 g	99	21.4	0.8	0.0	0.0	41.0
Halibut							
all types, broiled in butter	125.0 g	214	31.5	8.8	0.0	0.0	20.0
Atlantic or Pacific, raw	1 oz	31	5.9	0.6	0.0	0.0	13.3
cooked, broiled	85.0 g	119	22.7	2.5	0.0	0.0	51.0
Greenland, broiled	159.0 g	380	29.3	28.2	0.0		6.0
Greenland, raw	85.0 g	158	12.2	11.8	0.0	0.0	3.0
Indian	1 oz	23	5.5	0.1	0.1	0.0	12.2
raw	85.0 g	93	17.7	2.0	0.0	0.0	40.0
Herring							
air dried flesh, Alaska	6.5 g	286	44.7	10.6	0.0		
air dried, packed in oil, Alaska	43.5 g	286	44.5	34.6	0.0		
Atlantic, broiled	85.0 g	173	19.6	9.9	0.0	0.0	62.9
Atlantic, raw	85.0 g	134	15.3	7.7	0.0	0.0	49.0
canned, solids and liquids	100.0 g	208	19.9	13.6	0.0	0.0	147.0
herring eggs, dry, Alaska	1 cup	333	60.4	6.6	2.8		29.0
herring eggs on giant kelp, Alaska	1 cup	59	11.3	0.8	2.6		161.0
herring eggs, plain, Alaska	1 cup	56	9.6	1.9	4.4		19.0
Pacific, broiled	144.0 g	360	30.3	25.6	0.0		
Pacific, raw	184.0 g	359	30.2	25.5	0.0		
pickled, bismarck type	50.0 g	131	7.1	9.0	4.8	0.0	38.5
round	1 oz	34	6.1	1.0	0.0	0.0	21.8
wolf	1 oz	29	5.8	0.5	0.2	0.0	14.5
Inconnu							
coney, raw	1 oz	68	4.8	5.3	0.0	0.0	5.1
Jelawat	1 oz	62	4.9	4.7	0.0	0.0	9.1
Jewfish							
brown	1 oz	26	5.5	0.4	0.1	0.0	11.9
silver	1 oz	28	5.3	0.5	0.3	0.0	9.6
Kissing gouramy	1 oz	24	5.6	0.2	0.0	0.0	21.8
Ling							
broiled	151.0 g	168	36.8	1.2	0.0		66.0
raw	193.0 g	168	36.4	1.2	0.0		65.0
Lingcod							
broiled	1 oz	31	6.4	0.4	0.0		5.0
flesh, Alaska	1 oz	84	17.9	0.8	0.0		
liver, Alaska	1 oz	400	5.6	42.0	6.0		5.0
raw	193.0 g	164	34.1	2.0	0.0		27.0
Lobster							
American, boiled or steamed	1 oz	28	5.8	0.2	0.4	0.0	17.3
American, raw	1 oz	26	5.3	0.3	0.1	0.0	13.6
cooked, moist heat	1 oz	28	5.8	0.2	0.4	0.0	17.3
northern, raw	150.0 g	136	28.2	1.4	0.8		
newburg	1 cup	485	46.3	26.5	12.8	0.0	218.0

FOOD	IRON (mg)	POTAS-SIUM (mg)	SODIUM (mg)	CHOLES-TEROL (mg)	MAGNE-SIUM (mg)	DHA3 (gm)	EPA3 (gm)	% OF CALORIES FROM FAT
Haddock								
baked or broiled	3.51	1037	226	192	130.0			7
breaded, fried	1.00	296	150	42				32
broiled	1.15	339	74	63	42.5			7
raw	0.30	88	19	16	11.1			7
raw	0.89	264	58	49	33.0			7
smoked	1.19	353	649	65	46.0			7
Halibut								
all types, broiled in butter	1.00	656	168	75		0.40	0.11	37
Atlantic or Pacific, raw	0.24	128	15	9	23.5			19
cooked, broiled	0.91	490	59	35	91.0	0.32	0.08	19
Greenland, broiled	1.35	546	163	94		0.80	1.07	67
Greenland, raw	0.56	228	68	39	26.4			67
Indian	0.11	119	29	0		0.00	0.00	2
raw	0.71	382	46	27	71.0			19
Herring								
air dried flesh, Alaska								33
air dried, packed in oil, Alaska								100
Atlantic, broiled	1.20	356	98	66	34.9			51
Atlantic, raw	0.94	278	76	51	27.0	0.73	0.60	52
canned, solids and liquids	1.80			98		0.51	0.47	59
herring eggs, dry, Alaska								18
herring eggs on giant kelp, Alaska	3.40		61					12
herring eggs, plain, Alaska	2.70		61	40				31
Pacific, broiled	2.07	781	137	142		1.27	1.79	64
Pacific, raw	2.06	778	136	141		1.27	1.78	64
pickled, bismarck type	0.61	35	435	7	4.0	0.27	0.42	62
round	0.37	90	28					27
wolf	0.22	78	19					17
Inconnu								
coney, raw	0.10	93	10	12	8.8			70
Jelawat	0.17	84	10					68
Jewfish								
brown	0.11	96	37					14
silver	0.11	115	26					18
Kissing gouramy	0.23	86	5					6
Ling								
broiled	1.26	734	261		122.0			7
raw	1.25	732	261		121.0			7
Lingcod								
broiled	0.12	159	21	19	9.3	0.04	0.05	11
flesh, Alaska		433	59					9
liver, Alaska	1.00							95
raw	0.62	844	113	100	51.0	0.20	0.20	11
Lobster								
American, boiled or steamed	0.11	100	108	20	9.9			5
American, raw	0.09	78	84	27	7.7			9
cooked, moist heat	0.11	100	108	20	9.9	0.01	0.02	5
northern, raw				143				9
newburg	2.30	428	573	376	56.4	0.08	0.13	49

FISH

FOOD	AMOUNT	CALORIES (kcal)	PROTEIN (g)	FAT (g)	CARBO-HYDRATES (g)	FIBER (g)	CALCIUM (mg)
Lobster (continued)							
spiny, cooked/moist	163.0 g	233	43.0	3.2	5.1		102.0
spiny, raw	209.0 g	233	43.0	3.2	5.1		102.0
thermidor	157.0 g	405	28.5	26.6	14.8	0.0	290.0
Lobster salad w/tomato and egg	256.0 g	211	13.2	13.0	11.1	2.10	64.8
Long tongue sole	1 oz	22	5.1	0.1	0.1	0.0	9.4
Mackerel							
Atlantic, raw	112.0 g	229	20.8	15.6	0.0		13.0
Atlantic, canned	1 cup	296	44.0	12.0	0.0	0.0	458.0
barred Spanish	1 oz	31	6.1	0.7	0.0	0.0	7.1
cooked, dry heat	85.0 g	223	20.3	15.1	0.0	0.0	13.0
Indian	1 oz	35	5.9	1.1	0.2	0.0	13.6
king, broiled	1 oz	38	7.4	0.7	0.0		11.3
king, raw	1 oz	30	5.8	0.6	0.0		8.7
Pacific, broiled	176.0 g	354	45.3	17.8	0.0		52.0
Pacific, cooked, dry heat	176.0 g	354	45.3	17.8	0.0		52.0
Pacific, raw	225.0 g	355	45.2	17.8	0.0		52.0
raw, all varieties	85.0 g	133	17.1	6.7	0.0	0.0	19.0
Spanish	1 oz	29	5.4	0.5	0.5	0.0	5.1
Spanish, cooked, dry heat	85.0 g	134	20.1	5.4	0.0	0.0	11.0
Spanish, raw	85.0 g	118	16.4	5.4	0.0	0.0	10.0
Milkfish							
broiled	1 oz	54	7.5	2.4	0.0		18.7
raw	1 oz	42	5.8	1.9	0.0		14.3
Monkfish							
broiled	1 oz	27	5.3	0.6	0.0		3.0
goosefish/anglerfish, raw	1 oz	22	4.1	0.4	0.0	0.0	2.3
raw	1 oz	21	4.1	0.4	0.0		2.3
Mullet							
bluetail	1 oz	34	5.4	1.2	0.3	0.0	11.1
cooked, dry heat	85.0 g	128	21.1	4.1	0.0	0.0	26.4
striped, raw	85.0 g	99	16.5	3.2	0.0	0.0	34.0
Mussels							
Atlantic/Pacific, meat only	1 oz	27	4.1	0.6	0.9	0.0	25.0
blue, cooked, moist heat	85.0 g	147	20.2	3.8	6.3	0.0	28.0
blue, raw	1 cup	129	17.8	3.4	5.5		39.0
Needlefish, Alaska	1 oz	101	9.9	6.3	1.1		93.0
Ocean perch							
breaded, fried	85.0 g	195	16.0	11.0	6.0	0.1	28.0
cooked, dry heat	85.0 g	103	20.3	1.8	0.0	0.0	117.0
White perch, fried filet	65.0 g	108	12.5	5.3	0.0	0.0	9.0
Ocean fish almondine, efficiency entree	113.0 g	236	16.0	17.0	3.0		22.0
Ocean fish w/lemon sauce, efficiency entree	113.0 g	262	14.0	21.0	3.0	0.9	15.0
Octopus							
cooked/moist	1 oz	47	8.5	1.0	1.3		30.0
raw	85.0 g	70	12.7	0.9	1.9	0.0	45.1
Oyster							
breaded, fried	23.2 g	61	2.1	3.0	6.7		4.5

FOOD	IRON (mg)	POTAS-SIUM (mg)	SODIUM (mg)	CHOLES-TEROL (mg)	MAGNE-SIUM (mg)	DHA3 (gm)	EPA3 (gm)	% OF CALORIES FROM FAT
Lobster (continued)								
spiny, cooked/moist	2.29		370	146		0.23	0.56	12
spiny, raw	2.55		370	146		0.23	0.55	12
thermidor	1.90	388	360	236	35.4			59
Lobster salad w/tomato and egg	1.71	468	637	176	31.5			55
Long tongue sole	0.11	58	65	30	4.8			5
Mackerel								
Atlantic, raw	1.82	352	101	78	85.0	1.57	1.01	61
Atlantic, canned	3.88	369	720	150	70.0			36
barred Spanish	0.14	92	19					21
cooked, dry heat	1.33	341	71	64	82.5	0.59	0.43	61
Indian	0.51	105	17	20	21.5			29
king, broiled	0.65	158	57	19	11.7	0.06	0.05	17
king, raw	0.50	123	45	15	9.0	0.05	0.04	17
Pacific, broiled	2.62	916	194	106	63.0	2.10	1.15	45
Pacific, cooked, dry heat	2.62	916	194	106	63.0	2.10	1.15	45
Pacific, raw	2.61	914	194	106	63.0	2.10	1.14	45
raw, all varieties	0.99	345	73	40	24.0			45
Spanish	0.31	48	21	20	21.5			17
Spanish, cooked, dry heat	0.63	471	56	62	32.0			36
Spanish, raw	0.37	379	50	65	28.0			41
Milkfish								
broiled	0.12			19				41
raw	0.09			15				41
Monkfish								
broiled	0.12		7	9	7.7			18
goosefish/anglerfish, raw	0.09	113	5	7	6.0			18
raw	0.09		5	7	6.0			18
Mullet								
bluetail	0.34	92	16	14	8.2			32
cooked, dry heat	1.20	389	60	54	28.1			29
striped, raw	0.87	304	55	42	24.0			29
Mussels								
Atlantic/Pacific, meat only	0.97	90	81	16	7.1			21
blue, cooked, moist heat	5.71	228	313	48	32.0	0.43	0.24	23
blue, raw	5.92	479	429	42	51.0	0.38	0.28	23
Needlefish, Alaska	6.20							56
Ocean perch								
breaded, fried	1.10	242	128	32				51
cooked, dry heat	1.00	298	82	46	33.0	0.23	0.09	16
White perch, fried filet	0.70							44
Ocean fish almondine, efficiency entree	0.70	229	388			0.00	0.00	65
Ocean fish w/lemon sauce, efficiency entree	0.70	224	370	16	21.8	0.00	0.00	72
Octopus								
cooked/moist	2.70			27		0.05	0.04	11
raw	4.51	298	196	41	25.5			11
Oyster								
breaded, fried	0.74	30	113	18	4.0			44

FISH

FOOD	AMOUNT	CALORIES (kcal)	PROTEIN (g)	FAT (g)	CARBO-HYDRATES (g)	FIBER (g)	CALCIUM (mg)
Oyster (continued)							
Pacific, cooked/moist	25.0 g	41	4.7	1.1	2.5		4.0
Pacific, raw	50.0 g	41	4.7	1.1	2.5		4.0
sauce, fish	1 oz	24	0.9	0.1	4.9	0.0	4.8
shelled	1 oz	18	2.6	0.6	0.7	0.0	39.7
Oyster, eastern							
canned	1 cup	171	17.5	6.1	9.7	0.0	112.0
cooked, dry heat	1 oz	22	2.0	0.6	2.1		
cooked, moist heat	85.0 g	117	12.0	4.2	6.7	0.0	76.0
raw	1 oz	17	1.4	0.4	1.6		
Oyster, eastern, wild							
breaded/fried	1 oz	56	2.5	3.6	3.3		17.7
canned	1 cup	170	17.5	6.1	9.7		111.0
cooked, dry	1 oz	20	2.3	0.5	1.0		
cooked, moist	1 oz	39	4.0	1.4	2.2		25.3
raw	1 cup	169	17.5	6.1	9.7		112.0
Painted sweetlip	1 oz	24	5.6	0.1	0.1	0.0	11.1
Perch							
Atlantic, raw	85.0 g	80	15.8	1.4	0.0	0.0	91.0
climbing	1 oz	42	5.2	2.3	0.0	0.0	25.2
cooked, dry heat	85.0 g	100	21.1	1.0	0.0	0.0	86.7
giant sea	1 oz	24	5.5	0.0	0.3	0.0	7.9
raw, all varieties	85.0 g	77	16.5	0.8	0.0	0.0	68.0
sea	1 oz	31	5.7	0.9	0.1	0.0	7.3
Pickerel							
walleye, yellow pike, raw	1 oz	26	5.4	0.3	0.0	0.0	31.2
Pike							
air dried flesh, Alaska	12.0 g	300	68.7	2.8	0.0		32.0
broiled	124.0 g	147	30.4	1.9	0.0		175.0
cooked, dry heat	85.0 g	96	21.0	0.8	0.0	0.0	62.1
flesh, Alaska	1 oz	88	18.3	1.1	0.0		
liver, Alaska	1 oz	156	16.6	8.0	4.3		28.0
northern, raw	85.0 g	75	16.4	0.6	0.0	0.0	48.0
walleye, raw	159.0 g	147	30.4	1.9	0.0		175.0
Pollock							
Atlantic, broiled	1 oz	33	7.1	0.4	0.0		21.7
Atlantic, raw	1 oz	26	5.5	0.3	0.0		17.0
cooked, dry heat	85.0 g	96	20.0	1.0	0.0	0.0	5.1
walleye, raw	85.0 g	68	14.6	1.0	0.0	0.0	4.0
Pomfret							
black	1 oz	27	5.8	0.4	0.1	0.0	11.1
Chinese	1 oz	27	5.0	0.8	0.0	0.0	7.9
white	1 oz	32	5.5	1.1	0.0	0.0	4.5
Pompano							
cooked, dry heat	85.0 g	179	20.1	10.3	0.0	0.0	36.0
Florida, raw	85.0 g	140	15.7	8.1	0.0	0.0	19.0
Ponyfish, greater	1 oz	22	5.5	0.0	0.0	0.0	15.3
Pout							
ocean, broiled	1 oz	29	6.0	0.3	0.0		3.7
ocean, raw	1 oz	22	4.7	0.3	0.0		2.7

FOOD	IRON (mg)	POTAS- SIUM (mg)	SODIUM (mg)	CHOLES- TEROL (mg)	MAGNE- SIUM (mg)	DHA3 (gm)	EPA3 (gm)	% OF CALORIES FROM FAT
Oyster (continued)								
Pacific, cooked/moist	2.30	76	53		11.0	0.13	0.22	25
Pacific, raw	2.56	84	53		11.0	0.13	0.22	25
sauce, fish	0.14	20	1110	9	9.5			5
shelled	1.73	4	5					28
Oyster, eastern								
canned	16.60	568	278	136	134.0			32
cooked, dry heat	2.20	43	46	11	9.3	0.06	0.07	24
cooked, moist heat	11.40	389	190	93	92.7	0.39	0.36	32
raw	1.64	35	50	7	9.3	0.06	0.05	24
Oyster, eastern, wild								
breaded/fried	1.97	69	118	23	16.3	0.06	0.06	58
canned	16.60	568	277	136	135.0	0.57	0.52	33
cooked, dry	1.23	47	69	14	13.0	0.08	0.07	24
cooked, moist	3.40	80	120	30	27.0	0.17	0.15	32
raw	16.50	387	523	130	118.0	0.72	0.66	32
Painted sweetlip	0.11	103	24	0		0.00	0.00	2
Perch								
Atlantic, raw	0.78	232	64	36	26.0			16
climbing	0.51	76	7	12	8.5			50
cooked, dry heat	0.99	292	67	98	32.3			9
giant sea	0.11	118	22	0		0.00	0.00	1
raw, all varieties	0.77	228	52	76	26.0			9
sea	0.14	85	10					26
Pickerel								
walleye, yellow pike, raw	0.37	110	15	24	8.5			12
Pike								
air dried flesh, Alaska	0.90							8
broiled	2.07	618	81	137	48.0	0.36	0.14	12
cooked, dry heat	0.60	281	42	43	34.0			7
flesh, Alaska	0.60							11
liver, Alaska	2.10							46
northern, raw	0.47	220	33	33	26.4			7
walleye, raw	2.07	619	81	137	48.0	0.36	0.14	12
Pollock								
Atlantic, broiled	0.17	129	31	46	24.3	0.13	0.00	10
Atlantic, raw	0.13	101	24	20	19.0	0.10	0.02	10
cooked, dry heat	0.24	329	99	82	62.1			9
walleye, raw	0.20	277	84	61	26.4			9
Pomfret								
black	0.14	64	16					13
Chinese	0.06	80	43					26
white	0.14	89	35					32
Pompano								
cooked, dry heat	0.57	541	65	54	27.0	0.03	0.21	52
Florida, raw	0.51	324	55	43	23.0			52
Ponyfish, greater	0.17	64	28	0		0.00	0.00	0
Pout								
ocean, broiled	0.10		22	19	4.7			10
ocean, raw	0.08		17	15	3.7			10

FISH

FOOD	AMOUNT	CALORIES (kcal)	PROTEIN (g)	FAT (g)	CARBO-HYDRATES (g)	FIBER (g)	CALCIUM (mg)
Prawn							
pink	1 oz	21	4.9	0.1	0.6	0.0	17.0
salted, dried	1 oz	65	14.7	0.5	0.4	0.0	58.1
Prawn paste	1 oz	44	8.5	1.1	8.9	0.0	95.8
Queenfish	1 oz	27	5.8	0.3	0.2	0.0	41.4
Rabbitfish, streaked	1 oz	26	5.7	0.2	0.1	0.0	6.5
Ribbonfish	1 oz	25	5.4	0.3	0.0	0.0	9.1
Red snapper							
cooked, dry heat	85.0 g	109	22.4	1.5	0.0	0.0	34.0
raw	85.0 g	85	17.4	1.1	0.0	0.0	27.0
Rockfish							
cooked, dry heat	100.0 g	121	24.0	2.0	0.0	0.0	12.0
Pacific, raw	191.0 g	180	35.8	3.0	0.0	-	18.0
Roe							
broiled	1 oz	19	2.7	0.8	0.0		
Rohu	1 oz	25	4.8	0.4	0.4	0.0	5.4
Roughy							
orange, broiled	1 oz	25	5.3	0.3	0.0		
orange, raw	1 oz	20	4.2	0.2	0.0		
Sablefish							
broiled	1 oz	71	4.9	5.6	0.0		
raw	1 oz	55	3.8	4.3	0.0		
smoked	1 oz	72	4.9	5.6	0.0		
SALMON							
broiled or baked, with butter	100.0 g	182	27.0	7.4	0.0	0.0	17.6
cooked, moist heat	85.0 g	157	23.3	6.4	0.0	0.0	39.1
red/sockeye, kip, can, Alaska	1 oz	190	29.5	7.7	0.7		68.0
silver/coho, raw, Alaska	1 oz	146	21.6	6.0	0.0		
smoked	100.0 g	117	18.3	4.3	0.0	0.0	11.0
Atlantic							
broiled	1 oz	52	7.2	2.3	0.0		4.3
cooked, dry heat	1 oz	58	6.3	3.5	0.0		
raw	1 oz	52	5.6	3.1	0.0		
wild, cooked, dry	1 oz	52	7.2	2.3	0.0		4.3
Chinook							
broiled	1 oz	65	7.3	3.8	0.0		8.0
raw	1 oz	51	5.7	3.0	0.0		6.3
smoked	1 oz	33	5.2	1.2	0.0		3.0
Chum							
broiled	1 oz	44	7.3	1.4	0.0		4.0
canned	85.0 g	120	18.2	4.5	0.0	0.0	212.0
dog, cooked, Alaska	1 oz	152	25.5	4.8	0.0		13.0
keta, fresh, frozen, raw	1 oz	36	6.6	1.1	0.0	0.0	12.5
keta, poached	1 cup	294	57.9	6.8	0.0	0.0	131.0
raw	85.0 g	102	17.1	3.2	0.0	0.0	9.0
Coho							
cooked, dry heat	143.0 g	255	34.8	11.8	0.0		18.0
dried/seal oil, Alaska	10.4 g	350	51.4	19.4	0.0		
fresh, frozen, raw	1 oz	34	5.7	1.3	0.0	0.0	11.6

FOOD	IRON (mg)	POTAS-SIUM (mg)	SODIUM (mg)	CHOLES-TEROL (mg)	MAGNE-SIUM (mg)	DHA3 (gm)	EPA3 (gm)	% OF CALORIES FROM FAT
Prawn								
pink	0.28	53	30	0		0.00	0.00	4
salted, dried	4.00	179	724					7
Prawn paste	6.97	94	494					23
Queenfish	0.20	94	23					11
Rabbitfish, streaked	0.09	97	19					8
Ribbonfish	0.14	79	30					12
Red snapper								
cooked, dry heat	0.20	444	48	40	31.0	0.23	0.04	12
raw	0.15	355	54	31	27.0	0.22	0.04	12
Rockfish								
cooked, dry heat	0.53	520	77	44	34.0	0.26	0.18	15
Pacific, raw	0.78	774	114	66	50.0	0.39	0.27	15
Roe								
broiled				136		0.50	0.36	36
Rohu	0.34	24	9					15
Roughy								
orange, broiled	0.07		23	7			0.00	9
orange, raw	0.05		21	6			0.00	9
Sablefish								
broiled	0.46	130	20	18		0.26	0.25	70
raw	0.36	101	16	14		0.20	0.19	71
smoked		132	206	18		0.27	0.20	71
SALMON								
broiled or baked, with butter	1.20	443	116	47	31.6	0.62	0.41	37
cooked, moist heat	0.76	454	50	42	31.5	0.52	0.35	37
red/sockeye, kip, can, Alaska	1.30							36
silver/coho, raw, Alaska	0.70	422	46	39				37
smoked	0.85	175	784	23	18.0	0.27	0.18	33
Atlantic								
broiled	0.29	178	16	20		0.41	0.12	40
cooked, dry heat	0.10	109	17	18	8.7	0.41	0.20	54
raw	0.10	103	17	17	8.0	0.37	0.18	53
wild, cooked, dry	0.29	178	16	20		0.41	0.12	40
Chinook								
broiled	0.26	143	17	24		0.21	0.29	52
raw	0.20	112	13	19		0.16	0.22	52
smoked	0.24	49	220	7	5.0	0.08	0.05	33
Chum								
broiled	0.20	156	18	27		0.14	0.09	28
canned	0.75	285	414	33	27.9			35
dog, cooked, Alaska	0.70	543	64	94				28
keta, fresh, frozen, raw	0.18	107	26	11	8.8			26
keta, poached	1.86	969	206	74	83.9			21
raw	0.47	365	42	63	20.4			28
Coho								
cooked, dry heat	0.56	658	74	91	49.0	1.24	0.58	42
dried/seal oil, Alaska								50
fresh, frozen, raw	0.23	100	21	14	9.8			34

FISH

FOOD	AMOUNT	CALORIES (kcal)	PROTEIN (g)	FAT (g)	CARBO-HYDRATES (g)	FIBER (g)	CALCIUM (mg)
SALMON (continued)							
Coho (continued)							
poached	1 cup	327	61.1	9.1	0.0	0.0	116.0
raw	159.0 g	254	33.8	12.2	0.0		19.0
silver, cooked, Alaska	1 oz	185	27.4	7.5	0.0		
silver, dried, Alaska	6.0 g	578	58.2	37.3	0.0		
Coho, wild							
cooked, dry	1 oz	39	6.6	1.2	0.0		
cooked, moist	1 oz	52	7.8	2.1	0.0		13.0
raw	1 oz	41	6.1	1.7	0.0		10.3
King or Chinook							
brined, Alaska	6.5			25.0			
cooked, Alaska	1 oz	214	23.3	13.1	0.3		39.0
dried, Alaska	6.5 g	428	51.0	36.3	0.0		28.0
kipp, canned, Alaska	1 oz	266	30.7	15.9	0.0		38.0
liver, Alaska	1 oz	156	16.6	8.0	4.3		28.0
raw, Alaska	1 oz	217	22.5	13.4	0.0		79.0
smoked brand, Alaska	6.5 g	420	39.9	30.0	2.9	2.0	23.0
smoked cannned, Alaska	1 oz	150	23.2	5.9	1.0		23.0
Pink							
broiled	1 oz	42	7.2	1.3	0.0		
canned, solids & liquids	85.0 g	118	16.8	5.1	0.0	0.0	181.0
humpback, cooked, Alaska	28.3 g	149	25.6	4.4	0.0		
dried, Alaska	6.0 g	256	53.6	5.8	0.0		
raw, Alaska	1 oz	116	19.9	3.5	0.0		
raw	85.0 g	99	17.0	2.9	0.0	0.0	5.1
Pink humpback							
frozen, raw	1 oz	40	5.7	1.9	0.0	0.0	8.1
poached	1 cup	374	62.6	13.8	0.0	0.0	77.4
no salt, canned	1 cup	314	37.6	17.1	0.0	0.0	487.0
salt, canned	1 cup	314	37.4	17.1	0.0	0.0	487.0
Sockeye							
canned	369.0 g	566	75.5	27.0	0.0		883.0
cooked, dry heat	85.0 g	183	23.2	9.3	0.0	0.0	6.0
raw	1 oz	48	6.0	2.4	0.0		1.7
raw	85.0 g	143	18.1	7.3	0.0	0.0	5.0
Sockeye/red							
cooked, dry, Alaska	1 oz	216	27.3	11.0	0.0		7.0
dried, Alaska	6.5 g	313	42.7	14.4	3.2		84.0
no salt, canned	1 cup	376	38.8	23.3	0.0	0.0	527.0
raw, Alaska	1 oz	168	21.3	9.0	0.0		6.0
salt, canned	1 cup	376	38.8	23.3	0.0	0.0	527.0
solids/liquids, Alaska	1 oz	171	20.3	9.3	0.0		259.0
Salmon eggs, king, raw, Alaska	1 cup	250	29.2	14.0	2.9		
Salmon eggs, pink, canned w/salt, Alaska	1 cup			8.8			
Salmon patty	100.0 g	239	15.8	12.4	16.1	1.0	78.0
Salmon rice loaf	100.0 g	122	12.0	4.5	7.3	0.7	180.0
Salmon tipnuk, Alaska	92.0 g	174	15.9	10.6	2.7		

FOOD	IRON (mg)	POTAS-SIUM (mg)	SODIUM (mg)	CHOLES-TEROL (mg)	MAGNE-SIUM (mg)	DHA3 (gm)	EPA3 (gm)	% OF CALORIES FROM FAT
SALMON (continued)								
Coho (continued)								
poached	1.67	876	153	172	92.5			25
raw	0.54	716	74	82	49.0	1.31	0.61	43
silver, cooked, Alaska	0.89	534	59	49				37
silver, dried, Alaska	1.50			120				58
Coho, wild								
cooked, dry	0.17	123	16	16	9.3	0.19	0.11	28
cooked, moist	0.20	129	15	16	10.0	0.24	0.15	37
raw	0.16	120	13	13	8.7	0.19	0.12	37
King or Chinook								
brined, Alaska			1820	128				
cooked, Alaska	2.00	399	62	65				55
dried, Alaska	2.00		139	139				76
kipp, canned, Alaska	1.70							54
liver, Alaska	2.60							46
raw, Alaska	0.90							56
smoked brand, Alaska	4.50	700	693	107				64
smoked cannned, Alaska	4.50							35
Pink								
broiled	0.28	117	24	19		0.21	0.15	27
canned, solids & liquids	0.72	277	471	47	29.0	0.69	0.72	39
humpback, cooked, Alaska	0.99	414	86					27
dried, Alaska	3.12							20
raw, Alaska	0.77	323	67	52				27
raw	0.65	274	57	44	20.4			27
Pink humpback								
frozen, raw	0.22	105	19	15	9.1			42
poached	2.13	928	149	169	90.7			33
no salt, canned	2.47	769	173	53	71.6			49
salt, canned	2.47	769	1081	53	71.6			49
Sockeye								
canned	3.90	1392	1987	161	107.0	2.45	1.82	43
cooked, dry heat	0.47	319	56	74	26.0			46
raw	0.13	111	13	18	6.7	0.19	0.15	46
raw	0.40	332	40	53	20.0			46
Sockeye/red								
cooked, dry, Alaska	0.55	375	66	87	31.0			46
dried, Alaska	3.30	846	166					41
no salt, canned	2.06	806	142	58	64.7			56
raw, Alaska	0.50	391	47	62	24.0			48
salt, canned	2.06	808	959	58	64.7			56
solids/liquids, Alaska	1.20	344	522					49
Salmon eggs, king, raw, Alaska				174				50
Salmon eggs, pink, canned w/salt, Alaska				72				
Salmon patty	1.24	89	96	64	34.0			47
Salmon rice loaf	1.23	275	753	116	28.9			33
Salmon tipnuk, Alaska								55

FISH

FOOD	AMOUNT	CALORIES (kcal)	PROTEIN (g)	FAT (g)	CARBO-HYDRATES (g)	FIBER (g)	CALCIUM (mg)
Sardine							
Atlantic, canned in oil	12.0 g	25	3.0	1.4	0.0	0.0	45.8
canned (sardine tin)	1 oz	33	4.4	1.5	0.5	0.0	66.3
canned in tomato sauce	38.0 g	68	6.2	4.6	0.0	0.1	91.2
Sardine sandwich	1 oz	71	2.1	1.6	12.1	0.2	26.6
Sauger							
walleye, yellow, raw	1 oz	24	4.9	0.3	0.0	0.0	2.2
Scad							
hairtail	1 oz	29	5.8	0.4	0.6	0.0	18.1
hairtail, dried	1 oz	47	10.3	0.6	0.0	0.0	27.8
one finlet	1 oz	26	5.8	0.3	0.1	0.0	21.8
yellowtail	1 oz	29	6.1	0.5	0.0	0.0	22.7
Scallops							
bay and sea, steamed	1 oz	32	6.6	0.4	0.5	0.0	32.7
frozen, breaded, fried	15.0 g	32	2.7	1.6	1.5	0.1	6.3
mixed species, raw	1 cup	119	22.6	1.0	3.2	0.0	32.4
raw	30.0 g	26	5.0	0.2	0.7		7.0
Mrs.Paul's® fried	1 oz	53	2.7	2.3	6.0	0.1	6.7
Surimi® imitation	85.0 g	84	10.9	0.4	9.0		7.0
Scallops/clams/linguine							
Budget Light®	269.0 g	290	15.0	11.0	32.0	3.6	173.0
Scallops and shrimp mariner							
Stouffer®	291.0 g	400	23.0	16.0	40.0		
Scallops/vegetables/rice							
Lean Cuisine®	312.0 g	220	17.0	3.0	32.0		
Scup							
broiled	50.0 g	67	12.1	1.8	0.0		26.0
raw	85.0 g	89	16.0	2.3	0.0	0.0	34.0
Sea bass							
cooked, dry heat	85.0 g	105	20.1	2.2	0.0	0.0	11.0
raw, all varieties	85.0 g	82	15.7	1.7	0.0	0.0	9.0
Sea cucumber	1 oz	68	13.0	0.4	3.1		30.0
Seafood gumbo, entree, Hormel®	1 oz	10	1.3	0.1	0.8		8.1
Seafood lasagna, light, Mrs.Paul's®	1 oz	31	1.5	0.8	4.1		26.3
Seafood newburg, Healthy Choice®	227.0 g	200	13.0	3.0	30.0	1.2	60.4
Seafood rotini, light, Mrs.Paul's®	28.4 g	27	1.3	1.0	3.8		22.2
Sea pike, blunt jawed	1 oz	25	5.7	0.2	0.0	0.0	8.5
Sea slug/cucumber, washed	1 oz	6	1.3	0.6	0.0	0.0	5.7
Seatrout							
broiled	186.0 g	248	39.9	8.6	0.0		41.0
raw	238.0 g	248	39.8	8.6	0.0		41.0
Shad							
American, broiled	144.0 g	363	31.3	25.4	0.0		87.0
American, raw	184.0 g	362	31.2	25.3	0.0		87.0
baked, butter/margarine & bacon	100.0 g	201	23.2	11.3	0.0	0.0	24.0
gizzard	1 oz	37	5.6	1.7	0.0	0.0	29.8
longtail	1 oz	56	5.2	3.9	0.0	0.0	15.6
slender	1 oz	24	5.4	0.3	0.0	0.0	15.9

FOOD	IRON (mg)	POTAS-SIUM (mg)	SODIUM (mg)	CHOLES-TEROL (mg)	MAGNE-SIUM (mg)	DHA3 (gm)	EPA3 (gm)	% OF CALORIES FROM FAT
Sardine								
Atlantic, canned in oil	0.35	48	61	17	4.5	0.06	0.06	50
canned (sardine tin)	0.77	464	87	40	11.0			41
canned in tomato sauce	0.87	130	157	23	12.9			61
Sardine sandwich	0.45	26	130	29	6.3			21
Sauger								
walleye, yellow, raw	0.13	90	25	16	8.8			12
Scad								
hairtail	0.71	75	20					11
hairtail, dried	0.94	65	1679					11
one finlet	0.31	85	15					11
yellowtail	0.23	86	16					17
Scallops								
bay and sea, steamed	0.85	135	75	15				11
frozen, breaded, fried	0.12	50	70	9	8.9			46
mixed species, raw	0.39	435	217	45	75.6			8
raw	0.09	97	48	10	17.0	0.01	0.03	8
Mrs.Paul's® fried	0.00	95	107	3	16.6			39
Surimi® imitation	0.26	88	676	18				4
Scallops/clams/linguine								
Budget Light®	21.40	270	710	45	52.0			34
Scallops and shrimp mariner								
Stouffer®		355	1120			0.00	0.00	36
Scallops/vegetables/rice								
Lean Cuisine®		360	1200	20		0.00	0.00	12
Scup								
broiled	0.34	184	27		15.0			24
raw	0.45	244	36	41	19.0			23
Sea bass								
cooked, dry heat	0.32	279	74	45	45.0	0.47	0.18	19
raw, all varieties	0.25	218	58	35	35.0			19
Sea cucumber	0.60							5
Seafood gumbo, entree, Hormel®	0.20	82	146	6	4.7	0.00	0.00	9
Seafood lasagna, light, Mrs.Paul's®	0.15		79	6				25
Seafood newburg, Healthy Choice®	1.52	270	440	55	40.2	0.00	0.00	14
Seafood rotini, light, Mrs.Paul's®	0.20		63	2				22
Sea pike, blunt jawed	0.11	108	27					8
Sea slug/cucumber, washed	0.11	7	5	0		0.00	0.00	9
Seatrout								
broiled	0.64	813	138	198	74.0	0.49	0.39	31
raw	0.63	812	138	198	75.0	0.49	0.39	31
Shad								
American, broiled	1.79	709	94		55.0			63
American, raw	1.78	706	95		55.0			63
baked, butter/margarine & bacon	0.60	377	79	69				51
gizzard	0.23	101	35					40
longtail	0.31	64	19					63
slender	0.11	89	52					11

FISH

FOOD	AMOUNT	CALORIES (kcal)	PROTEIN (g)	FAT (g)	CARBO-HYDRATES (g)	FIBER (g)	CALCIUM (mg)
Shark							
dog	1 oz	30	7.3	0.1	0.0	0.0	3.7
fin	1 oz	108	27.1	0.0	0.0	0.0	120.0
raw	85.0 g	111	17.8	3.8	0.0	0.0	29.0
cooked in batter	85.0 g	194	15.8	11.8	5.4	50.6	42.0
Sheepshead							
cooked, dry heat	85.0 g	107	22.1	1.4	0.0	0.0	32.0
raw	85.0 g	92	17.2	2.1	0.0	0.0	18.0
Shrimp							
canned meat	1 cup	154	29.6	2.5	1.3	0.0	75.0
cooked, moist heat	85.0 g	84	17.8	0.9	0.0	0.0	33.2
fermented	1 oz	15	2.6	0.2	0.7	0.0	132.0
smooth shell	1 oz	23	5.2	0.1	0.2	0.0	16.7
french fried	85.0 g	206	18.2	10.4	9.8	0.5	57.0
mixed species, boiled/steamed	1 cup	127	26.8	1.4	0.0	0.0	49.9
mixed species, raw	1 oz	30	5.6	0.5	0.3	0.0	14.7
raw, mixed species	7.0 g	8	1.4	0.1	0.1	0.0	3.8
imitation, Surimi®	85.0 g	86	10.5	1.3	7.8		16.0
Shrimp creole, Ultra Slim Fast®	340.0 g	240	12.0	4.0	45.0	2.6	45.5
Shrimp marinara, Healthy Choice	298.0 g	260	10.0	1.0	51.0		60.0
Shrimp marinara, Ultra Slim Fast®	340.0 g	290	17.0	3.0	53.0	4.6	73.2
Shrimp paste	1 oz	46	8.1	0.6	1.9	0.0	514.0
Shrimp & clams/linguine, light, Mrs.Paul's®	1 oz	24	1.2	0.5	3.6	0.4	4.0
Shrimp & tomato/linguine, Healthy Choice®	269.0 g	230	12.0	2.0	40.0	3.5	92.9
Shrimp or lobster, paste, canned	1 cup	608	70.3	31.8	5.1		389.0
Shrimp primavera, Right Course®	273.0 g	240	12.0	7.0	32.0		80.0
Shrimp tail-on cooked, harvest	1 oz	23	5.7	0.0	0.0	0.0	22.7
Shrimp tail-on large cooked, harvest	1 oz	23	5.7	0.0	0.0	0.0	22.7
Sicklefish, spotted	1 oz	26	5.6	0.1	0.6	0.0	9.6
Smelt							
Atlantic, canned	20.0 g	40	3.7	2.7	0.0	0.0	71.6
breaded, fried	1 cup	652	55.7	32.5	31.5	8.6	101.0
cooked, dry heat	85.0 g	105	19.2	2.6	0.0	0.0	65.5
flesh and small bones, Alaska	63.0 g	117	16.7	5.1	0.0		74.0
rainbow, dry flesh, Alaska	1 oz	361	59.3	11.9	0.0		
rainbow, raw	85.0 g	83	15.0	2.1	0.0	0.0	51.0
Snakehead	1 oz	25	5.2	0.4	0.0	0.0	10.2
Snapper							
golden stripped	1 oz	29	6.0	0.5	0.0	0.0	6.0
red	1 oz	30	5.9	0.7	0.0	0.0	5.7
russell's	1 oz	25	5.7	0.1	0.4	0.0	22.7
Sole/flounder, baked	127.0 g	148	30.7	1.9	0.0	0.0	23.0
Sole/lemon butter sauce, Healthy Choice®	234.0 g	230	16.0	4.0	33.0	0.2	18.7
Sole, light, frozen dinner, Van de Kamp's®	142.0 g	293	16.0	18.0	17.0	1.9	39.1

FOOD	IRON (mg)	POTAS-SIUM (mg)	SODIUM (mg)	CHOLES-TEROL (mg)	MAGNE-SIUM (mg)	DHA3 (gm)	EPA3 (gm)	% OF CALORIES FROM FAT
Shark								
dog	0.11	85	21	18	15.8	0.00	0.00	2
fin	0.71	6	8	0		0.00	0.00	0
raw	0.71	136	67	43	42.0	0.45	0.27	31
cooked in batter	0.94	132	103	50	37.0			55
Sheepshead								
cooked, dry heat	0.57	435	62	58	30.0			12
raw	0.39	344	61	41	27.0			20
Shrimp								
canned meat	3.50	269	216	222	53.0	0.00	0.00	15
cooked, moist heat	2.63	155	190	166	28.9			10
fermented	0.88	25	1271					13
smooth shell	0.43	53	38					6
french fried	1.07	191	292	150	34.0	0.11	0.09	45
mixed species, boiled/steamed	3.96	233	287	250	43.5			10
mixed species, raw	0.68	52	42	43	10.5			15
raw, mixed species	0.17	13	11	11	2.5			14
imitation, Surimi®	0.51	76	599	31				13
Shrimp creole, Ultra Slim Fast®	4.21	470	430	80	46.4			15
Shrimp marinara, Healthy Choice	2.70	390	320	60				4
Shrimp marinara, Ultra Slim Fast®	3.75	500	280	55	50.6			9
Shrimp paste	3.26	200	405	30	4.5			12
Shrimp & clams/linguine, light, Mrs.Paul's®	0.27	78	75	4	5.3			19
Shrimp & tomato/linguine, Healthy Choice®	13.20	280	390	55	50.5			47
Shrimp or lobster, paste, canned	10.50	412	473	581				47
Shrimp primavera, Right Course®	1.80	150	590	50				26
Shrimp tail-on cooked, harvest			198	43		0.00	0.00	0
Shrimp tail-on large cooked, harvest			198	43		0.00	0.00	0
Sicklefish, spotted	0.14	85	23					5
Smelt								
Atlantic, canned	0.34							61
breaded, fried	3.20	1078	1393	257	98.7			45
cooked, dry heat	0.98	316	66	77	32.3			23
flesh and small bones, Alaska	0.60							39
rainbow, dry flesh, Alaska								30
rainbow, raw	0.77	247	51	60	26.0			22
Snakehead	0.40	92	6					15
Snapper								
golden stripped	0.14	93	23					17
red	0.17	77	24					20
russell's	0.14	91	24	0		0.00	0.00	3
Sole/flounder, baked	0.43	436	133	86	74.0	0.33	0.31	12
Sole/lemon butter sauce, Healthy Choice®	1.22	380	390	45	4.7	0.00	0.00	16
Sole, light, frozen dinner, Van de Kamp's®	0.93	453	412	45	38.5	0.00	0.00	55

FISH

FOOD	AMOUNT	CALORIES (kcal)	PROTEIN (g)	FAT (g)	CARBO-HYDRATES (g)	FIBER (g)	CALCIUM (mg)
Spot							
broiled	50.0 g	79	11.9	3.1	0.0		9.0
raw	64.0 g	79	11.8	3.1	0.0		9.0
Squid							
cooked, fried	85.0 g	149	15.3	6.4	6.6	0.3	33.0
raw	85.0 g	78	13.2	1.2	2.6	0.0	27.2
Sting ray	1 oz	28	6.9	0.1	0.0	0.0	2.8
Sturgeon							
cooked, dry heat	85.0 g	115	17.6	4.4	0.0	0.0	11.3
raw	1 oz	30	4.6	1.1	0.0		
smoked	85.0 g	147	26.5	3.7	0.0	0.0	19.1
steamed	100.0 g	135	20.7	5.2	0.0	0.0	40.0
Sucker							
white, broiled	124.0 g	147	26.6	4.0	0.0		111.0
white, raw	159.0 g	147	26.6	3.7	0.0		111.0
Sunfish							
pumpkinseed, broiled	37.0 g	42	9.2	0.3	0.0		38.0
pumpkinseed, raw	48.0 g	43	9.3	0.3	0.0		38.0
Swordfish							
broiled, butter/margarine	100.0 g	174	28.0	6.0	0.0	0.0	6.8
cooked, dry heat	85.0 g	132	21.6	4.4	0.0	0.0	5.0
raw	85.0 g	103	16.8	3.4	0.0	0.0	4.0
Threadfin	1 oz	26	5.6	0.3	0.1	0.0	4.0
dried	1 oz	51	11.4	0.5	0.0	0.0	
Tilefish							
cooked, dry heat	1 oz	42	6.9	1.3	0.0		7.3
raw	85.0 g	81	14.9	2.0	0.0	0.0	22.0
Toman	28.3 g	23	5.6	0.1	0.0	0.0	9.07
Tom cod							
dry flesh, Alaska	1 oz	293	64.3	2.0	0.0		
liver, Alaska	1 oz	448	8.0	45.1	1.9		6.0
Trevally							
malabar	1 oz	28	5.9	0.5	0.0	0.0	13.0
yellow	1 oz	30	6.1	0.6	0.0	0.0	15.0
yellow, dried	1 oz	45	10.0	0.6	0.0	0.0	42.5
Triggerfish, starry	1 oz	21	5.2	0.0	0.0	0.0	6.5
Trout							
broiled	62.0 g	118	16.5	5.3	0.0		34.0
brook, cooked	100.0 g	196	23.5	11.2	0.4	0.0	218.0
dolly varden, Alaska	1 oz	100	19.7	2.0	0.5	0.6	13.0
mixed species, raw	1 oz	42	5.9	1.9	0.0	0.0	12.2
mixed species, raw, USDA	79.0 g	117	16.4	5.2	0.0		34.0
raw, all varieties	85.0 g	126	17.7	5.6	0.0	0.0	36.0
Trout, rainbow							
baked or broiled	1 cup	392	68.4	11.2	0.0	0.0	223.0
cooked, dry heat	71.0 g	120	17.2	5.1	0.0		
raw	79.0 g	109	16.5	4.3	0.0		
raw	1 oz	34	5.8	1.0	0.0	0.0	19.0

FOOD	IRON (mg)	POTAS-SIUM (mg)	SODIUM (mg)	CHOLES-TEROL (mg)	MAGNE-SIUM (mg)	DHA3 (gm)	EPA3 (gm)	% OF CALORIES FROM FAT
Spot								
broiled	0.21	318	19		27.0	0.26	0.14	36
raw	0.20	318	18		27.0	0.26	0.14	36
Squid								
cooked, fried	0.86	237	260	221	33.0	0.32	0.14	38
raw	0.58	209	37	198	28.1			13
Sting ray	0.20	68	25	0		0.00	0.00	3
Sturgeon								
cooked, dry heat	0.59	309	291	63	29.6			34
raw		80				0.03	0.06	34
smoked	1.01	409	412	86	50.4			23
steamed	2.00	364	108	75	34.8	0.12	0.25	35
Sucker								
white, broiled	2.07	604	64	65	48.0	0.46	0.30	23
white, raw	2.07	604	64	66	48.0	0.46	0.30	23
Sunfish								
pumpkinseed, broiled	0.57	166	38	32	14.0	0.03	0.02	7
pumpkinseed, raw	0.58	168	38	32	14.0	0.04	0.02	7
Swordfish								
broiled, butter/margarine	1.30	354	478	4	32.8	0.68	0.14	31
cooked, dry heat	0.88	314	98	43	29.0	0.58	0.12	30
raw	0.69	245	76	33	23.0			30
Threadfin	0.26	81	15					10
dried								10
Tilefish								
cooked, dry heat	0.09	145	17		9.3	0.21	0.05	29
raw	0.21	368	45	41	24.0			22
Toman	0.11	95	5	0		0.00	0.00	2
Tom cod								
dry flesh, Alaska								6
liver, Alaska	3.80							91
Trevally								
malabar	0.17	61	23					17
yellow	0.26	111	12					20
yellow, dried	0.48	73	1957					12
Triggerfish, starry	0.20	88	49	0		0.00	0.00	1
Trout								
broiled	1.19	287	41	46	17.0	0.42	0.16	40
brook, cooked	1.10	602	79	69	35.0	0.55	0.18	51
dolly varden, Alaska	1.30	285	102	53				18
mixed species, raw	0.43	102	15	16	6.2			40
mixed species, raw, USDA	1.18	285	41	46	17.0	0.42	0.16	40
raw, all varieties	1.27	307	44	49	19.0			40
Trout, rainbow								
baked or broiled	6.34	1647	88	190	101.0			26
cooked, dry heat	0.23	313	30	48	23.0	0.58	0.24	38
raw	0.22	356	28	47	26.0	0.53	0.21	35
raw	0.54	140	8	16	8.8			26

FISH

FOOD	AMOUNT	CALORIES (kcal)	PROTEIN (g)	FAT (g)	CARBO-HYDRATES (g)	FIBER (g)	CALCIUM (mg)
Trout, rainbow, wild							
cooked, dry	143.0 g	215	32.8	8.3	0.0		
raw	159.0 g	189	32.6	5.5	0.0		107.0
Tuna							
bluefin, cooked, dry heat	85.0 g	156	25.4	5.3	0.0	0.0	8.5
bluefin, fresh, raw	85.0 g	122	19.8	4.2	0.0	0.0	13.6
dietetic, low sodium, drained	1 oz	36	7.7	0.5	0.0	0.0	1.4
little/bonito	1 oz	33	6.6	0.8	0.0	0.0	5.7
skipjack, broiled	1 oz	37	8.0	0.4	0.0		10.7
skipjack, raw	1 oz	29	6.2	0.3	0.0		8.0
yellow, broiled	1 oz	39	8.5	0.3	0.0		5.7
yellowfin, raw	1 oz	31	6.6	0.3	0.0		4.7
white, albacore, canned in water	85.0 g	116	22.7	2.1	0.0	0.0	3.4
white, canned with oil	85.0 g	158	22.6	6.9	0.0	0.0	4.0
Starkist® canned, water pack	56.7 g	65	14.0	1.0	1.0	0.0	6.8
Tuna, light, canned							
in oil, drained	1 oz	56	8.3	2.3	0.0		3.7
in oil, no salt	1 oz	56	8.3	2.3	0.0	0.0	3.7
in oil, salt	1 oz	56	8.3	2.3	0.0	0.0	3.7
in water, drained	1 oz	33	7.2	0.2	0.0		3.3
Tuna Helper®							
au gratin	41.1 g	180	6.0	5.0	27.0		40.0
buttery rice, dry	42.5 g	160	4.0	2.0	32.0		60.0
cheesy noodle, dry	41.1 g	160	7.0	3.0	26.0		60.0
creamy mushroom, dry	38.3 g	140	5.0	1.0	28.0		20.0
creamy noodle, dry	46.8 g	220	6.0	9.0	28.0		20.0
fettucini alfredo, dry	41.1 g	160	6.0	3.0	28.0		40.0
romanoff, dry	52.4 g	210	7.0	3.0	38.0		40.0
tuna pot pie, dry	55.5 g	290	4.0	17.0	31.0	0.6	20.0
tuna salad, dry	35.4 g	140	5.0	1.0	28.0	0.2	O.O
tetrazzini, dry	39.7 g	160	6.0	3.0	26.0		40.0
Tuna noodle casserole, Stouffer® dinner	163.0 g	200	10.0	9.0	18.0	0.5	97.7
Tuna salad sandwich w/mayonnaise	1 oz	64	4.8	2.6	5.3	0.3	9.9
Turbot							
European, broiled	1 oz	35	5.8	1.1	0.0		6.7
European, raw	85.0 g	81	13.6	2.5	0.0	0.0	15.0
Whelk							
raw, all varieties	85.0 g	117	20.3	0.3	6.6	0.0	48.0
steamed, all varieties	85.0 g	233	40.5	0.7	13.2	0.0	96.0
White							
lake, mixed species, raw	1 oz	38	5.4	1.7	0.0	0.0	7.4
Whitefish							
broiled	1 oz	49	6.9	2.1	0.0		
dry flesh, Alaska	20.0 g	412	69.0	12.5	0.9		65.0
Head, eyes, bones, Alaska	1 oz	112	18.6	3.6	0.0		
lake, baked, stuffed	100.0 g	215	15.2	14.0	5.8	0.6	
liver, Alaska	1 oz	104	11.0	4.4	5.1		53.0
raw	1 oz	38	5.4	1.7	0.0		

FOOD	IRON (mg)	POTAS-SIUM (mg)	SODIUM (mg)	CHOLES-TEROL (mg)	MAGNE-SIUM (mg)	DHA3 (gm)	EPA3 (gm)	% OF CALORIES FROM FAT
Trout, rainbow, wild								
cooked, dry	0.54	641	80	99	44.0	0.74	0.67	35
raw	1.11	765	50	94	49.0	0.67	0.27	26
Tuna								
bluefin, cooked, dry heat	1.11	275	43	42	54.4			31
bluefin, fresh, raw	0.87	214	33	32	0.0			31
dietetic, low sodium, drained	0.34	74	11	10	9.1			14
little/bonito	0.45	98	15					21
skipjack, broiled	0.45	148	13	17	12.3	0.07	0.03	9
skipjack, raw	0.35	115	10	13	9.7	0.05	0.02	9
yellow, broiled	0.27		13	16		0.07	0.01	8
yellowfin, raw	0.21		10	13		0.05	0.01	8
white, albacore, canned in water	0.51	241	333	35	28.9	0.44	0.16	16
white, canned with oil	0.56	283	336	26	29.0			39
Starkist® canned, water pack	0.72	85	35	10	16.4			14
Tuna, light, canned								
in oil, drained	0.39	59	100	5	8.7	0.03	0.01	37
in oil, no salt	0.39	59	14	5	8.8			37
in oil, salt	0.39	59	100	5	8.8			37
in water, drained	0.43	67	96	8	7.7	0.06	0.01	6
Tuna Helper®								
au gratin	1.08	100	800					25
buttery rice, dry	0.72	125	830					11
cheesy noodle, dry	1.08	140	810					17
creamy mushroom, dry	1.08	180	580					6
creamy noodle, dry	1.08	140	790					37
fettucini alfredo, dry	1.08	120	760					17
romanoff, dry	1.08	180	660					13
tuna pot pie, dry	1.44	120	730	7				53
tuna salad, dry	1.08	110	580	5				7
tetrazzini, dry	0.72	90	620					17
Tuna noodle casserole, Stouffer® dinner	1.15	210	670			0.00	0.00	41
Tuna salad sandwich w/mayonnaise	1.39	31	93	3	5.4			37
Turbot								
European, broiled		86	54		18.7			28
European, raw	0.31	202	127	41	44.0			28
Whelk								
raw, all varieties	4.28	295	175	55	73.0			3
steamed, all varieties	8.55	590	350	110	147.0			3
White								
lake, mixed species, raw	0.11	90	15	17	9.4			39
Whitefish								
broiled	0.13	115	19	22	12.0	0.34	0.12	39
dry flesh, Alaska	0.90			284				27
Head, eyes, bones, Alaska	3.90							29
lake, baked, stuffed	0.50	291	195					59
liver, Alaska	8.60							38
raw	0.10	90	14	17	9.3	0.27	0.09	39

FISH

FOOD	AMOUNT	CALORIES (kcal)	PROTEIN (g)	FAT (g)	CARBO-HYDRATES (g)	FIBER (g)	CALCIUM (mg)
Whitefish (continued)							
raw, mixed species, Alaska	1 oz	136	18.9	6.1	0.0		
roe, Alaska	1 oz	87	8.0	5.0	2.4		54.0
smoked	1 oz	30	6.6	0.3	0.0		5.0
Whiting							
cooked, dry heat	85.0 g	98	20.0	1.4	0.0	0.0	53.0
raw, all varieties	85.0 g	77	15.6	1.1	0.0	0.0	41.0
silver	1 oz	25	5.8	0.2	0.0	0.0	17.0
trumpeter	1 oz	23	5.6	0.1	0.0	0.0	14.2
Wolffish							
Atlantic, broiled	1 oz	35	6.4	0.9	0.0		
Atlantic, raw	1 oz	27	5.0	0.7	0.0		
Yellowtail							
broiled	1 oz	53	8.4	1.9	0.0		
raw	1 oz	41	6.6	1.5	0.0		0.0

FOOD	IRON (mg)	POTAS- SIUM (mg)	SODIUM (mg)	CHOLES- TEROL (mg)	MAGNE- SIUM (mg)	DHA3 (gm)	EPA3 (gm)	% OF CALORIES FROM FAT
Whitefish (continued)								
raw, mixed species, Alaska	0.29	317	51	55	33.0			40
roe, Alaska	0.90							52
smoked	0.14	118	285	9	6.0	0.04	0.01	8
Whiting								
cooked, dry heat	0.36	369	113	71	23.0	0.33	0.40	13
raw, all varieties	0.29	212	61	57	18.0			13
silver	0.09	99	22					6
trumpeter	0.11	95	28	0		0.00	0.00	2
Wolffish								
Atlantic, broiled	0.03		31	17		0.12	0.11	22
Atlantic, raw	0.03		24	13		0.09	0.01	22
Yellowtail								
broiled	0.18		14					32
raw	0.14	0	11	0	0.0			32

POULTRY PRODUCTS

FOOD	AMOUNT	CALORIES (kcal)	PROTEIN (g)	FAT (g)	MONO-UN-SATURATED FAT (g)	POLY-UN-SATURATED FAT (g)	SATURATED FAT (g)
CHICKEN, Broilers or fryers							
Flesh, skin, giblets, & neck, raw	1 chicken	2223	191.76	155.12	44.34	63.57	33.39
cooked, fried, batter dipped	308 g	895	70.36	53.98	14.38	21.95	12.77
cooked, fried, flour coated	212 g	577	60.56	32.37	8.81	12.71	7.44
cooked, roasted	205 g	480	54.90	27.20	7.59	10.59	5.94
cooked, stewed	225 g	487	55.10	27.84	7.76	10.85	6.08
Flesh & skin, w/out neck, raw	276 g	594	51.34	41.55	11.89	17.22	8.91
cooked, fried, batter dipped	280 g	810	63.10	48.57	12.92	19.85	11.47
cooked, fried, flour coated	188 g	505	53.69	28.05	7.63	11.08	6.40
cooked, roasted	178 g	426	48.60	24.21	6.74	9.50	5.29
cooked, stewed	200 g	437	49.35	25.13	6.99	9.86	5.49
Flesh only, w/out neck, raw	197 g	235	42.14	6.06	1.56	1.78	1.47
cooked, fried	155 g	340	47.38	14.14	3.81	5.20	3.33
cooked, roasted	146 g	278	42.24	10.81	2.98	3.88	2.47
cooked, stewed	157 g	278	42.84	10.53	2.89	3.75	2.41
Skin only, w/out neck skin, raw	47 g	164	6.26	15.20	4.27	6.36	3.20
cooked, fried, batter dipped	114 g	449	11.76	32.86	8.67	14.08	7.78
cooked, fried, flour coated	33 g	166	6.30	14.05	3.85	5.94	3.11
cooked, roasted	34 g	154	6.92	13.83	3.88	5.79	2.91
cooked, stewed	44 g	160	6.70	14.54	4.08	6.08	3.06
Giblets, raw	23 g	28	4.11	1.03	0.31	0.26	0.25
cooked, fried, flour coated	13 g	36	4.23	1.75	0.49	0.57	0.44
cooked, simmered	14 g	22	3.62	0.67	0.21	0.17	0.15
Gizzard, raw	11 g	13	2.00	0.46	0.13	0.12	0.13
cooked, simmered	7 g	11	1.90	0.26	0.07	0.07	0.07
Heart, raw	1.8 g	3	0.28	0.17	0.05	0.04	0.05
cooked, simmered	1 g	2	0.26	0.08	0.02	0.02	0.02
Liver, raw	10 g	12	1.80	0.39	0.13	0.09	0.06
cooked, simmered	6 g	9	1.46	0.33	0.11	0.08	0.05
Light meat w/skin, raw	116 g	216	23.51	12.84	3.66	5.24	2.72
cooked, fried, batter dipped	113 g	312	26.61	17.44	4.66	7.19	4.07
cooked, fried, flour coated	78 g	192	23.75	9.43	2.59	3.74	2.10
cooked, roasted	79 g	175	22.93	8.57	2.41	3.36	1.82
cooked, stewed	90 g	181	23.53	8.97	2.52	3.53	1.91
Dark meat w/skin, w/out neck, raw	160 g	379	26.70	29.34	8.41	12.24	6.33
cooked, fried, batter dipped	167 g	497	36.49	31.13	8.26	12.66	7.40
cooked, fried, flour coated	110 g	313	29.94	18.60	5.03	7.32	4.30
cooked, roasted	101 g	256	26.23	15.93	4.41	6.25	3.51
cooked, stewed	110 g	256	25.84	16.13	4.46	6.32	3.57
Light meat w/out skin, raw	88 g	100	20.42	1.45	0.38	0.35	0.33
cooked, fried	64 g	123	21.00	3.55	0.97	1.26	0.80
cooked, roasted	64 g	110	19.78	2.89	0.81	0.99	0.63
cooked, stewed	71 g	113	20.50	2.83	0.80	0.96	0.63
Dark meat w/out skin, w/out neck							
raw	109 g	136	21.89	4.70	1.20	1.46	1.1
cooked, fried	91 g	217	26.38	10.58	2.84	3.93	2.5
cooked, roasted	81 g	166	22.17	7.88	2.15	2.88	1.8
cooked, stewed	86 g	165	22.33	7.72	2.10	2.80	1.8

FOOD	CARBO-HYDRATES (mg)	FIBER (mg)	CALCIUM (mg)	IRON (mg)	POTAS-SIUM (mg)	SODIUM (mg)	CHOLES-TEROL (mg)	% OF CALORIES FROM FAT
CHICKEN, Broilers or fryers								
Flesh, skin, giblets, & neck, raw	1.3	0.00	119	13.67	1980	732	940	63
cooked, fried, batter dipped	27.8	0.11	65	5.50	584	875	316	54
cooked, fried, flour coated	6.9	0.03	37	4.21	503	182	238	50
cooked, roasted	0.1	0.00	32	3.41	435	161	219	51
cooked, stewed	0.1	0.00	31	3.45	367	148	218	51
Flesh & skin, w/out neck, raw	0.0	0.00	31	2.50	522	192	208	63
cooked, fried, batter dipped	26.3	0.10	58	3.82	518	817	243	54
cooked, fried, flour coated	5.9	0.02	31	2.59	440	158	169	50
cooked, roasted	0.0	0.00	27	2.25	397	146	157	51
cooked, stewed	0.0	0.00	26	2.32	333	134	157	52
Flesh only, w/out neck, raw	0.0	0.00	24	1.76	452	152	138	23
cooked, fried	2.6	0.01	26	2.09	399	140	145	37
cooked, roasted	0.0	0.00	22	1.76	355	125	130	35
cooked, stewed	0.0	0.00	21	1.83	283	110	130	34
Skin only, w/out neck skin, raw	0.0	0.00	5	0.51	48	30	51	83
cooked, fried, batter dipped	26.3	0.10	29	1.63	86	663	84	66
cooked, fried, flour coated	3.0	0.01	5	0.50	41	18	24	76
cooked, roasted	0.0	0.00	5	0.51	46	22	28	81
cooked, stewed	0.0	0.00	5	0.50	52	25	28	82
Giblets, raw	0.4	0.00	2	1.35	52	18	60	33
cooked, fried, flour coated	0.5	0.00	2	1.34	43	15	58	44
cooked, simmered	0.1	0.00	2	0.90	22	8	55	27
Gizzard, raw	0.0	0.00	1	0.39	26	8	14	32
cooked, simmered	0.0	0.00	1	0.29	12	5	14	21
Heart, raw	0.0	0.00	0	0.11	3	1	2	51
cooked, simmered	0.0	0.00	0	0.09	1	0	2	36
Liver, raw	0.3	0.00	1	0.86	23	8	44	29
cooked, simmered	0.0	0.00	1	0.51	8	3	38	33
Light meat w/skin, raw	0.0	0.00	13	0.92	237	76	78	54
cooked, fried, batter dipped	10.7	0.04	22	1.42	209	324	94	50
cooked, fried, flour coated	1.4	0.01	12	0.94	186	60	68	44
cooked, roasted	0.0	0.00	12	0.90	179	59	67	44
cooked, stewed	0.0	0.00	11	0.88	150	57	66	45
Dark meat w/skin, w/out neck, raw	0.0	0.00	18	1.57	285	117	130	70
cooked, fried, batter dipped	15.6	0.06	36	2.40	309	493	149	56
cooked, fried, flour coated	4.4	0.02	19	1.65	254	98	101	53
cooked, roasted	0.0	0.00	15	1.37	222	88	92	56
cooked, stewed	0.0	0.00	15	1.44	182	77	90	57
Light meat w/out skin, raw	0.0	0.00	10	0.64	210	60	51	13
cooked, fried	0.2	0.00	10	0.73	168	52	57	26
cooked, roasted	0.0	0.00	10	0.68	158	49	54	24
cooked, stewed	0.0	0.00	9	0.66	128	46	54	23
Dark meat w/out skin, w/out neck raw	0.0	0.00	13	1.12	241	93	87	31
cooked, fried	2.3	0.01	16	1.36	230	88	88	44
cooked, roasted	0.0	0.00	12	1.07	195	75	75	43
cooked, stewed	0.0	0.00	12	1.17	155	64	76	42

POULTRY PRODUCTS

FOOD	AMOUNT	CALORIES (kcal)	PROTEIN (g)	FAT (g)	MONO-UN-SATURATED FAT (g)	POLY-UN-SATURATED FAT (g)	SATU-RATED FAT (g)
CHICKEN, Broilers or fryers (continued)							
Separable fat, raw	32 g	201	1.19	21.74	6.48	9.70	4.54
Back, meat & skin, raw	59 g	188	8.29	16.95	4.92	7.22	3.62
cooked, fried, batter dipped	72 g	238	15.82	15.77	4.19	6.42	3.74
cooked, fried, flour coated	44 g	146	12.23	9.12	2.47	3.60	2.12
cooked, roasted	32 g	96	8.30	6.71	1.86	2.65	1.48
cooked, stewed	36 g	93	7.99	6.53	1.81	2.57	1.44
Back, meat only, raw	31 g	42	6.06	1.83	0.47	0.57	0.46
cooked, fried	35 g	101	10.50	5.36	1.44	2.01	1.27
cooked, roasted	24 g	57	6.77	3.16	0.86	1.16	0.73
cooked, stewed	26 g	54	6.58	2.91	0.79	1.04	0.68
Breast, meat & skin, raw	87 g	150	18.14	8.05	2.32	3.33	1.70
cooked, fried, batter dipped	84 g	218	20.87	11.08	2.96	4.58	2.59
cooked, fried, flour coated	59 g	131	18.78	5.23	1.44	2.06	1.16
cooked, roasted	58 g	115	17.28	4.51	1.27	1.76	0.96
cooked, stewed	66 g	121	18.08	4.90	1.37	1.91	1.04
Breast, meat only, raw	71 g	78	16.39	0.88	0.23	0.21	0.20
cooked, fried	52 g	97	17.39	2.45	0.67	0.89	0.56
cooked, roasted	52 g	86	16.13	1.86	0.52	0.64	0.40
cooked, stewed	57 g	86	16.52	1.73	0.49	0.59	0.38
Drumstick, meat & skin, raw	44 g	71	8.48	3.82	1.05	1.48	0.85
cooked, fried, batter dipped	43 g	115	9.44	6.77	1.78	2.76	1.63
cooked, fried, flour coated	29 g	71	7.82	3.98	1.06	1.57	0.94
cooked, roasted	31 g	67	8.38	3.46	0.94	1.32	0.78
cooked, stewed	34 g	69	8.61	3.62	0.99	1.38	0.81
Drumstick, meat only, raw	37 g	44	7.62	1.27	0.32	0.39	0.31
cooked, fried	25 g	49	7.15	2.02	0.53	0.74	0.49
cooked, roasted	26 g	45	7.35	1.47	0.39	0.49	0.36
cooked, stewed	28 g	47	7.70	1.60	0.42	0.54	0.38
Leg, meat & skin, raw	101 g	189	18.33	12.24	3.45	4.94	2.68
cooked, fried, batter dipped	95 g	259	20.68	15.37	4.07	6.25	3.66
cooked, fried, flour coated	67 g	170	17.98	9.67	2.62	3.80	2.23
cooked, roasted	69 g	160	17.91	9.29	2.57	3.61	2.02
cooked, stewed	75 g	165	18.12	9.69	2.68	3.78	2.15
Leg, meat only, raw	78 g	94	15.70	2.97	0.76	0.92	0.74
cooked, fried	56 g	116	15.89	5.22	1.40	1.92	1.24
cooked, roasted	57 g	109	15.40	4.80	1.31	1.74	1.12
cooked, stewed	60 g	111	15.76	4.84	1.32	1.76	1.13
Neck, meat & skin, raw	15 g	45	2.11	3.94	1.09	1.58	0.83
cooked, fried, batter dipped	16 g	53	3.17	3.76	1.00	1.57	0.89
cooked, fried, flour coated	11 g	37	2.64	2.60	0.70	1.07	0.60
cooked, simmered	11 g	27	2.16	1.99	0.55	0.79	0.4
Neck, meat only, raw	6 g	9	1.05	0.53	0.14	0.16	0.1
cooked, fried	7 g	16	1.88	0.83	0.21	0.32	0.2
cooked, simmered	5 g	9	1.23	0.41	0.10	0.13	0.1
Thigh, meat & skin, raw	57 g	120	9.85	8.69	2.47	3.58	1.8
cooked, fried, batter dipped	52 g	144	11.24	8.60	2.29	3.49	2.0
cooked, fried, flour coated	38 g	99	10.17	5.69	1.56	2.23	1.3
cooked, roasted	37 g	91	9.27	5.73	1.60	2.27	1.2
cooked, stewed	41 g	95	9.54	6.04	1.68	2.40	1.3

FOOD	CARBO-HYDRATES (mg)	FIBER (mg)	CALCIUM (mg)	IRON (mg)	POTAS-SIUM (mg)	SODIUM (mg)	CHOLES-TEROL (mg)	% OF CALORIES FROM FAT
CHICKEN, Broilers or fryers (continued)								
Separable fat, raw	0.0	0.00	2	0.22	20	10	19	97
Back, meat & skin, raw	0.0	0.00	8	0.56	85	38	47	81
cooked, fried, batter dipped	7.3	0.03	19	1.07	130	228	63	60
cooked, fried, flour coated	2.8	0.01	10	0.71	100	40	39	56
cooked, roasted	0.0	0.00	7	0.46	67	28	28	63
cooked, stewed	0.0	0.00	7	0.44	52	23	28	63
Back, meat only, raw	0.0	0.00	5	0.32	63	25	25	39
cooked, fried	1.9	0.01	9	0.58	88	35	32	48
cooked, roasted	0.0	0.00	6	0.33	57	23	21	50
cooked, stewed	0.0	0.00	6	0.33	41	18	22	49
Breast, meat & skin, raw	0.0	0.00	9	0.64	192	54	55	48
cooked, fried, batter dipped	7.5	0.03	17	1.05	169	231	72	46
cooked, fried, flour coated	0.9	0.00	9	0.70	153	45	53	36
cooked, roasted	0.0	0.00	8	0.62	142	41	49	35
cooked, stewed	0.0	0.00	8	0.61	117	41	50	36
Breast, meat only, raw	0.0	0.00	8	0.51	181	46	41	10
cooked, fried	0.2	0.00	8	0.59	143	41	47	23
cooked, roasted	0.0	0.00	8	0.54	133	38	44	19
cooked, stewed	0.0	0.00	7	0.50	107	36	44	18
Drumstick, meat & skin, raw	0.0	0.00	5	0.45	91	37	35	48
cooked, fried, batter dipped	3.5	0.01	7	0.58	80	116	37	53
cooked, fried, flour coated	0.4	0.00	4	0.39	66	26	26	50
cooked, roasted	0.0	0.00	4	0.41	71	28	28	46
cooked, stewed	0.0	0.00	4	0.45	63	26	28	47
Drumstick, meat only, raw	0.0	0.00	4	0.38	84	32	28	26
cooked, fried	0.0	0.00	3	0.33	62	24	24	37
cooked, roasted	0.0	0.00	3	0.34	64	25	24	29
cooked, stewed	0.0	0.00	3	0.38	56	23	25	31
Leg, meat & skin, raw	0.0	0.00	10	1.02	200	80	83	58
cooked, fried, batter dipped	8.2	0.03	17	1.33	180	265	85	53
cooked, fried, flour coated	1.6	0.01	9	0.95	156	59	63	51
cooked, roasted	0.0	0.00	9	0.92	155	60	64	52
cooked, stewed	0.0	0.00	9	1.01	132	55	63	53
Leg, meat only, raw	0.0	0.00	8	0.80	178	67	62	28
cooked, fried	0.3	0.00	7	0.78	142	54	55	41
cooked, roasted	0.0	0.00	7	0.74	138	52	53	40
cooked, stewed	0.0	0.00	7	0.84	114	47	53	39
Neck, meat & skin, raw	0.0	0.00	3	0.29	21	10	15	79
cooked, fried, batter dipped	1.3	0.01	5	0.34	24	44	15	64
cooked, fried, flour coated	0.4	0.00	3	0.27	20	9	10	63
cooked, simmered	0.0	0.00	3	0.25	12	6	8	66
Neck, meat only, raw	0.0	0.00	2	0.12	11	5	5	53
cooked, fried	0.1	0.00	3	0.21	15	7	7	47
cooked, simmered	0.0	0.00	2	0.13	7	3	4	41
Thigh, meat & skin, raw	0.0	0.00	6	0.56	110	43	48	65
cooked, fried, batter dipped	4.7	0.02	9	0.75	100	150	48	54
cooked, fried, flour coated	1.2	0.00	5	0.57	90	33	37	52
cooked, roasted	0.0	0.00	5	0.49	82	31	34	57
cooked, stewed	0.0	0.00	5	0.56	70	29	35	57

POULTRY PRODUCTS

FOOD	AMOUNT	CALO- RIES (kcal)	PROTEIN (g)	FAT (g)	MONO-UN- SATURATED FAT (g)	POLY-UN- SATURATED FAT (g)	SATU- RATED FAT (g)
CHICKEN, Broilers or fryers (continued)							
Thigh, meat only, raw	41 g	49	8.06	1.60	0.41	0.50	0.40
cooked, fried	31 g	68	8.74	3.19	0.86	1.19	0.75
cooked, roasted	31 g	65	8.04	3.37	0.94	1.29	0.77
cooked, stewed	33 g	64	8.25	3.23	0.89	1.22	0.74
Wing, meat & skin, raw	29 g	64	5.31	4.63	1.30	1.84	0.98
cooked, fried, batter dipped	29 g	94	5.76	6.32	1.69	2.60	1.47
cooked, fried, flour coated	19 g	61	4.96	4.21	1.15	1.69	0.94
cooked, roasted	21 g	61	5.64	4.09	1.14	1.60	0.87
cooked, stewed	24 g	60	5.47	4.04	1.13	1.58	0.86
Wing, meat only, raw	17 g	21	3.73	0.60	0.16	0.14	0.14
cooked, fried	12 g	25	3.62	1.10	0.30	0.37	0.25
cooked, roasted	13 g	26	3.96	1.06	0.29	0.34	0.23
cooked, stewed	14 g	25	3.80	1.00	0.28	0.32	0.22
Tyson® split broilers	100 g	245	27.10	14.70	1.20		2.60
CHICKEN, Roasting							
Flesh, skin, giblets, & neck, raw	1 chicken	3210	257.92	233.22	66.56	96.41	50.23
cooked, roasted	235 g	518	56.31	30.72	8.59	12.27	6.70
Flesh & skin, raw	293 g	633	50.22	46.45	13.26	19.44	9.96
cooked, roasted	210 g	469	50.33	28.13	7.85	11.35	6.12
Flesh only, raw	209 g	232	42.49	5.63	1.40	1.73	1.40
cooked, roasted	171 g	285	42.76	11.34	3.10	4.27	2.59
Giblets, raw	25 g	32	4.54	1.26	0.39	0.32	0.31
cooked, simmered	15 g	25	4.02	0.78	0.25	0.20	0.18
Light meat w/out skin, raw	96 g	105	21.31	1.56	0.36	0.46	0.39
cooked, roasted	78 g	119	21.16	3.17	0.84	1.18	0.72
Dark meat w/out skin, raw	113 g	127	21.17	4.07	1.05	1.27	1.01
cooked, roasted	94 g	168	21.86	8.23	2.28	3.12	1.88
CHICKEN, Stewing							
Flesh, skin, giblets, & neck, raw	1 chicken	2275	158.17	176.61	49.60	9.52	38.60
cooked, stewed	202 g	557	53.58	36.43	9.90	13.80	8.12
Flesh & skin, raw	271 g	700	47.57	55.10	15.47	22.32	12.02
cooked, stewed	178 g	507	47.85	33.58	9.10	12.79	7.52
Flesh only, raw	194 g	287	41.24	12.27	3.04	3.76	3.04
cooked, stewed	137 g	325	41.68	16.28	4.24	5.55	3.88
Giblets, raw	28 g	47	5.01	2.58	0.74	0.77	0.59
cooked, simmered	17 g	33	4.37	1.58	0.45	0.50	0.32
Light meat w/out skin, raw	89 g	122	20.55	3.75	0.86	1.11	0.92
cooked, stewed	64 g	136	21.14	5.11	1.27	1.72	1.21
Dark meat w/out skin, raw	105 g	165	20.68	8.52	2.19	2.65	2.12
cooked, stewed	73 g	188	20.54	11.16	2.97	3.83	2.67
CHICKEN ENTREES							
A la king, cooked, home recipe	245 g	470	27.00	34.00	12.90	134	6.20
Bryan® puree	28.35 g	27	2.13	1.33			
Le Menu®	28.4 g	32	32.20	1.27	0.50	0.51	0.27
Legout®	28.4 g	30	2.83	1.33			

FOOD	CARBO-HYDRATES (mg)	FIBER (mg)	CALCIUM (mg)	IRON (mg)	POTAS-SIUM (mg)	SODIUM (mg)	CHOLES-TEROL (mg)	% OF CALORIES FROM FAT
CHICKEN, Broilers or fryers (continued)								
Thigh, meat only, raw	0.0	0.00	4	0.43	95	35	34	29
cooked, fried	0.3	0.00	4	0.45	80	30	32	42
cooked, roasted	0.0	0.00	4	0.41	74	27	29	47
cooked, stewed	0.0	0.00	4	0.47	60	25	30	45
Wing, meat & skin, raw	0.0	0.00	3	0.28	45	21	22	65
cooked, fried, batter dipped	3.1	0.01	6	0.37	40	93	23	61
cooked, fried, flour coated	0.4	0.00	3	0.24	34	15	15	62
cooked, roasted	0.0	0.00	3	0.27	39	17	18	60
cooked, stewed	0.0	0.00	3	0.27	33	16	17	61
Wing, meat only, raw	0.0	0.00	2	0.15	33	14	10	26
cooked, fried	0.0	0.00	2	0.14	25	11	10	40
cooked, roasted	0.0	0.00	2	0.15	27	12	11	37
cooked, stewed	0.0	0.00	2	0.16	21	10	10	36
Tyson® split broilers	0.0	0.00	11	1.80	275	70	58	54
CHICKEN, Roasting								
Flesh, skin, giblets, & neck, raw	1.2	0.00	151	20.67	2951	1040	1295	65
cooked, roasted	0.1	0.00	30	3.78	479	167	220	53
Flesh & skin, raw	0.0	0.00	28	2.95	573	200	212	66
cooked, roasted	0.0	0.00	25	2.65	444	152	160	54
Flesh only, raw	0.0	0.00	21	2.15	497	156	136	22
cooked, roasted	0.0	0.00	20	2.08	392	128	128	36
Giblets, raw	0.2	0.00	2	1.35	57	19	59	35
cooked, simmered	0.1	0.00	2	0.91	24	9	54	28
Light meat w/out skin, raw	0.0	0.00	10	0.85	241	49	54	13
cooked, roasted	0.0	0.00	10	0.84	184	40	58	24
Dark meat w/out skin, raw	0.0	0.00	10	1.30	256	107	81	29
cooked, roasted	0.0	0.00	10	1.25	210	89	70	44
CHICKEN, Stewing								
Flesh, skin, giblets, & neck, raw	1.7	0.00	93	13.63	1846	647	786	70
cooked, stewed	0.0	0.00	27	3.69	358	143	205	59
Flesh & skin, raw	0.0	0.00	27	2.82	553	193	192	71
cooked, stewed	0.0	0.00	22	2.43	325	130	140	60
Flesh only, raw	0.0	0.00	20	2.11	486	154	123	38
cooked, stewed	0.0	0.00	18	1.96	276	107	114	45
Giblets, raw	0.6	0.00	3	1.66	63	22	67	49
cooked, simmered	0.0	0.00	2	1.09	26	9	60	43
Light meat w/out skin, raw	0.0	0.00	10	0.82	232	47	42	28
cooked, stewed	0.0	0.00	9	0.76	128	37	45	34
Dark meat w/out skin, raw	0.0	0.00	10	1.29	254	106	81	46
cooked, stewed	0.0	0.00	9	1.20	149	70	69	53
CHICKEN ENTREES								
A la king, cooked, home recipe	12.0	1.20	127	2.50	404	759	186	65
Bryan® puree	1.6				37	56		45
Le Menu®	2.8	0.19	7.8	0.14	52	81	22	35
Legout®	1.6		3.33	0.60	63	183		40

POULTRY PRODUCTS

FOOD	AMOUNT	CALO-RIES (kcal)	PROTEIN (g)	FAT (g)	MONO-UN-SATURATED FAT (g)	POLY-UN-SATURATED FAT (g)	SATU-RATED FAT (g)
CHICKEN, ENTREES (continued)							
A la king, cooked, home recipe (continued)							
Stouffer® with rice	269 g	290	19.00	9.00	3.52	3.59	1.90
Swanson® canned	28.4 g	36	1.90	2.29			
& broccoli, Light & Elegant®	270 g	290	19.00	11.00			
A l'orange, Healthy Choice®	255 g	260	23.00	2.00	1.00		1.00
A l'orange, Lean Cuisine® with almonds	227 g	260	24.00	5.00	0.72	3.56	0.72
& dumplings							
Hormel® with gravy	28.4 g	31	2.80	1.30	0.41	0.62	0.24
Legout®	28.4 g	17	1.50	0.67			
Luck's®	206 g	260	15.00	12.00	3.76	5.32	2.93
microwave	213 g	170	17.00	2.00	0.67	0.67	0.67
Swanson® canned	28.4 g	30	1.52	1.52	0.48	0.67	0.37
& noodles, cooked, home recipe	240 g	365	22.00	18.00	5.90	7.10	3.50
Stouffer® homestyle	284 g	310	23.00	15.00	3.41	5.63	3.40
& potatoes, microwave, Luck's®	213 g	190	16.00	4.00	1.00	1.00	1.00
& rice, microwave, Luck's®	213 g	150	17.00	2.00	0.67	0.67	0.67
& vegetables, Healthy Choice®	326 g	280	24.00	3.00	1.00		2.00
Au gratin, Budget Gourmet Light®	258 g	250	17.00	11.00	6.67	3.41	0.92
Barbecued, Light & Elegant®	227 g	300	26.00	6.00			
Barbecue sauce, Healthy Choice®	362 g	380	24.00	6.00	2.00		2.00
Batter gold, cooked, Tyson®	100 g	285	19.40	18.70	1.90		3.90
Boneless, Swanson® Hungry Man	28.4 g	39	2.70	1.58	0.50	0.70	0.39
Burgundy, Classic Lite® dinner	319 g	240	23.00	5.00			
Buttermilk, cooked, Tyson®	100 g	285	17.60	19.50	0.60		4.30
Cacciatore							
Healthy Choice® with pasta	354 g	310	26.00	3.00	1.00		1.00
Light Balance®	234 g	200	12.00	1.00	0.21	0.57	0.21
Stouffer® dinner	319 g	310	25.00	11.00			
Swanson® homestyle	28.4 g	24	1.37	0.73	0.20	0.30	0.23
Cashew, with rice, Stouffer®	269 g	380	31.00	16.00	2.22	3.23	6.33
Chic-ketts, frozen, Worthington®	168 g	320	38.00	14.00			
Chicken helper, Skillet®							
cheesy broccoli	43.9 g	160	4.00	2.00			
creamy chicken	41 g	170	6.00	5.00			
creamy mushroom	41 g	170	5.00	4.00			
fettucine alfredo	41 g	170	6.00	4.00			
stir-fried chicken	46.8 g	170	4.00	1.00			
Chik'n g'rilla, Pierce Foods®	75.4 g	99	12.70	5.23	1.39	2.48	1.36
Chikstiks, frozen, Worthington®	47 g	110	9.00	7.00			
Cordon bleu							
Le Menu®	28.4 g	42	2.09	1.82	1.03	0.63	0.15
Tyson®	100 g	225	22.30	12.80	0.70	3.94	2.40
Cornish & split Cornish, Tyson®	100 g	240	27.70	14.20	1.00	5.31	2.40
Chow mein, home recipe	250 g	255	31.00	10.00	2.40	3.40	3.10
canned	250 g	95	7.00	0.00	0.00	0.00	0.00
Healthy Choice®	255 g	240	20.00	5.00	2.00		2.00
La Choy® frozen	300 g	228	17.70	9.00			
canned	300 g	132	6.90	5.70	1.29	2.95	1.45
Le Menu® light	284 g	260	18.00	4.00	1.57	1.64	0.79

FOOD	CARBO-HYDRATES (mg)	FIBER (mg)	CALCIUM (mg)	IRON (mg)	POTAS-SIUM (mg)	SODIUM (mg)	CHOLES-TEROL (mg)	% OF CALORIES FROM FAT
CHICKEN, Roasting (continued)								
A la king, cooked, home recipe (continued)								
Stouffer® with rice	34.0	1.08	80	0.72	260	890	122	28
Swanson® canned	1.7		7.62	0.07		131		57
& broccoli, Light & Elegant®	30.0		204	1.60	180	805		34
A l'orange, Healthy Choice®	38.0		20	1.44	430	340	40	7
A l'orange, Lean Cuisine® with almonds	30.0	3.63	20	0.72	420	430	55	17
& dumplings								
Hormel® with gravy	2.0	0.31	5	0.15	45	116	9	38
Legout®	1.3		0	0.30	25	125		36
Luck's®	22.0	4.00	60	1.08	253	680	65	42
microwave	20.0	2.00	20	1.08	261	1550	25	11
Swanson® canned	2.6	0.08	2.76	0.10	35	135	11	45
& noodles, cooked, home recipe	26.0	1.30	26	2.20	149	600	96	44
Stouffer® homestyle	21.0	2.38	150	1.08	430	1090	50	44
& potatoes, microwave, Luck's®	22.0	3.00	20	1.08	373	1085	20	19
& rice, microwave, Luck's®	17.0	2.00	40	0.72	169	1170	30	12
& vegetables, Healthy Choice®	39.0		40	2.70	390	380	25	10
Au gratin, Budget Gourmet Light®	21.0	1.89	279	3.00	440	870	50	40
Barbecued, Light & Elegant®	35.0	3.20	22	1.50	450	900	97	18
Barbecue sauce, Healthy Choice®	57.0		60	2.70	670	560	60	14
Batter gold, cooked, Tyson®	9.7		33	1.20	120	312	85	59
Boneless, Swanson® Hungry Man	3.6	0.00	4.51	0.30	63	86	25	36
Burgundy, Classic Lite® dinner	24.0							19
Buttermilk, cooked, Tyson®	9.7		56	1.50	154	500	71	62
Cacciatore								
Healthy Choice® with pasta	47.0		40	2.70	660	430	35	9
Light Balance®	37.0	2.54	24.4	1.80	453	730	25	5
Stouffer® dinner	29.0	2.87	75.4	3.87	300	1135	166	32
Swanson® homestyle	3.0	0.26	7.31	0.25	80	94	15	28
Cashew, with rice, Stouffer®	29.0	1.62	20	1.80	530	1140	68	38
Chic-ketts, frozen, Worthington®	12.0		40	3.60	70	1280		39
Chicken helper, Skillet®								
cheesy broccoli	32.0		40	1.08	160	720		11
creamy chicken	26.0		20	1.08	150	720		26
creamy mushroom	28.0		20	1.08	150	720		21
fettucine alfredo	27.0		40	1.08	105	730		21
stir-fried chicken	36.0		40	1.08	130	800		5
Chik'n g'rilla, Pierce Foods®	0.0	0.00	1.04	0.32	168	401	33	48
Chikstiks, frozen, Worthington®	4.0		20	0.36	85	390		57
Cordon bleu								
Le Menu®	4.2	0.08	9.09	0.13	61	77	24	39
Tyson®	4.1	0.27	96	0.94	235	500	38	51
Cornish & split Cornish, Tyson®	0.0	0.00	11	1.80	256	65	52	53
Chow mein, home recipe	10.0	0.50	58	2.50	473	717	98	35
canned	18.0	0.90	45	1.30	418	722	98	0
Healthy Choice®	29.0		20	1.44	290	530	45	19
La Choy® frozen	19.2	0.45	37.2		360	47		36
canned	15.0	0.63	48	3.15	491	999	18	39
Le Menu® light	37.0	1.45	38.1	2.48	274	830	50	14

POULTRY PRODUCTS

FOOD	AMOUNT	CALORIES (kcal)	PROTEIN (g)	FAT (g)	MONO-UN-SATURATED FAT (g)	POLY-UN-SATURATED FAT (g)	SATURATED FAT (g)
CHICKEN ENTREES (continued)							
Chow mein, home recipe (continued)							
Lean Cuisine® dinner	319 g	250	14.00	5.00			
Stouffer®	227 g	130	13.00	4.00	1.23	1.67	1.01
Chow mein/chop suey with noodles	28.4 g	37	2.63	1.67	0.35	0.79	0.39
Chunk style mixin, canned, Swanson®	28.4 g	52	5.20	3.20			
Creamed, Stouffer®	184 g	300	19	21	3.07	2.4	1.43
Crepes, in mushroom sauce, Stouffer®	234 g	390	30.00	22.00	7.33	3.78	0.91
Curry	28.35 g	58	4.83	3.89	0.40	0.79	0.58
Delecta delicious, cooked, Tyson®	100 g	305	19.10	19.10	2.40		4.00
Dijon, Healthy Choice®	312 g	250	21.00	3.00	1.00		1.00
Dijon, Le Menu® light	241 g	240	22.00	7.00	2.00		1.00
Dinner, Swanson® frozen dinner	326 g	660	26.00	33.00	7.38	10.50	6.91
Dinner plate, w/fried potatoes	28.4 g	49	3.63	2.41			
Divan, Healthy Choice® with pasta	343 g	300	25.00	4.00	2.00		1.00
Divan, Stouffer® frozen dinner	241 g	335	21.00	22.00	9.23	8.16	3.26
Dumpling	28.3 g	68	3.46	0.74	0.23	0.33	0.18
Empress, Le Menu® light	28.4 g	26	1.94	0.61			
Enchanadas, Lean Cuisine®	280 g	270	17.00	9.00	2.00		2.00
Enchiladas							
Healthy Choice®	380 g	320	13.00	6.00	3.00		2.00
Le Menu® light	234 g	280	21.00	8.00	2.00		2.00
Stouffer®	284 g	490	22.00	29.00	10.20	5.24	1.60
Fajitas, Healthy Choice®	198 g	200	17.00	3.00	1.00		1.00
Fiesta, Lean Cuisine®	241 g	250	21.00	6.00	1.00		2.00
Fiesta, Light Balance®	234 g	210	10.00	3.00	1.00		1.00
Florentine, Le Menu® frozen dinner	354 g	510	28.00	28.00	8.01	11.40	7.50
French, w/vegetables, Budget Light®	284 g	240	18.00	9.00	2.84	3.94	2.21
Fried, w/potatoes, plate dinner	28.4 g	49	3.63	2.41	0.85	0.85	0.28
La Loma®							
w/gravy, canned	42.5 g	70	4.50	5.00			
frozen	57	180	11.00	14.00			
Swanson® dinner							
barbecue	28.4 g	54	2.50	2.20	0.68	0.97	0.56
dark	28.4 g	57	2.26	2.87	0.84	1.28	0.75
homestyle	28.4 g	56	2.57	3.00	0.92	1.32	0.76
white	28.4 g	55	2.20	2.50	0.76	1.10	0.64
Swanson Hungry Man® dark	28.4 g	60	2.53	3.16	0.95	1.39	0.81
white	28.4 g	61	2.46	3.23	0.71	1.01	0.57
Glazed							
Lean Cuisine® w/rice	241 g	270	26.00	8.00			
Light & Elegant®	227 g	230	24.00	4.00			
Heat n'serve, cooked, Tyson®	100 g	270	18.10	16.70	0.40	3.01	3.80
Herb roasted							
Healthy Choice®	326 g	380	26.00	7.00	3.00		1.00
Le Menu® light	262 g	220	21.00	6.00	1.53	3.96	0.51
Honey mustard, Healthy Choice®	269 g	250	24.00	3.00	1.00		1.00

FOOD	CARBO-HYDRATES (mg)	FIBER (mg)	CALCIUM (mg)	IRON (mg)	POTAS-SIUM (mg)	SODIUM (mg)	CHOLES-TEROL (mg)	% OF CALORIES FROM FAT
CHICKEN ENTREES (continued)								
Chow mein, home recipe (continued)								
Lean Cuisine® dinner	36.0				270	1030	25	18
Stouffer®	11.0	1.16	20	0.72	230	1080	34	28
Chow mein/chop suey with noodles	2.8	0.29	5.09	0.30	46	147	6	41
Chunk style mixin, canned, Swanson®	0.4		8	0.29		92		55
Creamed, Stouffer®		2.4	80	0.72	200	670	60.3	63
Crepes, in mushroom sauce, Stouffer®	19.0	2.33	53.8	2.62	420	1040	76	51
Curry	0.8	0.03	13	0.74	55	33	10	61
Delecta delicious, cooked, Tyson®	12.9		31	1.10	146	496	82	56
Dijon, Healthy Choice®	40.0		20	1.80	350	470	40	11
Dijon, Le Menu® light	21.0					500	40	26
Dinner, Swanson® frozen dinner	64.0	6.18	112	2.70	602	1610	111	45
Dinner plate, w/fried potatoes	3.2	0.31	11.6	0.34	32	98	14	44
Divan, Healthy Choice® with pasta	41.0		150	1.80	500	520	50	12
Divan, Stouffer® frozen dinner	14.0	0.98	269	1.72	415	830	86	59
Dumpling	11.8	0.20	5.95	0.79	4	28	11	10
Empress, Le Menu® light	3.1		2.42	0.13		84	4	21
Enchanadas, Lean Cuisine®	31.0		150	2.70	420	850	65	30
Enchiladas								
Healthy Choice®	58.0		100	3.60	430	550	30	17
Le Menu® light	32.0					530	35	26
Stouffer®	34.0	2.89	300	1.08	490	910	89	53
Fajitas, Healthy Choice®	25.0		80	2.70	360	310	35	14
Fiesta, Lean Cuisine®	29.0		20	1.08	450	880	45	22
Fiesta, Light Balance®	37.0			1.80		640	15	13
Florentine, Le Menu® frozen dinner	35.0	6.72	122	2.93	653	985	121	49
French, w/vegetables, Budget Light®	21.0	4.24	113	2.75	720	1000	50	34
Fried, w/potatoes, plate dinner La Loma®	3.2	0.31	11.6	0.34	32	98	14	44
w/gravy, canned	2.0		10	0.72	125	170		64
frozen	2.0		20	1.08	80	570		70
Swanson® dinner								
barbecue	6.1	0.29	8	0.40	64	116	21	37
dark	5.6	0.08	6.15	0.28	54	116	26	45
homestyle	4.7	0.00	5.71	0.26	68	157	26	48
white	6.0	0.00	6	0.27	68	146	26	41
Swanson Hungry Man® dark	5.4	0.00	4.21	0.25	67	116	27	47
white	5.6	0.00	5.61	0.25	74	151	26	48
Glazed								
Lean Cuisine® w/rice	23.0				380	810	55	27
Light & Elegant®	25.0		18	4.80	300	655		16
Heat n'serve, cooked, Tyson®	11.5	0.00	14	1.20	152	588	74	56
Herb roasted								
Healthy Choice®	56.0		60	1.44	650	470	60	17
Le Menu® light	21.0	0.00	113	2.54	513	610	55	25
Honey mustard, Healthy Choice®	37.0		20	1.44	110	480	40	11

POULTRY PRODUCTS

FOOD	AMOUNT	CALO-RIES (kcal)	PROTEIN (g)	FAT (g)	MONO-UN-SATURATED FAT (g)	POLY-UN-SATURATED FAT (g)	SATU-RATED FAT (g)
CHICKEN ENTREES (continued)							
Honey stung, cooked, Tyson®	100 g	260	21.40	14.20	0.90		3.50
Hum dinger, Pierce Foods®	100 g	225	16.00	13.70	0.00	0.00	0.00
Italiano, Right Course®	273 g	280	24.00	8.00	2.00		2.00
Kiev, Le Menu® frozen dinner	234 g	500	21.00	30.00	5.30	7.57	4.96
Kiev, Tyson®	100 g	290	19.50	21.50	2.30	4.01	4.96
Lightly breaded, cooked, Tyson®	100 g	255	21.60	14.20	1.20	7.97	3.30
Liver paté, canned	13 g	26	1.75	1.70	0.52	0.69	0.32
Mandarin							
Budget Gourmet Light®	284 g	300	20.00	7.00			
Healthy Choice®	284 g	240	21.00	2.00	1.00		1.00
Mesquite							
Con Agra® frozen dinner	298 g	340	23.00	1.00	0.09	0.83	0.09
Healthy Choice®	298 g	300	21.00	3.00	1.00		1.00
Ultra Slim Fast® with rice	340 g	360	29.00	1.00			
Nibbles, Swanson®	28.35 g	92	3.68	5.84			
homestyle	28.4 g	80	2.35	4.71			
Nuggets							
La Loma® frozen	17 g	54	3.00	4.00			
Swanson®	28.35 g	77	4.32	4.66	1.36	2.09	1.21
dinner	28.4 g	54	2.17	2.63	0.77	1.18	0.68
Orange glazed, Budget Light®	255 g	250	14.00	3.00	0.85	1.42	0.73
Oriental							
Healthy Choice®	319 g	200	19.00	1.00	1.00		1.00
with peanut sauce	269 g	280	29.00	5.00	1.00		2.00
Lean Cuisine®	266 g	230	22.00	6.00	0.97	3.09	1.94
Parmigiana							
Healthy Choice®	326 g	290	23.00	6.00	3.00		1.00
Le Menu®	28.4 g	35	2.21	1.70	0.65	0.53	0.52
frozen dinner	333 g	390	26.00	19.00			
Light & Elegant®	227 g	260	28.00	6.00			
Parts, pre-fried, Swanson®	28.35 g	83	4.61	4.91	1.19	1.72	0.99
Patties, Tyson®	100 g	275	17.70	18.60	3.20		3.60
heat n'serve	100 g	280	17.20	18.90	1.20		4.40
school lunch	100 g	290	16.20	19.70	1.60		4.80
Worthington® frozen crispychik	71 g	220	8.00	15.00			
Pie, Stouffer®	284 g	530	22.00	33.00	11.60	14.00	7.39
homestyle	28.4 g	51	1.88	2.63	0.93	1.12	0.59
Pieces w/fried rice	28.3 g	51	1.90	1.50	0.23	0.34	0.67
Potpie, baked, home recipe	232 g	545	23.00	31.00	11.00	13.50	5.50
Swanson®	28.4 g	54	1.57	3.14	1.10	1.33	0.70
Swanson Hungry Man®	28.4 g	39	1.38	2.19	0.77	0.93	0.49
Pre-breaded, marinated, Tyson®	100 g	285	23.30	17.30	1.00		3.20
Roasted, Ultra Slim Fast®	340 g	300	27.00	5.00			
Salsa, Healthy Choice®	319 g	240	20.00	2.00	2.00		2.00
Satay	28.35 g	65	11.72	1.73			
Scalloped	284 g	420	21.00	25.00	4.52	4.57	2.15
Sesame, Right Course®	24 g	320	25.00	9.00	2.00		4.00
Southwestern, Healthy Choice®	354 g	340	25.00	5.00	2.00		2.00
Stir fry, w/pasta, Healthy Choice®	340 g	300	23.00	5.00	1.00		2.00

FOOD	CARBO-HYDRATES (mg)	FIBER (mg)	CALCIUM (mg)	IRON (mg)	POTAS-SIUM (mg)	SODIUM (mg)	CHOLES-TEROL (mg)	% OF CALORIES FROM FAT
CHICKEN ENTREES (continued)								
Honey stung, cooked, Tyson®	10.9		12	1.50	215	622	90	49
Hum dinger, Pierce Foods®	9.4			0.75	348	762	0	55
Italiano, Right Course®	29.0		100	1.80	520	560	45	26
Kiev, Le Menu® frozen dinner	35.0	4.44	80.3	1.94	432	745	80	54
Kiev, Tyson®	3.6	0.19	8.8	0.67	238	432	73	67
Lightly breaded, cooked, Tyson®	10.2	0.30	13	1.30	244	724	94	50
Liver paté, canned	0.8	0.00	1	1.19	12	50	51	59
Mandarin								
Budget Gourmet Light®	40.0				430	670	40	21
Healthy Choice®	35.0		20	1.80	360	370	45	8
Mesquite								
Con Agra® frozen dinner	58.0	5.65	40	1.80	570	290	45	3
Healthy Choice®	54.0		60	1.80	460	390	40	9
Ultra Slim Fast® with rice	61.0	0.44	38.4	4.41	1010	170	65	3
Nibbles, Swanson®	5.8		6.14	0.44		212		57
homestyle	6.8		4.71	0.34		172		53
Nuggets								
La Loma® frozen	1.6			0.29	34	106		67
Swanson®	4.6	0.09	0	0.24	79	120	19	55
dinner	5.3	0.09	2.29	0.21	79	74	19	44
Orange glazed, Budget Light®	41.0	1.00	44.6	1.53	340	350	10	11
Oriental								
Healthy Choice®	32.0		40	1.44	400	440	35	5
with peanut sauce	31.0		40	0.72	340	400	45	16
Lean Cuisine®	23.0	1.60	40	1.80	400	790	100	23
Parmigiana								
Healthy Choice®	41.0		100	1.80	530	340	55	19
Le Menu®	2.6	0.21	8.51	0.23	72	88	22	44
frozen dinner	28.0					900		44
Light & Elegant®	23.0	1.69	73	2.80	310	685	172	21
Parts, pre-fried, Swanson®	4.9	0.00	0	0.33	67	200	26	53
Patties, Tyson®	8.6		18	0.85	237	364	58	61
heat n'serve	9.8		8.7	0.83	180	331	53	61
school lunch	11.3		42	2.30	314	690	33	61
Worthington® frozen crispychik	13.0		20	0.72	70	620		61
Pie, Stouffer®	35.0	3.28	100	1.80	290	1260	78	56
homestyle	5.1	0.33	5	0.23	43	129	8	46
Pieces w/fried rice	7.3	0.45	4.54	0.57	38	36	7	27
Potpie, baked, home recipe	42.0	4.20	70	3.00	343	593	72	51
Swanson®	5.0	0.33	2.86	0.26	43	109	8	52
Swanson Hungry Man®	3.5	0.33	3.75	0.23	43	100	8	50
Pre-breaded, marinated, Tyson®	8.9		20	1.50	169	520	65	55
Roasted, Ultra Slim Fast®	36.0	0.00	51.6	4.26	470	640	65	15
Salsa, Healthy Choice®	36.0		80	1.08	540	450	50	8
Satay	0.5	0.00	4.83	0.63	60	34		24
Scalloped	27.0	4.29	100	1.44	250	1230	64	54
Sesame, Right Course®	34.0		40	1.80	400	590	50	25
Southwestern, Healthy Choice®	51.0		40	1.80	560	550	60	13
Stir fry, w/pasta, Healthy Choice®	42.0		20	0.72	290	550	30	15

POULTRY PRODUCTS

FOOD	AMOUNT	CALORIES (kcal)	PROTEIN (g)	FAT (g)	MONO-UN-SATURATED FAT (g)	POLY-UN-SATURATED FAT (g)	SATURATED FAT (g)
CHICKEN ENTREES (continued)							
Sweet & sour							
Budget Gourmet®	284 g	350	18.00	7.00	1.26	1.72	3.25
Healthy Choice®	326 g	280	20.00	2.00	1.00		1.00
Le Menu®	28.4 g	36	1.69	1.60	0.13	0.17	0.33
dinner	298 g	450	20.00	22.00	1.32	1.80	3.41
Ultra Slim Fast®	340 g	330	20.00	2.00	0.49	1.01	0.49
Taco filling, McCarty®	28.35 g	113	8.51	7.37			
Tenders, Right Course®							
barbecue	248 g	270	20.00	6.00	1.00		2.00
peanut	262 g	330	27.00	10.00	2.00		3.00
Teriyaki, Healthy Choice®	347 g	290	24.00	4.00	1.00		2.00
w/pasta	357 g	350	24.00	3.00	1.00		2.00
Thighs & drumsticks, Swanson®	28.35 g	89	4.61	5.53	0.86	1.20	0.71
Vegetable, w/vermicelli, Lean Cuisine®	333 g	270	20.00	8.00	2.00	3.76	2.00
White & dark, canned, Swanson®	28.35 g	40	6.39	1.60	0.50	0.71	0.39
White, canned, Swanson®	28.4 g	40	6.00	1.60	0.50	0.71	0.39
Wine sauce, Le Menu®	28.4 g	28	2.60	0.70			
CHICKEN BREAST							
Boneless, Tyson®	100 g	205	22.60	12.50	0.70	5.31	2.00
Fried, Swanson®	28.35 g	80	5.10	4.43	0.71	1.01	0.57
Glazed							
Healthy Choice®	241 g	220	21.00	3.00	1.00		1.00
Le Menu® light	28.4 g	23	2.50	0.30	0.10	0.12	0.08
Herbed, Light & Healthy®	312 g	240	23.00	7.00	1.57	4.91	0.52
Herb sauce, Lean Cuisine®	269 g	260	26.00	10.00	2.29	6.18	1.53
Marsala, Lean Cuisine®	230 g	190	25.00	5.00	0.56	3.88	0.56
Parmigiana							
Lean Cuisine®	284 g	260	27.00	8.00	1.27	5.45	1.27
Light & Healthy®	312 g	260	22.00	8.00	1.91	4.81	1.27
Roasted, Healthy Choice®	10 g	10	2.00	0.17			
Strips, Tyson®	100 g	270	25.60	13.30	1.20	3.01	1.60
Stuffed, Tyson®	100 g	160	12.70	6.70	1.30	2.15	1.10
CHICKEN, Capons							
Flesh, skin, giblets, & neck, raw	1 chicken	4987	398.25	363.67	105.15	154.00	77.36
cooked, roasted	218 g	494	61.79	25.43	7.15	10.27	5.49
Flesh & skin, raw	297 g	695	55.74	50.71	14.69	21.72	10.76
cooked, roasted	196 g	448	56.75	22.83	6.40	9.31	4.93
Giblets, raw	18 g	23	3.29	0.93	0.30	0.24	0.21
cooked, simmered	11 g	18	2.90	0.59	0.19	0.15	0.12
DUCK, Domesticated							
Flesh & skin, raw	287 g	1159	32.97	112.90	37.94	53.64	14.57
cooked, roasted	173 g	583	32.86	49.05	16.73	22.32	6.32
Flesh only, raw	137 g	180	25.04	8.15	3.18	2.11	1.03
cooked, roasted	100 g	201	23.48	11.20	4.17	3.70	1.43
Liver, raw	10 g	14	1.87	0.46	0.14	0.07	0.06

FOOD	CARBO-HYDRATES (mg)	FIBER (mg)	CALCIUM (mg)	IRON (mg)	POTAS-SIUM (mg)	SODIUM (mg)	CHOLES-TEROL (mg)	% OF CALORIES FROM FAT
CHICKEN ENTREES (continued)								
Sweet & sour								
Budget Gourmet®	53.0	1.74	60	0.72	429	640	40	18
Healthy Choice®	52.0		40	1.80	480	320	35	6
Le Menu®	3.6	0.17	5.33	0.16	43	91	5	40
dinner	42.0	1.82	36.7	1.95	450	1170	53	44
Ultra Slim Fast®	57.0	2.08	41.8	2.22	350	160	35	5
Taco filling, McCarty®	3.3		51	1.70	74	320		59
Tenders, Right Course®								
barbecue	35.0		60	1.44	590	590	40	20
peanut	32.0		80	1.80	470	570	50	27
Teriyaki, Healthy Choice®	39.0		40	1.44	520	560	55	12
w/pasta	58.0		60	2.70	390	370	45	8
Thighs & drumsticks, Swanson®	5.2	0.00	0	0.44	65	188	26	56
Vegetable, w/vermicelli, Lean Cuisine®	29.0	3.97	100	1.44	400	980	45	27
White & dark, canned, Swanson®	0.0	0.00	0	0.29	39	96	18	36
White, canned, Swanson®	0.0	0.00	0	0.14	39	94	18	36
Wine sauce, Le Menu®	2.7		6	0.18		68		23
CHICKEN BREAST								
Boneless, Tyson®	0.0	0.00	3.9	0.75	213	59	50	55
Fried, Swanson®	4.6	0.00	8.87	0.32	74	178	26	50
Glazed								
Healthy Choice®	27.0		20	1.08	370	510	45	12
Le Menu® light	2.5	0.00	6	0.14	72	48	6	12
Herbed, Light & Healthy®	28.0	6.00	44.3	1.80	490	430	55	26
Herb sauce, Lean Cuisine®	17.0	0.00	100	1.08	460	910	80	35
Marsala, Lean Cuisine®	11.0	0.00	20	1.08	850	400	80	24
Parmigiana								
Lean Cuisine®	19.0	0.00	150	1.44	700	870	80	28
Light & Healthy®	29.0	5.00	323	1.44	440	420	50	28
Roasted, Healthy Choice®	0.1				33	100	5	15
Strips, Tyson®	10.9	0.00	8	1.00	281	295	43	44
Stuffed, Tyson®	12.4	0.20	23	1.20	165	284	34	38
CHICKEN, Capons								
Flesh, skin, giblets, & neck, raw	1.6	0.00	234	30.32	4594	1020	1882	66
cooked, roasted	0.0	0.00	32	3.91	529	108	224	46
Flesh & skin, raw	0.0	0.00	31	3.25	644	133	222	66
cooked, roasted	0.0	0.00	28	2.91	500	96	169	46
Giblets, raw	0.2	0.00	2	1.12	41	14	52	36
cooked, simmered	0.0	0.00	1	0.75	17	6	48	30
DUCK, Domesticated								
Flesh & skin, raw	0.0	0.00	30	6.89	600	181	218	88
cooked, roasted	0.0	0.00	20	4.67	353	103	145	76
Flesh only, raw	0.0	0.00	15	3.29	371	101	105	41
cooked, roasted	0.0	0.00	12	2.70	252	65	89	50
Liver, raw	0.3	0.00	1	3.05			51	30

POULTRY PRODUCTS

FOOD	AMOUNT	CALO-RIES (kcal)	PROTEIN (g)	FAT (g)	MONO-UN-SATURATED FAT (g)	POLY-UN-SATURATED FAT (g)	SATU-RATED FAT (g)
DUCK, Wild							
Flesh & skin, raw	239 g	505	41.63	36.32	12.04	16.26	4.82
Breast, meat only	73 g	90	14.49	3.10	0.96	0.88	0.42
GOOSE, Domesticated							
Flesh & skin, raw	320 g	1187	50.76	107.58	31.30	56.86	12.02
cooked, roasted	188 g	574	47.29	41.22	12.92	19.28	4.74
Flesh only, raw	185 g	299	42.09	13.19	5.15	3.42	1.67
cooked, roasted	143 g	340	41.42	18.11	6.52	6.20	2.21
Liver, raw	11 g	15	1.80	0.47	0.17	0.09	0.03
GUINEA							
Flesh & skin, raw	359 g	568	84.01	23.16			
Flesh only, raw	275 g	304	56.77	6.80			
PHEASANT							
Flesh & skin, raw	371 g	670	84.20	34.47	10.01	16.02	4.38
Flesh only, raw	326 g	435	76.83	11.87	4.03	3.80	2.02
Breast, meat only, raw	169 g	225	41.19	5.50	1.86	1.76	0.93
Leg, meat only, raw	99 g	132	21.98	4.26	1.45	1.36	0.72
QUAIL							
Flesh & skin, raw	405 g	780	79.48	48.80	13.70	16.93	12.06
Flesh only, raw	342 g	457	74.42	15.49	4.51	4.36	3.98
Breast, meat only	208 g	257	46.99	6.22	1.81	1.75	1.60
SQUAB (pigeon)							
Flesh & skin, raw	297 g	872	54.85	70.69	25.04	28.88	9.13
Flesh only, raw	251 g	357	43.93	18.83	4.92	6.69	4.02
Breast, meat only, raw	151 g	202	32.86	6.83	1.78	2.43	1.46
TURKEY, all classes							
Flesh, skin, giblets, & neck, raw	1 turkey	8738	1131.18	431.43	122.35	153.07	107.25
cooked, roasted	260 g	533	72.76	24.56	7.20	7.93	6.29
Flesh & skin, raw	332 g	530	67.80	26.62	7.51	9.62	6.59
cooked, roasted	240 g	498	67.43	23.34	6.81	7.66	5.96
Flesh only, raw	281 g	334	61.17	8.03	2.66	1.70	2.33
cooked, roasted	208 g	354	60.98	10.33	3.40	2.15	2.97
Skin only, raw	51 g	197	6.48	18.82	4.91	8.02	4.31
cooked, roasted	32 g	141	6.30	12.69	3.31	5.41	2.91
Giblets, raw	16 g	21	3.10	0.67	0.20	0.15	0.16
cooked, simmered	10 g	17	2.66	0.51	0.15	0.11	0.12
Gizzard, raw	7 g	8	1.34	0.26	0.07	0.05	0.07
cooked, simmered	4 g	7	1.18	0.16	0.04	0.03	0.04
Heart, raw	1.9 g	3	0.34	0.13	0.04	0.03	0.04
cooked, simmered	1.0 g	2	0.27	0.06	0.02	0.01	0.02
Liver, raw	7 g	10	1.40	0.28	0.09	0.07	0.05
cooked, simmered	5 g	8	1.20	0.30	0.09	0.07	0.05

FOOD	CARBO-HYDRATES (mg)	FIBER (mg)	CALCIUM (mg)	IRON (mg)	POTAS-SIUM (mg)	SODIUM (mg)	CHOLES-TEROL (mg)	% OF CALORIES FROM FAT
DUCK, Wild								
Flesh & skin, raw	0.0	0.00	11	9.94	594	135	191	65
Breast, meat only	0.0	0.00	2	3.29	196	42		31
GOOSE, Domesticated								
Flesh & skin, raw	0.0	0.00	38	8.00	985	234	256	82
cooked, roasted	0.0	0.00	25	5.32	618	132	172	65
Flesh only, raw	0.0	0.00	25	4.76	777	162	155	40
cooked, roasted	0.0	0.00	20	4.10	554	108	138	48
Liver, raw	0.6	0.00	5		25	15		28
GUINEA								
Flesh & skin, raw	0.0	0.00						37
Flesh only, raw	0.0	0.00					173	20
PHEASANT								
Flesh & skin, raw	0.0	0.00	46	4.25	900	150		46
Flesh only, raw	0.0	0.00	42	3.76	853	121		25
Breast, meat only, raw	0.0	0.00	5	1.33	409	55		22
Leg, meat only, raw	0.0	0.00	29	1.76	293	44		29
QUAIL								
Flesh & skin, raw	0.0	0.00	52	16.08	874	215		56
Flesh only, raw	0.0	0.00	46	15.42	811	175		31
Breast, meat only	0.0	0.00	20	4.81	542	114		22
SQUAB (pigeon)								
Flesh & skin, raw	0.0	0.00						73
Flesh only, raw	0.0	0.00						47
Breast, meat only, raw	0.0	0.00					136	30
TURKEY, all classes								
Flesh, skin, giblets, & neck, raw	4.3	0.00	841	93.70	14965	3705	4323	44
cooked, roasted	0.1	0.00	68	5.22	707	175	248	41
Flesh & skin, raw	0.0	0.00	49	4.74	885	215	227	45
cooked, roasted	0.0	0.00	63	4.29	673	164	196	42
Flesh only, raw	0.0	0.00	40	4.06	832	195	181	22
cooked, roasted	0.0	0.00	52	3.70	621	147	159	26
Skin only, raw	0.0	0.00	9	0.69	52	19	46	86
cooked, roasted	0.0	0.00	11	0.57	51	17	36	81
Giblets, raw	0.3	0.00	1	1.09	51	14	45	29
cooked, simmered	0.2	0.00	1	0.67	20	6	42	27
Gizzard, raw	0.0	0.00	1	0.27	24	6	11	29
cooked, simmered	0.0	0.00	1	0.22	8	2	9	21
Heart, raw	0.0	0.00	0	0.09	5	2	2	39
cooked, simmered	0.0	0.00	0	0.07	2	1	2	27
Liver, raw	0.2	0.00	1	0.75	21	7	33	25
cooked, simmered	0.1	0.00	1	0.39	10	3	31	34

POULTRY PRODUCTS

FOOD	AMOUNT	CALO-RIES (kcal)	PROTEIN (g)	FAT (g)	MONO-UN-SATURATED FAT (g)	POLY-UN-SATURATED FAT (g)	SATU-RATED FAT (g)
TURKEY, all classes (continued)							
Neck, meat only, raw	12 g	16	2.42	0.65	0.22	0.15	0.20
cooked, simmered	10 g	18	2.68	0.73	0.24	0.16	0.22
Light meat w/skin, raw	180 g	286	38.96	13.25	3.59	5.06	3.12
cooked, roasted	136 g	268	38.85	11.32	3.18	3.86	2.74
Dark meat w/ skin, raw	152 g	243	28.76	13.37	3.92	4.56	3.47
cooked, roasted	104 g	230	28.59	12.00	3.63	3.79	3.22
Light meat w/out skin, raw	150 g	172	35.33	2.35	0.75	0.41	0.62
cooked, roasted	117 g	183	34.99	3.76	1.20	0.66	1.00
Dark meat w/out skin, raw	132 g	165	26.50	5.78	1.94	1.31	1.73
cooked, roasted	91 g	170	26.00	6.57	2.20	1.49	1.97
Back, meat & skin, raw	47 g	92	8.51	6.16	1.72	2.32	1.52
cooked, roasted	34 g	83	9.04	4.89	1.42	1.70	1.26
Breast, meat & skin, raw	146 g	229	31.96	10.26	2.79	3.88	2.42
cooked, roasted	112 g	212	32.16	8.30	2.35	2.75	2.02
Leg, meat & skin, raw	105 g	151	20.51	7.06	2.16	2.16	1.92
cooked, roasted	71 g	147	19.78	6.97	2.17	2.04	1.93
Wing, meat & skin, raw	33 g	65	6.67	4.07	1.08	1.64	0.94
cooked, roasted	24 g	55	6.57	2.98	0.81	1.12	0.71
TURKEY, Fryer-roasters							
Flesh, skin, giblets, & neck, raw	1 turkey	3207	533.77	102.30	29.35	35.35	25.79
cooked, roasted	251 g	429	70.48	14.16	4.12	4.73	3.61
Flesh & skin, raw	310 g	415	69.35	13.18	3.75	4.72	3.30
cooked, roasted	229 g	395	64.72	13.11	3.78	4.50	3.32
Flesh only, raw	272 g	298	60.71	4.29	1.43	0.94	1.26
cooked, roasted	195 g	292	57.63	5.13	1.70	1.10	1.50
Skin only, raw	38 g	108	6.31	8.94	2.33	3.81	2.05
cooked, roasted	34 g	102	7.12	7.92	2.06	3.37	1.81
Light meat w/ skin, raw	159 g	211	36.71	6.05	1.62	2.41	1.41
cooked, roasted	123 g	202	35.38	5.63	1.54	2.09	1.34
Dark meat w/ skin, raw	151 g	195	30.30	7.23	2.16	2.35	1.91
cooked, roasted	106 g	193	29.35	7.48	2.24	2.41	1.99
Light meat w/out skin, raw	136 g	146	32.89	0.67	0.21	0.12	0.18
cooked, roasted	104 g	145	31.39	1.23	0.39	0.21	0.33
Dark meat w/out skin, raw	136 g	152	27.82	3.63	1.22	0.82	0.88
cooked, roasted	91 g	147	26.25	3.92	1.32	0.89	1.18
Back, meat & skin, raw	52 g	78	10.34	3.78	1.10	1.30	0.98
cooked, roasted	37 g	76	9.68	3.79	1.10	1.30	0.98
Back, meat only, raw	43 g	52	8.88	1.51	0.51	0.34	0.45
cooked, roasted	27 g	46	7.56	1.52	0.51	0.35	0.46
Breast, meat & skin, raw	123 g	154	29.22	3.26	0.89	1.23	0.77
cooked, roasted	98 g	150	28.48	3.14	0.86	1.18	0.74
Breast, meat only, raw	111 g	123	27.30	0.72	0.23	0.13	0.19
cooked, roasted	87 g	117	26.15	0.64	0.20	0.11	0.17
Leg, meat & skin, raw	99 g	117	19.93	3.53	1.09	1.07	0.96
cooked, roasted	70 g	119	19.95	3.78	1.17	1.13	1.04

FOOD	CARBO-HYDRATES (mg)	FIBER (mg)	CALCIUM (mg)	IRON (mg)	POTAS-SIUM (mg)	SODIUM (mg)	CHOLES-TEROL (mg)	% OF CALORIES FROM FAT
TURKEY, all classes (continued)								
Neck, meat only, raw	0.0	0.00	4	0.24	36	11	9	37
cooked, simmered	0.0	0.00	4	0.23	15	6	12	37
Light meat w/skin, raw	0.0	0.00	23	2.18	489	106	117	42
cooked, roasted	0.0	0.00	29	1.92	388	85	103	38
Dark meat w/ skin, raw	0.0	0.00	26	2.57	396	108	109	50
cooked, roasted	0.0	0.00	34	2.36	285	79	93	47
Light meat w/out skin, raw	0.0	0.00	18	1.78	458	95	90	12
cooked, roasted	0.0	0.00	23	1.57	356	75	81	18
Dark meat w/out skin, raw	0.0	0.00	22	2.30	377	101	91	32
cooked, roasted	0.0	0.00	29	2.12	264	72	78	35
Back, meat & skin, raw	0.0	0.00	8	0.77	111	31	35	60
cooked, roasted	0.0	0.00	11	0.75	89	25	31	53
Breast, meat & skin, raw	0.0	0.00	19	1.76	401	86	95	40
cooked, roasted	0.0	0.00	24	1.56	323	70	83	35
Leg, meat & skin, raw	0.0	0.00	18	1.81	287	78	74	42
cooked, roasted	0.0	0.00	23	1.63	199	55	61	43
Wing, meat & skin, raw	0.0	0.00	5	0.42	79	18	23	56
cooked, roasted	0.0	0.00	6	0.35	64	15	19	49
TURKEY, Fryer-roasters								
Flesh, skin, giblets, & neck, raw	1.2	0.00	322	42.10	5936	1467	2215	29
cooked, roasted	0.1	0.00	58	5.58	606	163	297	30
Flesh & skin, raw	0.0	0.00	39	4.40	753	179	252	29
cooked, roasted	0.0	0.00	51	4.46	573	151	241	30
Flesh only, raw	0.0	0.00	32	3.91	707	165	199	13
cooked, roasted	0.0	0.00	39	3.82	512	130	192	16
Skin only, raw	0.0	0.00	7	0.49	46	13	53	75
cooked, roasted	0.0	0.00	12	0.63	61	21	49	70
Light meat w/ skin, raw	0.0	0.00	19	1.96	403	79	121	26
cooked, roasted	0.0	0.00	22	1.98	322	70	117	25
Dark meat w/ skin, raw	0.0	0.00	21	2.44	350	100	131	33
cooked, roasted	0.0	0.00	29	2.47	251	81	124	35
Light meat w/out skin, raw	0.0	0.00	14	1.66	375	71	89	4
cooked, roasted	0.0	0.00	15	1.63	288	59	90	8
Dark meat w/out skin, raw	0.0	0.00	18	2.25	332	94	110	21
cooked, roasted	0.0	0.00	24	2.19	224	72	102	24
Back, meat & skin, raw	0.0	0.00	10	0.73	106	31	45	44
cooked, roasted	0.0	0.00	13	0.68	77	26	40	45
Back, meat only, raw	0.0	0.00	8	0.62	96	28	32	26
cooked, roasted	0.0	0.00	10	0.50	59	20	26	30
Breast, meat & skin, raw	0.0	0.00	14	1.46	339	59	86	19
cooked, roasted	0.0	0.00	15	1.53	274	52	88	19
Breast, meat only, raw	0.0	0.00	11	1.30	325	55	69	5
cooked, roasted	0.0	0.00	11	1.33	254	45	73	5
Leg, meat & skin, raw	0.0	0.00	11	1.72	244	69	86	27
cooked, roasted	0.0	0.00	16	1.81	176	56	49	29

POULTRY PRODUCTS

FOOD	AMOUNT	CALO-RIES (kcal)	PROTEIN (g)	FAT (g)	MONO-UN-SATURATED FAT (g)	POLY-UN-SATURATED FAT (g)	SATU-RATED FAT (g)
TURKEY, Fryer-roasters (continued)							
Leg, meat only, raw	93 g	101	18.93	2.21	0.74	0.50	0.66
cooked, roasted	64 g	102	18.68	2.41	0.81	0.55	0.72
Wing, meat & skin, raw	36 g	57	7.50	2.78	0.74	1.11	0.65
cooked, roasted	25 g	52	6.91	2.47	0.68	0.91	0.59
Wing, meat only, raw	26 g	28	5.85	0.29	0.09	0.05	0.08
cooked, roasted	17 g	28	5.24	0.59	0.19	0.10	0.16
TURKEY, Young hens							
Flesh, skin, giblets, & neck, raw	1 turkey	7384	898.13	391.46	110.85	139.41	97.16
cooked, roasted	263 g	565	73.65	27.74	8.15	8.91	7.10
Flesh & skin, raw	327 g	550	66.00	29.73	8.37	10.78	7.35
cooked, roasted	243 g	530	68.25	26.43	7.72	8.61	6.75
Flesh only, raw	276 g	336	60.06	8.78	2.91	1.87	2.55
cooked, roasted	212 g	370	62.01	11.69	3.85	2.42	3.35
Skin only, raw	51 g	213	6.01	20.71	5.40	8.83	4.75
cooked, roasted	31 g	149	5.90	13.78	3.59	5.87	3.16
Light meat w/ skin, raw	175 g	289	37.64	14.17	3.84	5.42	3.34
cooked, roasted	137 g	284	39.24	12.87	3.63	4.31	3.12
Dark meat w/ skin, raw	152 g	262	28.35	15.58	4.54	5.37	3.45
cooked, roasted	106 g	246	29.01	13.55	4.09	4.30	3.63
Light meat w/out skin, raw	147 g	170	34.75	2.44	0.78	0.43	0.65
cooked, roasted	119 g	192	35.57	4.45	1.42	0.78	1.19
Dark meat w/out skin, raw	130 g	169	26.09	6.35	2.13	1.44	1.90
cooked, roasted	93 g	178	26.43	7.24	2.43	1.64	2.17
Back, meat & skin, raw	47 g	103	8.23	7.49	2.07	2.87	1.61
cooked, roasted	35 g	89	9.24	5.48	1.59	1.91	1.40
Breast, meat & skin, raw	139 g	232	30.05	11.54	3.12	4.44	2.71
cooked, roasted	109 g	211	31.39	8.56	2.45	2.73	2.10
Leg, meat & skin, raw	105 g	158	20.43	7.87	2.41	2.41	2.14
cooked, roasted	71 g	151	19.69	7.46	2.33	2.16	2.07
Wing, meat & skin, raw	36 g	76	7.17	4.99	1.33	2.02	1.16
cooked, roasted	28 g	67	7.64	3.77	1.03	1.41	0.89
TURKEY, Young toms							
Flesh, skin, giblets, & neck, raw	1 turkey	12799	1712.56	605.23	171.76	214.26	150.51
cooked, roasted	258 g	514	72.16	22.74	6.66	7.37	5.82
Flesh & skin, raw	338 g	522	69.13	25.12	7.09	9.04	6.22
cooked, roasted	239 g	482	67.14	21.64	6.31	7.13	5.52
Flesh only, raw	286 g	335	62.12	7.72	2.55	1.63	2.24
cooked, roasted	206 g	345	60.47	9.64	3.18	2.01	2.78
Skin only, raw	51 g	188	6.75	17.63	4.60	7.51	4.04
cooked, roasted	32 g	135	6.44	11.92	3.11	5.08	2.73
Light meat w/ skin, raw	185 g	288	40.02	13.02	3.53	4.96	3.07
cooked, roasted	136 g	260	38.74	10.47	2.93	3.62	2.52
Dark meat w/ skin, raw	152 g	232	28.95	11.99	3.53	4.04	3.12
cooked, roasted	103 g	222	28.41	11.17	3.38	3.51	3.00

FOOD	CARBO-HYDRATES (mg)	FIBER (mg)	CALCIUM (mg)	IRON (mg)	POTAS-SIUM (mg)	SODIUM (mg)	CHOLES-TEROL (mg)	% OF CALORIES FROM FAT
TURKEY, Fryer-roasters (continued)								
Leg, meat only, raw	0.0	0.00	10	1.64	236	66	78	20
cooked, roasted	0.0	0.00	14	1.70	165	52	76	21
Wing, meat & skin, raw	0.0	0.00	5	0.50	64	20	35	44
cooked, roasted	0.0	0.00	7	0.45	49	18	29	43
Wing, meat only, raw	0.0	0.00	3	0.37	52	17	21	9
cooked, roasted	0.0	0.00	4	0.30	35	13	17	19
TURKEY, Young hens								
Flesh, skin, giblets, & neck, raw	4.7	0.00	705	84.15	11914	2826	3254	48
cooked, roasted	0.1	0.00	69	5.19	715	166	246	44
Flesh & skin, raw	0.0	0.00	50	5.24	862	201	206	49
cooked, roasted	0.0	0.00	64	4.33	684	156	190	45
Flesh only, raw	0.0	0.00	41	4.47	809	182	165	24
cooked, roasted	0.0	0.00	53	3.72	633	141	155	28
Skin only, raw	0.0	0.00	9	0.78	54	16	42	88
cooked, roasted	0.0	0.00	10	0.56	48	14	33	83
Light meat w/ skin, raw	0.0	0.00	23	2.46	467	96	108	44
cooked, roasted	0.0	0.00	31	1.91	391	80	101	41
Dark meat w/ skin, raw	0.0	0.00	27	2.78	394	102	98	54
cooked, roasted	0.0	0.00	33	2.42	293	76	89	50
Light meat w/out skin, raw	0.0	0.00	18	2.03	439	88	85	13
cooked, roasted	0.0	0.00	25	1.56	361	71	81	21
Dark meat w/out skin, raw	0.0	0.00	23	2.46	373	96	80	34
cooked, roasted	0.0	0.00	28	2.16	272	70	74	37
Back, meat & skin, raw	0.0	0.00	8	0.84	109	28	32	65
cooked, roasted	0.0	0.00	11	0.78	92	24	30	55
Breast, meat & skin, raw	0.0	0.00	19	1.96	370	76	86	45
cooked, roasted	0.0	0.00	24	1.48	315	64	78	37
Leg, meat & skin, raw	0.0	0.00	19	1.96	287	74	66	45
cooked, roasted	0.0	0.00	22	1.63	200	52	58	44
Wing, meat & skin, raw	0.0	0.00	5	0.51	86	18	23	59
cooked, roasted	0.0	0.00	7	0.40	75	16	22	51
TURKEY, Young toms								
Flesh, skin, giblets, & neck, raw	7.0	0.00	1237	126.24	23025	5895	6826	43
cooked, roasted	0.2	0.00	68	5.16	711	185	249	40
Flesh & skin, raw	0.0	0.00	49	4.32	917	231	243	43
cooked, roasted	0.0	0.00	64	4.25	675	173	197	40
Flesh only, raw	0.0	0.00	40	3.71	865	210	194	21
cooked, roasted	0.0	0.00	52	3.67	621	153	159	25
Skin only, raw	0.0	0.00	9	0.61	49	21	49	84
cooked, roasted	0.0	0.00	12	0.56	51	19	37	79
Light meat w/ skin, raw	0.0	0.00	24	1.92	512	116	125	41
cooked, roasted	0.0	0.00	28	1.92	390	91	103	36
Dark meat w/ skin, raw	0.0	0.00	25	2.38	402	114	117	47
cooked, roasted	0.0	0.00	36	2.33	284	82	94	45

POULTRY PRODUCTS

FOOD	AMOUNT	CALO-RIES (kcal)	PROTEIN (g)	FAT (g)	MONO-UN-SATURATED FAT (g)	POLY-UN-SATURATED FAT (g)	SATU-RATED FAT (g)
TURKEY, Young toms (continued)							
Light meat w/out skin, raw	154 g	176	36.08	2.42	0.77	0.42	0.64
cooked, roasted	117 g	180	34.96	3.41	1.09	0.60	0.91
Dark meat w/out skin, raw	133 g	163	26.66	5.47	1.83	1.24	1.64
cooked, roasted	90 g	167	25.81	6.28	2.11	1.43	1.88
Back, meat & skin, raw	45 g	81	8.31	5.01	1.41	1.85	1.25
cooked, roasted	33 g	78	8.84	4.51	1.31	1.56	1.16
Breast, meat & skin, raw	155 g	234	34.03	9.82	2.68	3.66	2.33
cooked, roasted	115 g	217	32.90	8.50	2.39	2.89	2.06
Leg, meat & skin, raw	107 g	150	20.91	6.78	2.07	2.08	1.84
cooked, roasted	70 g	144	19.55	6.74	2.09	1.98	1.86
Wing, meat & skin, raw	30 g	57	6.13	3.36	0.90	1.35	0.78
cooked, roasted	21 g	46	5.76	2.42	0.66	0.91	0.57
TURKEY ENTREES							
A la king							
Budget Gourmet® w/rice	284 g	390	20.00	18.00	3.89	7.84	6.27
Legout®	1 oz	30	16.70	1.50			
& gravy, frozen	240 g	160	14.10	6.30	2.04	2.33	1.13
Healthy Choice® gravy/dressing	284 g	270	27.00	4.00	2.00		1.00
Breast							
Healthy Choice®	298 g	260	21.00	3.00	2.00		1.00
roasted, w/gravy & mushrooms	241 g	200	18.00	3.00	1.00		1.00
Le Menu® frozen dinner	319 g	470	27.00	24.00			
w/gravy, sliced	28.4 g	29	2.10	0.67	0.14	0.29	0.23
Lean Cuisine® w/mushroom	227 g	240	23.00	7.00	1.44	4.83	0.72
Breast chub, barbecue, Mr.	28.35 g	29	6.19	0.50			
Turkey®							
Curry sauce, Right Course®	248 g	320	23.00	8.00	2.00		1.00
Dijon, Lean Cuisine®	269 g	270	24.00	10.00	3.00		1.00
Dinner plate, w/potatoes & peas	28.4 g	32	2.38	0.85	3.60		7.37
Dinner, Swanson® frozen dinner	326 g	340	20.00	10.00	2.54	4.23	3.23
w/dressing & potato, homestyle	28.4 g	32	2.00	1.22	0.34	0.46	0.42
Divan, Le Menu® light	284 g	280	22.00	9.00	4.00		1.00
Glazed							
Budget Gourmet® light	255 g	270	16.00	5.00	1.63	1.98	1.40
Le Menu® light	234 g	260	18.00	6.00	0.62	4.13	1.25
Ground							
Mr. Turkey®	28.35 g	42	5.09	2.50	0.80	0.90	0.70
Louis Rich® pure ground	28.35 g	60	6.99	3.99	0.80	0.90	0.70
Medallions							
Healthy Choice® w/vegetables	354 g	350	29.00	6.00	3.00		2.00
Ultra Slim Fast® w/herbs	340 g	320	28.00	5.00	2.00		2.00
Pot pie							
frozen, unheated, commercial	240 g	473	13.90	25.00			
baked/home prepared	240 g	569	25.00	32.40			
Stouffer® frozen dinner	284 g	460	20.00	26.00			
Swanson®	28.4 g	54	1.57	3.00	1.05	1.27	0.67
Swanson Hungry Man®	28.4 g	41	1.50	2.25	0.79	0.96	0.50

FOOD	CARBO-HYDRATES (mg)	FIBER (mg)	CALCIUM (mg)	IRON (mg)	POTAS-SIUM (mg)	SODIUM (mg)	CHOLES-TEROL (mg)	% OF CALORIES FROM FAT
TURKEY, Young toms (continued)								
Light meat w/out skin, raw	0.0	0.00	18	1.56	483	104	95	12
cooked, roasted	0.0	0.00	21	1.59	360	80	81	17
Dark meat w/out skin, raw	0.0	0.00	22	2.16	385	107	99	30
cooked, roasted	0.0	0.00	31	2.10	264	74	79	34
Back, meat & skin, raw	0.0	0.00	8	0.69	110	32	36	56
cooked, roasted	0.0	0.00	12	0.73	87	26	31	52
Breast, meat & skin, raw	0.0	0.00	20	1.61	437	98	103	38
cooked, roasted	0.0	0.00	24	1.62	332	77	87	35
Leg, meat & skin, raw	0.0	0.00	18	1.70	295	83	81	41
cooked, roasted	0.0	0.00	24	1.60	197	56	63	42
Wing, meat & skin, raw	0.0	0.00	4	0.32	75	18	22	53
cooked, roasted	0.0	0.00	5	0.31	57	14	17	47
TURKEY ENTREES								
A la king								
Budget Gourmet®w/rice	36.0	2.41	150	1.08	451	740	75	42
Legout®	1.3	1.67		3.33	1	63	183	45
& gravy, frozen	11.1	2.70	33	2.22	146	1328	43	35
Healthy Choice®gravy/dressing	30.0		60	1.80	590	530	50	13
Breast								
Healthy Choice®	41.0		40	1.80	560	560	40	10
roasted, w/gravy & mushrooms	26.0		20	1.44	260	380	40	14
Le Menu®frozen dinner	36.0					1165		46
w/gravy, sliced	3.6	0.24	3.81	0.14	45	97	5	21
Lean Cuisine®w/mushroom	20.0	1.93	20	0.72	350	790	50	26
Breast chub, barbecue, Mr. Turkey®	0.1	0.00				208	5	16
Curry sauce, Right Course®	40.0		100	1.44	550	570	50	23
Dijon, Lean Cuisine®	22.0		150	1.08	470	900	60	33
Dinner plate, w/potatoes & peas	0.3	###	113	9.07				24
Dinner, Swanson®frozen dinner	42.0	3.60	83.5	2.67	635	1295	74	26
w/dressing & potato, homestyle	3.3	0.19	4.44	0.20	47	112	4	34
Divan, Le Menu®light	26.0				499	840	40	29
Glazed								
Budget Gourmet®light	39.0	0.00	53.9	3.58	190	760	40	17
Le Menu®light	34.0	0.00	49.5	3.28	663	720	35	21
Ground								
Mr. Turkey®	0.0	0.00	7.41	0.51	79	26	21	54
Louis Rich®pure ground	0.0	0.00	7.41	0.51	79	35	23	60
Medallions								
Healthy Choice®w/vegetables	45.0		150	2.70	450	480	60	15
Ultra Slim Fast®w/herbs	40.0				380	830	50	14
Pot pie								
frozen, unheated, commercial	48.2	2.65	28.8	2.16	274	886	22	48
baked/home prepared	44.4	2.77	64.8	3.36	475	655	74	51
Stouffer®frozen dinner	35.0				270	1735		51
Swanson®	5.1	0.33	2.86	0.26	43	103	8	50
Swanson Hungry Man®	3.5	0.33	3.75	0.23	43	92	8	50

POULTRY PRODUCTS

FOOD	AMOUNT	CALO-RIES (kcal)	PROTEIN (g)	FAT (g)	MONO-UN-SATURATED FAT (g)	POLY-UN-SATURATED FAT (g)	SATU-RATED FAT (g)
TURKEY ENTREES (continued)							
Roasted, light & dark meat, frozen	100 g	155	21.30	5.78	1.93	2.17	1.68
Sliced							
Le Menu®light	28.4 g	21	2.10	0.50	0.16	0.20	0.14
Light & Elegant®	227 g	230	20.00	5.00			
Stuffed, Light & Healthy®	312 g	230	22.00	6.00	2.00	1.15	2.00
Tetrazzini							
Healthy Choice®	357 g	340	23.00	6.00	3.00		2.00
Stouffer®frozen dinner	170 g	240	12.00	14.00			
Traditional, Le Menu®light	234 g	200	19.00	5.00	0.52	3.44	1.04
Vegetables, homestyle, Healthy Choice®	269 g	230	24.00	3.00	1.00		1.00
White, canned, Swanson®	28.35 g	32	6.79	0.40	0.13	0.15	0.12
POULTRY FOOD PRODUCTS (For more poultry food products, also see section on luncheon meats)							
Chicken, canned, boned, w/broth	5-oz can	234	30.91	11.29	3.12	4.47	2.48
Gravy & turkey, frozen	5-oz pkg	95	8.35	3.73	1.21	1.38	0.67
Turkey, canned, boned, w/broth	5-oz can	231	33.62	9.74	2.84	3.21	2.49
Turkey, diced, light & dark, seasoned	$\frac{1}{2}$ lb	313	42.41	13.61	3.97	4.48	3.47
Turkey loaf, breast meat	2 slices	47	9.56	0.67	0.21	0.19	0.12
Turkey patties, breaded, battered, fried	1 patty	181	8.96	11.52			
Turkey, pre-basted products							
breast, meat & skin, cooked, roasted	1 breast	2175	382.94	59.81	16.93	19.73	14.55
thigh, meat & skin, cooked, roasted	1 thigh	494	59.03	26.82	8.31	7.93	7.38
Turkey roasts, boneless, frozen, seasoned – light & dark meat							
raw	$\frac{1}{4}$ box	340	49.98	6.25			
cooked, roasted	$\frac{1}{4}$ box	304	41.78	11.33			
Turkey sticks, breaded, battered, fried	1 stick	178	9.09	10.82			

FOOD	CARBO-HYDRATES (mg)	FIBER (mg)	CALCIUM (mg)	IRON (mg)	POTAS-SIUM (mg)	SODIUM (mg)	CHOLES-TEROL (mg)	% OF CALORIES FROM FAT
TURKEY ENTREES (continued)								
Roasted, light & dark meat, frozen	3.0	0.00	5	1.63	298	680	53	34
Sliced								
Le Menu® light	2.1	0.00	6	0.11	81	54	3	21
Light & Elegant®	25.0		18	1.00	280	1020		20
Stuffed, Light & Healthy®	29.0	8.00	116	1.44	560	520	40	23
Tetrazzini								
Healthy Choice®	49.0		100	1.80	510	490	40	16
Stouffer® frozen dinner	17.0		72	0.60	200	620		53
Traditional, Le Menu® light	19.0	0.00	49.5	3.28	663	610	25	23
Vegetables, homestyle, Healthy Choice®	28.0		60	1.44	160	470	35	12
White, canned, Swanson®	0.4	0.00	0	0.14	63	104	19	11
POULTRY FOOD PRODUCTS (For more poultry food products, also see section on luncheon meats)								
Chicken, canned, boned, w/broth	0.0	0.00	20	2.25	196	714		43
Gravy & turkey, frozen	6.5	0.42	20	1.31		786		35
Turkey, canned, boned, w/broth	0.0	0.00	17	2.64		663		38
Turkey, diced, light & dark, seasoned	2.2		2	4.08	703	1928		39
Turkey loaf, breast meat	0.0	0.00	3	0.17	118	608	17	13
Turkey patties, breaded, battered, fried	10.0		9	1.41	176	512		57
Turkey, pre-basted products								
breast, meat & skin, cooked, roasted	0.0	0.00	149	11.42	4281	6868	718	25
thigh, meat & skin, cooked, roasted	0.0	0.00	25	4.74	758	1371	194	49
Turkey roasts, boneless, frozen, seasoned – light & dark meat								
raw	18.1		3	5.96	1022	1926		17
cooked, roasted	6.0		10	3.19	584	1334	103	34
Turkey sticks, breaded, battered, fried	10.8		9	1.41	166	536		55

BEEF PRODUCTS

FOOD	AMOUNT	CALO-RIES (kcal)	PROTEIN (g)	FAT (g)	SATU-RATED FAT (g)	MONO-UN-SATURATED FAT (g)	POLY-UN-SATURATED FAT (g)
Carcass, lean & fat, choice raw	1 lb	1320	78.58	109.10	47.48	4.18	44.22
Carcass, lean & fat, select raw	1 lb	1261	79.31	102.30	44.56	3.92	41.56
Composite of trimmed retail cuts, separable lean & fat, all grades							
raw, trimmed to ¼" fat	1 lb	1140	82.74	87.26	37.78	3.22	35.37
cooked, trimmed to ¼" fat	3 oz	259	22.05	18.31	7.84	0.67	7.26
cooked, trimmed to 0" fat	3 oz	232	23.23	14.76	6.30	0.53	5.82
Composite of trimmed retail cuts, separable lean & fat, choice							
raw, trimmed to ¼" fat	1 lb	1177	82.40	91.45	39.57	3.37	37.01
cooked, trimmed to ¼" fat	3 oz	274	21.66	20.08	8.60	0.73	7.97
cooked, trimmed to 0" fat	3 oz	241	23.13	15.75	6.72	0.57	6.21
raw, trimmed to 0" fat	1 lb	1070	83.77	79.00	34.22	2.91	32.06
Composite of trimmed retail cuts, separable lean & fat, select							
cooked, trimmed to ¼" fat	3 oz	247	22.24	16.90	7.22	0.61	6.70
cooked, trimmed to 0" fat	3 oz	222	23.35	13.53	5.76	0.49	5.33
Composite of trimmed retail cuts, separable lean & fat, prime							
raw, trimmed to ¼" fat	1 lb	1307	82.91	105.68	45.94	3.95	43.36
cooked, trimmed to ¼" fat	3 oz	273	21.77	20.01	8.57	0.73	8.07
Composite of trimmed retail cuts, separable lean only, all grades							
raw, trimmed to ¼" fat	1 lb	655	94.25	27.96	11.82	1.09	10.51
cooked, trimmed to ¼" fat	3 oz	183	25.14	8.42	3.54	0.29	3.22
cooked, trimmed to 0" fat	3 oz	180	25.40	7.89	3.31	0.27	3.01
Composite of trimmed retail cuts, separable lean only, choice							
raw, trimmed to ¼" fat	1 lb	682	94.27	30.96	13.08	1.20	11.63
cooked, trimmed to ¼" fat	3 oz	189	25.14	9.06	3.81	0.31	3.46
cooked, trimmed to 0" fat	3 oz	180	25.40	7.89	3.31	0.27	3.01
Composite of trimmed retail cuts, separable lean only, select							
raw, trimmed to ¼" fat	1 lb	639	93.76	26.51	11.25	1.02	10.09
cooked, trimmed to ¼" fat	3 oz	175	25.15	7.44	3.13	0.25	2.85
cooked, trimmed to 0" fat	3 oz	170	25.41	6.87	2.89	0.23	2.63
Composite of trimmed retail cuts, separable lean only, prime							
raw, trimmed to ¼" fat	1 lb	806	95.98	43.93	18.93	1.76	17.55
cooked, trimmed to ¼" fat	3 oz	205	24.69	11.04	4.68	0.39	4.42
Retail cuts, separable fat, raw	4 oz	762	9.28	80.11	34.96	2.89	33.28
cooked	3 oz	578	9.05	59.78	25.88	2.26	24.23
Brisket, whole, separable lean & fat, all grades							
raw, trimmed to ¼" fat	1 lb	1414	76.86	120.39	53.31	4.23	48.51
cooked, braised, trimmed to ¼" fat	3 oz	327	19.98	26.82	11.82	0.96	10.5
cooked, braised, trimmed to 0" fat	3 oz	247	22.77	16.60	7.38	0.57	6.40
Brisket, whole, separable lean only, all grades							
cooked, braised, trimmed to ¼" fat	3 oz	206	25.29	10.85	4.99	0.33	3.8

FOOD	CARBO-HYDRATES (mg)	FIBER (mg)	CALCIUM (mg)	IRON (mg)	POTAS-SIUM (mg)	SODIUM (mg)	CHOLES-TEROL (mg)	% OF CALORIES FROM FAT
Carcass, lean & fat, choice raw	0.0	0.00	36	8.30	1212	267	337	74
Carcass, lean & fat, select raw	0.0	0.00	34	8.38	1230	267	334	73
Composite of trimmed retail cuts, separable lean & fat, all grades								
raw, trimmed to 1/4" fat	0.0	0.00	32	8.41	1349	256	306	69
cooked, trimmed to 1/4" fat	0.0	0.00	8	2.23	266	52	75	64
cooked, trimmed to 0" fat	0.0	0.00	8	2.32	275	53	74	57
Composite of trimmed retail cuts, separable lean & fat, choice								
raw, trimmed to 1/4" fat	0.0	0.00	32	8.37	1342	255	307	70
cooked, trimmed to 1/4" fat	0.0	0.00	8	2.18	260	52	75	66
cooked, trimmed to 0" fat	0.0	0.00	8	2.31	274	53	74	59
raw, trimmed to 0" fat	0.0	0.00	32	8.52	1373	259	303	66
Composite of trimmed retail cuts, separable lean & fat, select								
cooked, trimmed to 1/4" fat	0.0	0.00	8	2.25	268	53	73	62
cooked, trimmed to 0" fat	0.0	0.00	8	2.34	276	53	73	55
Composite of trimmed retail cuts, separable lean & fat, prime								
raw, trimmed to 1/4" fat	0.0	0.00	30	8.11	1349	239	307	73
cooked, trimmed to 1/4" fat	0.0	0.00	8	2.08	295	53	71	66
Composite of trimmed retail cuts, separable lean only, all grades								
raw, trimmed to 1/4" fat	0.0	0.00	29	9.68	1615	288	270	38
cooked, trimmed to 1/4" fat	0.0	0.00	7	2.54	306	57	73	41
cooked, trimmed to 0" fat	0.0	0.00	7	2.54	301	56	73	39
Composite of trimmed retail cuts, separable lean only, choice								
raw, trimmed to 1/4" fat	0.0	0.00	29	9.68	1616	288	270	41
cooked, trimmed to 1/4" fat	0.0	0.00	7	2.54	306	57	73	43
cooked, trimmed to 0" fat	0.0	0.00	7	2.54	301	56	73	39
Composite of trimmed retail cuts, separable lean only, select								
raw, trimmed to 1/4" fat	0.0	0.00	29	9.64	1604	287	271	37
cooked, trimmed to 1/4" fat	0.0	0.00	7	2.54	305	57	73	38
cooked, trimmed to 0" fat	0.0	0.00	7	2.54	301	56	73	36
Composite of trimmed retail cuts, separable lean only, prime								
raw, trimmed to 1/4" fat	0.0	0.00	26	9.45	1649	270	267	49
cooked, trimmed to 1/4" fat	0.0	0.00	7	2.41	338	57	69	48
Retail cuts, separable fat, raw	0.0	0.00	11	0.85	75	33	112	95
cooked	0.0	0.00	12	0.90	101	35	81	93
Brisket, whole, separable lean & fat, all grades								
raw, trimmed to 1/4" fat	0.0	0.00	30	7.11	1136	289	330	77
cooked, braised, trimmed to 1/4" fat	0.0	0.00	7	1.91	196	52	80	74
cooked, braised, trimmed to 0" fat	0.0	0.00	6	2.15	220	55	79	60
Brisket, whole, separable lean only, all grades								
cooked, braised, trimmed to 1/4" fat	0.0	0.00	5	2.39	242	60	79	47

BEEF PRODUCTS

FOOD	AMOUNT	CALO-RIES (kcal)	PROTEIN (g)	FAT (g)	SATU-RATED FAT (g)	MONO-UN-SATURATED FAT (g)	POLY-UN-SATURATED FAT (g)
Brisket, whole (continued)							
cooked, braised, trimmed to 0" fat	3 oz	185	25.29	8.56	3.96	0.25	3.09
Brisket, flat half, separable lean & fat, all grades							
raw, trimmed to $\frac{1}{4}$" fat	4 oz	327	20.20	26.74	11.68	0.97	10.62
cooked, braised, trimmed to $\frac{1}{4}$" fat	3 oz	309	21.29	24.22	10.56	0.92	9.37
cooked, braised, trimmed to 0" fat	3 oz	183	25.90	8.00	3.53	0.30	2.85
Brisket, flat half, separable lean only, all grades							
cooked, braised, trimmed to $\frac{1}{4}$" fat	3 oz	189	26.79	8.24	3.68	0.31	2.70
cooked, braised, trimmed to 0" fat	3 oz	162	26.79	5.27	2.35	0.20	1.72
Brisket, point half, separable lean & fat, all grades							
raw, trimmed to $\frac{1}{4}$" fat	1 lb	1502	73.11	131.95	59.02	4.52	53.71
cooked, braised, trimmed to $\frac{1}{4}$" fat	3 oz	343	18.81	29.13	12.93	1.00	11.54
cooked, braised, trimmed to 0" fat	3 oz	304	20.00	24.22	10.80	0.81	9.56
Brisket, point half, separable lean only, all grades							
cooked, braised, trimmed to $\frac{1}{4}$" fat	3 oz	222	23.84	13.34	6.25	0.34	5.01
cooked, braised, trimmed to 0" fat	3 oz	208	23.84	11.73	5.50	0.30	4.40
Chuck, arm pot roast, separable lean & fat, all grades							
raw, trimmed to $\frac{1}{4}$" fat	1 lb	1110	84.02	83.29	35.42	3.23	33.75
cooked, braised, trimmed to $\frac{1}{4}$" fat	3 oz	282	23.31	20.24	8.68	0.77	7.98
cooked, braised, trimmed to 0" fat	3 oz	238	25.21	14.46	6.18	0.55	5.63
Chuck, arm pot roast, separable lean & fat, choice							
raw, trimmed to $\frac{1}{4}$" fat	1 lb	1157	83.42	88.79	37.69	3.47	35.91
cooked, braised, trimmed to $\frac{1}{4}$" fat	3 oz	296	22.93	21.91	9.40	0.84	8.63
cooked, braised, trimmed to 0" fat	3 oz	249	25.02	15.78	6.74	0.60	6.13
Chuck, arm pot roast, separable lean & fat, select							
raw, trimmed to $\frac{1}{4}$" fat	1 lb	1059	84.61	77.37	33.00	2.98	31.44
cooked, braised, trimmed to $\frac{1}{4}$" fat	3 oz	268	23.69	18.46	7.92	0.70	7.28
cooked, braised, trimmed to 0" fat	3 oz	221	25.59	12.43	5.31	0.48	4.84
Chuck, arm pot roast, separable lean only, all grades							
cooked, braised, trimmed to $\frac{1}{4}$" fat	3 oz	183	28.07	7.05	2.95	0.28	2.56
cooked, braised, trimmed to 0" fat	3 oz	178	28.07	6.46	2.70	0.25	2.34
Chuck, arm pot roast, separable lean only, choice							
cooked, braised, trimmed to $\frac{1}{4}$" fat	3 oz	191	28.07	7.90	3.30	0.31	2.87
cooked, braised, trimmed to 0" fat	3 oz	187	28.07	7.39	3.09	0.29	2.68
Chuck, arm pot roast, separable lean only, select							
cooked, braised, trimmed to $\frac{1}{4}$" fat	3 oz	175	28.07	6.12	2.56	0.24	2.22
cooked, braised, trimmed to 0" fat	3 oz	168	28.07	5.35	2.24	0.21	1.94
Chuck, blade roast, separable lean & fat, all grades							
raw, trimmed to $\frac{1}{4}$" fat	1 lb	1152	77.30	91.16	40.00	3.33	36.81

FOOD	CARBO-HYDRATES (mg)	FIBER (mg)	CALCIUM (mg)	IRON (mg)	POTAS-SIUM (mg)	SODIUM (mg)	CHOLES-TEROL (mg)	% OF CALORIES FROM FAT
Brisket, whole (continued)								
cooked, braised, trimmed to 0" fat	0.0	0.00	5	2.39	242	60	79	42
Brisket, flat half, separable lean & fat, all grades								
raw, trimmed to $\frac{1}{4}$" fat	0.0	0.00	7	1.80	307	70	79	74
cooked, braised, trimmed to $\frac{1}{4}$" fat	0.0	0.00	7	1.94	206	48	81	71
cooked, braised, trimmed to 0" fat	0.0	0.00	5	2.34	246	53	81	39
Brisket, flat half, separable lean only, all grades								
cooked, braised, trimmed to $\frac{1}{4}$" fat	0.0	0.00	4	2.41	253	54	81	39
cooked, braised, trimmed to 0" fat	0.0	0.00	4	2.41	253	54	81	29
Brisket, point half, separable lean & fat, all grades								
raw, trimmed to $\frac{1}{4}$" fat	0.0	0.00	30	6.99	1050	296	343	79
cooked, braised, trimmed to $\frac{1}{4}$" fat	0.0	0.00	7	1.87	188	55	79	76
cooked, braised, trimmed to 0" fat	0.0	0.00	7	1.99	198	57	78	72
Brisket, point half, separable lean only, all grades								
cooked, braised, trimmed to $\frac{1}{4}$" fat	0.0	0.00	5	2.37	232	65	77	54
cooked, braised, trimmed to 0" fat	0.0	0.00	5	2.37	232	65	77	51
Chuck, arm pot roast, separable lean & fat, all grades								
raw, trimmed to $\frac{1}{4}$" fat	0.0	0.00	31	9.57	1396	268	309	68
cooked, braised, trimmed to $\frac{1}{4}$" fat	0.0	0.00	9	2.64	210	51	85	65
cooked, braised, trimmed to 0" fat	0.0	0.00	8	2.87	224	53	85	55
Chuck, arm pot roast, separable lean & fat, choice								
raw, trimmed to $\frac{1}{4}$" fat	0.0	0.00	31	9.49	1382	266	311	69
cooked, braised, trimmed to $\frac{1}{4}$" fat	0.0	0.00	9	2.59	207	50	84	67
cooked, braised, trimmed to 0" fat	0.0	0.00	8	2.85	223	53	85	57
Chuck, arm pot roast, separable lean & fat, select								
raw, trimmed to $\frac{1}{4}$" fat	0.0	0.00	31	9.64	1410	269	308	66
cooked, braised, trimmed to $\frac{1}{4}$" fat	0.0	0.00	9	2.69	212	51	85	62
cooked, braised, trimmed to 0" fat	0.0	0.00	8	2.92	227	53	85	51
Chuck, arm pot roast, separable lean only, all grades								
cooked, braised, trimmed to $\frac{1}{4}$" fat	0.0	0.00	8	3.22	246	56	86	35
cooked, braised, trimmed to 0" fat	0.0	0.00	8	3.22	246	56	86	33
Chuck, arm pot roast, separable lean only, choice								
cooked, braised, trimmed to $\frac{1}{4}$" fat	0.0	0.00	8	3.22	246	56	86	37
cooked, braised, trimmed to 0" fat	0.0	0.00	8	3.22	246	56	86	36
Chuck, arm pot roast, separable lean only, select								
cooked, braised, trimmed to $\frac{1}{4}$" fat	0.0	0.00	8	3.22	246	56	86	31
cooked, braised, trimmed to 0" fat	0.0	0.00	8	3.22	246	56	86	29
Chuck, blade roast, separable lean & fat, all grades								
raw, trimmed to $\frac{1}{4}$" fat	0.0	0.00	45	9.17	1217	306	326	71

FOOD	AMOUNT	CALO-RIES (kcal)	PROTEIN (g)	FAT (g)	SATU-RATED FAT (g)	MONO-UN-SATURATED FAT (g)	POLY-UN-SATURATED FAT (g)
Chuck, blade roast (continued)							
cooked, braised, trimmed to ¼" fat	3 oz	293	22.59	21.84	9.44	0.78	8.70
cooked, braised, trimmed to 0" fat	3 oz	284	23.11	20.52	8.86	0.73	8.15
Chuck, blade roast, separable lean & fat, choice							
raw, trimmed to ¼" fat	1 lb	1235	76.30	100.82	44.23	3.68	40.69
cooked, braised, trimmed to ¼" fat	3 oz	308	22.24	23.65	10.22	0.85	9.42
cooked, braised, trimmed to 0" fat	3 oz	296	22.93	21.95	9.49	0.78	8.72
Chuck, blade roast, separable lean & fat, select							
raw, trimmed to ¼" fat	1 lb	1068	78.31	81.31	35.67	2.97	32.85
cooked, braised, trimmed to ¼" fat	3 oz	277	22.93	19.84	8.58	0.71	7.90
cooked, braised, trimmed to 0" fat	3 oz	266	23.45	18.42	7.96	0.65	7.32
Chuck, blade roast, separable lean only, all grades							
cooked, braised, trimmed to ¼" fat	3 oz	213	26.40	11.13	4.80	0.36	4.32
cooked, braised, trimmed to 0" fat	3 oz	215	26.40	11.30	4.87	0.37	4.38
Chuck, blade roast, separable lean only, choice							
cooked, braised, trimmed to ¼" fat	3 oz	223	26.40	12.24	5.28	0.40	4.75
cooked, braised, trimmed to 0" fat	3 oz	225	26.40	12.49	5.39	0.41	4.85
Chuck, blade roast, separable lean only, select							
cooked, braised, trimmed to ¼" fat	3 oz	202	26.40	9.86	4.25	0.32	3.82
cooked, braised, trimmed to 0" fat	3 oz	202	26.40	9.94	4.29	0.33	3.86
Flank, trimmed to 0" fat, choice							
raw, separable lean & fat	4 oz	203	22.26	12.00	4.96	0.46	5.10
cooked, braised, lean & fat	3 oz	224	22.93	13.97	5.90	0.45	5.88
cooked, broiled, lean & fat	3 oz	192	22.45	10.65	4.36	0.42	4.52
cooked, braised, lean only	3 oz	201	23.82	11.05	4.63	0.33	4.71
cooked, broiled, lean only	3 oz	176	23.01	8.60	3.46	0.34	3.70
Rib, whole (ribs 6-12), trimmed to ¼" fat, all grades							
raw, separable lean & fat	1 lb	1421	74.23	122.40	52.74	4.41	50.47
cooked, broiled, lean & fat	3 oz	291	18.90	23.32	9.93	0.85	9.46
cooked, roasted, lean & fat	3 oz	304	19.12	24.66	10.60	0.88	9.94
cooked, broiled, lean only	3 oz	189	22.39	10.39	4.27	0.35	4.22
cooked, roasted, lean only	3 oz	195	23.16	10.62	4.49	0.32	4.23
Rib, whole (ribs 6-12), trimmed to ¼" fat, choice							
raw, separable lean & fat	1 lb	1513	72.86	133.22	57.41	4.80	54.92
cooked, broiled, lean & fat	3 oz	306	18.68	25.10	10.68	0.92	10.18
cooked, roasted, lean & fat	3 oz	320	18.84	26.54	11.41	0.94	10.71
cooked, broiled, lean only	3 oz	201	22.39	11.74	4.83	0.40	4.72
cooked, roasted, lean only	3 oz	206	23.16	11.92	5.05	0.36	4.76
Rib, whole (ribs 6-12), trimmed to ¼" fat, select							
raw, separable lean & fat	1 lb	1346	75.08	113.68	49.03	4.10	46.96
cooked, broiled, lean & fat	3 oz	274	19.12	21.37	9.09	0.78	8.6
cooked, roasted, lean & fat	3 oz	286	19.43	22.50	9.67	0.80	9.0

FOOD	CARBO-HYDRATES (mg)	FIBER (mg)	CALCIUM (mg)	IRON (mg)	POTAS-SIUM (mg)	SODIUM (mg)	CHOLES-TEROL (mg)	% OF CALORIES FROM FAT
Chuck, blade roast (continued)								
cooked, braised, trimmed to ¼" fat	0.0	0.00	11	2.64	197	55	88	67
cooked, braised, trimmed to 0" fat	0.0	0.00	11	2.70	200	56	88	65
Chuck, blade roast, separable lean & fat, choice								
raw, trimmed to ¼" fat	0.0	0.00	45	9.03	1195	301	329	73
cooked, braised, trimmed to ¼" fat	0.0	0.00	11	2.59	194	54	88	69
cooked, braised, trimmed to 0" fat	0.0	0.00	11	2.68	199	55	88	67
Chuck, blade roast, separable lean & fat, select								
raw, trimmed to ¼" fat	0.0	0.00	45	9.32	1240	310	323	69
cooked, braised, trimmed to ¼" fat	0.0	0.00	11	2.68	199	55	88	64
cooked, braised, trimmed to 0" fat	0.0	0.00	11	2.75	203	56	89	62
Chuck, blade roast, separable lean only, all grades								
cooked, braised, trimmed to ¼" fat	0.0	0.00	11	3.13	224	60	90	47
cooked, braised, trimmed to 0" fat	0.0	0.00	11	3.13	224	60	90	47
Chuck, blade roast, separable lean only, choice								
cooked, braised, trimmed to ¼" fat	0.0	0.00	11	3.13	224	60	90	49
cooked, braised, trimmed to 0" fat	0.0	0.00	11	3.13	224	60	90	50
Chuck, blade roast, separable lean only, select								
cooked, braised, trimmed to ¼" fat	0.0	0.00	11	3.13	224	60	90	44
cooked, braised, trimmed to 0" fat	0.0	0.00	11	3.13	224	60	90	44
Flank, trimmed to 0" fat, choice								
raw, separable lean & fat	0.0	0.00	6	2.22	396	80	59	53
cooked, braised, lean & fat	0.0	0.00	6	2.83	287	60	62	56
cooked, broiled, lean & fat	0.0	0.00	6	2.13	342	69	58	50
cooked, braised, lean only	0.0	0.00	5	2.95	298	61	60	49
cooked, broiled, lean only	0.0	0.00	6	2.19	352	70	57	44
Rib, whole (ribs 6-12), trimmed to ¼" fat, all grades								
raw, separable lean & fat	0.0	0.00	40	7.82	1215	245	322	78
cooked, broiled, lean & fat	0.0	0.00	10	1.85	265	53	70	72
cooked, roasted, lean & fat	0.0	0.00	9	1.99	256	54	72	73
cooked, broiled, lean only	0.0	0.00	9	2.18	324	60	66	49
cooked, roasted, lean only	0.0	0.00	8	2.43	318	61	68	49
Rib, whole (ribs 6-12), trimmed to ¼" fat, choice								
raw, separable lean & fat	0.0	0.00	40	7.66	1182	241	326	79
cooked, broiled, lean & fat	0.0	0.00	10	1.83	262	53	70	74
cooked, roasted, lean & fat	0.0	0.00	9	1.96	252	53	72	75
cooked, broiled, lean only	0.0	0.00	9	2.18	324	60	66	53
cooked, roasted, lean only	0.0	0.00	8	2.43	318	61	68	52
Rib, whole (ribs 6-12), trimmed to ¼" fat, select								
raw, separable lean & fat	0.0	0.00	39	7.92	1236	248	319	76
cooked, broiled, lean & fat	0.0	0.00	10	1.87	269	54	69	70
cooked, roasted, lean & fat	0.0	0.00	9	2.02	260	54	71	71

BEEF PRODUCTS

FOOD	AMOUNT	CALO-RIES (kcal)	PROTEIN (g)	FAT (g)	SATU-RATED FAT (g)	MONO-UN-SATURATED FAT (g)	POLY-UN-SATURATED FAT (g)
Rib, whole (continued)							
cooked, broiled, lean only	3 oz	175	22.38	8.86	3.61	0.30	3.60
cooked, roasted, lean only	3 oz	181	23.16	9.12	3.85	0.28	3.62
Rib, whole (ribs 6-12), trimmed to $\frac{1}{4}$" fat, prime							
raw, separable lean & fat	1 lb	1653	72.15	149.07	64.84	5.43	62.24
cooked, broiled, lean & fat	3 oz	333	18.46	28.18	12.30	0.98	11.67
cooked, roasted, lean & fat	3 oz	348	18.88	29.60	12.90	1.03	12.25
cooked, broiled, lean only	3 oz	238	22.12	15.89	7.01	0.48	6.78
cooked, roasted, lean only	3 oz	248	23.13	16.54	7.28	0.50	7.06
Rib, eye, small end (ribs 10-12), trimmed to 0" fat, choice							
raw, separable lean & fat	1 lb	1242	79.42	100.11	43.46	3.50	40.81
cooked, broiled, lean & fat	3 oz	261	21.17	18.92	8.10	0.64	7.66
cooked, broiled, lean only	3 oz	191	23.83	9.94	4.20	0.28	4.02
Rib, large end (ribs 6-9), separable lean & fat, all grades							
raw, trimmed to $\frac{1}{4}$" fat	1 lb	1465	72.99	127.85	54.81	4.66	52.89
cooked, broiled, trimmed to $\frac{1}{4}$" fat	3 oz	295	18.06	24.16	10.24	0.91	9.82
cooked, roasted, trimmed to $\frac{1}{4}$" fat	3 oz	310	19.24	25.30	10.84	0.88	10.21
cooked, roasted, trimmed to 0" fat	3 oz	300	19.67	23.97	10.25	0.83	9.67
Rib, large end (ribs 6-9), separable lean & fat, choice							
raw, trimmed to $\frac{1}{4}$" fat	1 lb	1567	71.44	139.87	59.97	5.10	57.86
cooked, broiled, trimmed to $\frac{1}{4}$" fat	3 oz	312	17.81	26.18	11.09	0.99	10.64
cooked, roasted, trimmed to $\frac{1}{4}$" fat	3 oz	326	18.95	27.15	11.63	0.95	10.95
cooked, roasted, trimmed to 0" fat	3 oz	317	19.38	25.92	11.09	0.90	10.45
Rib, large end (ribs 6-9), separable lean & fat, select							
raw, trimmed to $\frac{1}{4}$" fat	1 lb	1378	74.03	117.73	50.52	4.29	48.71
cooked, broiled, trimmed to $\frac{1}{4}$" fat	3 oz	276	18.31	21.90	9.25	0.83	8.88
cooked, roasted, trimmed to $\frac{1}{4}$" fat	3 oz	289	19.67	22.71	9.73	0.79	9.1
cooked, roasted, trimmed to 0" fat	3 oz	281	19.96	21.71	9.29	0.75	8.7
Rib, large end (ribs 6-9), separable lean & fat, prime							
raw, trimmed to $\frac{1}{4}$" fat	1 lb	1712	70.40	156.49	67.65	5.78	65.6
cooked, broiled, trimmed to $\frac{1}{4}$" fat	3 oz	351	17.26	30.78	13.45	1.07	12.7
cooked, roasted, trimmed to $\frac{1}{4}$" fat	3 oz	342	19.10	28.85	12.59	1.00	11.9

FOOD	CARBO-HYDRATES (mg)	FIBER (mg)	CALCIUM (mg)	IRON (mg)	POTAS-SIUM (mg)	SODIUM (mg)	CHOLES-TEROL (mg)	% OF CALORIES FROM FAT
Rib, whole (continued)								
cooked, broiled, lean only	0.0	0.00	9	2.18	324	60	66	46
cooked, roasted, lean only	0.0	0.00	8	2.43	318	61	68	45
Rib, whole (ribs 6-12), trimmed to ¼" fat, prime								
raw, separable lean & fat	0.0	0.00	40	7.57	1164	239	329	81
cooked, broiled, lean & fat	0.0	0.00	9	1.79	260	52	72	76
cooked, roasted, lean & fat	0.0	0.00	10	1.82	254	54	72	77
cooked, broiled, lean only	0.0	0.00	9	2.14	322	59	69	60
cooked, roasted, lean only	0.0	0.00	9	2.22	320	63	69	60
Rib, eye, small end ribs 10-12), trimmed to 0" fat, choice								
raw, separable lean & fat	0.0	0.00	45	8.46	1386	252	308	73
cooked, broiled, lean & fat	0.0	0.00	11	1.95	293	54	70	65
cooked, broiled, lean only	0.0	0.00	11	2.18	335	59	68	47
Rib, large end (ribs 6-9), separable lean & fat, all grades								
raw, trimmed to ¼" fat	0.0	0.00	36	7.66	1160	247	324	79
cooked, broiled, trimmed to ¼" fat	0.0	0.00	9	1.84	258	54	69	74
cooked, roasted, trimmed to ¼" fat	0.0	0.00	8	1.96	245	54	72	73
cooked, roasted, trimmed to 0" fat	0.0	0.00	8	2.01	251	55	72	72
Rib, large end (ribs 6-9), separable lean & fat, choice								
raw, trimmed to ¼" fat	0.0	0.00	36	7.47	1123	242	329	80
cooked, broiled, trimmed to ¼" fat	0.0	0.00	9	1.81	254	54	69	76
cooked, roasted, trimmed to ¼" fat	0.0	0.00	8	1.93	241	54	73	75
cooked, roasted, trimmed to 0" fat	0.0	0.00	8	1.98	247	54	72	74
Rib, large end (ribs 6-9), separable lean & fat, select								
raw, trimmed to ¼" fat	0.0	0.00	36	7.78	1185	251	320	77
cooked, broiled, trimmed to ¼" fat	0.0	0.00	9	1.86	262	55	68	71
cooked, roasted, trimmed to ¼" fat	0.0	0.00	8	2.01	251	55	72	71
cooked, roasted, trimmed to 0" fat	0.0	0.00	8	2.04	255	56	72	70
Rib, large end (ribs 6-9), separable lean & fat, prime								
raw, trimmed to ¼" fat	0.0	0.00	37	7.35	1098	239	333	82
cooked, broiled, trimmed to ¼" fat	0.0	0.00	8	1.73	248	52	73	79
cooked, roasted, trimmed to ¼" fat	0.0	0.00	8	1.95	243	54	72	76

FOOD	AMOUNT	CALO-RIES (kcal)	PROTEIN (g)	FAT (g)	SATU-RATED FAT (g)	MONO-UN-SATURATED FAT (g)	POLY-UN-SATURATED FAT (g)
Rib, large (continued)							
Rib, large end (ribs 6-9), separable lean only, all grades							
cooked, broiled, trimmed to 1/4" fat	3 oz	190	21.39	10.98	4.45	0.41	4.49
cooked, roasted, trimmed to 1/4" fat	3 oz	201	23.40	11.22	4.69	0.32	4.48
cooked, roasted, trimmed to 0" fat	3 oz	203	23.40	11.39	4.76	0.33	4.55
Rib, large end (ribs 6-9), separable lean only, choice							
cooked, broiled, trimmed to 1/4" fat	3 oz	204	21.39	12.45	5.04	0.47	5.08
cooked, roasted, trimmed to 1/4" fat	3 oz	213	23.40	12.49	5.22	0.36	4.99
cooked, roasted, trimmed to 0" fat	3 oz	215	23.40	12.75	5.33	0.37	5.09
Rib, large end (ribs 6-9), separable lean only, select							
cooked, broiled, trimmed to 1/4" fat	3 oz	175	21.39	9.28	3.70	0.35	3.78
cooked, roasted, trimmed to 1/4" fat	3 oz	187	23.40	9.69	4.05	0.28	3.87
cooked, roasted, trimmed to 0" fat	3 oz	187	23.40	9.69	4.05	0.28	3.87
Rib, large end (ribs 6-9), separable lean only, prime							
cooked, broiled, trimmed to 1/4" fat	3 oz	250	20.94	17.75	7.86	0.54	7.60
cooked, roasted, trimmed to 1/4" fat	3 oz	241	23.40	15.59	6.89	0.47	6.69
Rib, small end (ribs 10-12), separable lean & fat, all grades							
raw, trimmed to 1/4" fat	1 lb	1352	76.18	113.88	49.51	4.02	46.62
cooked, broiled, trimmed to 1/4" fat	3 oz	285	20.14	22.09	9.48	0.77	8.94
cooked, broiled, trimmed to 0" fat	3 oz	252	21.17	17.94	7.69	0.61	7.26
cooked, roasted, trimmed to 1/4" fat	3 oz	295	18.96	23.77	10.28	0.87	9.52
Rib, small end (ribs 10-12), separable lean & fat, choice							
raw, trimmed to 1/4" fat	1 lb	1429	75.10	122.82	53.40	4.33	50.3
cooked, broiled, trimmed to 1/4" fat	3 oz	297	19.99	23.47	10.07	0.81	9.5
cooked, broiled, trimmed to 0" fat	3 oz	265	21.02	19.41	8.32	0.66	7.8
cooked, roasted, trimmed to 1/4" fat	3 oz	312	18.69	25.70	11.12	0.94	10.3
Rib, small end (ribs 10-12), separable lean & fat, select							
raw, trimmed to 1/4" fat	1 lb	1296	76.72	107.35	46.69	3.80	44.0
cooked, broiled, trimmed to 1/4" fat	3 oz	273	20.28	20.61	8.86	0.72	8.3

FOOD	CARBO-HYDRATES (mg)	FIBER (mg)	CALCIUM (mg)	IRON (mg)	POTAS-SIUM (mg)	SODIUM (mg)	CHOLES-TEROL (mg)	% OF CALORIES FROM FAT
Rib, large (continued)								
Rib, large end (ribs 6-9), separable lean only, all grades								
cooked, broiled, trimmed to ¼" fat	0.0	0.00	8	2.18	316	61	64	52
cooked, roasted, trimmed to ¼" fat	0.0	0.00	7	2.40	303	62	69	50
cooked, roasted, trimmed to 0" fat	0.0	0.00	7	2.40	303	62	69	50
Rib, large end (ribs 6-9), separable lean only, choice								
cooked, broiled, trimmed to ¼" fat	0.0	0.00	8	2.18	316	61	64	55
cooked, roasted, trimmed to ¼" fat	0.0	0.00	7	2.40	303	62	69	53
cooked, roasted, trimmed to 0" fat	0.0	0.00	7	2.40	303	62	69	53
Rib, large end (ribs 6-9), separable lean only, select								
cooked, broiled, trimmed to ¼" fat	0.0	0.00	8	2.18	316	61	64	48
cooked, roasted, trimmed to ¼" fat	0.0	0.00	7	2.40	303	62	69	47
cooked, roasted, trimmed to 0" fat	0.0	0.00	7	2.40	303	62	69	47
Rib, large end (ribs 6-9), separable lean only, prime								
cooked, broiled, trimmed to ¼" fat	0.0	0.00	7	2.11	314	59	70	64
cooked, roasted, trimmed to ¼" fat	0.0	0.00	7	2.40	303	62	69	58
Rib, small end (ribs 10-12), separable lean & fat, all grades								
raw, trimmed to ¼" fat	0.0	0.00	45	8.07	1302	243	318	76
cooked, broiled, trimmed to ¼" fat	0.0	0.00	11	1.86	276	53	71	70
cooked, broiled, trimmed to 0" fat	0.0	0.00	11	1.95	293	54	70	64
cooked, roasted, trimmed to ¼" fat	0.0	0.00	11	2.03	272	53	71	73
Rib, small end (ribs 10-12), separable lean & fat, choice								
raw, trimmed to ¼" fat	0.0	0.00	45	7.94	1274	240	322	77
cooked, broiled, trimmed to ¼" fat	0.0	0.00	11	1.85	274	52	71	71
cooked, broiled, trimmed to 0" fat	0.0	0.00	11	1.94	290	54	70	66
cooked, roasted, trimmed to ¼" fat	0.0	0.00	11	2.00	267	53	71	74
Rib, small end (ribs 10-12), separable lean & fat, select								
raw, trimmed to ¼" fat	0.0	0.00	45	8.14	1316	244	317	75
cooked, broiled, trimmed to ¼" fat	0.0	0.00	11	1.88	279	53	71	68

FOOD	AMOUNT	CALO-RIES (kcal)	PROTEIN (g)	FAT (g)	SATU-RATED FAT (g)	MONO-UN-SATURATED FAT (g)	POLY-UN-SATURATED FAT (g)
Rib, small (continued)							
cooked, broiled, trimmed to 0" fat	3 oz	242	21.17	16.82	7.22	0.58	6.81
cooked, roasted, trimmed to 1/4" fat	3 oz	282	19.10	22.19	9.59	0.81	8.92
Rib, small end (ribs 10-12), separable lean & fat, prime							
raw, trimmed to 1/4" fat	1 lb	1551	75.10	136.44	60.02	4.85	56.47
cooked, broiled, trimmed to 1/4" fat	3 oz	307	20.28	24.38	10.61	0.85	10.07
cooked, roasted, trimmed to 1/4" fat	3 oz	354	18.62	30.48	13.26	1.06	12.59
Rib, small end (ribs 10-12), separable lean only, all grades							
cooked, broiled, trimmed to 1/4" fat	3 oz	188	23.83	9.52	4.02	0.27	3.85
cooked, broiled, trimmed to 0" fat	3 oz	181	23.83	8.75	3.69	0.25	3.54
cooked, roasted, trimmed to 1/4" fat	3 oz	185	22.82	9.76	4.21	0.33	3.87
Rib, small end (ribs 10-12), separable lean only, choice							
cooked, broiled, trimmed to 1/4" fat	3 oz	198	23.83	10.71	4.52	0.31	4.33
cooked, broiled, trimmed to 0" fat	3 oz	191	23.83	9.94	4.20	0.28	4.02
cooked, roasted, trimmed to 1/4" fat	3 oz	198	22.82	11.10	4.79	0.37	4.42
Rib, small end (ribs 10-12), separable lean only, select							
cooked, broiled, trimmed to 1/4" fat	3 oz	176	23.83	8.24	3.48	0.24	3.33
cooked, broiled, trimmed to 0" fat	3 oz	168	23.83	7.39	3.12	0.21	2.99
cooked, roasted, trimmed to 1/4" fat	3 oz	172	22.82	8.29	3.56	0.27	3.26
Rib, small end (ribs 10-12), separable lean only, prime							
cooked, broiled, trimmed to 1/4" fat	3 oz	221	23.83	13.20	5.78	0.40	5.6
cooked, roasted, trimmed to 1/4" fat	3 oz	259	22.73	17.93	7.84	0.54	7.6
Rib, shortribs, choice							
raw, separable lean & fat	1 lb	1761	65.30	164.33	74.33	6.00	71.4
cooked, braised, separable lean & fat	3 oz	400	18.33	35.69	16.05	1.30	15.1
cooked, braised, separable lean only	3 oz	251	26.14	15.41	6.78	0.47	6.5
Round, full cut, trimmed to 1/4" fat, choice							
raw, separable lean & fat	1 lb	919	92.41	58.11	25.09	2.23	22.7
cooked, broiled, separable lean & fat	3 oz	204	23.25	11.57	4.96	0.46	4.3
cooked, broiled, separable lean only	3 oz	162	24.83	6.22	2.63	0.26	2.1

FOOD	CARBO-HYDRATES (mg)	FIBER (mg)	CALCIUM (mg)	IRON (mg)	POTAS-SIUM (mg)	SODIUM (mg)	CHOLES-TEROL (mg)	% OF CALORIES FROM FAT
Rib, small (continued)								
cooked, broiled, trimmed to 0" fat	0.0	0.00	11	1.95	293	54	70	63
cooked, roasted, trimmed to 1/4" fat	0.0	0.00	11	2.05	274	54	71	71
Rib, small end (ribs 10-12), separable lean & fat, prime								
raw, trimmed to 1/4" fat	0.0	0.00	45	7.94	1274	240	322	79
cooked, broiled, trimmed to 1/4" fat	0.0	0.00	11	1.88	279	53	71	71
cooked, roasted, trimmed to 1/4" fat	0.0	0.00	11	1.64	271	55	72	77
Rib, small end (ribs 10-12), separable lean only, all grades								
cooked, broiled, trimmed to 1/4" fat	0.0	0.00	11	2.18	335	59	68	46
cooked, broiled, trimmed to 0" fat	0.0	0.00	11	2.18	335	59	68	44
cooked, roasted, trimmed to 1/4" fat	0.0	0.00	10	2.47	338	61	67	47
Rib, small end (ribs 10-12), separable lean only, choice								
cooked, broiled, trimmed to 1/4" fat	0.0	0.00	11	2.18	335	59	68	49
cooked, broiled, trimmed to 0" fat	0.0	0.00	11	2.18	335	59	68	47
cooked, roasted, trimmed to 1/4" fat	0.0	0.00	10	2.47	338	61	67	50
Rib, small end (ribs 10-12), separable lean only, select								
cooked, broiled, trimmed to 1/4" fat	0.0	0.00	11	2.18	335	59	68	42
cooked, broiled, trimmed to 0" fat	0.0	0.00	11	2.18	335	59	68	40
cooked, roasted, trimmed to 1/4" fat	0.0	0.00	10	2.47	338	61	67	43
Rib, small end (ribs 10-12), separable lean only, prime								
cooked, broiled, trimmed to 1/4" fat	0.0	0.00	11	2.18	335	59	68	54
cooked, roasted, trimmed to 1/4" fat	0.0	0.00	11	1.95	343	64	68	62
Rib, shortribs, choice								
raw, separable lean & fat	0.0	0.00	41	7.03	1053	224	345	84
cooked, braised, separable lean & fat	0.0	0.00	10	1.96	191	43	80	80
cooked, braised, separable lean only	0.0	0.00	9	2.86	266	50	79	55
Round, full cut, trimmed to 1/4" fat, choice								
raw, separable lean & fat	0.0	0.00	20	8.96	1533	241	285	57
cooked, broiled, separable lean & fat	0.0	0.00	5	2.15	333	52	68	51
cooked, broiled, separable lean only	0.0	0.00	4	2.29	359	54	66	35

BEEF PRODUCTS

FOOD	AMOUNT	CALO-RIES (kcal)	PROTEIN (g)	FAT (g)	SATU-RATED FAT (g)	MONO-UN-SATURATED FAT (g)	POLY-UN-SATURATED FAT (g)
Round, full cut, trimmed to ¼" fat, select							
raw, separable lean & fat	1 lb	869	92.39	52.55	22.77	1.99	20.80
cooked, broiled, separable lean & fat	3 oz	189	23.28	9.97	3.94	0.35	3.51
cooked, broiled, separable lean only	3 oz	146	24.87	4.44	1.89	0.19	1.55
Round, bottom round, separable lean & fat, all grades							
raw, trimmed to ¼" fat	1 lb	942	91.76	60.94	26.96	2.26	23.65
cooked, braised, trimmed to ¼" fat	3 oz	234	24.36	14.36	6.25	0.55	5.42
cooked, braised, trimmed to 0" fat	3 oz	181	26.49	7.53	3.29	0.29	2.62
cooked, roasted, trimmed to ¼" fat	3 oz	211	22.61	12.69	5.60	0.49	4.79
cooked, roasted, trimmed to 0" fat	3 oz	160	24.30	6.24	2.83	0.24	2.13
Round, bottom round, separable lean & fat, choice							
raw, trimmed to ¼" fat	1 lb	990	91.14	66.66	29.50	2.48	25.84
cooked, braised, trimmed to ¼" fat	3 oz	241	24.36	15.24	6.63	0.58	5.71
cooked, braised, trimmed to 0" fat	3 oz	193	26.32	8.97	3.92	0.34	3.15
cooked, roasted, trimmed to ¼" fat	3 oz	221	22.46	13.90	6.14	0.53	5.24
cooked, roasted, trimmed to 0" fat	3 oz	172	24.15	7.66	3.45	0.30	2.66
Round, bottom round, separable lean & fat, select							
raw, trimmed to ¼" fat	1 lb	885	92.38	54.35	24.03	2.02	21.60
cooked, braised, trimmed to ¼" fat	3 oz	220	24.54	12.80	5.57	0.49	4.85
cooked, braised, trimmed to 0" fat	3 oz	171	26.49	6.44	2.82	0.25	2.26
cooked, roasted, trimmed to ¼" fat	3 oz	199	22.76	11.25	4.97	0.43	4.26
cooked, roasted, trimmed to 0" fat	3 oz	150	24.30	5.14	2.33	0.20	1.74
Round, bottom round, separable lean only, all grades							
cooked, braised, trimmed to ¼" fat	3 oz	178	26.85	6.97	3.05	0.27	2.35
cooked, braised, trimmed to 0" fat	3 oz	173	26.85	6.46	2.83	0.25	2.18
cooked, roasted, trimmed to ¼" fat	3 oz	161	24.46	6.26	2.84	0.24	2.13
cooked, roasted, trimmed to 0" fat	3 oz	156	24.45	5.70	2.59	0.22	1.90
Round, bottom round, separable lean only, choice							
cooked, braised, trimmed to ¼" fat	3 oz	87	26.85	7.99	3.50	0.31	2.70
cooked, braised, trimmed to 0" fat	3 oz	181	26.85	7.39	3.24	0.28	2.50
cooked, roasted, trimmed to ¼" fat	3 oz	168	24.46	7.05	3.19	0.27	2.40
cooked, roasted, trimmed to 0" fat	3 oz	164	24.45	6.60	3.00	0.26	2.22

FOOD	CARBO-HYDRATES (mg)	FIBER (mg)	CALCIUM (mg)	IRON (mg)	POTAS-SIUM (mg)	SODIUM (mg)	CHOLES-TEROL (mg)	% OF CALORIES FROM FAT
Round, full cut, trimmed to ¼" fat, select								
raw, separable lean & fat	0.0	0.00	20	8.97	1533	242	285	54
cooked, broiled, separable lean & fat	0.0	0.00	5	2.16	334	52	47	47
cooked, broiled, separable lean only	0.0	0.00	4	2.30	359	54	66	27
Round, bottom round, separable lean & fat, all grades								
raw, trimmed to ¼" fat	0.0	0.00	21	9.91	1517	251	289	58
cooked, braised, trimmed to ¼" fat	0.0	0.00	5	2.66	239	42	81	55
cooked, braised, trimmed to 0" fat	0.0	0.00	4	2.90	259	43	82	37
cooked, roasted, trimmed to ¼" fat	0.0	0.00	5	2.45	304	54	68	54
cooked, roasted, trimmed to 0" fat	0.0	0.00	4	2.64	330	56	66	35
Round, bottom round, separable lean & fat, choice								
raw, trimmed to ¼" fat	0.0	0.00	22	9.83	1503	250	291	61
cooked, braised, trimmed to ¼" fat	0.0	0.00	5	2.66	239	42	81	57
cooked, braised, trimmed to 0" fat	0.0	0.00	4	2.88	257	43	82	42
cooked, roasted, trimmed to ¼" fat	0.0	0.00	5	2.43	302	53	68	57
cooked, roasted, trimmed to 0" fat	0.0	0.00	4	2.63	327	56	66	40
Round, bottom round, separable lean & fat, select								
raw, trimmed to ¼" fat	0.0	0.00	21	9.98	1531	253	288	55
cooked, braised, trimmed to ¼" fat	0.0	0.00	5	2.68	241	42	81	52
cooked, braised, trimmed to 0" fat	0.0	0.00	4	2.90	259	43	82	34
cooked, roasted, trimmed to ¼" fat	0.0	0.00	5	2.47	307	54	68	51
cooked, roasted, trimmed to 0" fat	0.0	0.00	4	2.64	330	56	66	31
Round, bottom round, separable lean only, all grades								
cooked, braised, trimmed to ¼" fat	0.0	0.00	4	2.94	262	43	82	35
cooked, braised, trimmed to 0" fat	0.0	0.00	4	2.94	262	43	82	34
cooked, roasted, trimmed to ¼" fat	0.0	0.00	4	2.66	332	56	66	35
cooked, roasted, trimmed to 0" fat	0.0	0.00	4	2.66	332	56	66	33
Round, bottom round, separable lean only, choice								
cooked, braised, trimmed to ¼" fat	0.0	0.00	4	2.94	262	43	82	83
cooked, braised, trimmed to 0" fat	0.0	0.00	4	2.94	262	43	82	37
cooked, roasted, trimmed to ¼" fat	0.0	0.00	4	2.66	332	56	66	38
cooked, roasted, trimmed to 0" fat	0.0	0.00	4	2.66	332	56	66	36

BEEF PRODUCTS

FOOD	AMOUNT	CALO-RIES (kcal)	PROTEIN (g)	FAT (g)	SATU-RATED FAT (g)	MONO-UN-SATURATED FAT (g)	POLY-UN-SATURATED FAT (g)
Round, bottom round, separable lean only, select							
cooked, braised, trimmed to 1/4" fat	3 oz	167	26.85	5.78	2.53	0.22	1.95
cooked, braised, trimmed to 0" fat	3 oz	163	26.85	5.35	2.35	0.21	1.81
cooked, roasted, trimmed to 1/4" fat	3 oz	152	24.46	5.26	2.38	0.20	1.79
cooked, roasted, trimmed to 0" fat	3 oz	146	24.45	4.59	2.09	0.18	1.51
Round, eye of round, separable lean & fat, all grades							
raw, trimmed to 1/4" fat	1 lb	967	89.45	64.81	27.92	2.44	25.74
cooked, roasted, trimmed to 1/4" fat	3 oz	195	22.77	10.84	4.66	0.39	4.24
cooked, roasted, trimmed to 0" fat	3 oz	146	24.48	4.55	1.93	0.15	1.68
Round, eye of round, separable lean & fat, choice							
raw, trimmed to 1/4" fat	1 lb	987	89.45	67.13	28.88	2.54	26.54
cooked, roasted, trimmed to 1/4" fat	3 oz	205	22.61	11.99	5.15	0.43	4.68
cooked, roasted, trimmed to 0" fat	3 oz	153	24.48	5.39	2.29	0.18	1.98
Round, eye of round, separable lean & fat, select							
raw, trimmed to 1/4" fat	1 lb	917	90.06	59.06	25.47	2.22	23.53
cooked, roasted, trimmed to 1/4" fat	3 oz	184	22.92	9.60	4.13	0.35	3.76
cooked, roasted, trimmed to 0" fat	3 oz	137	24.48	3.54	1.51	0.12	1.31
Round, eye of round, separable lean only, all grades							
cooked, roasted, trimmed to 1/4" fat	3 oz	143	24.64	4.16	1.76	0.13	1.51
cooked, roasted, trimmed to 0" fat	3 oz	141	24.64	3.99	1.69	0.13	1.45
Round, eye of round, separable lean only, choice							
cooked, roasted, trimmed to 1/4" fat	3 oz	149	24.64	4.84	2.05	0.16	1.76
cooked, roasted, trimmed to 0" fat	3 oz	149	24.64	4.84	2.05	0.16	1.76
Round, eye of round, separable lean only, select							
cooked, roasted, trimmed to 1/4" fat	3 oz	136	24.64	3.40	1.44	0.11	1.23
cooked, roasted, trimmed to 0" fat	3 oz	132	24.64	2.97	1.26	0.10	1.08
Round, tip round, separable lean & fat, all grades							
raw, trimmed to 1/4" fat	1 lb	914	87.57	59.84	25.68	2.34	23.75
cooked, roasted, trimmed to 1/4" fat	3 oz	199	22.87	11.26	4.69	0.44	4.27

FOOD	CARBO-HYDRATES (mg)	FIBER (mg)	CALCIUM (mg)	IRON (mg)	POTAS-SIUM (mg)	SODIUM (mg)	CHOLES-TEROL (mg)	% OF CALORIES FROM FAT
Round, bottom round, separable lean only, select								
cooked, braised, trimmed to 1/4" fat	0.0	0.00	4	2.94	262	43	82	31
cooked, braised, trimmed to 0" fat	0.0	0.00	4	2.94	262	43	82	30
cooked, roasted, trimmed to 1/4" fat	0.0	0.00	4	2.66	332	56	66	31
cooked, roasted, trimmed to 0" fat	0.0	0.00	4	2.66	332	56	66	28
Round, eye of round, separable lean & fat, all grades								
raw, trimmed to 1/4" fat	0.0	0.00	22	6.14	1522	224	276	60
cooked, roasted, trimmed to 1/4" fat	0.0	0.00	5	1.57	308	51	61	50
cooked, roasted, trimmed to 0" fat	0.0	0.00	4	1.65	333	53	59	28
Round, eye of round, separable lean & fat, choice								
raw, trimmed to 1/4" fat	0.0	0.00	22	6.14	1522	224	276	61
cooked, roasted, trimmed to 1/4" fat	0.0	0.00	5	1.56	305	50	62	53
cooked, roasted, trimmed to 0" fat	0.0	0.00	4	1.65	333	53	59	32
Round, eye of round, separable lean & fat, select								
raw, trimmed to 1/4" fat	0.0	0.00	22	6.17	1536	225	274	58
cooked, roasted, trimmed to 1/4" fat	0.0	0.00	5	1.57	310	51	61	47
cooked, roasted, trimmed to 0" fat	0.0	0.00	4	1.65	333	53	59	23
Round, eye of round, separable lean only, all grades								
cooked, roasted, trimmed to 1/4" fat	0.0	0.00	4	1.66	336	53	59	26
cooked, roasted, trimmed to 0" fat	0.0	0.00	4	1.66	336	53	59	25
Round, eye of round, separable lean only, choice								
cooked, roasted, trimmed to 1/4" fat	0.0	0.00	4	1.66	336	53	59	29
cooked, roasted, trimmed to 0" fat	0.0	0.00	4	1.66	336	53	59	29
Round, eye of round, separable lean only, select								
cooked, roasted, trimmed to 1/4" fat	0.0	0.00	4	1.66	336	53	59	23
cooked, roasted, trimmed to 0" fat	0.0	0.00	4	1.66	336	53	59	20
Round, tip round, separable lean & fat, all grades								
raw, trimmed to 1/4" fat	0.0	0.00	22	8.94	1462	260	297	59
cooked, roasted, trimmed to 1/4" fat	0.0	0.00	5	2.34	305	53	70	51

BEEF PRODUCTS

FOOD	AMOUNT	CALO-RIES (kcal)	PROTEIN (g)	FAT (g)	SATU-RATED FAT (g)	MONO-UN-SATURATED FAT (g)	POLY-UN-SATURATED FAT (g)
Round, tip round (continued)							
cooked, roasted, trimmed to 0" fat	3 oz	162	23.94	6.66	2.71	0.26	2.43
Round, tip round, separable lean & fat, choice							
raw, trimmed to $\frac{1}{4}$" fat	1 lb	960	86.99	65.20	27.95	2.56	25.81
cooked, roasted, trimmed to $\frac{1}{4}$" fat	3 oz	210	22.56	12.63	5.28	0.49	4.82
cooked, roasted, trimmed to 0" fat	3 oz	170	23.79	7.61	3.11	0.30	2.79
Round, tip round, separable lean & fat, select							
raw, trimmed to $\frac{1}{4}$" fat	1 lb	842	88.74	51.36	22.04	2.01	20.38
cooked, roasted, trimmed to $\frac{1}{4}$" fat	3 oz	191	23.02	10.33	4.30	0.40	3.91
cooked, roasted, trimmed to 0" fat	3 oz	158	23.94	6.16	2.51	0.24	2.25
Round, tip round, separable lean & fat, prime							
raw, trimmed to $\frac{1}{4}$" fat	1 lb	973	88.16	66.11	28.51	2.77	26.09
cooked, roasted, trimmed to $\frac{1}{4}$" fat	3 oz	233	22.41	15.21	6.43	0.60	5.88
Round, tip round, separable lean only, all grades							
cooked, roasted, trimmed to $\frac{1}{4}$" fat	3 oz	157	24.41	5.86	2.33	0.23	2.05
cooked, roasted, trimmed to 0" fat	3 oz	149	24.41	5.01	1.99	0.20	1.75
Round, tip round, separable lean only, choice							
cooked, roasted, trimmed to $\frac{1}{4}$" fat	3 oz	160	24.41	6.20	2.47	0.25	2.17
cooked, roasted, trimmed to 0" fat	3 oz	153	24.41	5.44	2.16	0.22	1.90
Round, tip round, separable lean only, select							
cooked, roasted, trimmed to $\frac{1}{4}$" fat	3 oz	153	24.41	5.44	2.16	0.22	1.90
cooked, roasted, trimmed to 0" fat	3 oz	145	24.41	4.50	1.79	0.18	1.58
Round, tip round, separable lean only, prime							
cooked, roasted, trimmed to $\frac{1}{4}$" fat	3 oz	181	24.41	8.55	3.52	0.35	3.14
Round, top round, separable lean & fat, all grades							
raw, trimmed to $\frac{1}{4}$" fat	1 lb	800	97.41	42.56	17.94	1.65	16.69
cooked, braised, trimmed to $\frac{1}{4}$" fat	3 oz	210	28.76	9.71	4.01	0.40	3.67
cooked, braised, trimmed to 0" fat	3 oz	178	30.27	5.36	2.14	0.23	1.92
cooked, broiled, trimmed to $\frac{1}{4}$" fat	3 oz	183	25.64	8.18	3.37	0.34	3.08

FOOD	CARBO-HYDRATES (mg)	FIBER (mg)	CALCIUM (mg)	IRON (mg)	POTAS-SIUM (mg)	SODIUM (mg)	CHOLES-TEROL (mg)	% OF CALORIES FROM FAT
Round, tip round (continued)								
cooked, roasted, trimmed to 0" fat	0.0	0.00	4	2.45	321	55	69	37
Round, tip round, separable lean & fat, choice								
raw, trimmed to $\frac{1}{4}$" fat	0.0	0.00	22	8.88	1448	259	299	61
cooked, roasted, trimmed to $\frac{1}{4}$" fat	0.0	0.00	5	2.31	301	53	70	54
cooked, roasted, trimmed to 0" fat	0.0	0.00	5	2.44	319	54	69	40
Round, tip round, separable lean & fat, select								
raw, trimmed to $\frac{1}{4}$" fat	0.0	0.00	21	9.07	1489	263		55
cooked, roasted, trimmed to $\frac{1}{4}$" fat	0.0	0.00	5	2.36	308	53	70	49
cooked, roasted, trimmed to 0" fat	0.0	0.00	4	2.45	321	55	69	35
Round, tip round, separable lean & fat, prime								
raw, trimmed to $\frac{1}{4}$" fat	0.0	0.00	22	9.01	1475	262	295	61
cooked, roasted, trimmed to $\frac{1}{4}$" fat	0.0	0.00	5	2.29	299	53	70	59
Round, tip round, separable lean only, all grades								
cooked, roasted, trimmed to $\frac{1}{4}$" fat	0.0	0.00	4	2.50	328	55	69	34
cooked, roasted, trimmed to 0" fat	0.0	0.00	4	2.50	328	55	69	30
Round, tip round, separable lean only, choice								
cooked, roasted, trimmed to $\frac{1}{4}$" fat	0.0	0.00	4	2.50	328	55	69	35
cooked, roasted, trimmed to 0" fat	0.0	0.00	4	2.50	328	55	69	32
Round, tip round, separable lean only, select								
cooked, roasted, trimmed to $\frac{1}{4}$" fat	0.0	0.00	4	2.50	328	55	69	32
cooked, roasted, trimmed to 0" fat	0.0	0.00	4	2.50	328	55	69	28
Round, tip round, separable lean only, prime								
cooked, roasted, trimmed to $\frac{1}{4}$" fat	0.0	0.00	4	2.50	328	55	69	43
Round, top round, separable lean & fat, all grades								
raw, trimmed to $\frac{1}{4}$" fat	0.0	0.00	16	8.93	1608	226	276	48
cooked, braised, trimmed to $\frac{1}{4}$" fat	0.0	0.00	4	2.65	267	38	77	42
cooked, braised, trimmed to 0" fat	0.0	0.00	3	2.78	280	38	77	27
cooked, broiled, trimmed to $\frac{1}{4}$" fat	0.0	0.00	6	2.34	356	51	72	40

BEEF PRODUCTS

FOOD	AMOUNT	CALO-RIES (kcal)	PROTEIN (g)	FAT (g)	SATU-RATED FAT (g)	MONO-UN-SATURATED FAT (g)	POLY-UN-SATURATED FAT (g)
Round, top round, separable lean & fat, choice							
raw, trimmed to $\frac{1}{4}$" fat	1 lb	822	97.41	45.04	18.91	1.77	17.54
cooked, braised, trimmed to $\frac{1}{4}$" fat	3 oz	221	28.54	10.95	4.52	0.45	4.13
cooked, braised, trimmed to 0" fat	3 oz	184	30.27	6.03	2.39	0.26	2.14
cooked, broiled, trimmed to $\frac{1}{4}$" fat	3 oz	190	25.64	8.97	3.68	0.37	3.35
cooked, pan-fried, trimmed to $\frac{1}{4}$" fat	3 oz	235	27.53	13.07	4.99	1.49	4.50
Round, top round, lean & fat, select							
raw, trimmed to $\frac{1}{4}$" fat	1 lb	745	98.07	36.16	15.30	1.40	14.26
cooked, braised, trimmed to $\frac{1}{4}$" fat	3 oz	199	28.97	8.38	3.47	0.34	3.17
cooked, braised, trimmed to 0" fat	3 oz	170	30.27	4.53	1.81	0.19	1.63
cooked, broiled, trimmed to $\frac{1}{4}$" fat	3 oz	175	25.64	7.23	3.00	0.29	2.75
Round, top round, lean & fat, prime							
raw, trimmed to $\frac{1}{4}$" fat	1 lb	814	100.06	42.92	17.88	1.83	16.46
cooked, broiled, trimmed to $\frac{1}{4}$" fat	3 oz	195	26.40	9.11	3.64	0.41	3.28
Round, top round, separable lean only, all grades							
cooked, braised, trimmed to $\frac{1}{4}$" fat	3 oz	174	30.71	4.76	1.85	0.21	1.64
cooked, braised, trimmed to 0" fat	3 oz	169	30.71	4.25	1.65	0.19	1.46
cooked, broiled, trimmed to $\frac{1}{4}$" fat	3 oz	153	26.93	4.16	1.62	0.19	1.43
Round, top round, separable lean only, choice							
cooked, braised, trimmed to $\frac{1}{4}$" fat	3 oz	181	30.71	5.52	2.15	0.25	1.90
cooked, braised, trimmed to 0" fat	3 oz	176	30.71	4.93	1.91	0.22	1.69
cooked, broiled, trimmed to $\frac{1}{4}$" fat	3 oz	160	26.93	5.01	1.95	0.22	1.72
cooked, pan-fried, trimmed to $\frac{1}{4}$" fat	3 oz	193	29.81	7.29	2.40	1.39	2.06
Round, top round, lean only, select							
cooked, braised, trimmed to $\frac{1}{4}$" fat	3 oz	166	30.71	3.91	1.52	0.18	1.34
cooked, braised, trimmed to 0" fat	3 oz	162	30.71	3.40	1.32	0.15	1.17
cooked, broiled, trimmed to $\frac{1}{4}$" fat	3 oz	143	26.93	3.14	1.22	0.14	1.08
Round, top round, separable lean only, prime							
cooked, broiled, trimmed to $\frac{1}{4}$" fat	3 oz	183	26.93	7.54	2.95	0.36	2.64
Shank crosscuts, trimmed to $\frac{1}{4}$" fat, choice							
raw, separable lean & fat	3 oz	150	17.45	8.40	3.73	0.31	3.24
cooked, simmered, separable lean & fat	3 oz	224	26.08	12.47	5.48	0.45	4.84
cooked, simmered, separable lean only	3 oz	171	28.63	5.41	2.43	0.18	1.94

FOOD	CARBO-HYDRATES (mg)	FIBER (mg)	CALCIUM (mg)	IRON (mg)	POTAS-SIUM (mg)	SODIUM (mg)	CHOLES-TEROL (mg)	% OF CALORIES FROM FAT
Round, top round, separable lean & fat, choice								
raw, trimmed to ¼" fat	0.0	0.00	16	8.93	1608	226	276	49
cooked, braised, trimmed to ¼" fat	0.0	0.00	4	2.63	266	38	77	45
cooked, braised, trimmed to 0" fat	0.0	0.00	3	2.78	280	38	77	29
cooked, broiled, trimmed to ¼" fat	0.0	0.00	6	2.34	356	51	72	42
cooked, pan-fried, trimmed to ¼" fat	0.0	0.00	5	2.48	399	58	82	50
Round, top round, lean & fat, select								
raw, trimmed to ¼" fat	0.0	0.00	16	8.99	1622	228	274	44
cooked, braised, trimmed to ¼" fat	0.0	0.00	4	2.67	269	38	77	38
cooked, braised, trimmed to 0" fat	0.0	0.00	3	2.78	280	38	77	24
cooked, broiled, trimmed to ¼" fat	0.0	0.00	6	2.34	356	51	72	37
Round, top round, lean & fat, prime								
raw, trimmed to ¼" fat	0.0	0.00	15	9.18	1665	231	268	47
cooked, broiled, trimmed to ¼" fat	0.0	0.00	5	2.40	367	51	72	42
Round, top round, separable lean only, all grades								
cooked, braised, trimmed to ¼" fat	0.0	0.00	3	2.82	284	38	76	25
cooked, braised, trimmed to 0" fat	0.0	0.00	3	2.82	284	28	76	23
cooked, broiled, trimmed to ¼" fat	0.0	0.00	5	2.45	376	52	71	24
Round, top round, separable lean only, choice								
cooked, braised, trimmed to ¼" fat	0.0	0.00	3	2.82	284	38	76	27
cooked, braised, trimmed to 0" fat	0.0	0.00	3	2.82	284	38	76	25
cooked, broiled, trimmed to ¼" fat	0.0	0.00	5	2.45	376	52	71	28
cooked, pan-fried, trimmed to ¼" fat	0.0	0.00	4	2.68	436	60	82	34
Round, top round, lean only, select								
cooked, braised, trimmed to ¼" fat	0.0	0.00	3	2.82	284	38	76	21
cooked, braised, trimmed to 0" fat	0.0	0.00	3	2.82	284	38	76	19
cooked, broiled, trimmed to ¼" fat	0.0	0.00	5	2.45	376	52	71	20
Round, top round, separable lean only, prime								
cooked, broiled, trimmed to ¼" fat	0.0	0.00	5	2.45	376	52	71	37
Shank crosscuts, trimmed to ¼" fat, choice								
raw, separable lean & fat	0.0	0.00	16	1.85	304	51	38	50
cooked, simmered, separable lean & fat	0.0	0.00	25	2.97	344	52	68	50
cooked, simmered, separable lean only	0.0	0.00	27	3.28	380	54	66	28

BEEF PRODUCTS

FOOD	AMOUNT	CALO-RIES (kcal)	PROTEIN (g)	FAT (g)	SATU-RATED FAT (g)	MONO-UN-SATURATED FAT (g)	POLY-UN-SATURATED FAT (g)
Short loin, porterhouse steak, trimmed to 1/4" fat, choice							
raw, separable lean & fat	1 lb	1230	80.20	98.41	42.63	3.69	40.50
cooked, broiled, separable lean & fat	3 oz	260	21.11	18.79	7.90	0.71	7.58
cooked, broiled, separable lean only	3 oz	185	23.94	9.18	3.68	0.34	3.67
Short loin, T-bone steak, trimmed to 1/4" fat, choice							
raw, separable lean & fat	1 lb	1235	79.84	99.15	42.94	3.72	40.78
cooked, broiled, separable lean & fat	3 oz	253	21.24	17.99	7.56	0.68	7.25
cooked, broiled, separable lean only	3 oz	182	23.91	8.81	3.54	0.33	3.53
Short loin, top loin, separable lean & fat, all grades							
raw, trimmed to 1/4" fat	1 lb	1101	86.19	81.30	35.30	2.92	33.05
cooked, broiled, trimmed to 1/4" fat	3 oz	244	21.73	16.79	7.06	0.60	6.65
cooked, broiled, trimmed to 0" fat	3 oz	181	23.87	8.72	3.56	0.29	3.37
Short loin, top loin, separable lean & fat, choice							
raw, trimmed to 1/4" fat	1 lb	1179	84.98	90.46	39.27	3.25	36.75
cooked, broiled, trimmed to 1/4" fat	3 oz	253	21.58	17.83	7.50	0.64	7.06
cooked, broiled, trimmed to 0" fat	3 oz	193	23.71	10.22	4.18	0.34	3.96
Short loin, top loin, separable lean & fat, select							
raw, trimmed to 1/4" fat	1 lb	1044	86.79	74.62	32.41	2.68	30.39
cooked, broiled, trimmed to 1/4" fat	3 oz	226	22.03	14.60	6.15	0.52	5.78
cooked, broiled, trimmed to 0" fat	3 oz	169	23.87	7.48	3.06	0.25	2.90
Short loin, top loin, separable lean & fat, prime							
raw, trimmed to 1/4" fat	1 lb	1385	83.17	114.16	50.27	4.13	46.85
cooked, broiled, trimmed to 1/4" fat	3 oz	275	21.58	20.25	8.61	0.73	8.16
Short loin, top loin, separable lean only, all grades							
cooked, broiled, trimmed to 1/4" fat	3 oz	176	24.33	7.99	3.21	0.26	3.05
cooked, broiled, trimmed to 0" fat	3 oz	168	24.33	7.14	2.87	0.23	2.72
Short loin, top loin, separable lean only, choice							
cooked, broiled, trimmed to 1/4" fat	3 oz	182	24.33	8.63	3.47	0.28	3.29
cooked, broiled, trimmed to 0" fat	3 oz	177	24.33	8.16	3.28	0.26	3.11
Short loin, top loin, separable lean only, select							
cooked, broiled, trimmed to 1/4" fat	3 oz	164	24.33	6.63	2.66	0.22	2.53
cooked, broiled, trimmed to 0" fat	3 oz	157	24.33	5.86	2.36	0.19	2.24

FOOD	CARBO-HYDRATES (mg)	FIBER (mg)	CALCIUM (mg)	IRON (mg)	POTAS-SIUM (mg)	SODIUM (mg)	CHOLES-TEROL (mg)	% OF CALORIES FROM FAT
Short loin, porterhouse steak, trimmed to ¼" fat, choice								
raw, separable lean & fat	0.0	0.00	28	8.00	1340	224	311	72
cooked, broiled, separable lean & fat	0.0	0.00	7	2.24	299	52	70	65
cooked, broiled, separable lean only	0.0	0.00	6	2.55	346	56	68	45
Short loin, T-bone steak, trimmed to ¼" fat, choice								
raw, separable lean & fat	0.0	0.00	28	8.00	1340	224	311	72
cooked, broiled, separable lean & fat	0.0	0.00	7	2.25	302	52	70	64
cooked, broiled, separable lean only	0.0	0.00	6	2.55	346	56	68	44
Short loin, top loin, separable lean & fat, all grades								
raw, trimmed to ¼" fat	0.0	0.00	27	7.19	1339	242	302	66
cooked, broiled, trimmed to ¼" fat	0.0	0.00	8	1.90	297	54	67	62
cooked, broiled, trimmed to 0" fat	0.0	0.00	7	2.06	330	57	65	43
Short loin, top loin, separable lean & fat, choice								
raw, trimmed to ¼" fat	0.0	0.00	27	7.09	1313	239	306	69
cooked, broiled, trimmed to ¼" fat	0.0	0.00	8	1.88	294	54	68	63
cooked, broiled, trimmed to 0" fat	0.0	0.00	7	2.05	327	57	65	48
Short loin, top loin, separable lean & fat, select								
raw, trimmed to ¼" fat	0.0	0.00	27	7.23	1352	243	300	64
cooked, broiled, trimmed to ¼" fat	0.0	0.00	8	1.92	301	54	67	58
cooked, broiled, trimmed to 0" fat	0.0	0.00	7	2.06	330	57	65	40
Short loin, top loin, separable lean & fat, prime								
raw, trimmed to ¼" fat	0.0	0.00	28	6.95	1275	235	311	74
cooked, broiled, trimmed to ¼" fat	0.0	0.00	8	1.88	294	54	68	66
Short loin, top loin, separable lean only, all grades								
cooked, broiled, trimmed to ¼" fat	0.0	0.00	7	2.10	337	58	65	41
cooked, broiled, trimmed to 0" fat	0.0	0.00	7	2.10	337	58	65	38
Short loin, top loin, separable lean only, choice								
cooked, broiled, trimmed to ¼" fat	0.0	0.00	7	2.10	337	58	65	43
cooked, broiled, trimmed to 0" fat	0.0	0.00	7	2.10	337	58	65	41
Short loin, top loin, separable lean only, select								
cooked, broiled, trimmed to ¼" fat	0.0	0.00	7	2.10	337	58	65	36
cooked, broiled, trimmed to 0" fat	0.0	0.00	7	2.10	337	58	65	34

BEEF PRODUCTS

FOOD	AMOUNT	CALO-RIES (kcal)	PROTEIN (g)	FAT (g)	SATU-RATED FAT (g)	MONO-UN-SATURATED FAT (g)	POLY-UN-SATURATED FAT (g)
Short loin, top loin, separable lean only, prime							
cooked, broiled, trimmed to ¼" fat	3 oz	208	24.33	11.57	4.82	0.40	4.63
Tenderloin, lean & fat, all grades							
raw, trimmed to ¼" fat	1 lb	1286	80.58	104.41	44.20	4.04	42.24
cooked, broiled, trimmed to ¼" fat	3 oz	247	21.47	17.22	7.06	0.65	6.76
cooked, broiled, trimmed to 0" fat	3 oz	200	23.11	11.18	4.42	0.42	4.29
cooked, roasted, trimmed to ¼" fat	3 oz	282	20.07	21.76	9.11	0.88	8.61
Tenderloin, lean & fat, choice							
raw, trimmed to ¼" fat	1 lb	1308	80.58	106.82	44.86	3.90	43.14
cooked, broiled, trimmed to ¼" fat	3 oz	259	21.32	18.57	7.60	0.70	7.28
cooked, broiled, trimmed to 0" fat	3 oz	208	22.97	12.17	4.82	0.46	4.68
cooked, roasted, trimmed to ¼" fat	3 oz	288	20.07	22.42	9.30	0.85	8.86
Tenderloin, lean & fat, select							
raw, trimmed to ¼" fat	1 lb	1261	80.58	101.65	43.13	3.91	41.21
cooked, broiled, trimmed to ¼" fat	3 oz	231	21.77	15.25	6.25	0.58	5.98
cooked, broiled, trimmed to 0" fat	3 oz	194	23.11	10.62	4.20	0.40	4.08
cooked, roasted, trimmed to ¼" fat	3 oz	275	20.07	21.01	8.81	0.84	8.33
Tenderloin, lean & fat, prime							
raw, trimmed to ¼" fat	1 lb	1290	81.21	104.59	44.48	4.13	42.96
cooked, broiled, trimmed to ¼" fat	3 oz	270	21.17	19.87	8.23	0.77	7.93
cooked, roasted, trimmed to ¼" fat	3 oz	300	20.12	23.70	9.82	0.91	9.46
Tenderloin, lean only, all grades							
cooked, broiled, trimmed to ¼" fat	3 oz	179	24.01	8.50	3.21	0.32	3.18
cooked, broiled, trimmed to 0" fat	3 oz	175	24.01	8.07	3.05	0.30	3.02
cooked, roasted, trimmed to ¼" fat	3 oz	189	23.55	9.76	3.81	0.44	3.68
Tenderloin, lean only, choice							
cooked, broiled, trimmed to ¼" fat	3 oz	188	24.01	9.52	3.59	0.36	3.56
cooked, broiled, trimmed to 0" fat	3 oz	180	24.01	8.58	3.24	0.32	3.21
cooked, roasted, trimmed to ¼" fat	3 oz	196	23.55	10.62	4.06	0.40	4.01
Tenderloin, lean only, select							
cooked, broiled, trimmed to ¼" fat	3 oz	169	24.01	7.39	2.79	0.28	2.76
cooked, broiled, trimmed to 0" fat	3 oz	170	24.01	7.48	2.82	0.28	2.80
cooked, roasted, trimmed to ¼" fat	3 oz	180	23.55	8.77	3.42	0.40	3.31
Tenderloin, lean only, prime							
cooked, broiled, trimmed to ¼" fat	3 oz	197	24.01	10.51	4.09	0.42	4.11
cooked, roasted, trimmed to ¼" fat	3 oz	217	23.41	12.98	5.05	0.51	5.07

FOOD	CARBO-HYDRATES (mg)	FIBER (mg)	CALCIUM (mg)	IRON (mg)	POTAS-SIUM (mg)	SODIUM (mg)	CHOLES-TEROL (mg)	% OF CALORIES FROM FAT
Short loin, top loin, separable lean only, prime								
cooked, broiled, trimmed to 1/4" fat	0.0	0.00	7	2.10	337	58	65	50
Tenderloin, lean & fat, all grades								
raw, trimmed to 1/4" fat	0.0	0.00	32	10.37	1337	218	322	73
cooked, broiled, trimmed to 1/4" fat	0.0	0.00	7	2.68	313	50	73	63
cooked, broiled, trimmed to 0" fat	0.0	0.00	6	2.91	341	52	72	50
cooked, roasted, trimmed to 1/4" fat	0.0	0.00	8	2.60	277	48	73	69
Tenderloin, lean & fat, choice								
raw, trimmed to 1/4" fat	0.0	0.00	32	10.37	1337	218	322	74
cooked, broiled, trimmed to 1/4" fat	0.0	0.00	7	2.66	310	50	73	65
cooked, broiled, trimmed to 0" fat	0.0	0.00	6	2.89	338	52	72	53
cooked, roasted, trimmed to 1/4" fat	0.0	0.00	8	2.60	340	55	73	70
Tenderloin, lean & fat, select								
raw, trimmed to 1/4" fat	0.0	0.00	32	10.37	1337	218	322	73
cooked, broiled, trimmed to 1/4" fat	0.0	0.00	7	2.72	318	51	73	59
cooked, broiled, trimmed to 0" fat	0.0	0.00	6	2.91	341	52	72	49
cooked, roasted, trimmed to 1/4" fat	0.0	0.00	8	2.60	277	48	73	69
Tenderloin, lean & fat, prime								
raw, trimmed to 1/4" fat	0.0	0.00	31	10.47	1352	219	320	73
cooked, broiled, trimmed to 1/4" fat	0.0	0.00	7	2.64	308	50	73	66
cooked, roasted, trimmed to 1/4" fat	0.0	0.00	7	2.60	281	47	75	71
Tenderloin, lean only, all grades								
cooked, broiled, trimmed to 1/4" fat	0.0	0.00	6	3.04	356	54	71	43
cooked, broiled, trimmed to 0" fat	0.0	0.00	6	3.04	356	54	71	42
cooked, roasted, trimmed to 1/4" fat	0.0	0.00	6	3.14	333	52	70	46
Tenderloin, lean only, choice								
cooked, broiled, trimmed to 1/4" fat	0.0	0.00	6	3.04	356	54	71	46
cooked, broiled, trimmed to 0" fat	0.0	0.00	6	3.04	356	54	71	43
cooked, roasted, trimmed to 1/4" fat	0.0	0.00	7	3.14	416	61	70	49
Tenderloin, lean only, select								
cooked, broiled, trimmed to 1/4" fat	0.0	0.00	6	3.04	356	54	71	39
cooked, broiled, trimmed to 0" fat	0.0	0.00	6	3.04	356	54	71	40
cooked, roasted, trimmed to 1/4" fat	0.0	0.00	6	3.14	333	52	70	44
Tenderloin, lean only, prime								
cooked, broiled, trimmed to 1/4" fat	0.0	0.00	6	3.04	356	54	71	48
cooked, roasted, trimmed to 1/4" fat	0.0	0.00	6	3.11	334	50	73	54

BEEF PRODUCTS

FOOD	AMOUNT	CALO-RIES (kcal)	PROTEIN (g)	FAT (g)	SATU-RATED FAT (g)	MONO-UN-SATURATED FAT (g)	POLY-UN-SATURATED FAT (g)
Top sirloin, lean & fat, all grades							
raw, trimmed to ¼" fat	1 lb	986	86.88	68.21	29.14	2.66	27.26
cooked, broiled, trimmed to ¼" fat	3 oz	219	23.63	13.10	5.63	0.50	5.22
cooked, broiled, trimmed to 0" fat	3 oz	183	24.98	8.48	3.63	0.33	3.35
Top sirloin, separable lean & fat, trimmed to ¼" fat, choice							
raw, trimmed to ¼" fat	1 lb	1031	86.29	73.49	31.36	2.87	29.32
cooked, broiled, trimmed to ¼" fat	3 oz	228	23.47	14.22	6.11	0.54	5.67
cooked, broiled, trimmed to 0" fat	3 oz	194	24.81	9.82	4.21	0.38	3.88
cooked, pan-fried, trimmed to ¼" fat	3 oz	277	23.90	19.42	8.19	1.48	7.58
Top sirloin, lean & fat, select							
raw, trimmed to ¼" fat	1 lb	937	87.47	62.50	26.74	2.42	25.05
cooked, broiled, trimmed to ¼" fat	3 oz	208	23.80	11.81	5.08	0.45	4.71
cooked, broiled, trimmed to 0" fat	3 oz	166	25.25	6.42	2.76	0.25	2.55
Top sirloin, lean only, all grades							
cooked, broiled, trimmed to ¼" fat	3 oz	165	25.81	6.12	2.61	0.24	2.38
cooked, broiled, trimmed to 0" fat	3 oz	162	25.81	5.78	2.46	0.23	2.25
Top sirloin, lean only, choice							
cooked, broiled, trimmed to ¼" fat	3 oz	172	25.81	6.80	2.90	0.26	2.65
cooked, broiled, trimmed to 0" fat	3 oz	170	25.81	6.63	2.82	0.26	2.58
cooked, pan-fried, trimmed to ¼" fat	3 oz	202	27.61	9.32	3.77	1.28	3.42
Top sirloin, separable lean only, select							
cooked, broiled, trimmed to ¼" fat	3 oz	158	25.81	5.27	2.24	0.21	2.05
cooked, broiled, trimmed to 0" fat	3 oz	153	25.81	4.76	2.03	0.19	1.85
Ground, extra lean, raw	4 oz	265	21.13	19.27	8.38	0.80	7.70
cooked, baked, medium	3 oz	213	20.80	13.72	6.01	0.51	5.39
cooked, baked, well done	3 oz	232	25.76	13.58	5.95	0.51	5.34
cooked, broiled, medium	3 oz	217	21.59	13.88	6.08	0.52	5.45
cooked, broiled, well done	3 oz	225	24.29	13.43	5.88	0.50	5.28
cooked, pan-fried, medium	3 oz	216	21.22	13.96	6.11	0.52	5.48
cooked, pan-fried, well done	3 oz	224	23.79	13.56	5.94	0.51	5.33
Ground, lean, raw	4 oz	298	19.98	23.35	10.18	0.96	9.39
cooked, baked, medium	3 oz	227	20.34	15.59	6.82	0.58	6.12
cooked, baked, well done	3 oz	248	25.16	15.60	6.83	0.58	6.13
cooked, broiled, medium	3 oz	231	21.01	15.69	6.87	0.58	6.16
cooked, broiled, well done	3 oz	238	23.97	14.99	6.56	0.56	5.89
cooked, pan-fried, medium	3 oz	234	20.60	16.20	7.09	0.60	6.36
cooked, pan-fried, well done	3 oz	235	23.43	15.02	6.58	0.56	5.90
Ground, regular, raw	4 oz	351	18.78	30.00	13.15	1.22	12.18
cooked, baked, medium	3 oz	244	19.57	17.79	7.79	0.66	6.99
cooked, baked, well done	3 oz	269	24.48	18.25	7.99	0.68	7.17
cooked, broiled, medium	3 oz	246	20.46	17.59	7.70	0.66	6.91
cooked, broiled, well done	3 oz	248	23.12	16.54	7.24	0.62	6.50
cooked, pan-fried, medium	3 oz	260	20.33	19.18	8.39	0.71	7.53
cooked, pan-fried, well done	3 oz	243	22.95	16.08	7.04	0.60	6.32
Ground patties, frozen, raw	4 oz	319	19.33	26.20	11.45	1.07	10.58
cooked, broiled, medium	3 oz	240	20.83	16.70	7.31	0.62	6.56

FOOD	CARBO-HYDRATES (mg)	FIBER (mg)	CALCIUM (mg)	IRON (mg)	POTAS-SIUM (mg)	SODIUM (mg)	CHOLES-TEROL (mg)	% OF CALORIES FROM FAT
Top sirloin, lean & fat, all grades								
raw, trimmed to 1/4" fat	0.0	0.00	34	10.79	1423	242	304	62
cooked, broiled, trimmed to 1/4" fat	0.0	0.00	10	2.60	311	53	76	54
cooked, broiled, trimmed to 0" fat	0.0	0.00	9	2.76	330	55	76	42
Top sirloin, separable lean & fat, trimmed to 1/4" fat, choice								
raw, trimmed to 1/4" fat	0.0	0.00	34	10.71	1410	241	306	64
cooked, broiled, trimmed to 1/4" fat	0.0	0.00	10	2.58	309	53	76	56
cooked, broiled, trimmed to 0" fat	0.0	0.00	10	2.74	328	55	76	46
cooked, pan-fried, trimmed to 1/4" fat	0.0	0.00	10	2.83	336	59	83	63
Top sirloin, lean & fat, select								
raw, trimmed to 1/4" fat	0.0	0.00	34	10.88	1437	243	303	60
cooked, broiled, trimmed to 1/4" fat	0.0	0.00	10	2.62	314	54	76	51
cooked, broiled, trimmed to 0" fat	0.0	0.00	9	2.79	334	55	76	35
Top sirloin, lean only, all grades								
cooked, broiled, trimmed to 1/4" fat	0.0	0.00	9	2.86	343	56	76	33
cooked, broiled, trimmed to 0" fat	0.0	0.00	9	2.86	343	56	76	32
Top sirloin, lean only, choice								
cooked, broiled, trimmed to 1/4" fat	0.0	0.00	9	2.86	343	56	76	36
cooked, broiled, trimmed to 0" fat	0.0	0.00	9	2.86	343	56	76	35
cooked, pan-fried, trimmed to 1/4" fat	0.0	0.00	9	3.31	395	65	84	42
Top sirloin, separable lean only, select								
cooked, broiled, trimmed to 1/4" fat	0.0	0.00	9	2.86	343	56	76	30
cooked, broiled, trimmed to 0" fat	0.0	0.00	9	2.86	343	56	76	28
Ground, extra lean, raw	0.0	0.00	7	2.20	321	75	78	65
cooked, baked, medium	0.0	0.00	6	1.94	190	42	70	58
cooked, baked, well done	0.0	0.00	7	2.52	247	54	91	53
cooked, broiled, medium	0.0	0.00	6	2.00	266	59	71	58
cooked, broiled, well done	0.0	0.00	7	2.35	314	70	84	54
cooked, pan-fried, medium	0.0	0.00	6	2.01	265	59	69	58
cooked, pan-fried, well done	0.0	0.00	7	2.32	306	69	79	54
Ground, lean, raw	0.0	0.00	9	1.99	295	78	85	71
cooked, baked, medium	0.0	0.00	8	1.78	190	47	66	62
cooked, baked, well done	0.0	0.00	10	2.26	243	61	84	57
cooked, broiled, medium	0.0	0.00	9	1.79	256	65	74	61
cooked, broiled, well done	0.0	0.00	10	2.08	296	76	86	57
cooked, pan-fried, medium	0.0	0.00	8	1.85	254	65	71	62
cooked, pan-fried, well done	0.0	0.00	9	2.11	289	74	81	58
Ground, regular, raw	0.0	0.00	10	1.96	258	77	96	77
cooked, baked, medium	0.0	0.00	8	2.05	188	51	74	66
cooked, baked, well done	0.0	0.00	10	2.54	233	63	92	61
cooked, broiled, medium	0.0	0.00	9	2.07	248	70	76	64
cooked, broiled, well done	0.0	0.00	10	2.33	278	79	86	60
cooked, pan-fried, medium	0.0	0.00	10	2.08	255	71	75	66
cooked, pan-fried, well done	0.0	0.00	11	2.30	283	79	83	60
Ground patties, frozen, raw	0.0	0.00	9	2.01	280	77	89	74
cooked, broiled, medium	0.0	0.00	9	1.79	250	66	80	63

BEEF PRODUCTS

FOOD	AMOUNT	CALO-RIES (kcal)	PROTEIN (g)	FAT (g)	SATU-RATED FAT (g)	MONO-UN-SATURATED FAT (g)	POLY-UN-SATURATED FAT (g)
Brain, raw	1 oz	36	2.78	2.63	0.53	0.30	0.61
cooked, pan-fried	3 oz	167	10.68	13.46	3.38	1.96	3.18
cooked, simmered	3 oz	136	9.41	10.65	2.13	1.23	2.48
Heart, raw	1 oz	33	4.83	1.07	0.24	0.26	0.32
cooked, simmered	3 oz	148	24.47	4.77	1.06	1.16	1.43
Kidneys, raw	1 oz	30	4.70	0.87	0.19	0.19	0.28
cooked, simmered	3 oz	122	21.66	2.92	0.63	0.63	0.93
Liver, raw	1 oz	40	5.67	1.09	0.14	0.24	0.42
cooked, braised	3 oz	137	20.72	4.16	0.55	0.91	1.62
cooked, pan-fried	3 oz	184	22.71	6.80	1.38	1.45	2.27
Lungs, raw	1 oz	26	4.59	0.71	0.18	0.10	0.24
cooked, braised	3 oz	102	17.34	3.15	0.81	0.43	0.83
Mechanically separated beef, raw	1 oz	78	4.24	6.67	2.39	0.22	3.34
Pancreas, raw	1 oz	67	4.45	5.27			
cooked, braised	3 oz	230	23.04	14.62			
Spleen, raw	1 oz	30	125.00	5.19			
cooked, braised	3 oz	123	21.34	3.57			
Suet, raw	1 oz	242	0.43	26.65	8.94	0.90	14.83
Tallow	1 tbsp	115	0.00	12.80	5.35	0.51	6.37
Thymus							
raw	1 oz	67	3.45	5.77			
cooked, braised	3 oz	271	18.57	21.23			
Tongue, raw	1 oz	63	4.22	4.56	2.09	0.25	1.95
cooked, simmered	3 oz	241	18.80	17.63	8.05	0.66	7.59
Tripe, raw	1 oz	28	4.13	1.12	0.37	0.02	0.58
Cured, breakfast strips							
raw or unheated	1 pkg	1381	42.50	131.92	63.52	7.45	54.23
cooked	3 slices	153	10.64	11.70	5.73	0.54	4.88
Cured, corned beef, brisket							
raw	1 lb	896	66.58	67.59	32.57	2.42	21.44
cooked	3 oz	213	15.44	16.13	7.83	0.57	5.39

ENTREES

FOOD	AMOUNT	CALO-RIES (kcal)	PROTEIN (g)	FAT (g)	SATU-RATED FAT (g)	MONO-UN-SATURATED FAT (g)	POLY-UN-SATURATED FAT (g)
Americana, Light Balance®	234 g	170	9.00	3.00		1.00	1.00
Beef pot pie, home recipe, 1/3 of 9" pie	210 g	515	21.00	30.00			
Beefsteak ranchero, Lean Cuisine®	262 g	270	16.00	9.00		1.00	3.00
Bordeaux, w/pasta, Light Balance®	234 g	180	12.00	1.00	0.67	0.16	0.16
Beef stew w/vegetables	1 cup	220	16.00	11.00			
home recipe	1 cup	221	22.60	5.25	2.10	0.32	1.85
Campbell's® Stroganoff	1 oz	30	1.40	1.49	0.48	0.29	0.60
Legout® chef style	1 oz	28	20.00	1.83			
Burgundy, efficiency frozen dinner	142 g	144	17.00	5.00			
Light & Elegant®	255 g	230	23.00	4.00			
Chili con Carne w/beans, canned	1 cup	340	19.00	16.00			
Chop suey w/beef & pork, home recipe	1 cup	300	26.00	17.00			

FOOD	CARBO-HYDRATES (mg)	FIBER (mg)	CALCIUM (mg)	IRON (mg)	POTAS-SIUM (mg)	SODIUM (mg)	CHOLES-TEROL (mg)	% OF CALORIES FROM FAT
Brain, raw	0.0	0.00	2	0.61	91	29	474	66
cooked, pan-fried	0.0	0.00	8	1.89	301	134	1696	73
cooked, simmered	0.0	0.00	8	1.88	204	102	1746	70
Heart, raw	0.7	0.00	1	1.31	75	18	40	29
cooked, simmered	0.3	0.00	5	6.38	198	54	164	29
Kidneys, raw	0.6	0.00	2	2.09	73	51	81	26
cooked, simmered	0.8	0.00	15	6.21	152	114	329	22
Liver, raw	1.6	0.00	2	1.93	92	21	100	25
cooked, braised	2.9	0.00	6	5.75	200	59	331	27
cooked, pan-fried	6.6	0.00	9	5.34	309	90	410	33
Lungs, raw	0.0	0.00	3	2.25	96	56	69	25
cooked, braised	0.0	0.00	9	4.59	147	86	236	28
Mechanically separated beef, raw	0.0	0.00	137	1.61			59	77
Pancreas, raw	0.0	0.00	2	0.63	78	19		71
cooked, braised	0.0	0.00	14	2.22	209	51		57
Spleen, raw	0.8	0.00	2	12.63	122	24	75	156
cooked, braised	0.0	0.00	10	33.46	242	48	295	26
Suet, raw	0.0	0.00			5		19	99
Tallow	0.0	0.00			0	0	14	100
Thymus								
raw	0.0	0.00		0.60	102	27	63	78
cooked, braised	0.0	0.00		1.27	368	99	250	71
Tongue, raw	1.0	0.00	2	0.84	89	20	25	65
cooked, simmered	0.2	0.00	6	2.88	153	51	91	66
Tripe, raw	0.0	0.00		0.55	77	13	27	36
Cured, breakfast strips								
raw or unheated	2.3	0.00		4.18	520	3247	279	86
cooked	0.4	0.00		1.07	140	766	40	69
Cured, corned beef, brisket								
raw	0.6	0.00	30	7.66	1348	5519	245	68
cooked	0.4	0.00	7	1.58	123	964	83	68
ENTREES								
Americana, Light Balance®	28.0			1.44		700	15	16
Beef pot pie, home recipe, 1/3 of 9" pie	39.0	3.90	29	3.80	334	596	44	52
Beefsteak ranchero, Lean Cuisine®	30.0		40	1.44	430	950	40	30
Bordeaux, w/pasta, Light Balance®	31.0	1.50	15.4	1.80	462	660	25	5
Beef stew w/vegetables	15.0	3.19	29	2.90	613	1006	72	45
home recipe	20.1		32	3.15	527	461	60	21
Campbell's® Stroganoff	2.6	0.17	5.57	0.25	39.73	113.8	5.95	45
Legout® chef style	1.6		0.3	73.30	125		0.667	58
Burgundy, efficiency frozen dinner	6.0		5	0.60	147	411		31
Light & Elegant®	25.0	1.61	14.2	3.10	200	1235	94.7	16
Chili con Carne w/beans, canned	31.0	5.00	82	4.30	594	1354	38	42
Chop suey w/beef & pork, home recipe	13.0		60	4.80	425	1052	64	51

BEEF PRODUCTS

FOOD	AMOUNT	CALO-RIES (kcal)	PROTEIN (g)	FAT (g)	SATU-RATED FAT (g)	MONO-UN-SATURATED FAT (g)	POLY-UN-SATURATED FAT (g)
ENTREES (continued)							
Chow mein/chop suey with noodles	28.4 g	53	3.00	2.83	1.50	0.44	0.65
Stouffers® chop suey & rice	340 g	300	16.00	9.00			
Corned beef hash, canned	1 cup	400	19.00	25.00			
Legout®	28.4 g	48	6.00	2.50			
Cream chipped beef, Stouffer® dinner	156 g	235	12.00	16.00	5.72	3.12	4.94
Creamed, sliced, cured, Legout®	28.4 g	25	1.33	1.17			
Cubes in wine sauce, Hormel®	28.4 g	52	4.00	3.61	1.60	0.14	1.87
Dijon, pasta, vegetable, Right Course®	269 g	290	20.00	9.00		1.00	2.00
Dinner, Swanson®	28.4 g	28	2.31	0.53	0.26	0.08	0.74
in barbecue sauce	28.4 g	42	2.73	1.55	0.72	0.08	0.74
frozen dinner	326 g	320	25.00	9.00	4.34	1.38	3.27
Enchilada							
Healthy Choice®	380 g	370	15.00	5.00		2.00	2.00
Swanson® dinner	28.4 g	35	1.24	1.53	0.64	0.43	0.46
Fajita	158 g	244	11.00	10.30	4.68	1.16	3.87
Fiesta, corn pasta, Right Course®	252 g	270	18.00	7.00		2.00	2.00
Green peppers, Stouffer®	220 g	225	10.00	11.00			
Julienne, Light & Elegant®	241 g	260	21.00	7.00			
Hamburger Helper®							
beef noodle, dry	1 cup	150	4.00	2.00	0.51	0.10	0.45
beef Romanoff, dry	1 cup	180	7.00	3.00			
beef taco, dry	1 cup	160	4.00	1.00	0.44	0.04	0.52
cheddar, bacon, dry	1 cup	190	6.00	6.00			
cheeseburger, macaroni, dry	1 cup	190	6.00	6.00			
cheesy Italian, dry	1 cup	170	6.00	4.00			
chili macaroni, dry	1 cup	150	4.00	1.00			
hamburger hash, dry	1 cup	140	3.00	2.00			
hamburger stew, dry	1 cup	120	3.00	1.00			
lasagna, dry	1 cup	160	4.00	1.00			
meat loaf, dry	17 g	70	2.00	1.00			
nacho cheese, dry	1 cup	160	4.00	2.00			
pizza dish, dry	1 cup	180	6.00	1.00			
pizzabake, dry	38.9 g	150	4.00	2.00			
potatoes au gratin, dry	1 cup	140	4.00	2.00			
potatoes Stroganoff, dry	1 cup	140	3.00	3.00			
rice oriental, dry	1 cup	180	4.00	1.00			
sloppy Joe bake, dry	44.9 g	180	5.00	3.00	1.48	0.16	1.36
spaghetti, dry	1 cup	160	6.00	1.00			
stroganoff, dry	1 cup	190	5.00	5.00			
tacobake, dry	42.5 g	170	4.00	4.00			
zesty Italian, dry	1 cup	170	6.00	1.00			
Meatballs							
Bernardi®	28.4 g	80	5.00	7.00	2.02	0.00	3.00
Chef Boyardee® stew	227 g	330	10.00	23.00			
La Loma® frozen	10 g	27	3.14	1.14			
Stouffer® dinner w/noodles	312 g	475	25.00	27.00			

FOOD	CARBO-HYDRATES (mg)	FIBER (mg)	CALCIUM (mg)	IRON (mg)	POTAS-SIUM (mg)	SODIUM (mg)	CHOLES-TEROL (mg)	% OF CALORIES FROM FAT
ENTREES (continued)								
Chow mein/chop suey with noodles	3.9	0.43	5.47	0.51	64.5	116	6.46	48
Stouffers® chop suey & rice	38.0	5.19	20	1.44	280	1170	77.5	27
Corned beef hash, canned	24.0		29	4.40	440	1188	50	56
Legout®	3.5		3.33	0.90	90	193		47
Cream chipped beef, Stouffer® dinner	10.0	0.16	127	1.65	290	900	27.6	61
Creamed, sliced, cured, Legout®	2.5		3.33	0.60	42.5	223		42
Cubes in wine sauce, Hormel®	1.0		2.8	0.47	71	106	15	62
Dijon, pasta, vegetable, Right Course®	31.0		40	2.70	270	580	40	28
Dinner, Swanson®	0.0	0.37	7.27	0.41	100	78.2	17.7	17
in barbecue sauce	0.0	0.37	7.27	0.41	100	78.2	17.7	33
frozen dinner	34.0	3.34	35.6	3.98	616	1085	83.8	25
Enchilada								
Healthy Choice®	66.0		150	1.80	600	450	30	12
Swanson® dinner	4.0	0.42	14.5	0.20	37	98.2	2.51	39
Fajita	27.5	2.15	69.2	2.32	296	247	26	38
Fiesta, corn pasta, Right Course®	33.0		60	2.70	430	590	30	23
Green peppers, Stouffer®	18.0		0	2.33	420	960		44
Julienne, Light & Elegant®	27.0		27	4.90	240	990		24
Hamburger Helper®								
beef noodle, dry	29.0	0.60	0	0.72	50	920	15.6	12
beef Romanoff, dry	31.0		60	1.44	200	1030		15
beef taco, dry	33.0	0.30	20	1.08	120	930	20.8	6
cheddar, bacon, dry	27.0		60	0.72	125	900		28
cheeseburger, macaroni, dry	28.0		60	1.08	190	980		28
cheesy Italian, dry	27.0		40	1.08	175	970		21
chili macaroni, dry	32.0		20	1.08	210	920		6
hamburger hash, dry	27.0		20	0.72	970			13
hamburger stew, dry	26.0		40	1.08	330	960		8
lasagna, dry	33.0		20	1.08	220	860		6
meat loaf, dry	13.0		20	0.72	120	620		13
nacho cheese, dry	32.0		20	0.72	80	980		11
pizza dish, dry	37.0		20	1.80	290	960		5
pizzabake, dry	29.0		40	1.44	180	800		12
potatoes au gratin, dry	27.0		40	0.72	340	820		13
potatoes Stroganoff, dry	26.0		40	0.36	350	930		19
rice oriental, dry	38.0		20	1.08	110	1070		5
sloppy Joe bake, dry	33.0	0.45	100	1.44	220	1060	14.4	15
spaghetti, dry	32.0		20	1.44	300	1060		6
stroganoff, dry	30.0		20	1.08	100	800		24
tacobake, dry	31.0		40	1.80	160	920		21
zesty Italian, dry	35.0		20	1.44	290	940		5
Meatballs								
Bernardi®	2.0	0.20	20	0.72	110	220	15	79
Chef Boyardee® stew	22.0	0.00	20	1.80	570	1470	40	63
La Loma® frozen	1.0		2.86	0.26	24.3	60		38
Stouffer® dinner w/noodles	33.0				395	1620		51

BEEF PRODUCTS

FOOD	AMOUNT	CALO-RIES (kcal)	PROTEIN (g)	FAT (g)	SATU-RATED FAT (g)	MONO-UN-SATURATED FAT (g)	POLY-UN-SATURATED FAT (g)
ENTREES (continued)							
Meatloaf							
w/celery & onions	87.6 g	213	15.80	13.90			
plate dinner w/potatoes & peas	28.4 g	37	2.27	1.90			
Banquet®frozen dinner	312 g	412	20.90	23.70	9.13	2.90	7.45
Healthy Choice®	340 g	340	17.00	8.00		1.00	3.00
La Loma ®savory loaf dinner mix, dry	1 cup	200	36.00	0.00			
Swanson®dinner	28.4 g	34	1.40	1.40	0.72	0.09	0.60
Oriental							
Budget Gourmet Light®	284 g	290	17.00	9.00	3.01	0.78	2.34
La Choy®pepper	300 g	216	17.70	4.50			
Lean Cuisine®frozen dinner	245 g	250	18.00	7.00			
Pepper steak							
Budget Gourmet®w/rice	284 g	300	15.00	9.00	2.85	4.13	2.02
Healthy Choice®	312 g	260	20.00	5.00		1.00	2.00
Le Menu®	28.4 g	32	2.26	1.13	0.36	0.52	0.25
frozen dinner	326 g	360	26.00	13.00			
Ultra Slim Fast®w/rice	340 g	310	23.00	5.00	2.98	0.67	1.34
Pie, Stouffers®	284 g	500	20.00	32.00	15.00	7.71	9.29
Pot roast							
beef w/potatoes & peas, plate dinner	1 oz	30	3.71	0.91			
Light & Healthy®budget	298 g	210	23.00	8.00			
Right Course®homestyle	262 g	220	17.00	7.00		1.00	2.00
Potpie, home recipe	210 g	515	21.00	30.00	12.90	7.40	7.90
Swanson®	28.4 g	53	1.71	2.71	0.82	0.43	0.52
Swanson Hungry Man®	28.4 g	38	1.50	1.94	0.82	0.43	0.52
Ragout & rice pilaf, Right Course®	284 g	300	19.00	8.00		1.00	2.00
Ribs, w/barbecue sauce, Healthy Choice®	312 g	330	28.00	6.00		2.00	2.00
Salisbury steak							
Banquet®frozen dinner	312 g	390	18.10	24.60	8.41	2.08	7.34
Budget Light®sirloin	241 g	260	15.00	13.00	5.20	0.72	7.08
Healthy Choice®	326 g	280	19.00	7.00		1.00	3.00
w/gravy	312 g	280	21.00	6.00		1.00	3.00
Le Menu®	28.4 g	35	1.90	1.90	0.77	0.19	0.67
light	298 g	220	18.00	7.00	4.09	0.58	2.33
Lean Cuisine®	269 g	280	25.00	15.00			
Light & Healthy®sirloin	312 g	260	21.00	9.00	5.35	0.73	2.92
Swanson®dinner	28.4 g	37	1.67	1.58	0.75	0.19	0.65
homestyle	28.4 g	32	2.10	1.60	0.76	0.19	0.66
Short ribs							
Hormel®in barbecue sauce	28.4 g	54	4.70	3.30	1.35	0.21	1.67
Stouffers®in gravy	255 g	350	30.00	20.00			
Sirloin							
Budget Gourmet Light®herb	269 g	270	20.00	10.00	3.28	0.44	3.86
Healthy Choice®w/barbecue sauce	312 g	280	17.00	4.00		1.00	2.00
Le Menu®chopped	28.4 g	35	2.04	1.96	0.83	0.13	1.00

FOOD	CARBO-HYDRATES (mg)	FIBER (mg)	CALCIUM (mg)	IRON (mg)	POTAS-SIUM (mg)	SODIUM (mg)	CHOLES-TEROL (mg)	% OF CALORIES FROM FAT
ENTREES (continued)								
Meatloaf								
w/celery & onions	5.2	0.11	22.8	1.91	182	103	107	59
plate dinner w/potatoes & peas	2.7	0.50	5.39	0.37	32.6	111	8.79	46
Banquet® frozen dinner	29.0	5.44	84	4.30	468	1991	79	52
Healthy Choice®	48.0		40	3.60	690	560	40	21
La Loma ® savory loaf dinner mix, dry	16.0		80	2.88	560	1520		0
Swanson® dinner	3.8	0.10	9.3	0.07	76.9	89.3	23.6	38
Oriental								
Budget Gourmet Light®	36.0	1.31	42.4	4.66	390	810	30	28
La Choy® pepper	29.4	0.12	49.5			480	34.2	19
Lean Cuisine® frozen dinner	28.0				270	1150	35	25
Pepper steak								
Budget Gourmet® w/rice	39.0	1.37	40	0.72	729	800	25	27
Healthy Choice®	40.0		20	1.08	230	500	40	17
Le Menu®	3.1	0.14	3.48	0.31	72.9	88.7	9.49	32
frozen dinner	34.0					1045		33
Ultra Slim Fast® w/rice	43.0	1.75	54	4.12	290	530	45	15
Pie, Stouffers®	33.0	2.93	40	2.70	300	1300	47.4	58
Pot roast								
beef w/potatoes & peas, plate dinner	1.7	0.31	2.83	0.45	69.2	73.4	14.2	27
Light & Healthy® budget	19.0	7.00	32	1.80	580	440	65	34
Right Course® homestyle	22.0		20	1.44	480	550	35	29
Potpie, home recipe	39.0	3.90	29	3.80	334	596	44	52
Swanson®	5.1	0.36	2.86	0.39	80.4	104	5.72	46
Swanson Hungry Man®	3.6	0.36	2.5	0.28	80.4	85	5.72	46
Ragout & rice pilaf, Right Course®	38.0		40	1.80	320	550	50	24
Ribs, w/barbecue sauce, Healthy Choice®	40.0		60	1.80	670	530	70	16
Salisbury steak								
Banquet® frozen dinner	24.0	5.34	90	3.50	387	2059	86.1	57
Budget Light® sirloin	20.0	3.15	28	2.21	400	700	65	45
Healthy Choice®	45.0		60	2.70	590	550	50	23
w/gravy	35.0		60	2.70	630	500	55	19
Le Menu®	2.6	0.49	9.52	0.26	86.2	83.8	7.84	49
light	21.0	3.40	147	3.30	535	830	45	29
Lean Cuisine®	11.0				650	800	95	48
Light & Healthy® sirloin	28.0	6.00	154	1.80	620	510	30	31
Swanson® dinner	4.0	0.49	5.58	0.25	86.2	81.9	7.84	38
homestyle	2.2	0.49	4	0.27	86.2	98	7.84	45
Short ribs								
Hormel® in barbecue sauce	1.3	0.80	3	0.73	92	176	15	55
Stouffers® in gravy	12.0	0.00	40	2.70	400	900	238	51
Sirloin								
Budget Gourmet Light® herb	25.0	3.27	43.7	2.98	540	720	60	33
Healthy Choice® w/barbecue sauce	44.0		40	1.80	630	240	25	13
Le Menu® chopped	2.2	0.44	12.2	0.29	64.3	82.4	11.4	50

BEEF PRODUCTS

FOOD	AMOUNT	CALORIES (kcal)	PROTEIN (g)	FAT (g)	SATURATED FAT (g)	MONO-UN-SATURATED FAT (g)	POLY-UN-SATURATED FAT (g)
ENTREES (continued)							
Sirloin (continued)							
Light & Healthy® in wine sauce	312 g	230	17.00	6.00	3.35	0.88	1.76
Swanson® chopped	28.4 g	32	1.86	1.49	0.63	0.10	0.76
Sirloin tips							
Budget Gourmet® w/vegetables	284 g	310	16.00	18.00	2.04	0.42	1.88
Healthy Choice®	319 g	270	22.00	7.00		2.00	3.00
Le Menu®	28.4 g	35	2.61	1.57	0.20	0.04	0.19
frozen dinner	326 g	400	29.00	19.00			
Swanson® homestyle, in sauce	28.4 g	23	1.71	0.71	0.20	0.04	0.19
Sizzle burger, La Loma® frozen	71 g	220	17.00	12.00			
Sliced, Swanson Hungry Man®	28.4 g	30	2.43	0.79	0.37	0.12	0.29
Smoked, slices, Worthington® frozen	9.33 g	20	1.67	1.00			
Stakelets, frozen, Worthington®	71 g	150	13.00	8.00			
Steak							
Stouffers® w/green peppers, rice	298 g	330	21.00	11.00	3.89	1.67	3.18
Swanson Hungry Man® chopped	28.4 g	38	2.09	2.21	1.09	0.09	1.02
Stew							
w/vegetables	1 cup	220	16.00	11.00	4.50	0.50	4.90
Chef Boyardee® w/meatballs	227 g	330	10.00	23.00			
Hormel®	28.4 g	29	2.20	1.30	0.46	0.04	0.46
Lean Cuisine® w/meatballs, frozen dinner	284 g	240	22.00	7.00			
Legout® chef style	1.8 g	28	20.00	1.83			
Stroganoff, frozen dinner	170 g	192	20.00	8.00			
Budget Gourmet Light®	248 g	290	19.00	12.00			
Le Menu®	28.4 g	43	2.60	2.40	0.72	0.64	1.04
Light & Elegant®	255 g	260	24.00	6.00			
Stouffers® w/noodles	278 g	390	24.00	20.00	5.91	5.24	8.35
Swedish meatballs							
Hormel® in sauce	28.4 g	44	2.70	3.01	1.13	0.18	1.70
Le Menu® light	241 g	260	18.00	8.00		2.00	3.00
Swiss steak							
Hormel® in gravy	28.4 g	34	3.50	1.90	0.99	0.20	0.66
Swanson® dinner	28.4 g	35	2.60	1.10	0.42	0.35	0.32
Szechwan, with noodles, Lean Cuisine®	262 g	260	20.00	10.00		2.00	3.00
Teriyaki							
Light & Elegant®	227 g	240	18.00	3.00			
Stouffers® w/rice, vegetable	276 g	290	22.00	8.00	3.57	1.44	2.70
Tips, country style, Ultra Slim Fast®	340 g	230	21.00	5.00			
Turf & surf, Classic Lite® frozen dinner	283 g	250	29.00	8.00			
Yankee pot roast							
Healthy Choice®	312 g	260	19.00	4.00		1.00	2.00
Le Menu®	28.4 g	33	2.60	1.30	0.66	0.05	0.59
frozen dinner	312 g	360	27.00	15.00			

FOOD	CARBO-HYDRATES (mg)	FIBER (mg)	CALCIUM (mg)	IRON (mg)	POTAS-SIUM (mg)	SODIUM (mg)	CHOLES-TEROL (mg)	% OF CALORIES FROM FAT
ENTREES (continued)								
Sirloin (continued)								
Light & Healthy® in wine sauce	33.0	6.00	50.7	1.80	430	570	30	23
Swanson® chopped	2.6	0.44	5.58	0.25	64.3	73.5	11.4	42
Sirloin tips								
Budget Gourmet® w/vegetables	21.0	2.62	60	0.36	504	570	40	52
Healthy Choice®	29.0		20	1.80	520	360	65	23
Le Menu®	2.5	0.26	5.22	0.31	50.4	66.1	5.74	41
frozen dinner	27.0					1100		43
Swanson® homestyle, in sauce	2.2	0.26	5.71	0.26	50.4	78.6	5.74	28
Sizzle burger, La Loma® frozen	10.0		0	0.18	310	420		49
Sliced, Swanson Hungry Man®	3.2	0.29	2.62	0.30	60.1	69.5	6.4	24
Smoked, slices, Worthington® frozen	1.1		0	0.18	11.7	132		45
Stakelets, frozen, Worthington®	7.0		40	1.08	105	460		48
Steak								
Stouffers® w/green peppers, rice	36.0	1.53	20	1.80	410	1440	69.9	30
Swanson Hungry Man® chopped	2.4	0.00	3.58	0.32	103	95.5	23.5	52
Stew								
w/vegetables	15.0	3.19	29	2.90	613	1006	72	45
Chef Boyardee® w/meatballs	22.0	0.00	20	1.80	570	1470	40	63
Hormel®	2.0		3.8	0.21	51	106	6.5	40
Lean Cuisine® w/meatballs, frozen dinner	21.0				410	1250	65	26
Legout® chef style	1.6		0.3	73.30	125		0.667	58
Stroganoff, frozen dinner	8.0		23	2.90	316	785		38
Budget Gourmet Light®	27.0	1.30	90.3	3.51	280	570	85	37
Le Menu®	2.8	0.15	10	0.27	61.2	98	9.31	50
Light & Elegant®	27.0	1.34	45	3.00	230	785	83.6	21
Stouffers® w/noodles	28.0	1.78	60	2.70	300	1090	78.2	46
Swedish meatballs								
Hormel® in sauce	1.6	0.09	14.9	0.49	87	165	8	62
Le Menu® light	30.0					700	40	28
Swiss steak								
Hormel® in gravy	0.9	0.45	5.2	0.46	86	110	8	50
Swanson® dinner	3.7	0.21	4	0.36	82.5	70	8.23	28
Szechwan, with noodles, Lean Cuisine®	22.0		40	1.80	320	680	100	35
Teriyaki								
Light & Elegant®	37.0		29.6	5.60	215	625		11
Stouffers® w/rice, vegetable	33.0	1.46	40	1.80	380	1450	52.4	25
Tips, country style, Ultra Slim Fast®	26.0	0.98	31.4	7.01	520	960	45	20
Turf & surf, Classic Lite® frozen dinner	15.0							29
Yankee pot roast								
Healthy Choice®	36.0		40	1.80	350	400	55	14
Le Menu®	2.7	0.00	4	0.36	71.3	70	28.4	35
frozen dinner	29.00					830		38

LAMB, VEAL & GAME PRODUCTS

FOOD	AMOUNT	CALORIES (kcal)	PROTEIN (g)	FAT (g)	MONO-UN-SATURATED FAT (g)	POLY-UN-SATURATED FAT (g)	SATURATED FAT (g)
LAMB, domestic							
Composite of trimmed retail cuts, separable lean & fat, choice							
raw	1 oz	76	4.79	6.13	2.52	0.48	2.69
cooked	3 oz	250	20.85	17.80	7.50	1.29	7.51
Composite of trimmed retail cuts, separable lean only, choice							
raw	1 oz	38	5.76	1.49	0.60	0.14	0.53
cooked	3 oz	175	23.99	8.09	3.55	0.53	2.89
Composite of trimmed retail cuts, separable fat, choice							
raw	1 oz	189	1.89	20.05	8.27	1.52	9.16
cooked	3 oz	498	10.33	50.30	20.74	3.81	22.96
Foreshank, separable lean & fat, choice							
raw	1 oz	57	5.37	3.80	1.56	0.30	1.66
cooked, braised	3 oz	206	24.12	11.44	4.83	0.82	4.79
Foreshank, separable lean only, choice							
raw	1 oz	34	5.99	0.93	0.38	0.09	0.33
cooked, braised	3 oz	159	26.36	5.12	2.24	0.34	1.83
Leg, whole (shank & sirloin), separable lean & fat, choice							
raw	1 oz	65	5.09	4.85	1.99	0.38	2.11
cooked, roasted	3 oz	219	21.72	14.01	5.92	1.01	5.85
Leg, whole (shank & sirloin), separable lean only, choice							
raw	1 oz	36	5.84	1.28	0.52	0.12	0.46
cooked, roasted	3 oz	162	24.05	6.58	2.88	0.43	2.35
Leg, shank half, separable lean & fat, choice							
raw	1 oz	57	5.28	3.83	1.57	0.31	1.65
cooked, roasted	3 oz	191	22.45	10.58	4.49	0.75	4.33
Leg, shank half, separable lean only, choice							
raw	1 oz	36	5.83	1.19	0.48	0.11	0.43
cooked, roasted	3 oz	153	23.94	5.67	2.49	0.37	2.03
Leg, sirloin half, separable lean & fat, choice							
raw	1 oz	77	4.81	6.28	2.58	0.49	2.76
cooked, roasted	3 oz	248	20.93	17.57	7.40	1.27	7.43
Leg, sirloin half, separable lean only, choice							
raw	1 oz	38	5.84	1.44	0.58	0.13	0.52
cooked, roasted	3 oz	173	24.1	7.80	3.42	0.51	2.79
Loin, separable lean & fat, choice							
raw	1 oz	88	4.64	7.56	3.11	0.59	3.34
cooked, broiled	3 oz	268	21.4	19.62	8.24	1.42	8.36
cooked, roasted	3 oz	263	19.17	20.05	8.22	1.59	8.71

FOOD	CARBO-HYDRATES (g)	CALCIUM (mg)	IRON (mg)	POTAS-SIUM (mg)	SODIUM (mg)	CHOLES-TEROL (mg)	% OF CALORIES FROM FAT
LAMB, domestic							
Composite of trimmed retail cuts, separable lean & fat, choice							
raw	0	3	0.45	65	16	20	73
cooked	0	14	1.59	263	61	83	64
Composite of trimmed retail cuts, separable lean only, choice							
raw	0	3	0.50	79	19	19	35
cooked	0	13	1.74	293	64	78	42
Composite of trimmed retail cuts, separable fat, choice							
raw	0	6	0.28	23	9	26	95
cooked	0	20	1.10	165	50	97	91
Foreshank, separable lean & fat, choice							
raw	0	3	0.47	61	20	20	60
cooked, braised	0	17	1.82	218	61	90	50
Foreshank, separable lean only, choice							
raw	0	3	0.51	67	22	19	25
cooked, braised	0	17	1.93	227	63	89	29
Leg, whole (shank & sirloin), separable lean & fat, choice							
raw	0	2	0.47	71	16	20	67
cooked, roasted	0	9	1.69	266	56	79	58
Leg, whole (shank & sirloin), separable lean only, choice							
raw	0	2	0.52	82	18	18	32
cooked, roasted	0	7	1.81	287	58	76	37
Leg, shank half, separable lean & fat, choice							
raw	0	2	0.48	74	16	19	60
cooked, roasted	0	8	1.68	277	55	77	50
Leg, shank half, separable lean only, choice							
raw	0	2	0.52	82	17	18	30
cooked, roasted	0	7	1.75	291	56	74	33
Leg, sirloin half, separable lean & fat, choice							
raw	0	3	0.46	66	16	20	73
cooked, roasted	0	10	1.70	256	58	82	64
Leg, sirloin half, separable lean only, choice							
raw	0	2	0.52	81	18	19	34
cooked, roasted	0	7	1.87	283	60	78	41
Loin, separable lean & fat, choice							
raw	0	4	0.46	61	16	21	77
cooked, broiled	0	17	1.54	278	65	85	66
cooked, roasted	0	16	1.80	209	54	80	69

LAMB, VEAL & GAME PRODUCTS

FOOD	AMOUNT	CALORIES (kcal)	PROTEIN (g)	FAT (g)	MONO-UN-SATURATED FAT (g)	POLY-UN-SATURATED FAT (g)	SATURATED FAT (g)
LAMB, domestic (continued)							
Loin, separable lean only, choice							
raw	1 oz	41	5.93	1.69	0.68	0.15	0.60
cooked, broiled	3 oz	183	25.49	8.27	3.62	0.54	2.95
cooked, roasted	3 oz	171	22.6	8.29	3.36	0.73	3.16
Rib, separable lean & fat, choice							
raw	1 oz	106	4.12	9.77	4.01	0.76	4.31
cooked, broiled	3 oz	307	18.81	25.15	10.30	2.02	10.80
cooked, roasted	3 oz	305	17.95	25.35	10.64	1.85	10.85
Rib, separable lean only, choice							
raw	1 oz	48	5.68	2.62	1.06	0.24	0.94
cooked, broiled	3 oz	200	23.57	11.00	4.43	1.01	3.95
cooked, roasted	3 oz	197	22.23	11.32	4.96	0.74	4.04
Shoulder, whole (arm & blade), separable lean & fat, choice							
raw	1 oz	75	4.71	6.09	2.50	0.48	2.63
cooked, braised	3 oz	292	24.38	20.87	8.53	1.70	8.79
cooked, broiled	3 oz	236	20.76	16.37	6.69	1.34	6.83
cooked, roasted	3 oz	235	19.13	16.97	6.94	1.38	7.17
Shoulder, whole (arm & blade), separable lean only, choice							
raw	1 oz	41	5.55	1.92	0.77	0.18	0.69
cooked, braised	3 oz	241	27.89	13.51	5.48	1.17	5.24
cooked, broiled	3 oz	179	23.05	8.92	3.60	0.80	3.29
cooked, roasted	3 oz	173	21.2	9.16	3.71	0.81	3.47
Shoulder, arm, separable lean & fat, choice, raw	1 oz	74	4.77	5.94	2.44	0.47	2.60
cooked, braised	3 oz	294	25.84	20.40	8.65	1.45	8.39
cooked, broiled	3 oz	239	20.78	16.62	6.81	1.33	7.12
cooked, roasted	3 oz	237	19.15	17.21	7.05	1.37	7.43
Shoulder, arm, separable lean only, choice, raw	1 oz	38	5.68	1.48	0.59	0.14	0.53
cooked, braised	3 oz	237	30.21	11.97	5.24	0.79	4.28
cooked, broiled	3 oz	170	23.55	7.67	3.10	0.68	2.90
cooked, roasted	3 oz	163	21.64	7.87	3.19	0.68	3.05
Shoulder, blade, separable lean & fat, choice, raw	1 oz	74	4.72	5.92	2.43	0.48	2.54
cooked, braised	3 oz	293	24.24	21.02	8.58	1.73	8.75
cooked, broiled	3 oz	237	19.62	16.95	7.19	1.20	6.95
cooked, roasted	3 oz	239	18.91	17.52	7.16	1.43	7.35
Shoulder, blade, separable lean only, choice, raw	1 oz	43	5.48	2.17	0.87	0.20	0.78
cooked, braised	3 oz	245	27.5	14.15	5.73	1.24	5.47
cooked, broiled	3 oz	179	21.66	9.62	4.22	0.63	3.44
cooked, roasted	3 oz	178	20.92	9.83	3.98	0.87	3.61
Cubed lamb for stew or kabob (leg & shoulder), separable lean only							
raw	1 oz	38	5.74	1.50	0.60	0.14	0.5
cooked, braised	3 oz	190	28.64	7.48	3.01	0.68	2.68
cooked, broiled	3 oz	158	23.86	6.23	2.51	0.57	2.2

FOOD	CARBO-HYDRATES (g)	CALCIUM (mg)	IRON (mg)	POTAS-SIUM (mg)	SODIUM (mg)	CHOLES-TEROL (mg)	% OF CALORIES FROM FAT
LAMB, domestic (continued)							
Loin, separable lean only, choice							
raw	0	4	0.54	78	19	19	37
cooked, broiled	0	16	1.70	320	71	80	41
cooked, roasted	0	14	2.07	227	56	74	44
Rib, separable lean & fat, choice							
raw	0	4	0.39	54	16	22	83
cooked, broiled	0	16	1.60	230	64	84	74
cooked, roasted	0	19	1.36	231	62	82	75
Rib, separable lean only, choice							
raw	0	3	0.47	75	21	19	49
cooked, broiled	0	14	1.88	266	73	78	50
cooked, roasted	0	18	1.50	268	69	74	52
Shoulder, whole (arm & blade), separable lean & fat, choice							
raw	0	4	0.43	65	17	20	73
cooked, braised	0	21	2.04	211	63	99	64
cooked, broiled	0	18	1.73	256	67	82	62
cooked, roasted	0	17	1.67	214	56	78	65
Shoulder, whole (arm & blade), separable lean only, choice							
raw	0	4	0.47	78	20	19	42
cooked, braised	0	22	2.27	222	67	99	50
cooked, broiled	0	17	1.87	276	70	79	45
cooked, roasted	0	16	1.81	225	58	74	48
Shoulder, arm, separable lean & fat, choice, raw	0	4	0.44	68	17	20	72
cooked, braised	0	21	2.03	260	61	102	62
cooked, broiled	0	16	1.78	263	65	82	63
cooked, roasted	0	15	1.72	220	55	78	65
Shoulder, arm, separable lean only, choice, raw	0	3	0.50	82	20	18	35
cooked, braised	0	22	2.30	287	64	103	45
cooked, broiled	0	15	1.96	289	70	78	41
cooked, roasted	0	14	1.90	236	57	73	43
Shoulder, blade, separable lean & fat, choice, raw	0	5	42.00	65	18	20	72
cooked, braised	0	23	2.00	206	64	99	65
cooked, broiled	0	20	1.46	286	70	81	64
cooked, roasted	0	18	1.63	209	56	79	66
Shoulder, blade, separable lean only, choice, raw	0	5	0.46	76	20	19	45
cooked, braised	0	24	2.21	216	67	99	52
cooked, broiled	0	21	1.54	312	75	78	48
cooked, roasted	0	18	1.76	220	58	74	50
Cubed lamb for stew or kabob (leg & shoulder), separable lean only							
raw	0	3	0.50	81	18	18	36
cooked, braised	0	13	2.38	221	60	92	35
cooked, broiled	0	11	1.99	285	65	77	35

LAMB, VEAL & GAME PRODUCTS

FOOD	AMOUNT	CALORIES (kcal)	PROTEIN (g)	FAT (g)	MONO-UN-SATURATED FAT (g)	POLY-UN-SATURATED FAT (g)	SATURATED FAT (g)
LAMB, domestic (continued)							
Lamb, ground, raw	1 oz	80	4.7	6.65	2.73	0.53	2.89
cooked, broiled	3 oz	240	21.04	16.70	7.07	1.19	6.90
LAMB, New Zealand, imported, frozen							
Composite of trimmed retail cuts, separable lean & fat, raw	1 oz	79	4.75	6.46	2.48	0.28	3.29
cooked	3 oz	259	20.76	18.92	7.30	0.88	9.39
Composite of trimmed retail cuts, separable lean only, raw	1 oz	36	5.89	1.25	0.48	0.06	0.53
cooked	3 oz	175	25.15	7.53	2.95	0.44	3.28
Composite of trimmed retail cuts, separable fat, raw	1 oz	182	1.97	19.21	7.36	0.80	10.02
cooked	3 oz	498	8.26	51.34	19.68	2.15	26.79
Foreshank, separable lean & fat							
raw	1 oz	63	5.12	4.59	1.76	0.20	2.32
cooked, braised	3 oz	219	22.93	13.45	5.18	0.62	6.64
Foreshank, separable lean, raw	1 oz	34	5.91	0.93	0.36	0.05	0.40
cooked, braised	3 oz	158	26.14	5.14	2.00	0.29	2.22
Leg, whole (shank & sirloin), separable lean & fat, raw	1 oz	61	5.21	4.34	1.66	0.19	2.18
cooked, roasted	3 oz	209	21.08	13.22	5.11	0.63	6.40
Leg, whole (shank & sirloin), separable lean only, raw	1 oz	35	5.92	1.08	0.41	0.05	0.40
cooked, roasted	3 oz	154	23.53	5.96	2.34	0.35	2.59
Loin, separable lean & fat, raw	1 oz	86	4.64	7.36	2.82	0.31	3.70
cooked, broiled	3 oz	268	19.92	20.30	7.82	0.93	10.10
Loin, separable lean only, raw	1 oz	37	6.01	1.25	0.48	0.06	0.5
cooked, broiled	3 oz	170	24.91	7.00	2.74	0.40	3.0
Rib, separable lean & fat, raw	1 oz	98	4.24	8.89	3.41	0.38	4.5
cooked, roasted	3 oz	289	16.13	24.44	9.42	1.11	12.2
Rib, separable lean only, raw	1 oz	40	5.82	1.72	0.66	0.09	0.7
cooked, roasted	3 oz	167	20.76	8.64	3.39	0.50	3.7
Shoulder, whole (arm & blade), separable lean & fat, raw	1 oz	77	4.73	6.31	2.42	0.27	3.1
cooked, braised	3 oz	299	24.4	21.57	8.40	1.10	10.4
Shoulder, whole (arm & blade), separable lean only, raw	1 oz	38	5.75	1.54	0.59	0.08	0.6
cooked, braised	3 oz	242	28.95	13.17	5.22	0.81	5.7
VEAL							
Composite of trimmed retail cuts, separable lean & fat, raw	1 oz	41	5.49	1.92	0.73	0.13	0.7
cooked	3 oz	197	25.58	9.68	3.74	0.68	3.6
Composite of trimmed retail cuts, separable lean only, raw	1 oz	32	5.74	0.81	0.26	0.08	0.2
cooked	3 oz	166	27.11	5.59	2.00	0.50	1.3

FOOD	CARBO-HYDRATES (g)	CALCIUM (mg)	IRON (mg)	POTAS-SIUM (mg)	SODIUM (mg)	CHOLES-TEROL (mg)	% OF CALORIES FROM FAT
LAMB, domestic (continued)							
Lamb, ground, raw	0	4	0.44	63	17	21	75
cooked, broiled	0	19	1.52	288	69	82	63
LAMB, New Zealand, imported, frozen							
Composite of trimmed retail cuts, separable lean & fat, raw	0	4	0.42	39	11	22	74
cooked	0	14	1.78	138	39	93	66
Composite of trimmed retail cuts, separable lean only, raw	0	2	0.46	49	13	21	31
cooked	0	11	2.00	160	43	93	39
Composite of trimmed retail cuts, separable fat, raw	0	6	0.32	15	6	25	95
cooked	0	23	1.18	74	29	93	93
Foreshank, separable lean & fat							
raw	0	3	0.42	37	13	20	66
cooked, braised	0	12	1.76	101	40	87	55
Foreshank, separable lean, raw	0	2	0.45	43	14	19	25
cooked, braised	0	9	1.88	106	42	85	29
Leg, whole (shank & sirloin), separable lean & fat, raw	0	2	0.45	44	11	22	64
cooked, roasted	0	8	1.79	142	37	86	57
Leg, whole (shank & sirloin), separable lean only, raw	0	1	0.48	51	12	21	28
cooked, roasted	0	6	1.90	155	38	85	35
Loin, separable lean & fat, raw	0	5	0.44	34	11	23	77
cooked, broiled	0	19	1.74	135	41	96	68
Loin, separable lean only, raw	0	4	0.50	45	13	23	30
cooked, broiled	0	18	1.99	161	46	97	37
Rib, separable lean & fat, raw	0	5	0.40	32	11	23	82
cooked, roasted	0	16	1.45	106	37	85	76
Rib, separable lean only, raw	0	3	0.45	44	15	22	39
cooked, roasted	0	12	1.61	124	41	80	47
Shoulder, whole (arm & blade), separable lean & fat, raw	0	5	0.38	38	12	21	74
cooked, braised	0	23	1.81	127	44	104	65
Shoulder, whole (arm & blade), separable lean only, raw	0	4	0.41	46	13	20	36
cooked, braised	0	23	1.99	141	48	108	49
VEAL							
Composite of trimmed retail cuts, separable lean & fat, raw	0	4	0.24	89	23	23	42
cooked	0	19	0.98	276	74	97	44
Composite of trimmed retail cuts, separable lean only, raw	0	4	0.24	93	24	23	23
cooked	0	20	0.99	288	76	100	30

LAMB, VEAL & GAME PRODUCTS

FOOD	AMOUNT	CALORIES (kcal)	PROTEIN (g)	FAT (g)	MONO-UN-SATURATED FAT (g)	POLY-UN-SATURATED FAT (g)	SATURATED FAT (g)
VEAL (continued)							
Composite of trimmed retail cuts, separable fat, raw	1 oz	181	1.71	19.26	8.08	0.93	9.35
cooked	3 oz	546	8.01	56.73	23.78	2.74	27.53
Leg (top round), separable lean & fat, raw	1 oz	33	5.96	0.87	0.32	0.07	0.33
cooked, braised	3 oz	180	30.74	5.38	2.01	0.40	2.15
cooked, pan-fried, breaded	3 oz	194	23.2	7.81	2.89	1.26	2.60
cooked, pan-fried, not breaded	3 oz	179	26.99	7.10	2.75	0.50	2.68
cooked, roasted	3 oz	136	23.54	3.96	0.17	0.30	1.57
Leg (top round), separable lean only, raw	1 oz	30	6.04	0.50	0.16	0.05	0.15
cooked, braised	3 oz	172	31.2	4.33	1.57	0.35	1.63
cooked, pan-fried, breaded	3 oz	175	24.15	5.33	1.84	1.15	1.36
cooked, pan-fried, not breaded	3 oz	156	28.2	3.93	1.40	0.35	1.10
cooked, roasted	3 oz	128	23.86	2.88	1.02	0.25	1.04
Loin, separable lean & fat, raw	1 oz	46	5.37	2.60	1.00	0.17	1.10
cooked, braised	3 oz	242	25.66	14.63	5.72	0.98	5.72
cooked, roasted	3 oz	184	21.08	10.47	4.07	0.69	4.47
Loin, separable lean only, raw	1 oz	33	5.73	0.95	0.30	0.10	0.29
cooked, braised	3 oz	192	28.53	7.78	2.78	0.70	2.17
cooked, roasted	3 oz	149	22.37	5.90	2.12	0.49	2.19
Rib, separable lean & fat, raw	1 oz	46	5.36	2.56	0.97	0.18	1.05
cooked, braised	3 oz	214	27.57	10.65	3.95	0.80	4.21
cooked, roasted	3 oz	194	20.37	11.87	4.63	0.81	4.60
Rib, separable lean only, raw	1 oz	34	5.67	1.11	0.36	0.11	0.33
cooked, braised	3 oz	185	29.27	6.64	2.23	0.63	2.18
cooked, roasted	3 oz	151	21.89	6.32	2.26	0.57	1.72
Shoulder, whole (arm & blade), separable lean & fat, raw	1 oz	37	5.47	1.50	0.55	0.12	0.58
cooked, braised	3 oz	194	27.25	8.62	3.31	0.62	3.19
cooked, roasted	3 oz	156	21.52	7.16	2.69	0.52	2.8
Shoulder, whole (arm & blade), separable lean only, raw	1 oz	32	5.62	0.85	0.27	0.09	0.2
cooked, braised	3 oz	169	28.62	5.19	1.85	0.47	1.4
cooked, roasted	3 oz	144	21.94	5.62	2.04	0.45	2.1
Shoulder, arm, separable lean & fat, raw	1 oz	37	5.49	1.55	0.59	0.11	0.6
cooked, braised	3 oz	201	28.58	8.71	3.39	0.59	3.3
cooked, roasted	3 oz	156	21.64	7.01	2.72	0.46	2.9
Shoulder, arm, separable lean only							
raw	1 oz	30	5.69	0.61	0.20	0.06	0.1
cooked, braised	3 oz	171	30.37	4.53	1.62	0.41	1.2
cooked, roasted	3 oz	139	22.21	4.94	1.84	0.37	1.9
Shoulder, blade, separable lean & fat, raw	1 oz	37	5.46	1.48	0.53	0.12	0.5
cooked, braised	3 oz	191	26.57	8.58	3.28	0.63	3.1
cooked, roasted	3 oz	158	21.38	7.37	2.75	0.55	2.9

FOOD	CARBO-HYDRATES (g)	CALCIUM (mg)	IRON (mg)	POTAS-SIUM (mg)	SODIUM (mg)	CHOLES-TEROL (mg)	% OF CALORIES FROM FAT
VEAL (continued)							
Composite of trimmed retail cuts, separable fat, raw	0	2	0.17	30	7	21	96
cooked	0	3	0.85	147	48	62	94
Leg (top round), separable lean & fat, raw	0	1	0.22	104	18	22	24
cooked, braised	0	7	1.12	325	57	114	27
cooked, pan-fried, breaded	8	33	1.40	315	386	95	36
cooked, pan-fried, not breaded	0	5	0.75	362	64	89	36
cooked, roasted	0	5	0.77	330	58	87	26
Leg (top round), separable lean only, raw	0	1	0.23	106	18	22	15
cooked, braised	0	7	1.13	329	57	115	23
cooked, pan-fried, breaded	8	33	1.39	326	387	96	27
cooked, pan-fried, not breaded	0	6	0.74	375	65	91	23
cooked, roasted	0	5	0.77	334	58	88	20
Loin, separable lean & fat, raw	0	5	0.21	86	24	23	51
cooked, braised	0	24	0.92	238	68	100	54
cooked, roasted	0	16	0.74	276	79	87	51
Loin, separable lean only, raw	0	5	0.21	92	26	23	26
cooked, braised	0	27	0.93	253	71	107	36
cooked, roasted	0	18	0.73	289	82	90	36
Rib, separable lean & fat, raw	0	4	0.24	82	25	23	50
cooked, braised	0	19	1.20	260	81	118	45
cooked, roasted	0	10	0.82	251	78	94	55
Rib, separable lean only, raw	0	4	0.25	87	27	24	29
cooked, braised	0	20	1.23	270	84	123	32
cooked, roasted	0	10	0.82	264	82	97	38
Shoulder, whole (arm & blade), separable lean & fat, raw	0	6	0.26	86	26	25	36
cooked, braised	0	29	1.21	263	80	107	40
cooked, roasted	0	23	0.87	274	81	96	41
Shoulder, whole (arm & blade), separable lean only, raw	0	6	0.26	88	26	25	24
cooked, braised	0	31	1.23	271	83	110	28
cooked, roasted	0	23	0.87	278	82	97	35
Shoulder, arm, separable lean & fat, raw	0	6	0.28	93	24	23	38
cooked, braised	0	24	1.17	283	74	126	39
cooked, roasted	0	22	0.98	296	76	92	40
Shoulder, arm, separable lean only raw	0	6	0.29	96	24	24	18
cooked, braised	0	26	1.20	295	76	132	24
cooked, roasted	0	23	0.98	302	77	93	32
Shoulder, blade, separable lean & fat, raw	0	6	0.25	82	27	25	36
cooked, braised	0	32	1.22	252	84	130	40
cooked, roasted	0	24	0.85	260	85	100	42

LAMB, VEAL & GAME PRODUCTS

FOOD	AMOUNT	CALORIES (kcal)	PROTEIN (g)	FAT (g)	MONO-UN-SATURATED FAT (g)	POLY-UN-SATURATED FAT (g)	SATURATED FAT (g)
VEAL (continued)							
Shoulder, blade, separable lean only, raw	1 oz	32	5.58	0.93	0.30	0.10	0.28
cooked, braised	3 oz	168	27.76	5.50	1.97	0.49	1.54
cooked, roasted	3 oz	146	21.79	5.84	2.10	0.48	2.18
Sirloin, separable lean & fat, raw	1 oz	43	5.41	2.22	0.86	0.14	0.95
cooked, braised	3 oz	214	26.57	11.17	4.38	0.74	4.40
cooked, roasted	3 oz	171	21.37	8.89	3.47	0.57	3.83
Sirloin, separable lean only, raw	1 oz	31	5.74	0.74	0.24	0.08	0.22
cooked, braised	3 oz	173	28.86	5.53	1.98	0.50	1.54
cooked, roasted	3 oz	143	22.38	5.29	1.94	0.41	2.04
Cubed for stew (leg & shoulder), separable lean only, raw	1 oz	31	5.76	0.71	0.23	0.07	0.21
cooked, braised	3 oz	160	29.7	3.66	1.18	0.38	1.10
Ground, raw	1 oz	41	5.49	1.92	0.73	0.13	0.79
cooked, broiled	3 oz	146	20.72	6.43	2.41	0.47	2.59
GAME MEAT							
Antelope, raw	1 oz	32	6.36	0.58	0.14	0.13	0.21
cooked, roasted	3 oz	127	25.03	2.27	0.54	0.49	0.83
Bear, raw	1 oz	46	5.71	2.36			
cooked, simmered	3 oz	220	27.56	11.38			
Beaver, raw	1 oz	41	6.83	1.36			
cooked, roasted	3 oz	141	23.23	4.64			
Beefalo, composite of cuts, raw	1 oz	41	6.62	1.36	0.58	0.04	0.58
cooked, roasted	3 oz	160	26.06	5.37	2.28	0.17	2.28
Bison, raw	1 oz	31	6.14	0.52	0.20	0.05	0.20
cooked, roasted	3 oz	122	24.18	2.05	0.80	0.21	0.72
Boar, wild, raw	1 oz	35	6.11	0.95	0.37	0.14	0.28
cooked, roasted	3 oz	136	24.05	3.72	1.45	0.54	1.10
Buffalo, water, raw	1 oz	28	5.79	0.39	0.12	0.08	0.1
cooked, roasted	3 oz	111	22.8	1.53	0.47	0.30	0.5
Caribou, raw	1 oz	36	6.43	0.95	0.29	0.13	0.3
cooked, roasted	3 oz	142	25.31	3.76	1.13	0.52	1.4
Deer, raw	1 oz	34	6.52	0.69	0.19	0.13	0.2
cooked, roasted	3 oz	134	25.68	2.71	0.74	0.53	1.0
Elk, raw	1 oz	32	6.52	0.41	0.10	0.09	0.1
cooked, roasted	3 oz	124	25.66	1.62	0.41	0.34	0.6
Goat, raw	1 oz	31	5.85	0.65	0.29	0.05	0.2
cooked, roasted	3 oz	122	23.04	2.58	1.16	0.19	0.7
Horse, raw	1 oz	38	6.07	1.31	0.46	0.18	0.4
cooked, roasted	3 oz	149	23.92	5.14	1.80	0.72	1.6
Moose, raw	1 oz	29	6.32	0.21	0.04	0.07	0.0
cooked, roasted	3 oz	114	24.88	0.82	0.17	0.27	0.2
Muskrat, raw	1 oz	46	5.9	2.30			
cooked, roasted	3 oz	156	20.05	7.82			
Opossum cooked, roasted	3 oz	188	25.67	8.67			

FOOD	CARBO-HYDRATES (g)	CALCIUM (mg)	IRON (mg)	POTAS-SIUM (mg)	SODIUM (mg)	CHOLES-TEROL (mg)	% OF CALORIES FROM FAT
VEAL (continued)							
Shoulder, blade, separable lean only, raw	0	7	0.25	84	27	26	26
cooked, braised	0	34	1.25	259	86	135	29
cooked, roasted	0	24	0.85	264	86	101	36
Sirloin, separable lean & fat, raw	0	3	0.22	93	22	22	46
cooked, braised	0	15	1.02	273	67	92	47
cooked, roasted	0	11	0.78	299	71	87	47
Sirloin, separable lean only, raw	0	3	0.23	99	23	22	21
cooked, braised	0	16	1.05	288	69	96	29
cooked, roasted	0	12	0.77	310	72	89	33
Cubed for stew (leg & shoulder), separable lean only, raw	0	5	0.25	94	24	24	21
cooked, braised	0	24	1.23	291	79	124	21
Ground, raw	0	4	0.24	89	23	23	42
cooked, broiled	0	14	0.84	287	70	87	40
GAME MEAT							
Antelope, raw	0	1	0.91	100	14	27	16
cooked, roasted	0	4	3.57	316	46	107	16
Bear, raw	0	1	1.89				46
cooked, simmered	0	4	9.12				47
Beaver, raw	0	4	1.96	99	14		30
cooked, roasted	0	14	6.66	269	39		30
Beefalo, composite of cuts, raw	0	5	0.66	124	22	13	30
cooked, roasted	0	21	2.59	390	70	49	30
Bison, raw	0	2	0.74	97	15	18	15
cooked, roasted	0	7	2.91	307	48	70	15
Boar, wild, raw	0	3					24
cooked, roasted	0	13					25
Buffalo, water, raw	0	3	0.46	84	15	13	13
cooked, roasted	0	13	1.81	266	48	52	12
Caribou, raw	0	5	1.33	84	16	24	24
cooked, roasted	0	19	5.25	264	51	93	24
Deer, raw	0	1	0.97	90	15	24	18
cooked, roasted	0	6	3.80	285	46	95	18
Elk, raw	0	1	0.78	89	16	16	12
cooked, roasted	0	4	3.08	279	52	62	12
Goat, raw	0	4	0.80	109	23	16	19
cooked, roasted	0	15	3.17	344	73	64	19
Horse, raw	0	2	1.09	102	15	15	31
cooked, roasted	0	7	4.28	322	47	58	31
Moose, raw	0	1	0.91	90	19	17	7
cooked, roasted	0	5	3.59	284	58	66	6
Muskrat, raw	0	7		78	23		45
cooked, roasted	0	24		213	63		45
Opossum							
cooked, roasted	0						42

LAMB, VEAL & GAME PRODUCTS

FOOD	AMOUNT	CALORIES (kcal)	PROTEIN (g)	FAT (g)	MONO-UN-SATURATED FAT (g)	POLY-UN-SATURATED FAT (g)	SATURATED FAT (g)
GAME MEAT (continued)							
Rabbit, domesticated, composite of cuts, raw	1 oz	39	5.69	1.58	0.43	0.31	0.47
cooked, roasted	3 oz	131	19.37	5.36	1.45	1.04	1.60
cooked, stewed	3 oz	175	25.82	7.15	1.93	1.39	2.13
Rabbit, wild							
raw	1 oz	32	6.19	0.66	0.18	0.13	0.20
cooked, stewed	3 oz	147	28.06	2.99	0.81	0.58	0.89
Raccoon							
cooked, roasted	3 oz	217	24.82	12.32			
Squirrel							
raw	1 oz	34	6.03	0.91	0.34	0.27	0.11
cooked, roasted	3 oz	116	20.51	3.10	1.14	0.91	0.37
VARIETY MEATS & BYPRODUCTS							
Brain, lamb							
raw	1 oz	35	2.95	2.44	0.44	0.25	0.62
cooked, braised	3 oz	124	10.66	8.64	1.57	0.89	2.21
cooked, pan-fried	3 oz	232	14.42	18.86	3.42	1.94	4.82
Brain, veal							
raw	1 oz	34	2.93	2.33			
cooked, braised	3 oz	115	9.76	8.18			
cooked, pan-fried	3 oz	181	12.31	14.24			
Heart, lamb							
raw	1 oz	35	4.68	1.61	0.45	0.16	0.64
cooked, braised	3 oz	158	21.22	6.73	1.89	0.66	2.67
Heart, veal							
raw	1 oz	31	4.88	1.13	0.24	0.30	0.30
cooked, braised	3 oz	158	24.76	5.74	1.21	1.52	1.54
Kidneys, lamb							
raw	1 oz	28	4.47	0.84	0.18	0.16	0.28
cooked, braised	3 oz	117	20.1	3.08	0.66	0.57	1.04
Kidneys, veal							
raw	1 oz	28	4.48	0.89	0.19	0.18	0.27
cooked, braised	3 oz	139	22.37	4.81	1.05	0.96	1.48
Liver, lamb							
raw	1 oz	40	5.79	1.43	0.30	0.21	0.55
cooked, braised	3 oz	187	25.98	7.49	1.56	1.12	2.90
cooked, pan-fried	3 oz	202	21.7	10.76	2.25	1.60	4.16
Liver, veal							
raw	1 oz	38	5.07	1.24	0.27	0.20	0.46
cooked, braised	3 oz	140	18.38	5.87	1.26	0.93	2.18
cooked, pan-fried	3 oz	208	25.3	9.68	2.09	1.53	3.59
Lungs, lamb							
raw	1 oz	27	4.74	0.74			
cooked, braised	3 oz	96	16.9	2.63			
Lungs, veal							
raw	1 oz	26	4.63	0.65			
cooked, braised	3 oz	88	15.93	2.25			

FOOD	CARBO-HYDRATES (g)	CALCIUM (mg)	IRON (mg)	POTAS-SIUM (mg)	SODIUM (mg)	CHOLES-TEROL (mg)	% OF CALORIES FROM FAT
GAME MEAT (continued)							
Rabbit, domesticated, composite of cuts, raw	0	4	0.44	94	12	16	36
cooked, roasted	0	13	1.51	255	31	55	37
cooked, stewed	0	17	2.02	255	31	73	37
Rabbit, wild							
raw	0	3	0.91	107	14	23	19
cooked, stewed	0	15	4.12	292	38	104	18
Raccoon							
cooked, roasted	0						51
Squirrel							
raw	0	1	1.33	86	29	24	24
cooked, roasted	0	2	4.54	235	80	80	24
VARIETY MEATS & BYPRODUCTS							
Brain, lamb							
raw	0	3	0.50	84	32	384	63
cooked, braised	0	10	1.43	175	114	1737	63
cooked, pan-fried	0	18	1.73	304	133	2128	73
Brain, veal							
raw	0	3	0.61	89	36	452	62
cooked, braised	0	13	1.42	181	133	2635	64
cooked, pan-fried	0	9	0.91	401	150	1802	71
Heart, lamb							
raw	0	2	1.31	90	25	38	41
cooked, braised	2	12	4.69	160	54	212	38
Heart, veal							
raw	0	1	1.21	74	22	30	33
cooked, braised	0	7	3.67	169	50	150	33
Kidneys, lamb							
raw	0	4	1.81	79	44	96	27
cooked, braised	1	15	10.54	151	128	481	24
Kidneys, veal							
raw	0	3	0.95	77	50	103	29
cooked, braised	0	25	2.58	135	93	672	31
Liver, lamb							
raw	1	2	2.09	89	20	105	32
cooked, braised	2	7	7.04	188	48	426	36
cooked, pan-fried	3	8	8.67	299	105	419	48
Liver, veal							
raw	1	3	1.36	83	18	88	29
cooked, braised	2	6	2.23	174	45	477	38
cooked, pan-fried	3	10	4.45	372	112	280	42
Lungs, lamb							
raw	0		1.82	68	45		25
cooked, braised	0		3.89	108	71		25
Lungs, veal							
raw	0	2	1.48	78	31		23
cooked, braised	0	6	3.06	120	47		23

323

LAMB, VEAL & GAME PRODUCTS

FOOD	AMOUNT	CALORIES (kcal)	PROTEIN (g)	FAT (g)	MONO-UN-SATURATED FAT (g)	POLY-UN-SATURATED FAT (g)	SATURATED FAT (g)
VARIETY MEATS & BYPRODUCTS (continued)							
Mechanically separated lamb							
raw	1 oz	78	4.25	6.69			
Pancreas, lamb							
raw	1 oz	43	4.21	2.79	1.01	0.14	1.26
cooked, braised	3 oz	199	19.4	12.85	4.64	0.63	5.81
Pancreas, veal							
raw	1 oz	52	4.26	3.72			
cooked, braised	3 oz	218	24.73	12.41			
Spleen, lamb							
raw	1 oz	29	4.88	0.88			
cooked, braised	3 oz	133	22.49	4.05			
Spleen, veal							
raw	1 oz	28	5.2	0.62			
cooked, braised	3 oz	110	20.47	2.46			
Thymus, veal							
raw	1 oz	28	5.11	0.69			
cooked, braised	3 oz	148	26.84	3.65			
Tongue, lamb							
raw	1 oz	63	4.46	4.88	2.40	0.30	1.88
cooked, braised	3 oz	234	18.34	17.24	8.50	1.06	6.66
Tongue, veal							
raw	1 oz	37	4.88	1.56			
cooked, braised	3 oz	171	21.98	8.59			
ENTREES							
Moose stew, Alaska®	1 cup	54	6.6	0.50	0.01	0.02	0.01
Reindeer, stewed, Alaska®	1 cup	44	3.6	0.60		0.01	0.01
Veal marsala, light, Le Menu®	1 item	260	20	6.00			
Veal parmigiana, frozen entree	1 item	296	24	14.00	4.96	3.15	5.89
Le Menu®	1 oz	34	2.09	1.48	0.52	0.33	0.62
Swanson® dinner	1 oz	35	1.63	1.63	0.58	0.37	0.69
homestyle	1 oz	33	1.9	1.30	0.46	0.29	0.55
Swanson Hungry Man®	1 oz	32	1.75	1.42	0.00	1.41	0.01
Veal steak, Classic Lite®	1 item	280	25	8.00	3.36	1.76	2.88

FOOD	CARBO-HYDRATES (g)	CALCIUM (mg)	IRON (mg)	POTAS-SIUM (mg)	SODIUM (mg)	CHOLES-TEROL (mg)	% OF CALORIES FROM FAT
VARIETY MEATS & BYPRODUCTS (continued)							
Mechanically separated lamb							
raw	0	46					77
Pancreas, lamb							
raw	0	2	0.65	119	21	74	58
cooked, braised	0	10	1.80	247	44	340	58
Pancreas, veal							
raw	0		0.60				64
cooked, braised	0		2.02				51
Spleen, lamb							
raw	0		11.90	102	24	71	27
cooked, braised	0		32.87	211	49	327	27
Spleen, veal							
raw	0	2	2.65	103	28	97	20
cooked, braised	0	6	6.26	182	49	380	20
Thymus, veal							
raw	0	0	0.54	123	24	76	22
cooked, braised	0	2	1.71	291	56	399	22
Tongue, lamb							
raw	0	3	0.75	73	22	44	70
cooked, braised	0	8	2.24	134	57	161	66
Tongue, veal							
raw	1	2	0.77	77	23		38
cooked, braised	0	8	1.78	138	54		45
ENTREES							
Moose stew, Alaska®	6	12	1.52	100	222		8
Reindeer, stewed, Alaska®	6	6	1.00	112	4	2	12
Veal marsala, light, Le Menu®	31	37	2.27	421	800	100	21
Veal parmigiana, frozen entree	17	97	2.30	466	973	162	43
Le Menu®	3	17	0.24	84	73	22	39
Swanson® dinner	3	12	0.22	84	82	22	42
homestyle	3	8	0.18	84	96	22	35
Swanson Hungry Man®	3	11	0.25	9	101	10	40
Veal steak, Classic Lite®	27	171	3.58	932	1738	60	26

PORK PRODUCTS

FOOD	AMOUNT	CALO-RIES (kcal)	PROTEIN (g)	FAT (g)	MONO-UN-SATURATED FAT (g)	POLY-UN-SATURATED FAT (g)	SATU-RATED FAT (g)
PORK, Fresh							
Carcass, separable lean & fat, raw	1 lb	1704	63.11	159.06	72.27	17.23	56.44
Composite of trimmed retail cuts (leg, loin, shoulder, & spareribs), separable lean & fat							
raw	1 lb	979	85.97	67.80	30.05	7.02	23.94
cooked	3 oz	232	23.44	14.60	6.49	1.23	5.28
Composite of trimmed retail cuts (leg, loin, & shoulder), separable lean only, raw	1 lb	649	95.57	26.68	12.05	2.87	9.21
cooked	3 oz	180	24.88	8.22	3.70	0.64	2.90
Composite of trimmed retail cuts (loin & shoulder blade), separable lean & fat, raw	1 lb	906	88.59	58.49	26.10	6.23	20.30
cooked	3 oz	214	23.61	12.54	5.57	1.00	4.51
Composite of trimmed retail cuts (loin & shoulder blade), separable lean only, raw	1 lb	652	96.31	26.66	12.04	2.87	9.20
cooked	3 oz	179	25.05	8.03	3.59	0.61	2.84
Backfat, raw	1 lb	3685	13.25	402.30	190.30	46.97	146.12
Belly, raw	1 lb	2350	42.37	240.45	112.02	25.62	87.66
Separable fat							
raw	4 oz	721	7.16	76.51	33.83	8.15	26.57
cooked	4 oz	710	13.79	72.22	30.91	7.21	27.68
Leg (ham), whole, separable lean & fat, raw	1 lb	1109	79.04	85.57	38.02	9.13	29.68
cooked, roasted	3 oz	232	22.80	14.97	6.70	1.43	5.50
Leg (ham), whole, separable lean only, raw	1 lb	618	92.90	24.54	11.09	2.64	8.47
cooked, roasted	3 oz	179	25.00	8.02	3.78	0.72	2.80
Leg (ham), rump half, separable lean & fat, raw	1 lb	1005	85.01	71.17	31.66	7.60	24.68
cooked, roasted	3 oz	214	24.55	12.13	5.41	1.17	4.46
Leg (ham), rump half, separable lean only, raw	1 lb	624	96.36	23.52	10.63	2.53	8.12
cooked, roasted	3 oz	175	26.30	6.92	3.21	0.65	2.44
Leg (ham), shank half, separable lean & fat, raw	1 lb	1191	77.47	95.37	42.35	10.18	33.08
cooked, roasted	3 oz	246	21.54	17.05	7.67	1.60	6.26
Leg (ham), shank half, separable lean only							
Leg (ham), shank half, separable lean only, raw	1 lb	630	93.53	25.54	11.54	2.75	8.82
cooked, roasted	3 oz	183	23.98	8.92	4.27	0.77	3.08
Loin, whole, separable lean & fat							
raw	1 lb	897	89.52	57.05	25.45	6.07	19.80
cooked, braised	3 oz	206	23.05	11.90	5.29	1.03	4.47
cooked, broiled	3 oz	210	23.05	12.43	5.51	1.08	4.67
cooked, roasted	3 oz	211	23.03	12.45	5.53	1.03	4.57

FOOD	CARBO-HYDRATES (mg)	FIBER (mg)	CALCIUM (mg)	IRON (mg)	POTAS-SIUM (mg)	SODIUM (mg)	CHOLES-TEROL (mg)	% OF CALORIES FROM FAT
PORK, Fresh								
Carcass, separable lean & fat, raw	0	0	87	3.13	1147	192	334	84
Composite of trimmed retail cuts (leg, loin, shoulder, & spareribs), separable lean & fat								
raw	0	0	86	3.88	1519	250	303	62
cooked	0	0	21	0.93	301	53	77	57
Composite of trimmed retail cuts (leg, loin, & shoulder), separable lean only, raw	0	0	71	4.12	1724	256	277	37
cooked	0	0	18	0.94	319	50	73	41
Composite of trimmed retail cuts (loin & shoulder blade), separable lean & fat, raw	0	0	86	3.73	1596	232	291	58
cooked	0	0	20	0.84	307	49	73	53
Composite of trimmed retail cuts (loin & shoulder blade), separable lean only, raw	0	0	78	3.97	1744	245	273	37
cooked	0	0	19	0.91	320	48	72	40
Backfat, raw	0	0	9	0.82	295	50	259	98
Belly, raw	0	0	23	2.36	839	145	327	92
Separable fat								
raw	0	0	51	0.33	135	21	105	96
cooked	0	0	60	0.41	266	39	105	92
Leg (ham), whole, separable lean & fat, raw	0	0	24	3.88	1430	214	333	69
cooked, roasted	0	0	6	0.85	299	51	80	58
Leg (ham), whole, separable lean only, raw	0	0	27	4.58	1674	249	308	36
cooked, roasted	0	0	6	0.95	317	54	80	40
Leg (ham), rump half, separable lean & fat, raw	0	0	25	3.51	1510	274	301	64
cooked, roasted	0	0	6	0.90	318	52	81	51
Leg (ham), rump half, separable lean only, raw	0	0	27	3.95	1706	313	277	34
cooked, roasted	0	0	6	0.97	332	55	82	36
Leg (ham), shank half, separable lean & fat, raw	0	0	27	3.53	1295	249	309	72
cooked, roasted	0	0	5	0.83	287	50	78	62
Leg (ham), shank half, separable lean only								
Leg (ham), shank half, separable lean only, raw	0	0	32	4.26	1542	304	272	36
cooked, roasted	0	0	6	0.94	306	54	78	44
Loin, whole, separable lean & fat								
raw	0	0	83	3.58	1616	226	287	57
cooked, braised	0	0	18	0.91	317	41	68	52
cooked, broiled	0	0	17	0.73	357	52	68	53
cooked, roasted	0	0	15	0.84	311	45	70	53

PORK PRODUCTS

FOOD	AMOUNT	CALO-RIES (kcal)	PROTEIN (g)	FAT (g)	MONO-UN-SATURATED FAT (g)	POLY-UN-SATURATED FAT (g)	SATU-RATED FAT (g)
Loin, whole, separable lean only							
raw	1 lb	646	97.19	25.66	11.59	2.76	8.86
cooked, braised	3 oz	174	24.28	7.76	3.53	0.60	2.87
cooked, broiled	3 oz	179	24.28	8.33	3.78	0.65	3.10
cooked, roasted	3 oz	178	24.33	8.19	3.67	0.65	2.98
Backribs, separable lean & fat, raw	1 lb	1277	73.12	106.96	48.33	8.89	39.58
cooked, roasted	3 oz	315	20.62	25.14	11.44	1.97	9.34
Loin, blade (chops or roasts) bone-in, lean & fat, raw	1 lb	1293	71.75	109.43	48.65	11.68	37.95
cooked, braised (chops)	3 oz	274	18.62	21.61	9.31	1.98	8.11
cooked, broiled (chops)	3 oz	272	19.10	21.12	9.10	1.93	7.92
cooked, pan-fried (chops)	3 oz	291	18.26	23.58	9.96	2.63	8.65
cooked, roasted (roasts)	3 oz	275	20.16	20.94	9.04	1.83	7.77
Loin, blade (chops or roasts) bone-in, lean only, raw	1 lb	711	87.41	37.42	16.91	4.03	12.92
cooked, braised (chops)	3 oz	191	21.27	11.11	4.83	0.88	4.03
cooked, broiled (chops)	3 oz	199	21.55	11.81	5.13	0.94	4.30
cooked, pan-fried (chops)	3 oz	205	21.03	12.81	5.31	1.66	4.38
cooked, roasted (roasts)	3 oz	210	22.61	12.59	5.49	0.94	4.51
Loin, center loin (loin chops or roasts) bone-in, lean & fat, raw	1 lb	909	91.28	57.55	25.64	6.15	19.95
cooked, braised (loin chops)	3 oz	210	23.75	12.03	5.27	1.06	4.52
cooked, broiled (loin chops)	3 oz	204	24.40	11.10	4.98	0.83	4.08
cooked, pan-fried (loin chops)	3 oz	235	25.42	14.08	6.00	1.62	5.11
cooked, roasted (loin roasts)	3 oz	199	22.36	11.44	5.01	1.01	4.30
Loin, center loin (loin chops or roasts) bone-in, lean only, raw	1 lb	633	99.97	22.87	10.33	2.46	7.89
cooked, braised (loin chops)	3 oz	172	25.32	7.07	3.16	0.54	2.61
cooked, broiled (loin chops)	3 oz	171	25.66	6.86	3.09	0.49	2.51
cooked, pan-fried (loin chops)	3 oz	197	27.36	8.90	3.78	1.13	3.09
cooked, roasted (loin roasts)	3 oz	169	23.42	7.66	3.40	0.62	2.84
Loin, center rib (rib chops or roasts) bone-in, lean & fat, raw	1 lb	947	91.50	61.68	27.50	6.60	21.37
cooked, braised (rib chops)	3 oz	212	22.67	12.81	5.84	1.08	4.96
cooked, broiled (rib chops)	3 oz	223	24.47	13.16	5.85	1.04	4.84
cooked, pan-fried (rib chops)	3 oz	225	22.34	14.42	6.37	1.63	5.39
cooked, roasted (rib roasts)	3 oz	217	23.31	12.98	5.93	1.09	5.03
Loin, center rib (rib chops or roasts) boneless, lean & fat, raw	1 lb	959	90.26	63.57	28.36	6.80	22.02
cooked, braised (rib chops)	3 oz	216	22.35	13.42	6.13	1.12	5.20
cooked, broiled (rib chops)	3 oz	221	23.49	13.40	5.96	1.06	4.92
cooked, pan-fried (rib chops)	3 oz	232	21.95	15.35	6.76	1.77	5.71
cooked, roasted (rib roasts)	3 oz	214	22.94	12.88	5.68	1.10	4.54
Loin, center rib (rib chops or roasts) bone-in, lean only, raw	1 lb	674	100	27.26	12.32	2.93	9.41
cooked, braised (rib chops)	3 oz	175	24.10	7.99	3.82	0.57	3.12
cooked, broiled (rib chops)	3 oz	186	26.14	8.28	3.79	0.52	2.94
cooked, pan-fried (rib chops)	3 oz	185	23.89	9.24	4.17	1.14	3.38
cooked, roasted (rib roasts)	3 oz	190	24.41	9.49	4.47	0.72	3.70

FOOD	CARBO-HYDRATES (mg)	FIBER (mg)	CALCIUM (mg)	IRON (mg)	POTAS-SIUM (mg)	SODIUM (mg)	CHOLES-TEROL (mg)	% OF CALORIES FROM FAT
Loin, whole, separable lean only								
raw	0	0	75	3.80	1764	237	270	36
cooked, braised	0	0	15	0.96	329	42	67	40
cooked, broiled	0	0	14	0.77	372	54	67	42
cooked, roasted	0	0	15	0.93	322	44	69	41
Backribs, separable lean & fat, raw	0	0	145	4.15	1055	339	367	75
cooked, roasted	0	0	38	1.18	268	85	100	72
Loin, blade (chops or roasts) bone-in, lean & fat, raw	0	0	130	3.75	1277	244	325	76
cooked, braised (chops)	0	0	26	0.94	258	47	73	71
cooked, broiled (chops)	0	0	25	0.79	292	60	73	70
cooked, pan-fried (chops)	0	0	26	0.75	282	57	72	73
cooked, roasted (roasts)	0	0	29	0.94	277	26	79	69
Loin, blade (chops or roasts) bone-in, lean only, raw	0	0	103	4.63	1544	303	290	47
cooked, braised (chops)	0	0	20	1.15	277	52	71	52
cooked, broiled (chops)	0	0	19	0.93	318	68	72	53
cooked, pan-fried (chops)	0	0	19	0.91	310	66	70	56
cooked, roasted (roasts)	0	0	25	1.10	296	25	79	54
Loin, center loin (loin chops or roasts) bone-in, lean & fat, raw	0	0	109	3.49	1508	272	302	57
cooked, braised (loin chops)	0	0	22	0.89	300	50	73	52
cooked, broiled (loin chops)	0	0	28	0.68	305	49	70	49
cooked, pan-fried (loin chops)	0	0	23	0.77	361	68	78	54
cooked, roasted (loin roasts)	0	0	23	0.84	299	54	68	52
Loin, center loin (loin chops or roasts) bone-in, lean only, raw	0	0	96	3.79	1642	298	286	33
cooked, braised (loin chops)	0	0	19	0.96	312	53	72	37
cooked, broiled (loin chops)	0	0	26	0.73	319	51	70	36
cooked, pan-fried (loin chops)	0	0	20	0.83	382	73	78	41
cooked, roasted (loin roasts)	0	0	21	0.89	308	56	67	41
Loin, center rib (rib chops or roasts) bone-in, lean & fat, raw	0	0	109	3.18	1741	191	271	59
cooked, braised (rib chops)	0	0	21	0.77	329	34	62	54
cooked, broiled (rib chops)	0	0	28	0.66	340	53	70	53
cooked, pan-fried (rib chops)	0	0	20	0.62	365	42	62	58
cooked, roasted (rib roasts)	0	0	24	0.80	358	39	62	54
Loin, center rib (rib chops or roasts) boneless, lean & fat, raw	0	0	23	3.23	1741	190	271	60
cooked, braised (rib chops)	0	0	5	0.79	329	34	62	56
cooked, broiled (rib chops)	0	0	24	0.66	340	53	70	55
cooked, pan-fried (rib chops)	0	0	9	0.62	364	42	62	60
cooked, roasted (rib roasts)	0	0	5	0.79	294	41	69	54
Loin, center rib (rib chops or roasts) bone-in, lean only, raw	0	0	96	3.44	1909	206	249	36
cooked, braised (rib chops)	0	0	18	0.83	344	35	60	41
cooked, broiled (rib chops)	0	0	26	0.70	357	55	69	40
cooked, pan-fried (rib chops)	0	0	17	0.66	387	44	59	45
cooked, roasted (rib roasts)	0	0	22	0.84	372	40	61	45

PORK PRODUCTS

FOOD	AMOUNT	CALO-RIES (kcal)	PROTEIN (g)	FAT (g)	MONO-UN-SATURATED FAT (g)	POLY-UN-SATURATED FAT (g)	SATU-RATED FAT (g)
Loin, center rib (rib chops or roasts) boneless, lean only, raw	1 lb	688	98.88	29.41	13.29	3.17	10.15
cooked, braised (rib chops)	3 oz	179	23.76	8.62	4.12	0.62	3.37
cooked, broiled (rib chops)	3 oz	184	25.04	8.54	3.91	0.54	3.04
cooked, pan-fried (rib chops)	3 oz	191	23.53	10.03	4.51	1.27	3.65
cooked, roasted (rib roasts)	3 oz	182	24.49	8.61	3.81	0.72	3.01
Loin, country-style ribs, separable lean & fat, raw	1 lb	1095	77.09	84.89	37.83	9.07	29.42
cooked, braised	3 oz	251	20.29	18.28	7.89	1.62	6.81
cooked, roasted	3 oz	279	19.89	21.54	9.36	1.71	7.83
Loin, country-style ribs, separable lean only, raw	1 lb	711	87.41	37.42	16.91	4.03	12.92
cooked, braised	3 oz	199	22.13	11.56	5.03	0.91	4.20
cooked, roasted	3 oz	210	22.61	12.59	5.49	0.94	4.51
Loin, sirloin (sirloin chops or roasts), bone-in, separable lean & fat, raw	1 lb	929	87.05	61.82	27.55	6.61	21.42
cooked, braised (sirloin chops)	3 oz	208	21.55	12.84	5.58	1.19	4.73
cooked, broiled (sirloin chops)	3 oz	220	22.66	13.68	5.94	1.27	5.04
cooked, roasted (sirloin roasts)	3 oz	222	23.15	13.62	5.97	1.17	4.83
Loin, sirloin (sirloin chops or roasts), boneless, separable lean & fat, raw	1 lb	657	93.32	28.64	12.84	3.07	9.91
cooked, braised (sirloin chops)	3 oz	161	22.56	7.12	3.11	0.64	2.58
cooked, broiled (sirloin chops)	3 oz	177	25.94	7.31	3.19	0.59	2.45
cooked, roasted (sirloin roasts)	3 oz	176	24.22	8.02	3.50	0.72	2.91
Loin, sirloin (sirloin chops or roasts), bone-in, separable lean only, raw	1 lb	644	95.53	26.14	11.81	2.81	9.02
cooked, braised (sirloin chops)	3 oz	167	22.95	7.66	3.37	0.67	2.72
cooked, broiled (sirloin chops)	3 oz	181	24.19	8.60	3.78	0.75	3.07
cooked, roasted (sirloin roasts)	3 oz	183	24.49	8.75	3.85	0.74	3.08
Loin, sirloin (sirloin chops or roasts), boneless, separable lean onlyraw	1 lb	581	95.53	19.14	8.65	2.06	6.61
cooked, braised (sirloin chops)	3 oz	149	22.95	5.61	2.47	0.49	1.99
cooked, broiled (sirloin chops)	3 oz	164	26.46	5.67	2.48	0.45	1.89
cooked, roasted (sirloin roasts)	3 oz	168	24.52	7.03	3.08	0.62	2.53
Loin, sirloin (sirloin chops or roasts), boneless, separable lean only, raw	1 lb	619	93.15	24.52	10.98	2.63	8.48
cooked, broiled	3 oz	171	25.38	6.90	2.84	0.63	2.49
cooked, roasted	3 oz	147	23.63	5.14	2.09	0.46	1.82
Loin, tenderloin, separable lean only, raw	1 lb	546	95.21	15.48	6.99	1.67	5.34
cooked, broiled	3 oz	159	25.86	5.38	2.19	0.48	1.90
cooked, roasted	3 oz	139	23.92	4.09	1.64	0.35	1.41
Loin, top loin (loin chops or roasts), boneless, separable lean & fat, raw (loin chops)	1 lb	839	92.64	49.16	21.95	5.26	17.03
raw (loin roasts)	1 lb	867	91.80	52.67	23.50	5.63	18.25

FOOD	CARBO-HYDRATES (mg)	FIBER (mg)	CALCIUM (mg)	IRON (mg)	POTAS-SIUM (mg)	SODIUM (mg)	CHOLES-TEROL (mg)	% OF CALORIES FROM FAT
Loin, center rib (rib chops or roasts) boneless, lean only, raw	0	0	24	3.50	1909	205	249	38
cooked, braised (rib chops)	0	0	5	0.84	344	34	60	43
cooked, broiled (rib chops)	0	0	26	0.70	357	55	69	42
cooked, pan-fried (rib chops)	0	0	4	0.67	386	44	59	47
cooked, roasted (rib roasts)	0	0	5	0.85	308	43	70	43
Loin, country-style ribs, separable lean & fat, raw	0	0	121	4.05	1368	264	313	70
cooked, braised	0	0	25	1.04	279	50	74	66
cooked, roasted	0	0	22	0.90	292	44	78	69
Loin, country-style ribs, separable lean only, raw	0	0	103	4.63	1544	303	290	47
cooked, braised	0	0	21	1.17	293	54	74	52
cooked, roasted	0	0	25	1.10	296	25	79	54
Loin, sirloin (sirloin chops or roasts), bone-in, separable lean & fat, raw	0	0	77	4.08	1453	246	303	60
cooked, braised (sirloin chops)	0	0	15	0.99	276	44	70	56
cooked, broiled (sirloin chops)	0	0	15	0.84	325	58	73	56
cooked, roasted (sirloin roasts)	0	0	20	0.89	298	51	74	55
Loin, sirloin (sirloin chops or roasts), boneless, separable lean & fat, raw	0	0	57	3.84	1640	228	290	39
cooked, braised (sirloin chops)	0	0	11	0.92	299	39	69	40
cooked, broiled (sirloin chops)	0	0	15	1.03	317	47	78	37
cooked, roasted (sirloin roasts)	0	0	14	0.99	341	47	73	41
Loin, sirloin (sirloin chops or roasts), bone-in, separable lean only, raw	0	0	58	3.93	1677	233	286	37
cooked, braised (sirloin chops)	0	0	11	1.08	286	45	69	41
cooked, broiled (sirloin chops)	0	0	11	0.91	341	61	72	43
cooked, roasted (sirloin roasts)	0	0	17	0.95	311	54	73	43
Loin, sirloin (sirloin chops or roasts), boneless, separable lean onlyraw	0	0	58	3.93	1677	233	286	30
cooked, braised (sirloin chops)	0	0	11	0.94	302	39	69	34
cooked, broiled (sirloin chops)	0	0	16	1.05	321	48	78	31
cooked, roasted (sirloin roasts)	0	0	14	1.01	344	48	73	38
Loin, sirloin (sirloin chops or roasts), boneless, separable lean only, raw	0	0	22	5.45	1627	220	299	36
cooked, broiled	0	0	4	1.19	378	54	80	36
cooked, roasted	0	0	5	1.23	368	47	67	31
Loin, tenderloin, separable lean only, raw	0	0	22	5.58	1661	225	295	26
cooked, broiled	0	0	5	1.21	383	55	80	30
cooked, roasted	0	0	5	1.25	372	48	67	26
Loin, top loin (loin chops or roasts), boneless, separable lean & fat, raw (loin chops)	0	0	89	3.25	1787	195	265	53
raw (loin roasts)	0	0	88	3.23	1771	193	267	55

PORK PRODUCTS

FOOD	AMOUNT	CALO-RIES (kcal)	PROTEIN (g)	FAT (g)	MONO-UN-SATURATED FAT (g)	POLY-UN-SATURATED FAT (g)	SATU-RATED FAT (g)
Loin, top loin (loin chops or roasts), boneless, separable lean & fat (continued)							
cooked, braised (loin chops)	3 oz	198	23.65	10.78	4.85	0.88	4.00
cooked, broiled (loin chops)	3 oz	195	25.47	9.55	4.39	0.62	3.36
cooked, pan-fried (loin chops)	3 oz	219	24.65	12.60	5.48	1.44	4.50
cooked, roasted (loin roasts)	3 oz	192	24.49	9.72	4.50	0.67	3.54
Loin, top loin (loin chops or roasts), boneless, separable lean only (loin chops)	1 lb	639	98.88	24.09	10.88	2.59	8.31
raw (loin roasts)	1 lb	638	98.88	23.96	10.82	2.58	8.27
cooked, braised (loin chops)	3 oz	171	24.71	7.30	3.38	0.52	2.66
cooked, broiled (loin chops)	3 oz	173	26.47	6.60	3.05	0.41	2.31
cooked, pan-fried (loin chops)	3 oz	191	25.91	8.93	3.91	1.09	3.06
cooked, roasted (loin roasts)	3 oz	165	25.70	6.13	2.86	0.40	2.22
Shoulder, whole, separable lean & fat, raw	1 lb	1069	77.93	81.62	36.34	8.72	28.29
cooked, roasted	3 oz	248	19.79	18.18	8.05	1.74	6.68
Shoulder, whole, separable lean only, raw	1 lb	671	88.67	32.39	14.63	3.49	11.18
cooked, roasted	3 oz	196	21.53	11.51	5.25	1.06	4.07
Shoulder, arm picnic, separable lean & fat, raw	1 lb	1149	75.72	91.59	40.71	9.78	31.77
cooked, braised	3 oz	280	23.79	19.74	8.82	1.93	7.22
cooked, roasted	3 oz	269	19.95	20.41	9.12	2.00	7.47
Shoulder, arm picnic, separable lean only, raw	1 lb	635	89.59	27.94	12.62	3.01	9.65
cooked, braised	3 oz	211	27.42	10.38	4.92	0.99	3.54
cooked, roasted	3 oz	194	22.68	10.73	5.08	1.02	3.66
Shoulder, blade, Boston (roasts or steaks), lean & fat, raw	1 lb	989	80.13	71.76	32.03	7.68	24.86
cooked, braised (steaks)	3 oz	271	24.37	18.48	8.16	1.68	6.75
cooked, broiled (steaks)	3 oz	220	21.74	14.12	6.31	1.24	5.06
cooked, roasted (roasts)	3 oz	228	19.64	16.03	7.03	1.49	5.92
Shoulder, blade, Boston (roasts or steaks), lean only, raw	1 lb	702	87.87	36.28	16.39	3.91	12.52
cooked, braised (steaks)	3 oz	232	26.43	13.21	5.94	1.13	4.69
cooked, broiled (steaks)	3 oz	193	22.73	10.66	4.79	0.91	3.78
cooked, roasted (roasts)	3 oz	198	20.58	12.15	5.39	1.09	4.41
Spareribs, separable lean & fat							
raw	1 lb	1297	77.52	107.05	46.29	9.74	40.53
cooked, braised	3 oz	338	24.70	25.75	11.46	2.32	9.45
Ground, raw	4 oz	297	19.07	23.94	10.67	2.16	8.90
cooked	3 oz	252	21.84	17.65	7.86	1.59	6.56
Brains, raw	4 oz	14	1.16	1.04	0.19	0.16	0.23
cooked, braised	3 oz	117	10.32	8.09	1.46	1.25	1.82
Chitterlings, raw	1 oz	71	2.85	6.53	2.23	1.66	2.25
cooked, simmered	3 oz	258	8.71	24.44	8.22	6.14	8.59
Ears, frozen, raw	1 ear	263	25.37	17.06			
cooked, simmered	1 ear	183	17.55	11.88			
Feet, raw	1/2 foot	251	20.97	17.89	8.39	1.94	6.18
cooked, simmered	2.5 oz	138	13.63	8.80	4.13	0.96	3.04

FOOD	CARBO-HYDRATES (mg)	FIBER (mg)	CALCIUM (mg)	IRON (mg)	POTAS-SIUM (mg)	SODIUM (mg)	CHOLES-TEROL (mg)	% OF CALORIES FROM FAT
Loin, top loin (loin chops or roasts), boneless, separable lean & fat (continued)								
cooked, braised (loin chops)	0	0	18	0.82	346	35	64	49
cooked, broiled (loin chops)	0	0	25	0.67	345	53	69	44
cooked, pan-fried (loin chops)	0	0	18	0.69	407	47	66	52
cooked, roasted (loin roasts)	0	0	4	0.68	291	38	66	46
Loin, top loin (loin chops or roasts), boneless, separable lean only, raw (loin chops)	0	0	96	3.44	1909	206	249	34
raw (loin roasts)	0	0	96	3.44	1909	206	249	34
cooked, braised (loin chops)	0	0	19	0.86	358	36	62	38
cooked, broiled (loin chops)	0	0	26	0.70	357	55	68	34
cooked, pan-fried (loin chops)	0	0	19	0.72	425	48	65	42
cooked, roasted (loin roasts)	0	0	4	0.90	301	38	66	33
Shoulder, whole, separable lean & fat, raw	0	0	68	4.78	1368	297	324	69
cooked, roasted	0	0	20	1.12	279	58	77	66
Shoulder, whole, separable lean only, raw	0	0	65	5.54	1548	343	302	43
cooked, roasted	0	0	15	1.27	294	63	76	53
Shoulder, arm picnic, separable lean & fat, raw	0	0	24	4.47	1318	306	324	72
cooked, braised	0	0	15	1.37	314	74	93	63
cooked, roasted	0	0	16	1.01	276	59	80	68
Shoulder, arm picnic, separable lean only, raw	0	0	27	5.40	1547	372	295	40
cooked, braised	0	0	7	1.66	344	87	97	44
cooked, roasted	0	0	8	1.21	298	68	81	50
Shoulder, blade, Boston (roasts or steaks), lean & fat, raw	0	0	112	5.10	1418	287	323	65
cooked, braised (steaks)	0	0	27	1.56	331	59	96	61
cooked, broiled (steaks)	0	0	30	1.19	277	59	81	58
cooked, roasted (roasts)	0	0	24	1.23	282	57	73	63
Shoulder, blade, Boston (roasts or steaks), lean only, raw	0	0	98	5.67	1550	318	308	47
cooked, braised (steaks)	0	0	25	1.74	350	64	99	51
cooked, broiled (steaks)	0	0	28	1.32	292	63	80	50
cooked, roasted (roasts)	0	0	22	1.33	290	60	72	55
Spareribs, separable lean & fat								
raw	0	0	141	4.49	1175	345	354	74
cooked, braised	0	0	40	1.57	272	79	103	69
Ground, raw	0	0	16	1.00	324	64	81	73
cooked	0	0	19	1.10	307	62	80	63
Brains, raw	0	0	1	0.18	29	14	248	67
cooked, braised	0	0	8	1.55	166	77	2169	62
Chitterlings, raw	0	0	6	0.54	33	10	45	83
cooked, simmered	0	0	23	3.15	7	33	122	85
Ears, frozen, raw	0	0	23	2.71	62	215	93	58
cooked, simmered	0	0	20	1.65	44	183	99	58
Feet, raw	0	0	56		216	49	101	64
cooked, simmered	0	0	32				71	57

PORK PRODUCTS

FOOD	AMOUNT	CALO-RIES (kcal)	PROTEIN (g)	FAT (g)	MONO-UN-SATURATED FAT (g)	POLY-UN-SATURATED FAT (g)	SATU-RATED FAT (g)
Heart, raw	1 heart	267	39.02	9.85	2.31	2.53	2.61
cooked, braised	1 heart	191	30.44	6.51	1.52	1.67	1.72
Jowl, raw	4 oz	740	7.20	78.66	37.17	9.16	28.54
Kidneys, raw	1 kidney	232	38.34	7.57	2.50	0.60	2.42
cooked, braised	1 cup	211	35.56	6.58	2.16	0.53	2.11
Lard	1 tbsp	115	0.00	12.80	5.77	1.43	5.02
Leaf fat, raw	1 oz	243	0.50	26.69	10.55	2.06	12.82
Liver, raw	4 oz	151	24.17	4.12	0.59	0.98	1.32
cooked, braised	3 oz	141	22.12	3.74	0.53	0.90	1.20
Lungs, raw	1 oz	24	3.99	0.77	0.17	0.10	0.27
cooked, braised	3 oz	84	14.11	2.64	0.59	0.33	0.93
Mechanically separated pork, raw	8 oz	690	34.12	60.25	27.83	5.53	22.29
Pancreas, raw	4 oz	225	20.97	14.96			
cooked, braised	3 oz	186	24.23	9.18			
Spleen							
raw	4 oz	113	20.18	2.93	0.78	0.21	0.97
cooked, braised	3 oz	127	23.97	2.72	0.73	0.20	0.90
Stomach, raw	4 oz	177	18.64	10.79			
Tail, raw	4 oz	427	20.06	37.86	17.85	4.16	13.15
cooked, simmered	3 oz	336	14.45	30.43	14.36	3.35	10.58
Tongue, raw	4 oz	254	18.42	19.44	9.19	2.01	6.74
cooked, braised	3 oz	230	20.48	15.81	7.45	1.64	5.48
PORK, Cured							
Bacon, raw	3 slices	378	5.89	39.12	17.90	4.59	14.45
cooked, broiled, pan-fried, or roasted	3 slices	109	5.79	9.36	4.50	1.10	3.31
Breakfast strips							
raw or unheated	3 slices	264	7.98	25.27	11.42	3.78	8.78
cooked	3 slices	156	9.84	12.48	5.57	1.92	4.34
Canadian-style bacon							
unheated	2 slices	89	11.70	3.95	1.79	0.36	1.26
grilled	2 slices	86	11.27	3.92	1.88	0.37	1.32
Feet, pickled	1 oz	58	3.83	4.58	2.15	0.50	1.58
Ham, boneless, extra lean & regular, unheated	1 cup	227	25.56	11.75	5.51	1.30	3.79
roasted	1 cup	231	30.75	10.73	5.23	1.50	3.65
Ham, boneless, extra lean (approx. 5% fat), unheated	1 cup	183	27.09	6.94	3.29	0.67	2.27
roasted	1 cup	203	29.31	7.74	3.67	0.75	2.53
Ham, boneless, regular (approx. 11% fat), unheated	1 cup	255	24.59	14.80	6.93	1.69	4.75
roasted	1 cup	249	31.67	12.62	6.22	1.98	4.36
Ham, extra lean & regular, canned							
unheated	1 cup	202	25.16	10.44	5.00	1.06	3.43
roasted	1 cup	234	29.31	11.80	5.69	1.26	3.94

FOOD	CARBO-HYDRATES (mg)	FIBER (mg)	CALCIUM (mg)	IRON (mg)	POTAS-SIUM (mg)	SODIUM (mg)	CHOLES-TEROL (mg)	% OF CALORIES FROM FAT
Heart, raw	3	0	12	10.57	664	127	296	33
cooked, braised	1	0	9	7.52	266	46	285	31
Jowl, raw	0	0	5	0.47	167	29	101	96
Kidneys, raw	0	0	22	11.38	534	283	742	29
cooked, braised	0	0	18	7.41	200	111	673	28
Lard	0	0	0		0	0	12	100
Leaf fat, raw	0	0	0	0.03		2	31	99
Liver, raw	3	0	10	26.33	308	98	341	25
cooked, braised	3	0	9	15.23	128	42	302	24
Lungs, raw	0	0	2	5.36	86	43	91	29
cooked, braised	0	0	7	13.95	129	68	329	28
Mechanically separated pork, raw	0	0	715	9.65			174	79
Pancreas, raw	0	0	12	2.40	223	50	218	60
cooked, braised	0	0	13	2.29	143	35	268	44
Spleen								
raw	0	0	11	25.22	447		410	23
cooked, braised	0	0	11	18.90	193		428	19
Stomach, raw	0	0	11	2.46	227	59	218	55
Tail, raw	0	0	20				110	80
cooked, simmered	0	0	12				110	82
Tongue, raw	0	0	18	3.79	274	124	114	69
cooked, braised	0	0	16	4.24	201	93	124	62
PORK, Cured								
Bacon, raw	0	0	5	0.41	95	466	46	93
cooked, broiled, pan-fried, or roasted	0	0	2	0.31	92	303	16	77
Breakfast strips								
raw or unheated	0	0	5	0.64	139	671	47	86
cooked	0	0	5	0.67	158	714	36	72
Canadian-style bacon								
unheated	1	0	5	0.38	195	799	28	40
grilled	1	0	5	0.38	181	719	27	41
Feet, pickled	0	0	9				26	71
Ham, boneless, extra lean & regular, unheated	3	0	10	1.26	415	1789	74	47
roasted	1	0	11	1.95	507	1938	80	42
Ham, boneless, extra lean (approx. 5% fat), unheated	1	0	10	1.07	489	2000	66	34
roasted	2	0	11	2.07	402	1684	74	34
Ham, boneless, regular (approx. 11% fat), unheated	4	0	10	1.39	465	1844	80	52
roasted	0	0	12	1.88	573	2100	83	46
Ham, extra lean & regular, canned								
unheated	0	0	8	1.26	468	1787	54	47
roasted	1	0	10	1.50	491	1495	57	45

PORK PRODUCTS

FOOD	AMOUNT	CALO-RIES (kcal)	PROTEIN (g)	FAT (g)	MONO-UN-SATURATED FAT (g)	POLY-UN-SATURATED FAT (g)	SATU-RATED FAT (g)
PORK, Cured (continued)							
Ham, extra lean (approx. 4% fat), canned							
unheated	1 cup	168	25.89	6.38	3.09	0.55	2.11
roasted	1 cup	191	29.62	6.83	3.48	0.61	2.25
Ham, regular (approx. 13% fat), canned							
unheated	1 cup	266	23.76	18.19	8.65	2.05	5.96
roasted	1 cup	317	28.74	21.28	9.90	2.50	7.06
Ham, center slice, country-style, separable lean only, raw	4 oz	220	31.41	9.40	4.32	1.10	3.14
Ham, center slice, separable lean & fat, unheated	4 oz	229	22.79	14.58	6.88	1.59	5.17
Ham, patties							
raw	1 patty	206	8.34	18.38	8.64	1.98	6.61
grilled	1 patty	203	7.91	18.36	8.73	1.98	6.60
Ham, steak, boneless, extra lean, unheated	1 slice	69	11.09	2.41	1.11	0.20	0.82
Ham, whole, separable lean & fat							
unheated	1 cup	345	25.89	25.93	12.18	2.29	9.27
roasted	1 cup	341	30.20	23.48	11.03	2.53	8.37
Ham, whole, separable lean only							
unheated	1 cup	206	31.24	8.00	3.67	0.92	2.68
roasted	1 cup	219	35.07	7.69	3.54	0.88	2.57
Salt pork, raw	8 oz	1697	11.46	182.74	86.12	21.34	66.68
Separable fat (from ham & arm picnic)							
unheated	3 oz	492	4.83	52.20	25.05	5.55	19.14
roasted	3 oz	502	6.49	52.58	25.23	5.59	19.28
Shoulder, arm picnic, separable lean & fat, roasted	1 cup	392	28.60	29.89	14.19	3.24	10.73
Shoulder, arm picnic, separable lean only, roasted	1 cup	238	34.92	9.86	4.53	1.14	3.31
Shoulder, blade roll, separable lean & fat							
unheated	4 oz	304	18.61	24.84	11.02	2.64	8.97
roasted	3 oz	244	14.69	19.95	9.37	2.13	7.12
ENTREES							
Ham, Banquet® frozen dinner	284 g	369	16.80	12.20	3.37	3.06	2.02
Ham & cheese on a bagel, Swanson®	1 oz	80	4.00	2.67	0.88	0.17	1.62
Ham & Swiss cheese crepes, Stouffer®	1 item	410	25.00	25.00			
Ham & asparagus, baked, Stouffer®	269 g	510	18.00	35.00			
Ham steak, Le Menu®	1 oz	30	1.90	1.10			
Pork, sweet & sour, La Choy®	300 g	378	15.30	14.10	5.03	3.86	3.73
Pork & beans							
baked, canned	1 cup	268	13.10	3.92	1.70	0.50	1.52
baked, canned w/tomato sauce	1 cup	248	13.10	2.61	1.12	0.33	1.00

336

FOOD	CARBO-HYDRATES (mg)	FIBER (mg)	CALCIUM (mg)	IRON (mg)	POTAS-SIUM (mg)	SODIUM (mg)	CHOLES-TEROL (mg)	% OF CALORIES FROM FAT
PORK, Cured (continued)								
Ham, extra lean (approx. 4% fat), canned								
unheated	0	0	8	1.32	510	1757	53	34
roasted	1	0	8	1.29	487	1589	41	32
Ham, regular (approx. 13% fat), canned								
unheated	0	0	8	1.16	442	1736	55	62
roasted	1	0	12	1.92	500	1317	86	60
Ham, center slice, country-style, separable lean only, raw	0	0						38
Ham, center slice, separable lean & fat, unheated	0	0	8	0.85	381	1566	61	57
Ham, patties								
raw	1	0	5	0.69	156	709	46	80
grilled	1	0	5	0.96	145	632	43	81
Ham, steak, boneless, extra lean, unheated	0	0	2	0.57	184	720	26	31
Ham, whole, separable lean & fat								
unheated	0	0	10	1.00	434	1797	78	68
roasted	0	0	10	1.22	400	1661	86	62
Ham, whole, separable lean only								
unheated	0	0	10	1.13	519	2122	73	35
roasted	0	0	10	1.31	443	1858	78	32
Salt pork, raw	0	0	13	0.99	149	3232	196	97
Separable fat (from ham & arm picnic)								
unheated	0	0	4	0.33	89	430	58	95
roasted	0	0	7	0.52	139	530	73	94
Shoulder, arm picnic, separable lean & fat, roasted	0	0	14	1.33	362	1501	82	69
Shoulder, arm picnic, separable lean only, roasted	0	0	15	1.51	409	1723	68	37
Shoulder, blade roll, separable lean & fat								
unheated	0	0	8	0.93	333	1412	60	74
roasted	0	0	6	0.75	165	827	57	74
ENTREES								
Ham, Banquet® frozen dinner	48	3	151	2.50	125	1590	36	30
Ham & cheese on a bagel, Swanson®	9	0	33	0.60	50	200	14	30
Ham & Swiss cheese crepes, Stouffer®	23				345	905		55
Ham & asparagus, baked, Stouffer®	31		200	1.44	360	900		62
Ham steak, Le Menu®	3		6	0.18		150		33
Pork, sweet & sour, La Choy®	48	0	38	1.98	504	1413	60	34
Pork & beans								
baked, canned	51	14	134	4.30	782	1047	18	13
baked, canned w/tomato sauce	49	11	142	8.30	759	1113		9

PORK PRODUCTS

FOOD	AMOUNT	CALO-RIES (kcal)	PROTEIN (g)	FAT (g)	MONO-UN-SATURATED FAT (g)	POLY-UN-SATURATED FAT (g)	SATU-RATED FAT (g)
ENTREES (continued)							
Pork & beans (continued)							
w/frankfurters, canned	1 cup	365	17.30	16.90	7.27	2.15	6.05
w/sweet sauce, canned	1 cup	281	13.40	3.69	1.60	0.47	1.42
w/tomato sauce, canned	1 cup	248	13.10	2.61	1.12	0.33	1.00
Campbell's® w/sauce	1 oz	25	1.25	0.38	5.38		12.50
Luck's®							
blackeye, seasoned	198 g	230	9.00	9.00	2.21	2.12	1.31
butter	213 g	230	10.00	4.00	0.95	0.28	0.84
crowder, seasoned	213 g	210	10.00	4.00			
giant Lima, seasoned	213 g	240	12.00	5.00	2.00	1.00	2.00
green Lima, seasoned	213 g	240	11.00	5.00	0.11	0.89	0.42
navy, seasoned	213 g	230	12.00	6.00	2.00	1.00	2.00
northern	213 g	230	11.00	5.00	2.00	1.00	2.00
October, seasoned	213 g	230	12.00	5.00	0.95	0.28	0.84
pinto, seasoned	198 g	200	10.00	4.00	1.60	0.80	1.60
pinto, seasoned, w/onions	213 g	250	11.00	6.00			
red kidney	213 g	240	11.00	7.00	3.31	1.08	2.60
tomato sauce	213 g	240	11.00	2.00	0.21	0.29	0.15
yelloweye	213 g	240	12.00	6.00	0.95	0.28	0.84
Pork loin & gravy, Hormel®	1 oz	40	4.60	2.20	0.70	0.32	0.90
Pork loin dinner, Swanson®	1 oz	26	1.86	1.12	0.55	0.13	0.43

FOOD	CARBO-HYDRATES (mg)	FIBER (mg)	CALCIUM (mg)	IRON (mg)	POTAS-SIUM (mg)	SODIUM (mg)	CHOLES-TEROL (mg)	% OF CALORIES FROM FAT
ENTREES (continued)								
Pork & beans (continued)								
w/frankfurters, canned	40	13	123	4.45	604	1105	15	42
w/sweet sauce, canned	53	14	154	4.20	673	850	18	12
w/tomato sauce, canned	49	14	141	8.30	759	1113	17	9
Campbell's® w/sauce	0		96					14
Luck's®								
blackeye, seasoned	28	6	20	2.70	805	600	0	35
butter	38	9	40	2.70	639	570	15	16
crowder, seasoned	33	7	20	1.80		600		17
giant Lima, seasoned	36	9	20	2.70	0	500	6	19
green Lima, seasoned	37	8	40	2.70	995	590	0	19
navy, seasoned	33	11	80	3.60		560	6	23
northern	34	10	80	2.70	639	550	9	20
October, seasoned	32	9	40	3.60	639	600	15	20
pinto, seasoned	29	9	40	2.70	216	550	0	18
pinto, seasoned, w/onions	37	15	60	3.60		560	6	22
red kidney	33	10	40	3.60	797	550	15	26
tomato sauce	44	11	80	2.70	1160	980	0	8
yelloweye	35	10	60	3.60	639	530	10	23
Pork loin & gravy, Hormel®	1		2	0.17	82	133	9	50
Pork loin dinner, Swanson®	3	0	4	0.10	136	74	26	39

SAUSAGES & LUNCHEON MEATS

FOOD	AMOUNT	CALO-RIES (kcal)	PROTEIN (g)	FAT (g)	MONO-UN-SATURATED FAT (g)	POLY-UN-SATURATED FAT (g)	SATU-RATED FAT (g)
Barbecue loaf – pork, beef	1 oz	49	4.49	2.52	1.17	0.23	0.90
Beef, corned, deli, Hillshire®	1 oz	31	5.99	0.40	0.23	0.02	0.16
Beef, cured, deli, Hillshire®	1 oz	31	5.99	0.50	0.25	0.02	0.23
Beef, smoked, deli, Hillshire®	1 oz	31	5.99	0.50	0.28	0.02	0.20
Beerwurst, beer salami							
beef	1 slice	76	2.90	6.90	3.23	0.26	3.00
pork	1 slice	55	3.27	4.32	2.06	0.54	1.44
Berliner – pork, beef	28.4 g	65	4.33	4.88	2.27	0.45	1.72
Blood sausage	1 oz	107	4.14	9.78	4.49	0.98	3.79
Bockwurst – pork, veal, milk, eggs	1 oz	87	3.78	7.82	3.68	0.84	2.87
Bologna							
beef	1 slice	88	3.50	8.10	3.91	0.31	3.42
beef & pork	1 slice	89	3.31	8.01	3.80	0.68	3.03
pork	1 slice	70	4.34	5.63	2.77	0.60	1.95
turkey	1 slice	57	3.89	4.31			
Hillshire®							
large	1 oz	90	3.00	7.99	3.79	0.68	3.04
ring	1 oz	89	3.00	7.99	3.79	0.68	3.04
Oscar Mayer® light	1 slice	60	3.00	5.00	2.56	0.20	2.24
Tyson® chicken	100 g	230	12.10	18.10		4.20	1.40
Bratwurst, cooked – pork	1 oz	85	3.99	7.33	3.46	0.78	2.64
Hillshire®							
smoked link	1 oz	95	3.99	8.49	0.00	0.00	0.00
spicy	1 oz	90	3.99	8.49	3.45	0.78	2.65
Braunschweiger – pork	1 oz	102	3.83	9.10	4.23	1.06	3.09
Bratwurst – pork, beef, nonfat dry milk added	1 oz	92	4.04	7.88	3.77	0.80	2.81
Cheddarwurst, link, bun size, Hillshire®	1 oz	100	3.99	8.98			
sausage	1 oz	95	3.99	8.49			
Cheesefurter, Cheese smokie – pork, beef	1 oz	93	3.98	8.21	3.87	0.86	2.97
Chicken breast							
Hillshire® smoked, deli	1 oz	31	5.99	0.20	0.09	0.05	0.06
Mr. Turkey® lunchmeat	1 oz	33	5.39	0.90	0.40	0.22	0.29
Tyson® roll, whole & diced	100 g	155	18.40	9.30		2.20	2.20
Chicken franks							
Grillmaster®	1 frankfurter	130	7.00	11.00	4.87	2.32	3.18
Mr. Turkey® w/cheese	1 oz	68	3.68	5.68			
Tyson®	100 g	285	12.40	24.90	8.55	4.80	1.60
Chicken, liberty roll, whole & diced, Tyson®	100 g	185	19.10	11.60		2.30	2.50
Chicken roll, light meat	2 slices	90	11.07	4.18	1.68	0.91	1.15
Chicken sandwich mate, Tyson®	100 g	315	20.60	19.60	5.64	4.40	1.60
Chicken, smoked, sliced, deli, Mr. Turkey®	1 oz	33	5.79	0.60	0.27	0.15	0.19
Chicken spread, canned	1 oz	55	4.37	3.32			
Chorizo – pork & beef, 4" links	1 item	265g	14.50	23.00	11.00	2.08	0.63
Corned beef loaf, jellied	1 oz	43	6.50	1.70	0.76	0.09	0.74
Dutch brand loaf – pork, beef	1 oz	68	3.80	5.05	2.36	0.54	1.80

FOOD	CARBO-HYDRATES (mg)	FIBER (mg)	CALCIUM (mg)	IRON (mg)	POTAS-SIUM (mg)	SODIUM (mg)	CHOLES-TEROL (mg)	% OF CALORIES FROM FAT
Barbecue loaf – pork, beef	1.8		15.00	0.33	93	378	11	46
Beef, corned, deli, Hillshire®	1.0	0.00	2.27	0.23	41	321	28	12
Beef, cured, deli, Hillshire®	1.0	0.00	2.10	0.66	96	270	22	15
Beef, smoked, deli, Hillshire®	1.0	0.00	2.55	0.54	65	270	26	15
Beerwurst, beer salami								
beef	0.4	0.00	2.00	0.35	40	237	14	82
pork	0.4	0.00	2.00	0.17	58	285	13	71
Berliner – pork, beef	0.7	0.00	3.00	0.33	80	368	13	68
Blood sausage	0.3						34	82
Bockwurst – pork, veal, milk, eggs	0.1							81
Bologna								
beef	0.2	0.00	3.00	0.47	44	278	16	83
beef & pork	0.7	0.00	3.00	0.43	51	289	16	81
pork	0.2	0.00	3.00	0.22	80	336	17	72
turkey	0.2		24.00	0.43	56	249	28	68
Hillshire®								
large	1.0	0.00	3.40	0.43	51	289	16	80
ring	1.0	0.00	3.40	0.43	51	289	16	81
Oscar Mayer® light	1.0	0.00	3.36	0.39	44	320	10	75
Tyson® chicken	4.7		49.00	2.30	200	1000	60	71
Bratwurst, cooked – pork	0.5		13.00	0.36	60	158	17	78
Hillshire®								
smoked link	0.5					270	0	81
spicy	0.5	0.00	12.48	0.37	60	158	17	85
Braunschweiger – pork	0.8	0.00	2.00	2.65	57	324	44	80
Bratwurst – pork, beef, nonfat dry milk added	0.8		14.00	0.29	80	315	18	77
Cheddarwurst, link, bun size, Hillshire®	0.5					240		81
sausage	0.5					240		81
Cheesefurter, Cheese smokie – pork, beef	0.4		16.00	0.30	58	307	19	79
Chicken breast								
Hillshire® smoked, deli	1.0	0.00	4.02	0.30	69	290	24	6
Mr. Turkey® lunchmeat	0.2	0.00	4.02	0.30	69	190	9	25
Tyson® roll, whole & diced	0.1	0.00	5.60	1.00	231	481	47	54
Chicken franks								
Grillmaster®	3.0	0.00	57.60	1.21	48	641	61	76
Mr. Turkey® w/cheese	0.5	0.00	16.47	0.31	58	328	18	75
Tyson®	1.7	0.00	35.00	1.80	170	1180	68	79
Chicken, liberty roll, whole & diced, Tyson®	0.2		9.60	1.40	167	697	53	56
Chicken roll, light meat	1.3		24.00	0.55	129	331	28	42
Chicken sandwich mate, Tyson®	14.4	0.97	13.00	1.70	187	1001	40	56
Chicken, smoked, sliced, deli, Mr. Turkey®	0.2	0.00	2.97	0.30	49	324	15	16
Chicken spread, canned	1.5		35.00	0.66				54
Chorizo – pork & beef, 4" links	0.0					260		78
Corned beef loaf, jellied	0.0	0.00	3.00	0.58	29	270	13	36
Dutch brand loaf – pork, beef	1.5		24.00	0.35	107	354	13	67

SAUSAGES & LUNCHEON MEATS

FOOD	AMOUNT	CALO-RIES (kcal)	PROTEIN (g)	FAT (g)	MONO-UN-SATURATED FAT (g)	POLY-UN-SATURATED FAT (g)	SATU-RATED FAT (g)
Frankfurter							
beef	1 frankfurter	142	5.40	12.80	6.13	0.62	5.42
beef & pork	1 frankfurter	144	5.08	13.12	6.15	1.23	4.84
chicken	1 frankfurter	116	5.82	8.76	3.81	1.82	2.49
turkey	1 frankfurter	102	6.43	7.96			
Ball Park® light, low-fat	1 frankfurter	140	7.00	12.00	6.04	0.61	5.35
Butterball® turkey	1 frankfurter	120	7.00	10.00	3.11	2.88	3.38
Hormel® light & lean	1 frankfurter	70	5.00	5.00	2.52	0.26	2.23
Louis Rich® bun length, turkey	1 frankfurter	130	7.00	11.00	4.00	3.00	3.00
Mr. Turkey® turkey franks	1 oz	66	3.43	5.55	1.56	1.44	1.69
Ham							
chopped, canned	1 oz	68	4.55	5.34	2.60	0.58	1.78
chopped, not canned	1 slice	65	4.85	4.89	2.32	0.60	1.62
minced	1 oz	75	4.61	5.86	2.71	0.70	2.03
sliced, extra lean (approx. 5% fat)	1 slice	37	5.49	1.41	0.67	0.14	0.46
sliced, regular (approx. 11% fat)	1 slice	52	4.98	3.00	1.40	0.34	0.96
Healthy Choice®							
baked	1 slice	12	1.83	0.33			0.16
honey	1 slice	10	1.83	0.33			0.00
smoked	1 slice	10	1.67	0.17			0.17
Hillshire®							
honey, deli	1 oz	31	5.99	0.90	0.00	0.00	0.00
smoked	1 oz	31	5.99	0.90	0.45	0.13	0.32
Oscar Mayer® natural juice, thin slice	1 slice	12	2.00	1.00	0.47	0.11	0.32
Ham & cheese loaf or roll	1 slice	73	4.71	5.73	2.62	0.62	2.13
Ham & cheese spread	1 oz	69	4.59	5.25	2.01	0.39	2.44
Headcheese – pork	1 oz	60	4.50	4.50	2.30	0.47	1.40
Honey loaf – pork, beef	1 oz	36	4.47	1.27	0.57	0.13	0.41
Honey roll sausage – beef	1 oz	52	5.27	2.98	1.37	0.14	1.16
Hot dog, no fat, light, Oscar Mayer®	1 item	130	7.00	11.00	5.57	1.13	4.31
Italian sausage, pork							
raw	1 link	391	16.10	35.40	16.21	4.55	12.74
cooked	1 link	268	16.62	21.33	9.91	2.73	7.53
Kielbasa, kolbassy – pork, beef, nonfat dry milk added	1 oz	88	3.76	7.70	3.67	0.87	2.81
Hillshire® polska links	28.4 g	95	3.50	8.50	3.95	1.08	3.07
beef	28.4 g	95	3.50	8.50	3.85	0.37	3.40
bun size link	28.4 g	90	4.00	8.00	0.00	0.00	0.00
flavor-seal	28.4 g	95	4.00	8.50			
lite	28.4 g	65	4.00	5.50			
mild	28.4 g	95	3.50	8.50			
Knackwurst, knockwurst – pork, beef	1 oz	87	3.37	7.87	3.63	0.83	2.89
Hillshire® sausage, link	28.4 g	90	3.50	8.00	3.94	1.01	3.04
Lebanon bologna – beef	1 oz	60	5.50	3.70	1.69	0.17	1.66
Liver cheese – pork	1 oz	86	4.30	7.25	3.48	0.97	2.54
Liver sausage, liverwurst – pork	1 oz	92	4.01	8.10	3.78	0.74	3.00
Luncheon meat							
loaved, beef	1 oz	87	4.10	7.40	3.47	0.25	3.17

FOOD	CARBO-HYDRATES (mg)	FIBER (mg)	CALCIUM (mg)	IRON (mg)	POTAS-SIUM (mg)	SODIUM (mg)	CHOLES-TEROL (mg)	% OF CALORIES FROM FAT
Frankfurter								
beef	0.8	0.00	9.00	0.64	75	462	27	81
beef & pork	1.1	0.00	5.00	0.52	75	504	22	82
chicken	3.0		43.00	0.90		617	45	68
turkey	0.6		48.00	0.83	80	642	48	70
Ball Park® light, low-fat	1.0	0.00	11.40	0.82	95	525	35	77
Butterball® turkey	1.0	0.00	63.90	1.11	103	620	64	75
Hormel® light & lean	2.0	0.00	9.00	0.64	75	510	20	64
Louis Rich® bun length, turkey	2.0	0.00	64.30	1.12	111	505	53	76
Mr. Turkey® turkey franks	0.5	0.00	31.94	0.56	51	275	19	75
Ham								
chopped, canned	0.0	0.00	2.00	0.27	81	387	14	71
chopped, not canned	0.0	0.00	2.00	0.24	91	389	15	68
minced	0.5	0.00	3.00	0.22	88	353	20	70
sliced, extra lean (approx. 5% fat)	0.2	0.00	2.00	0.22	99	405	13	34
sliced, regular (approx. 11% fat)	0.8	0.00	2.00	0.28	94	373	16	52
Healthy Choice®								
baked	0.3			0.06	32	88	5	25
honey	0.3			0.06	67	90	4	30
smoked	0.1			0.06	32	95	5	15
Hillshire®								
honey, deli	1.0					270	0	26
smoked	1.0	0.00	2.27	0.40	103	300	16	26
Oscar Mayer® natural juice, thin slice	1.0	0.00	0.84	0.11	34	170	5	75
Ham & cheese loaf or roll	0.4		16.00	0.26	83	381	16	71
Ham & cheese spread	0.6		62.00	0.22	46	339	17	68
Headcheese – pork	0.1	0.00	5.00	0.33	9	356	23	68
Honey loaf – pork, beef	1.5		5.00	0.38	97	374	10	32
Honey roll sausage – beef	0.6	0.00	3.00	0.62	83	375	14	52
Hot dog, no fat, light, Oscar Mayer®	1.0	0.00	6.67	0.70	99	630	30	76
Italian sausage, pork								
raw	0.7	0.00	20.00	1.33	286	826	86	81
cooked	1.2	0.00	20.00	1.24	253	765	65	72
Kielbasa, kolbassy – pork, beef, nonfat dry milk added	0.6	0.00	12.00	0.41	77	305	19	79
Hillshire® polska links	1.0	0.00	9.09	0.36	103	265	24	81
beef	0.5	0.00	5.07	0.43	47	275	17	81
bun size link	1.0					285	0	80
flavor-seal	1.0					270		81
lite	0.5							76
mild	1.0					265		81
Knackwurst, knockwurst – pork, beef	0.5	0.00	3.00	0.26	57	286	16	81
Hillshire® sausage, link	0.5	0.00	8.52	0.33	95	230	19	80
Lebanon bologna – beef	0.8	0.00	4.00	0.70	85	379	20	56
Liver cheese – pork	0.5		2.00	3.07	64	347	49	76
Liver sausage, liverwurst – pork	0.6		7.00	1.81			45	79
Luncheon meat								
loaved, beef	0.8	0.00	3.00	0.66	59	377	18	77

343

SAUSAGES & LUNCHEON MEATS

FOOD	AMOUNT	CALO-RIES (kcal)	PROTEIN (g)	FAT (g)	MONO-UN-SATURATED FAT (g)	POLY-UN-SATURATED FAT (g)	SATU-RATED FAT (g)
Luncheon meat (continued)							
thin sliced, beef	1 oz	35	6.20	0.89	0.39	0.04	0.37
pork, beef	1 slice	100	3.57	9.12	4.28	1.06	3.29
pork, canned	1 oz	95	3.50	8.60	4.05	1.01	3.06
Luncheon sausage – pork & beef	1 oz	74	4.36	5.93	2.82	0.58	2.16
Luxury loaf – pork	1 oz	40	5.20	1.40	0.66	0.14	0.45
Mortadella – beef, pork	1 oz	88	4.64	7.20	3.23	0.89	2.70
Mother's loaf – pork	1 oz	80	3.42	6.32	2.93	0.73	2.25
New England Brand sausage – pork, beef	1 oz	46	4.89	2.15	1.03	0.20	0.72
Olive loaf – pork	1 oz	67	3.40	4.70	2.23	0.55	1.66
Pastrami, turkey	2 slices	80	10.41	3.52	1.16	0.90	1.03
Pâté							
chicken liver, canned	1 oz	57	3.81	3.71			
goose liver, smoked, canned	1 oz	131	3.23	12.43			
liver, not specified, canned	1 oz	90	4.03	7.94			
Peppered loaf – pork, beef	1 oz	42	4.90	1.81	0.85	0.14	0.65
Pepperoni – pork, beef	1 slice	27	1.15	2.42	1.16	0.24	0.89
Pickle & pimento loaf – pork	1 oz	74	3.30	6.00	2.72	0.73	2.22
Picnic loaf – pork, beef	1 oz	66	4.23	4.72	2.18	0.54	1.72
Polish sausage – pork	1 oz	92	4.00	8.14	3.83	0.87	2.93
Pork & beef sausage, fresh, cooked	1 link	52	1.79	4.71	2.23	0.51	1.68
Pork sausage, fresh							
raw	1 link	118	3.31	11.42	5.25	1.48	4.10
cooked	1 link	48	2.55	4.05	1.81	0.50	1.40
Poultry salad sandwich spread	1 oz	57	3.30	3.83	0.92	1.76	0.98
Salami							
cooked, beef	1 oz	72	4.17	5.70	2.64	0.25	2.39
cooked, beef & pork	1 oz	71	3.95	5.70	2.61	0.57	2.29
cooked, turkey	2 slices	111	9.28	7.82			
dry or hard, pork	1 slice	41	2.26	3.37	1.60	0.37	1.19
dry or hard, pork, beef	1 slice	42	2.29	3.44	1.71	0.32	1.22
Sandwich spread – pork, beef	1 oz	67	2.17	4.92	2.16	0.73	1.70
Sausage, beef, Hillshire®							
& cheddar	1 oz	95	3.99	7.49			
hot links	1 oz	95	3.99	8.49	3.86	0.39	3.41
smoked, flavor-seal	1 oz	90	3.49	7.99	3.84	0.37	3.39
smoked, linked	1 oz	90	3.99	7.99	4.02	0.92	3.02
summer, semi-dry	1 oz	95	4.49	8.49	3.84	0.37	3.39
Sausage, brats, cooked, link, Hillshire®	1 oz	85	3.49	7.99	3.86	0.39	3.41
Sausage, country recipe, Hillshire®	1 oz	90	3.49	7.99	3.89	1.07	3.0
Sausage, hot links, Hillshire®	1 oz	95	3.99	7.99			
Sausage, Italian, hot, link, Hillshire®	1 oz	90	3.49	8.49	3.38	0.93	2.5
mild	1 oz	95	3.49	8.49	3.38	0.93	2.5
Sausage, Polish links, Hillshire®	1 oz	95	3.99	8.98	3.66	0.87	2.8
Sausage, smoked, Hillshire®							
flavor-seal	1 oz	95	3.49	8.49	3.84	0.37	3.3
hot	1 oz	90	3.49	7.99	3.84	0.37	3.3

FOOD	CARBO- HYDRATES (mg)	FIBER (mg)	CALCIUM (mg)	IRON (mg)	POTAS- SIUM (mg)	SODIUM (mg)	CHOLES- TEROL (mg)	% OF CALORIES FROM FAT
Luncheon meat (continued)								
thin sliced, beef	0.0	0.00		0.60	116	470	12	23
pork, beef	0.6	0.00	3.00	0.24	57	367	15	82
pork, canned	0.6	0.00	2.00	0.20	61	365	18	81
Luncheon sausage – pork & beef	0.4	0.00	4.00	0.40	70	335	18	72
Luxury loaf – pork	1.4		10.00	0.30	107	347	10	32
Mortadella – beef, pork	0.8		5.00	0.40	46	353	16	74
Mother's loaf – pork	2.1		12.00	0.38	64	320	13	71
New England Brand sausage – pork, beef	1.3	0.00	2.00	0.27	91	346	14	42
Olive loaf – pork	2.6		31.00	0.15	84	421	11	63
Pastrami, turkey	0.9		5.00	0.94	147	593		40
Pâté								
chicken liver, canned	1.8		3.00	2.60				59
goose liver, smoked, canned	1.3	0.00					43	85
liver, not specified, canned	0.4		20.00	1.56	39	198		79
Peppered loaf – pork, beef	1.3		15.00	0.30	112	432	13	39
Pepperoni – pork, beef	0.1	0.00	1.00	0.08	19	112		81
Pickle & pimento loaf – pork	1.7		27.00	0.29	96	394	10	73
Picnic loaf – pork, beef	1.3		13.00	0.29	76	330	11	64
Polish sausage – pork	0.4	0.00	3.00	0.41	67	248	20	80
Pork & beef sausage, fresh, cooked	0.3	0.00		0.15		105		82
Pork sausage, fresh								
raw	0.2	0.00	5.00	0.26	58	228	19	87
cooked	0.1	0.00	4.00	0.16	47	168	11	76
Poultry salad sandwich spread	2.1		3.00	0.17	52	107	9	60
Salami								
cooked, beef	0.7	0.00	2.00	0.57	64	328	17	71
cooked, beef & pork	0.6	0.00	4.00	0.76	56	302	18	72
cooked, turkey	0.3		11.00	0.91	138	569	46	63
dry or hard, pork	0.1	0.00	1.00	0.13		226		74
dry or hard, pork, beef	0.2	0.00	1.00	0.15	38	186	8	74
Sandwich spread – pork, beef	3.3		3.00	0.22	31	287	11	66
Sausage, beef, Hillshire®								
& cheddar	0.5					250		71
hot links	0.5	0.00	5.67	0.41	47	280	17	81
smoked, flavor-seal	1.0	0.00	5.06	0.43	47	245	17	80
smoked, linked	1.0	0.00	2.84	0.41	54	285	20	80
summer, semi-dry	0.5	0.00	5.06	0.43	47	289	17	81
Sausage, brats, cooked, link, Hillshire®	0.5	0.00	5.67	0.41	47	190	17	85
Sausage, country recipe, Hillshire®	1.0	0.00	9.07	0.35	103	245	24	80
Sausage, hot links, Hillshire®	1.0					265		76
Sausage, Italian, hot, link, Hillshire®	0.5	0.00	6.81	0.43	86	262	22	85
mild	0.5	0.00	6.81	0.43	86	262	22	81
Sausage, Polish links, Hillshire®	0.5	0.00	12.48	0.41	77	260	19	85
Sausage, smoked, Hillshire®								
flavor-seal	0.5	0.00	5.06	0.43	47	250	17	81
hot	1.0	0.00	5.06	0.43	47	255	17	80

SAUSAGES & LUNCHEON MEATS

FOOD	AMOUNT	CALO-RIES (kcal)	PROTEIN (g)	FAT (g)	MONO-UN-SATURATED FAT (g)	POLY-UN-SATURATED FAT (g)	SATU-RATED FAT (g)
Sausage, smoked, Hillshire® (continued)							
lite	1 oz	65	3.99	5.49			
w/Italian	1 oz	100	3.49	8.98	3.38	0.93	2.58
Sausage, smoked link							
pork	2" link	62	3.50	5.10	2.34	0.60	1.81
pork & beef	2" link	54	2.14	4.85	2.27	0.52	1.70
pork & beef, flour & nonfat dry milk added	2" link	43	2.24	3.43	1.59	0.36	1.25
pork & beef, nonfat dry milk added	2" link	50	2.12	4.42	2.02	0.48	1.55
Hillshire®	1 oz	95	3.99	8.98	4.15	1.07	3.20
bun size	1 oz	90	3.99	7.99			
Sausage, summer, semi-dry, Hillshire®	1 oz	90	4.49	7.99	3.67	0.34	3.41
cheese	1 oz	100	4.49	8.98	3.75	0.34	3.63
Thüringer, cervelat, summer sausage – beef, pork	1 oz	98	4.55	8.49	3.95	0.54	3.41
Hillshire® semi-dry	1 oz	90	4.49	7.49	3.67	0.34	3.41
Turkey breast chub, Mr. Turkey®							
barbecue	1 oz	29	6.19	0.50			
smoked	1 oz	30	6.29	0.50	0.13	0.08	0.14
Turkey breast meat	1 slice	23	4.73	0.33	0.09	0.06	0.10
Healthy Choice® honey roast/smoked	1 slice	12	1.83	0.33			
Hillshire® deli, roasted	1 oz	31	5.99	0.20	0.08	0.06	0.07
smoked	1 oz	31	5.99	0.20	0.07	0.05	0.08
Mr. Turkey®							
lunchmeat	1 oz	32	5.59	0.70	0.13	0.08	0.14
smoked	1 oz	33	6.29	0.50	0.13	0.08	0.14
smoked, honey	1 oz	31	5.89	0.90	0.13	0.08	0.14
Turkey ham – cured turkey thigh meat	2 slices	73	10.74	2.88	0.65	0.86	0.97
Mr. Turkey®							
honey cured	1 oz	30	4.59	1.10	0.28	0.38	0.43
lunchmeat, sliced	1 oz	36	5.19	1.20	0.32	0.42	0.42
smoked	1 oz	32	4.89	1.10	0.29	0.38	0.42
Turkey ham chub, Mr. Turkey®							
honey	1 oz	34	5.79	1.40	0.33	0.43	0.48
honey cured	1 oz	30	4.59	1.10	0.29	0.38	0.42
smoked	1 oz	36	4.79	1.40	0.33	0.43	0.48
smoke hardwood	1 oz	36	5.49	1.20	0.32	0.42	0.4
Turkey pastrami, Mr. Turkey®							
lunchmeat	1 oz	28	4.79	0.90	0.34	0.26	0.36
sliced, deli	1 oz	35	4.99	1.20	0.45	0.35	0.46
Turkey polska kielbasa							
Louis Rich®	1 oz	40	4.99	2.00	0.76	0.67	0.5
Mr. Turkey®	1 oz	54	4.40	3.70			
Turkey salami, lunchmeat, Mr. Turkey®	1 oz	45	4.29	2.90	1.09	0.84	0.9

346

FOOD	CARBO-HYDRATES (mg)	FIBER (mg)	CALCIUM (mg)	IRON (mg)	POTAS-SIUM (mg)	SODIUM (mg)	CHOLES-TEROL (mg)	% OF CALORIES FROM FAT
Sausage, smoked, Hillshire® (continued)								
lite	0.5							76
w/Italian	0.5	0.00	6.81	0.43	86	250	22	81
Sausage, smoked link								
pork	0.3	0.00	5.00	0.19	54	240	11	74
pork & beef	0.2	0.00	2.00	0.23	30	151	11	81
pork & beef, flour & nonfat dry milk added	0.6		3.00	0.25	25	174	14	72
pork & beef, nonfat dry milk added	0.3	0.00	6.00	0.23	46	188	10	80
Hillshire®	0.5	0.00	8.51	0.33	95	260	19	85
bun size	1.0					285		80
Sausage, summer, semi-dry, Hillshire®	0.5	0.00	3.68	0.72	77	334	21	80
cheese	0.5	0.00	21.56	0.41	46	297	18	81
Thüringer, cervelat, summer sausage – beef, pork	0.6	0.00	2.00	0.58	65	412	19	78
Hillshire® semi-dry	0.5	0.00	3.68	0.72	77	324	21	75
Turkey breast chub, Mr. Turkey®								
barbecue	0.1	0.00				208	5	16
smoked	0.1	0.00	1.99	0.11	79	204	5	15
Turkey breast meat	0.0	0.00	1.00	0.08	58	301	9	13
Healthy Choice® honey roast/smoked	0.3				25	78	4	25
Hillshire® deli, roasted	1.0	0.00	5.99	0.40	80	339	21	6
smoked	1.0	0.00	1.99	0.11	79	290	12	6
Mr. Turkey®								
lunchmeat	0.2	0.00	1.99	0.11	79	233	10	20
smoked	0.2	0.00	1.99	0.11	79	331	10	14
smoked, honey	0.3	0.00	1.99	0.11	79	247	10	26
Turkey ham – cured turkey thigh meat	0.2		5.00	1.57	184	565		36
Mr. Turkey®								
honey cured	0.6	0.00	2.84	0.78	92	336	18	33
lunchmeat, sliced	1.0	0.00	2.84	0.78	92	325	22	30
smoked	0.3	0.00	2.84	0.78	92	286	18	31
Turkey ham chub, Mr. Turkey®								
honey	0.4	0.00	2.84	0.78	92	339	17	37
honey cured	0.6	0.00	2.84	0.78	92	336	18	33
smoked	0.4	0.00	2.84	0.78	92	339	17	35
smoke hardwood	0.8	0.00	2.84	0.78	92	324	25	30
Turkey pastrami, Mr. Turkey®								
lunchmeat	0.1	0.00	2.56	0.47	74	382	17	29
sliced, deli	0.1	0.00	2.56	0.47	74	319	18	31
Turkey polska kielbasa								
Louis Rich®	1.0	0.00	7.46	0.50	56	246	19	45
Mr. Turkey®	0.5					264	15	62
Turkey salami, lunchmeat, Mr. Turkey®	0.4	0.00	5.67	0.46	69	368	16	58

SAUSAGES & LUNCHEON MEATS

FOOD	AMOUNT	CALO-RIES (kcal)	PROTEIN (g)	FAT (g)	MONO-UN-SATURATED FAT (g)	POLY-UN-SATURATED FAT (g)	SATU-RATED FAT (g)
Turkey sausage, breakfast							
Louis Rich®	1 oz	60	5.99	3.99	0.89	0.69	0.79
Mr. Turkey®	1 oz	58	4.59	4.29	0.89	0.69	0.79
Turkey sausage, smoked							
Louis Rich®	1 oz	43	4.99	2.00	0.91	0.54	0.54
w/cheese	1 oz	47	4.99	3.00	1.00	1.00	1.00
Mr. Turkey®	1 oz	51	4.49	3.39	1.15	1.03	1.22
Turkey roll							
light & dark meat	1 oz	42	5.14	1.98	0.65	0.51	0.58
light meat	1 oz	42	5.30	2.05	0.71	0.49	0.57
Vienna sausage, canned – beef &	1 sausage	45	1.65	4.03	2.01	0.27	1.48
pork							
Wieners, link, Hillshire®							
bun size	1 oz	90	3.49	7.99	3.99	0.81	3.10
bun size, beef	1 oz	90	3.49	7.99	3.86	0.39	3.41
bun size, cheese	1 oz	90	3.49	7.99			
natural casing	1 oz	90	3.00	8.49			

FOOD	CARBO-HYDRATES (mg)	FIBER (mg)	CALCIUM (mg)	IRON (mg)	POTAS-SIUM (mg)	SODIUM (mg)	CHOLES-TEROL (mg)	% OF CALORIES FROM FAT
Turkey sausage, breakfast								
Louis Rich®	1.0	0.00	7.46	0.50	78	220	25	60
Mr. Turkey®	0.4	0.00	7.46	0.50	78	181	16	67
Turkey sausage, smoked								
Louis Rich®	1.0	0.00	23.86	0.43	53	239	18	42
w/cheese	1.0	0.00	23.86	0.43	52	256	17	57
Mr. Turkey®	0.5	0.00	23.86	0.43	56	230	19	60
Turkey roll								
light & dark meat	0.6		9.00	0.38	77	166	16	42
light meat	0.1		11.00	0.36	71	139	12	44
Vienna sausage, canned – beef & pork	0.3	0.00	2.00	0.14	16	152	8	81
Wieners, link, Hillshire®								
bun size	1.0	0.00	3.31	0.35	48	275	15	80
bun size, beef	1.0	0.00	5.67	0.41	47	280	17	80
bun size, cheese	1.0					265		80
natural casing	1.0					235		85

THE GOOD-SENSE FOOD GUIDE PYRAMID
Your guide to daily food choices

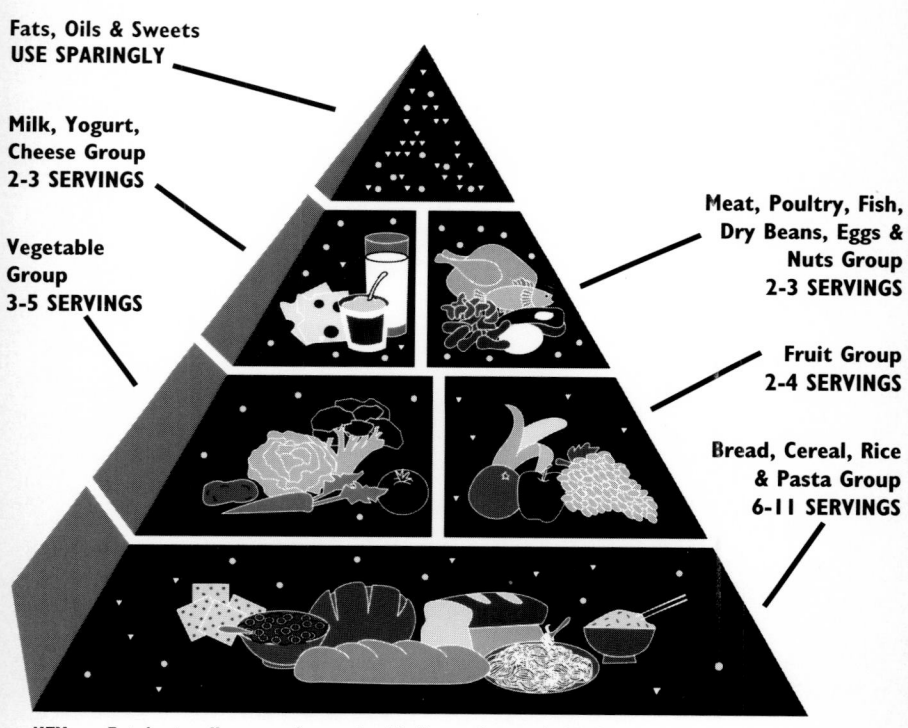

**Fats, Oils & Sweets
USE SPARINGLY**

**Milk, Yogurt,
Cheese Group
2-3 SERVINGS**

**Vegetable
Group
3-5 SERVINGS**

**Meat, Poultry, Fish,
Dry Beans, Eggs &
Nuts Group
2-3 SERVINGS**

**Fruit Group
2-4 SERVINGS**

**Bread, Cereal, Rice
& Pasta Group
6-11 SERVINGS**

KEY ● Fat (naturally occurring and added) ▼ Sugars (added)

FAST FOODS, FATS, OILS, SNACKS, AND SWEETS

The Food Guide Pyramid suggests using the foods in the top level sparingly. The dietary guidelines recommend that Americans limit their fat intake to 30 percent of total calories. This amounts to:

- 53 g of fat in a 1,600-calorie diet
- 73 g of fat in a 2,200-calorie diet
- 93 g of fat in a 2,800-calorie diet

All fats are mixtures of three types of fatty acids — saturated, monounsatured, and polyunsaturated. Saturated fats are the most harmful, and it is recommended that people limit their saturated-fat intake to less than 10 percent of total calories, or about one-third of total fat intake.

Snacks, sweets, and fast foods are a complex group. Most are multi-ingredient items that may include both plant and animal products. The snacks section gives information on corn-based snacks, fruit leathers, and pretzels. The sweets include candies, frostings, puddings, and frozen desserts. Sodium content of snacks ranges widely among types of snacks and the same snack produced by different manufacturers.

Only a select few fast-food companies disclose nutrition information. Given the frequency and volume with which we consume fast-food, it is important to know exactly what we are eating when we go to one of these restaurants. Fat, cholesterol, sodium, and sugar are the biggest problems in fast-foods. This category contains processed meats, deep-fried foods, sauces, and condiments high in sodium, and often high fat cheeses.

FAST FOODS

FOOD	AMOUNT	CALORIES (kcal)	PROTEIN (g)	FAT (g)	MONO-UN-SATURATED FAT (g)	POLY-UN-SATURATED FAT (g)	SATURATED FAT (g)
BREAKFAST ITEMS							
Big Country Breakfast, Hardees®							
w/bacon	1 serving	660	24.00	40.00	22.0	8.00	10.00
w/country ham	1 serving	670	29.00	38.00	21.0	8.00	9.00
w/ham	1 serving	620	28.00	33.00	18.4	7.76	6.79
w/sausage	1 serving	850	33.00	57.00	30.5	10.80	15.70
Biscuit							
plain	74 g	276	4.31	13.35	3.4	0.52	8.74
w/egg	136 g	315	11.12	20.20	8.1	4.22	6.18
w/egg & bacon	150 g	457	16.99	31.10	13.2	5.70	9.93
w/egg & ham	192 g	442	20.43	27.03	11.3	5.18	8.37
w/egg & sausage	180 g	582	19.15	38.69	16.4	4.45	14.98
w/egg & steak	148 g	474	17.94	28.43	11.7	5.84	8.61
w/egg, cheese & bacon	144 g	477	16.26	31.39	14.2	3.50	11.40
w/ham	113 g	387	13.39	18.42	4.8	1.04	11.41
w/sausage	124 g	485	12.12	31.78	12.8	3.03	14.22
w/steak	141 g	456	13.09	25.99	11.0	6.42	6.93
Hardees®							
w/egg & bacon	124 g	410	15.00	24.00	14.0	5.00	5.00
w/egg & ham	138 g	370	15.00	19.00	11.4	3.80	3.80
w/egg, ham & cheese	151 g	420	18.00	23.00	13.0	4.00	6.00
w/egg, cheese & bacon	137 g	460	17.00	28.00	15.0	5.00	8.00
McDonald's®							
w/egg & bacon	156 g	440	17.50	26.40	16.1	2.01	8.22
w/egg & sausage	175.7 g	505	19.00	33.00	3.0	10.00	20.00
w/sausage	118 g	420	12.00	28.00	3.0	8.00	17.00
w/spread	75 g	260	4.60	12.70	0.9	2.93	8.79
Swanson®							
bacon, egg & cheese	1 oz	80.8	3.08	4.23	1.5	0.41	1.54
sausage, egg & cheese	1 oz	83.6	3.27	5.09	2.3	0.77	1.98
Croissant							
w/egg & cheese	127 g	369	12.79	24.70	7.5	1.37	14.07
w/egg, cheese & bacon	129 g	413	16.23	28.35	9.1	1.76	15.43
w/egg, cheese & ham	152 g	475	18.93	33.58	11.3	2.36	17.48
w/egg, cheese & sausage	160 g	524	20.30	38.16	14.2	3.01	18.23
Burger King®							
w/egg & cheese	127 g	369	12.80	24.70	7.5	1.37	14.10
w/egg, cheese & ham	152 g	475	18.90	33.60	11.4	2.36	17.50
Danish pastry							
cheese	91 g	353	5.83	24.62	15.6	2.42	5.1.
cinnamon	88 g	349	4.80	16.72	10.5	1.65	3.48
fruit	94 g	335	4.76	15.94	10.1	1.57	3.32
McDonald's®							
apple	115 g	390	5.80	17.90	2.0	4.00	11.00
cheese, iced	110 g	390	7.40	21.80	2.0	6.00	13.00
cinnamon w/raisins	110 g	440	6.40	21.00	2.0	5.00	13.00
raspberry	117 g	410	6.10	15.90	2.0	3.00	11.00
Egg, scrambled	2 eggs	200	13.01	15.21	5.5	1.85	5.78
McDonald's®	100 g	140	12.40	9.80	1.9	2.94	4.90

354

FOOD	CARBO-HYDRATES (mg)	FIBER (mg)	CALCIUM (mg)	IRON (mg)	POTAS-SIUM (mg)	SODIUM (mg)	CHOLES-TEROL (mg)	% OF CALORIES FROM FAT
BREAKFAST ITEMS								
Big Country Breakfast, Hardees®								
w/bacon	51	0.00	78	2.46	530	1540	305	55
w/country ham	52				710	2870	345	51
w/ham	51				620	1780	325	48
w/sausage	51				670	1980	340	60
Biscuit								
plain	34	0.30	90	1.63	86	584	5	44
w/egg	24	0.12	154	3.13	160	655	232	58
w/egg & bacon	29	0.12	189	3.73	250	999	353	61
w/egg & ham	30	0.13	221	4.55	319	1381	299	55
w/egg & sausage	41	0.18	155	3.96	319	1142	302	60
w/egg & steak	37	0.10	138	5.30	306	888	272	54
w/egg, cheese & bacon	33	0.29	164	2.55	230	1261	261	59
w/ham	44	0.28	161	2.73	197	1433	25	43
w/sausage	40	0.31	128	2.59	198	1071	34	59
w/steak	44	0.21	115	4.31	233	795	26	51
Hardees®								
w/egg & bacon	35	0.63	253	2.18	180	990	155	53
w/egg & ham	35	1.06	95	2.75	210	1050	160	46
w/egg, ham & cheese	35	0.76	308	2.65	230	1270	170	49
w/egg, cheese & bacon	35	0.69	279	2.41	200	1220	165	55
McDonald's®								
w/egg & bacon	33	0.79	185	2.56	237	1230	253	54
w/egg & sausage	33		116	3.16	319	1210	260	59
w/sausage	32	1.35	83	1.98	196	1040	44	60
w/spread	32	0.98	75	1.31	100	730	1	44
Swanson®								
bacon, egg & cheese	7	0.14	48	0.87	43	355	31	47
sausage, egg & cheese	6	0.12	36	0.33	53	238	27	55
Croissant								
w/egg & cheese	24	0.22	244	2.20	174	551	216	60
w/egg, cheese & bacon	24	0.21	151	2.19	201	889	215	62
w/egg, cheese & ham	24	0.21	144	2.13	272	1080	213	64
w/egg, cheese & sausage	25	0.22	144	3.04	283	1115	216	66
Burger King®								
w/egg & cheese	24	2.05	244	2.20	174	551	216	60
w/egg, cheese & ham	24		144	2.13	272	1080	213	64
Danish pastry								
cheese	29	0.18	70	1.85	116	320	20	63
cinnamon	47	0.70	37	1.80	96	326	28	43
fruit	45	0.38	22	1.40	110	333	19	43
McDonald's®								
apple	51	1.57	14	1.37	69	370	26	41
cheese, iced	42		33	1.42		420	47	50
cinnamon w/raisins	58		35	1.81		430	35	43
raspberry	62		14	1.47		310	26	35
Egg, scrambled	2	0.19	54	2.43	138	211	400	68
McDonald's®	1	0.00	57	2.08	102	290	425	63

FAST FOODS

FOOD	AMOUNT	CALO- RIES (kcal)	PROTEIN (g)	FAT (g)	MONO-UN- SATURATED FAT (g)	POLY-UN- SATURATED FAT (g)	SATU- RATED FAT (g)
BREAKFAST ITEMS (continued)							
Egg, scrambled (continued)							
Swanson®							
w/cheese & pancakes	1 oz	85.3	2.06	6.76			
w/home fries	1 oz	56.5	1.52	4.13			
w/bacon & home fries	1 oz	60.7	1.96	4.64			
w/sausage & hash browns	1 oz	66.2	2.00	5.23	1.8	1.28	1.48
Muffin, McDonald's® apple bran	1 muffin	180	5.00	0.00	0.0	0.00	0.00
English muffin							
w/butter	63 g	189	4.87	5.76	1.5	1.35	2.43
w/cheese & sausage	115 g	394	15.34	24.26	10.0	2.69	9.85
w/egg, cheese & Canadian bacon	146 g	383	19.81	19.76	6.7	2.06	9.05
w/egg, cheese & sausage	165 g	487	21.66	30.85	12.7	3.32	12.42
McDonald's®	58 g	170	5.00	4.00	1.0	1.00	2.00
egg McMuffin	1 item	280	18.00	11.00	1.0	4.00	6.00
sausage McMuffin	1 item	345	15.00	20.00	2.0	7.00	11.00
sausage McMuffin w/egg	1 item	430	21.00	25.00	3.0	8.00	14.00
Swanson®							
egg, bacon & cheese	1 oz	70.7	3.66	3.66	1.5	0.60	1.52
egg, beefsteak & cheese	1 oz	73.5	3.47	4.08	1.7	0.66	1.69
French toast w/butter	2 slices	356	10.34	18.76	7.0	2.45	7.75
Swanson® w/sausage	1 oz	69.1	2.18	3.82	1.4	0.50	1.14
w/cinnamon	1 oz	70.9	2.18	3.82	1.4	0.50	1.14
mini	1 oz	76	2.40	3.60	1.4	0.50	1.14
oatmeal French toast w/lite links	1 oz	66.7	2.80	2.80			
French toast sticks	5 sticks	479	8.27	29.05	12.6	9.95	4.71
Arby's® toastix	1 serving	420	8.00	25.00	17.3	3.20	4.60
Pancakes w/butter & syrup	3 cakes	519	8.26	13.99	5.2	1.96	5.85
Hardees®	137 g	280	8.00	2.00	0.6	0.67	0.67
McDonald's®	174 g	440	8.00	12.00	5.0	2.00	5.00
Swanson®							
w/bacon	1 oz	88.9	2.44	4.44			
w/sausages	1 oz	76.7	2.50	3.67			
silver dollar w/sausage	1 oz	82.7	2.67	3.73	1.7	0.85	1.12
whole wheat w/lite links	1 oz	63.6	2.73	2.91	0.8	1.32	0.76
Platters, Arby's®							
bacon	1 serving	593	21.80	33.00	14.7	6.40	9.20
egg	1 serving	460	15.00	24.00	11.0	5.10	7.20
ham	1 serving	518	24.40	26.20	12.2	5.40	7.90
sausage	1 serving	640	21.00	41.00	20.2	6.80	13.30
Potatoes, hashed brown	½ cup	151	1.94	9.22	3.8	0.47	4.32
McDonald's®	53 g	130	1.40	7.30	2.0	1.00	4.00
Sandwiches, Jack in the Box® breakfast Jack	1 sandwich	307	18.00	13.00	5.0	2.50	5.10
Sausage	1 patty	100	5.31	8.41	3.7	1.03	2.9
McDonald's®	48 g	180	8.40	16.30	8.5	1.90	5.88
Waffle, w/bacon, Swanson®	1 oz	105	3.18	6.36			
Waffles, Belgian, Swanson®							
w/sausage	1 oz	98.2	2.46	6.67			
w/strawberries	1 oz	60	0.86	2.29			

FOOD	CARBO-HYDRATES (mg)	FIBER (mg)	CALCIUM (mg)	IRON (mg)	POTAS-SIUM (mg)	SODIUM (mg)	CHOLES-TEROL (mg)	% OF CALORIES FROM FAT
BREAKFAST ITEMS (continued)								
Egg, scrambled (continued)								
Swanson®								
w/cheese & pancakes	4		18	0.53		112		71
w/home fries	3		13	0.31		83		66
w/bacon & home fries	3		11	0.32		123		69
w/sausage & hash browns	3	0.17	9	0.28	74	117	41	71
Muffin, McDonald's® apple bran	40	4.47	31	0.60	202	200	0	0
English muffin								
w/butter	30	0.13	103	1.59	69	386	13	27
w/cheese & sausage	29	0.46	168	2.25	215	1036	58	55
w/egg, cheese & Canadian bacon	31	0.29	207	3.28	213	785	234	46
w/egg, cheese & sausage	31	0.49	196	3.46	294	1135	274	57
McDonald's®	26	1.56	151	1.61	74	285	0	21
egg McMuffin	28	1.38	256	2.77	213	710	235	35
sausage McMuffin	27	1.10	235	2.30	179	770	57	52
sausage McMuffin w/egg	27	1.56	263	3.34	255	920	270	52
Swanson®								
egg, bacon & cheese	6	0.34	37	0.66	52	188	37	47
egg, beefsteak & cheese	0	0.34	20	0.06	52	149	37	50
French toast w/butter	36	0.13	73	1.89	177	513	117	47
Swanson® w/sausage	6	0.19	18	0.49	57	100	39	50
w/cinnamon	7	0.19	18	0.49	57	96	39	48
mini	9	0.19	16	0.58	57	128	39	43
oatmeal French toast w/lite links	8		17	0.39		108		38
French toast sticks	49	0.18	78	2.96	126	499	74	55
Arby's® toastix	43			2.70	110	440	20	54
Pancakes w/butter & syrup	91	0.23	128	2.61	250	1103	57	24
Hardees®	56	1.35	341	1.86	240	890	15	6
McDonald's®	74		114	2.08	187	685	8	25
Swanson®								
w/bacon	10		13	0.40		222		45
w/sausages	9		13	0.45		153		43
silver dollar w/sausage	10	0.18	11	0.48	48	181	15	41
whole wheat w/lite links	7	1.11	7	0.49	65	109	18	41
Platters, Arby's®								
bacon	51		60	3.60	491	880	458	50
egg	45		60	3.60	412	591	346	47
ham	45		60	3.60	578	1177	374	46
sausage	46		80	3.60	507	861	406	58
Potatoes, hashed brown	16	0.36	7	0.48	267	290	9	55
McDonald's®	15	1.09	6	0.27	238	330	0	51
Sandwiches, Jack in the Box® breakfast Jack	30		177	2.50	190	871	203	38
Sausage	0	0.00	9	0.34	97	349	22	76
McDonald's®	0	0.00	8	0.67		350	48	82
Waffle, w/bacon, Swanson®	9		18	0.49		323		55
Waffles, Belgian, Swanson®								
w/sausage	7		14	0.38		147		61
w/strawberries	9		11	0.31		69		34

FAST FOODS

FOOD	AMOUNT	CALO-RIES (kcal)	PROTEIN (g)	FAT (g)	MONO-UN-SATURATED FAT (g)	POLY-UN-SATURATED FAT (g)	SATU-RATED FAT (g)
ENTREES							
Bacon cheddar deluxe, Arby's®	1 serving	512	21.20	31.50	12.7	10.10	8.70
Chicken, breaded & fried							
dark meat (drumstick or thigh)	2 pieces	430	30.07	26.71	10.9	6.32	7.05
light meat (breast or wing)	2 pieces	494	35.71	29.51	12.2	6.79	7.84
boneless pieces, plain	6 pieces	290	16.90	17.71	8.7	2.25	5.55
boneless pieces w/barbecue sauce	6 pieces	330	17.14	17.96	8.7	2.39	5.57
boneless pieces w/honey	6 pieces	329	16.77	17.54	8.6	2.23	5.49
boneless pieces w/mustard sauce	6 pieces	323	17.42	18.94	9.0	2.91	5.72
boneless pieces w/sweet & sour sauce	6 pieces	346	16.96	17.95	8.6	2.23	5.52
Burger King® chicken tenders	1 piece	39.3	2.67	2.17	0.8	0.50	0.50
Church's® chicken	100 g	327	21.00	23.00			
KFC® crispy chicken							
breast	110 g	343	21.70	22.30	14.5	2.30	5.50
drumstick	69 g	204	13.60	13.90	8.8	1.70	3.40
thigh	119 g	406	20.00	30.00	6.9	4.00	8.00
wing	65 g	254	12.40	18.60	10.6	3.99	3.99
Kentucky nuggets	1 piece	46	2.80	2.90		0.30	0.70
Long John Silver's® chicken plank	1 piece	120	8.00	6.00	4.3	0.10	1.60
chicken, light herb	100 g	120	22.00	4.00	1.7	1.10	1.20
McDonald's® chicken McNuggets	6 pieces	270	20.00	15.00	1.5	3.50	10.00
barbecue sauce, sauce only	32 g	50	0.00	0.50	0.2	0.10	0.20
honey sauce, sauce only	14 g	45	0.00	0.00	0.0	0.00	0.00
hot mustard sauce, sauce only	30 g	70	0.00	3.60	1.9	0.50	1.20
sweet & sour sauce, sauce only	32 g	60	0.00	0.20	0.1	0.00	0.10
Chili							
w/beans, canned	1 cup	286	14.60	14.00			
Chef Boyardee®							
beef & beans	1 serving	330	15.00	17.00			
chili mac	1 serving	230	8.00	11.00			
Chili Bowl®							
homestyle	1 oz	50	2.00	4.00			
w/beans	1 oz	30	2.00	2.00			
Gebhardt®							
beans	35 g	76	4.00	3.00			
beans longhorn	35 g	85	4.00	4.00			
plain	32 g	59	3.00	5.00			
Health Valley®							
mild vegetarian, beans	1 oz	28	2.20	0.20			
mild vegetarian, lentils	1 oz	28	1.60	0.60			
mild vegetarian, low-fat	1 oz	28	2.20	0.20			
mild vegetarian, 3 bean	1 oz	18	2.00	0.20			
spicy vegetarian, beans	1 oz	28	2.20	0.20			
Hunt's®							
beans	35 g	45	3.00	2.00			
no beans	32 g	53	3.00	4.00			
Legout®							
mild	1 oz	28.8	2.00	1.00			

FOOD	CARBO-HYDRATES (mg)	FIBER (mg)	CALCIUM (mg)	IRON (mg)	POTAS-SIUM (mg)	SODIUM (mg)	CHOLES-TEROL (mg)	% OF CALORIES FROM FAT
ENTREES								
Bacon cheddar deluxe, Arby's®	39		110	4.32	491	1094	38	55
Chicken, breaded & fried								
dark meat (drumstick or thigh)	16	0.00	36	1.60	446	756	165	56
light meat (breast or wing)	20	0.00	60	1.49	566	975	149	54
boneless pieces, plain	15	0.17	16	1.27	251	542	62	55
boneless pieces w/barbecue sauce	25	0.25	21	1.46	319	830	61	49
boneless pieces w/honey	27	0.16	17	1.32	255	537	61	48
boneless pieces w/mustard sauce	21	0.22	25	1.48	280	791	62	53
boneless pieces w/sweet & sour sauce	29	0.25	20	1.48	277	677	61	47
Burger King® chicken tenders	2	0.27	9	1.03	249	90	8	50
Church's® chicken	10		94	1.00	186	498		63
KFC® crispy chicken								
breast	14	0.08	30	0.80	347	748	81	59
drumstick	6	0.04	13	0.70	157	324	71	61
thigh	14	0.14	16	1.77	280	688	129	67
wing	9	0.06	18	0.60	115	422	67	66
Kentucky nuggets	2	0.00	2	0.10		140	12	57
Long John Silver's® chicken plank	11			0.72	160	400	15	45
chicken, light herb	1	0.00		0.72	270	570	60	30
McDonald's® chicken McNuggets	17		13	1.00		580	55	50
barbecue sauce, sauce only	12	1.89	13	0.31	56	340	0	9
honey sauce, sauce only	12			0.07		0	0	0
hot mustard sauce, sauce only	8	0.25	15	0.22	26	250	5	46
sweet & sour sauce, sauce only	14	0.02	11	0.17	10	190	0	3
Chili								
w/beans, canned	30	6.93	119	8.75	932	1330	43	44
Chef Boyardee®								
beef & beans	30	4.50	60	3.60	587	1005	50	46
chili mac	26	4.00	0	1.80	501	1410	20	43
Chili Bowl®								
homestyle	2	0.60	0	0.00	90	135	10	72
w/beans	3	0.60	0	0.72	110	100	5	60
Gebhardt®								
beans	8		17	1.00	136	163		36
beans longhorn	8		18	1.00	148	155		42
plain	2	0.68	7	0.50	70	157	8	76
Health Valley®								
mild vegetarian, beans	5	2.44	0	0.54	116	58	0	6
mild vegetarian, lentils	3	1.30	12	0.72	98	58	0	19
mild vegetarian, low-fat	5	2.44	0	0.36	116	6	0	6
mild vegetarian, 3 bean	2	1.80	8	0.36	88	36	0	10
spicy vegetarian, beans	5	2.44	0	0.54	116	58	0	6
Hunt's®								
beans	3		11	0.70	76	164		40
no beans	2	0.46	10	0.60	46	153	10	68
Legout®								
mild	3		5	0.45	89	129		31

FAST FOODS

FOOD	AMOUNT	CALO-RIES (kcal)	PROTEIN (g)	FAT (g)	MONO-UN-SATURATED FAT (g)	POLY-UN-SATURATED FAT (g)	SATU-RATED FAT (g)
ENTREES (continued)							
Chili (continued)							
Italian	1 oz	31.3	1.75	1.88			
spicy	1 oz	25	1.63	0.75			
con carne, w/beans	1 oz	43.3	2.33	1.83			
Natural Touch® vegetarian, canned	1 cup	345	18.00	18.00			
Right Course® vegetarian	276 g	280	9.00	7.00	1.6	2.00	1.00
Worthington® canned	1 cup	285	15.00	15.00			
Chili Con Carne	8 fl oz cup	254	24.61	8.28	3.4	0.53	3.43
Stouffer® w/beans	248 g	260	19.00	10.00	4.4	0.91	3.90
Swanson® homestyle	1 oz	32.7	2.42	1.21	0.5	0.11	0.51
Wendy's® chili, small	227 g	190	19.00	6.00	1.0	1.00	2.00
Clams, breaded & fried	¾ cup	451	12.82	26.40	11.4	6.77	6.60
Crab							
baked	1 crab	160	28.54	2.32	0.5	0.77	0.42
soft shell, fried	1 crab	334	10.99	17.86	7.6	4.88	4.40
Crab cake	1 cake	160	11.25	10.35	4.3	3.08	2.24
Fish fillet, battered or breaded, & fried	1 fillet	211	13.34	11.18	2.3	5.71	2.57
Oysters, battered or breaded, & fried	6 oysters	368	12.54	17.93	6.9	4.64	4.58
Tofu, Health Valley® fast menu							
baked beans	1 oz	18.7	1.47	0.40			
black beans	1 oz	21.3	2.13	0.40			
lentils	1 oz	22.7	2.00	0.40			
PIZZA							
Canadian bacon							
Jenos® crisp & tasty	109 g	250	11.00	11.00			
Stouffer® French bread	165 g	360	18.00	14.00			
Totinos® party	142 g	370	11.00	20.00			
Cheese	1 slice	140	7.68	3.21	0.9	0.49	1.54
w/cheese, meat, vegetables	1 slice	184	13.00	5.37			
Healthy Choice® French bread	159 g	290	19.00	4.00		1.00	2.00
Jenos®	63 g	160	6.00	8.00	2.3	0.82	2.66
crisp & tasty	105 g	270	10.00	14.00	3.9	1.36	4.43
rolls	85 g	240	8.00	12.00	4.9	1.52	4.58
Lean Cuisine®	145 g	310	16.00	10.00	5.2	1.91	2.87
extra cheese	156 g	350	21.00	12.00		2.00	4.00
Pappalos® French bread	161 g	360	16.00	15.00			
Pillsbury® microwave	102 g	240	10.00	10.00	3.8	1.32	4.30
French bread	161 g	370	18.00	15.00	2.6	1.74	2.95
Stouffer®	120 g	320	14.00	15.00	4.5	1.56	5.06
extra cheese	131 g	370	17.00	19.00	4.9	1.70	5.52
French bread	147 g	340	15.00	13.00	5.2	1.82	5.91
French bread, double cheese	167 g	410	19.00	18.00			
Totinos® slices	1 slice	170	7.00	7.00	2.7	0.94	3.04
microwave	110 g	250	10.00	8.00	3.2	1.12	3.64
my classic deluxe	87 g	210	10.00	9.00	3.2	1.13	3.62
party	139 g	340	13.00	17.00	5.2	1.80	5.86
three cheese	111 g	290	15.00	10.00	4.0	1.79	3.94

FOOD	CARBO-HYDRATES (mg)	FIBER (mg)	CALCIUM (mg)	IRON (mg)	POTAS-SIUM (mg)	SODIUM (mg)	CHOLES-TEROL (mg)	% OF CALORIES FROM FAT
ENTREES (continued)								
Chili (continued)								
Italian	2		5	0.34	66	148		54
spicy	3		5	0.45	81	125		27
con carne, w/beans	4		7	1.50	133	193		38
Natural Touch®vegetarian, canned	29		120	4.05	705	1335		47
Right Course®vegetarian	45	10.20	80	1.80	600	590	0	23
Worthington®canned	23		0	1.62	270	825		47
Chili Con Carne	22	1.86	67	5.19	691	1008	133	29
Stouffer®w/beans	24	4.65	80	3.60	700	1270	47	35
Swanson®homestyle	3	0.60	7	0.44	78	90	7	33
Wendy's® chili, small	21	6.00	80	5.40	440	670	40	28
Clams, breaded & fried	39	0.15	21	3.04	265	833	87	53
Crab								
baked	4	0.01	415	1.38	598	550	184	13
soft shell, fried	31	0.20	55	1.81	163	1118	45	48
Crab cake	5	0.02	202	1.12	162	452	82	58
Fish fillet, battered or breaded, & fried	15	0.04	17	1.92	292	484	31	48
Oysters, battered or breaded, & fried	40	0.11	27	4.46	182	677	109	44
Tofu, Health Valley® fast menu								
baked beans	2	2.11	13	0.60	35	19	0	19
black beans	2	1.81	20	1.20	35	33	0	17
lentils	2	1.96	5	1.92	45	35	0	16
PIZZA								
Canadian bacon								
Jenos®crisp & tasty	27		150	1.80	150	880		40
Stouffer®French bread	41		200	1.80	290	960		35
Totinos®party	35		200	2.70	220	1030		49
Cheese	21	0.23	116	0.58	110	336	9	21
w/cheese, meat, vegetables	21		101	1.53	178	382	21	26
Healthy Choice®French bread	46		300	3.60	310	390	15	12
Jenos®	17	1.24	100	1.08	85	460	9	45
crisp & tasty	28	2.07	200	1.80	140	770	16	47
rolls	23	1.57	150	1.80	95	350	19	45
Lean Cuisine®	40	2.85	250	2.70	300	750	15	29
extra cheese	39		500	3.60	300	850	20	31
Pappalos®French bread	40		350	1.80	200	830		38
Pillsbury®microwave	28	2.01	200	1.44	160	540	15	38
French bread	41	2.91	300	1.80	260	680	10	36
Stouffer®	32	2.36	250	1.80	180	640	18	42
extra cheese	33	2.58	300	1.80	190	720	20	46
French bread	41	2.89	200	2.70	270	840	22	34
French bread, double cheese	43		350	2.70	280	950		40
Totinos®slices	20	1.42	100	0.72	90	350	11	37
microwave	34	2.16	200	1.80	310	760	16	29
my classic deluxe	23	1.71	200	1.44	135	420	13	39
party	34	2.73	250	2.70	190	1000	21	45
three cheese	33	2.35	300	1.44	170	510	11	31

FAST FOODS

FOOD	AMOUNT	CALO-RIES (kcal)	PROTEIN (g)	FAT (g)	MONO-UN-SATURATED FAT (g)	POLY-UN-SATURATED FAT (g)	SATU-RATED FAT (g)
PIZZA (continued)							
Combination							
Jenos®	68 g	180	7.00	9.00	3.5	0.98	3.19
Mr. P®	102 g	260	10.00	13.00			
Pappalos® thin crust	106 g	260	13.00	10.00	4.5	1.27	4.13
French bread	184 g	430	19.00	21.00			
pan	126 g	340	17.00	15.00	6.7	2.38	6.01
Pillsbury® microwave	128 g	310	14.00	15.00	6.6	1.85	6.01
Totinos® slices	1 slice	200	7.00	10.00	3.9	1.09	3.55
my classic	91.3 g	270	13.00	14.00	4.7	1.32	4.28
party	149 g	380	13.00	21.00	7.7	2.15	6.99
Weight Watchers® frozen	205 g	340	20.00	12.00			
Deluxe							
Healthy Choice® French bread	180 g	330	23.00	7.00		1.00	3.00
Lean Cuisine®	174 g	350	20.00	12.00		2.00	3.00
Stouffer®	142 g	370	16.00	19.00			
French bread	176 g	430	18.00	21.00			
Tombstone® original	86 g	182	10.00	8.00	2.0	1.00	3.00
Golden topping							
Fox Deluxe®	96 g	240	9.00	11.00	4.8	1.53	4.54
Mr. P®	96 g	240	9.00	11.00	4.8	1.53	4.54
Hamburger							
Fox Deluxe®	108 g	260	11.00	12.00	5.2	0.60	6.18
Jenos®	70.8 g	180	8.00	9.00	3.9	0.45	4.64
crisp & tasty	115 g	290	12.00	15.00	6.5	0.76	7.72
rolls	85 g	240	9.00	13.00	4.9	1.52	4.58
Mr. P®	108 g	260	11.00	12.00	5.2	0.60	6.18
Pappalos® thin crust	104 g	240	14.00	8.00	3.5	1.01	3.47
pan	124 g	310	17.00	12.00	5.3	0.71	5.96
Stouffer® French bread	174 g	410	19.00	19.00	8.2	0.96	9.79
Totinos® party	150 g	370	15.00	19.00	8.2	0.95	9.80
Mexican style							
Taco Bell®	1 pizza	575	21.30	36.80			
Totinos® party	145 g	380	13.00	21.00			
Pepperoni	1 slice	181	10.13	6.96	3.1	1.17	2.2
w/pepperoni, beef, salami, mushroom, etc.	28.3 g	83.3	5.07	4.96			
Fox Deluxe®	99 g	250	8.00	13.00	5.7	1.64	5.5
Healthy Choice® French bread	170 g	310	20.00	7.00		1.00	2.0
Jenos®	65 g	170	6.00	9.00	3.9	1.11	3.7
crisp & tasty	108 g	280	10.00	15.00			
rolls, baked	85 g	230	7.00	13.00	4.9	1.52	4.5
rolls, microwave	85 g	240	7.00	13.00	4.9	1.52	4.5
La Choy® rolls	12.3 g	36	1.07	1.93			
Lean Cuisine®	149 g	340	18.00	12.00		2.00	4.0
Mr. P®	99	250	8.00	13.00	5.7	1.64	5.5
Pappalos®							
French bread	170 g	410	16.00	20.00			
pan	119 g	330	16.00	14.00	6.2	2.21	5.5
thin crust	104 g	270	13.00	11.00	4.9	1.38	4.7

FOOD	CARBO-HYDRATES (mg)	FIBER (mg)	CALCIUM (mg)	IRON (mg)	POTAS-SIUM (mg)	SODIUM (mg)	CHOLES-TEROL (mg)	% OF CALORIES FROM FAT
PIZZA (continued)								
Combination								
Jenos®	17	1.24	100	1.44	110	470	14	45
Mr. P®	26		100	1.80	150	640		45
Pappalos® thin crust	29	1.93	250	1.08	190	590	21	35
French bread	41		300	1.80	300	1120		44
pan	34	2.45	250	1.80	210	700	23	40
Pillsbury® microwave	29	2.34	200	1.80	200	780	26	44
Totinos® slices	20	1.38	80	1.08	105	630	15	45
my classic	23	1.67	200	1.44	210	630	18	47
party	35	2.72	4	1.44	220	1230	30	50
Weight Watchers® frozen	38							32
Deluxe								
Healthy Choice® French bread	41		250	4.50	350	500	35	19
Lean Cuisine®	40		250	3.60	370	990	35	31
Stouffer®	33		200	1.80	240	590		46
French bread	41		200	2.70	360	1130		44
Tombstone® original	18	1.57	147	1.61	189	442	22	40
Golden topping								
Fox Deluxe®	25	1.51	200	1.80	90	600	27	41
Mr. P®	25	1.51	200	1.80	90	600	27	41
Hamburger								
Fox Deluxe®	26	0.73	100	1.80	135	700	65	42
Jenos®	17	0.48	100	1.44	100	500	43	45
crisp & tasty	28	0.78	150	1.80	160	810	69	47
rolls	21	1.57	60	2.70	75	280	19	49
Mr. P®	26	0.73	100	1.80	135	700	65	42
Pappalos® thin crust	28	1.81	200	1.08	200	470	26	30
pan	34	1.09	250	1.80	230	580	62	35
Stouffer® French bread	40	1.17	200	2.70	340	1010	104	42
Totinos® party	35	1.01	200	2.70	220	1060	90	46
Mexican style								
Taco Bell®	40	5.75	257	3.74	408	1031	52	58
Totinos® party	35		200	3.60	270	970		50
Pepperoni	20	0.70	65	0.94	153	267	14	35
w/pepperoni, beef, salami, mushroom, etc.	5	0.09	76	0.23	61	367		54
Fox Deluxe®	26	1.72	100	1.80	115	640	25	47
Healthy Choice® French bread	38		200	4.50	350	470	30	20
Jenos®	17	1.13	100	1.08	85	460	17	48
crisp & tasty	27		150	1.80	140	760		48
rolls, baked	22	1.57	40	2.70	120	390	19	51
rolls, microwave	23	1.57	40	2.70	130	440	19	49
La Choy® rolls	4	0.18	11	0.27	27	58	1	48
Lean Cuisine®	40		250	3.60	340	970	30	32
Mr. P®	26	1.72	100	1.80	115	640	25	47
Pappalos®								
French bread	41		250	1.80	260	1130		44
pan	34	2.31	250	1.44	220	710	22	38
thin crust	28	1.81	250	0.72	210	600	26	37

FAST FOODS

FOOD	AMOUNT	CALO-RIES (kcal)	PROTEIN (g)	FAT (g)	MONO-UN-SATURATED FAT (g)	POLY-UN-SATURATED FAT (g)	SATU-RATED FAT (g)
PIZZA (continued)							
Pepperoni (continued)							
Pillsbury®							
French bread	170 g	430	19.00	19.00			
microwave	120 g	300	13.00	15.00	6.6	1.89	6.42
Stouffer®	124 g	350	15.00	18.00	6.5	2.44	4.67
French bread	160 g	410	17.00	20.00			
French bread w/mushrooms	174 g	430	18.00	22.00	9.0	2.51	8.17
Tombstone® original	76 g	196	9.00	10.00	4.0	1.00	4.00
light	113 g	272	15.00	10.00	4.0	1.94	3.00
single thin	116 g	306	14.00	18.00	7.0	2.00	7.00
thin	65 g	170	8.00	10.00	4.0	1.00	4.00
Totinos® slices	74.5 g	190	7.00	9.00	4.0	1.14	3.86
microwave	113 g	280	10.00	12.00	5.3	1.51	5.14
my classic deluxe	99.6 g	260	12.00	13.00	5.8	1.64	5.57
pan	119 g	330	16.00	14.00	6.2	2.21	5.56
party	145 g	370	13.00	20.00	8.8	2.49	8.46
Pepperoni & sausage							
Fox Deluxe®	102 g	260	10.00	13.00	5.7	1.64	5.57
Jenos® crisp	111 g	300	10.00	16.00			
rolls, baked	85 g	230	7.00	13.00	4.9	1.52	4.58
Stouffer®	133 g	380	16.00	21.00	8.0	2.28	7.76
French bread	177 g	450	20.00	23.00			
Tombstone® light	116 g	260	14.00	10.00			
Totinos®							
microwave	119 g	310	12.00	15.00	6.6	1.89	6.43
pan	126 g	340	16.00	15.00			
Sausage							
Fox Deluxe®	102 g	260	10.00	13.00	5.7	1.64	5.57
Healthy Choice® Italian turkey	180 g	330	23.00	5.00		1.00	2.00
sausage, French bread							
Jenos®	68 g	180	7.00	9.00	4.0	1.14	3.85
crisp & tasty	111 g	300	11.00	16.00	6.7	1.90	6.48
rolls	85 g	250	8.00	13.00	4.9	1.52	4.58
Lean Cuisine®	170 g	350	23.00	11.00		1.00	3.00
Mr. P®	102 g	260	10.00	13.00	5.7	1.64	5.57
Pappalos® thin crust	104 g	250	12.00	9.00	4.0	1.13	3.86
French bread	178 g	410	18.00	18.00			
pan	124 g	360	14.00	18.00			
Pillsbury®							
French bread	178 g	410	18.00	16.00			
microwave	124 g	280	13.00	13.00	5.7	1.64	5.57
Stouffer®	133 g	360	16.00	18.00	8.0	2.28	7.76
French bread	170 g	420	18.00	20.00			
French bread, w/mushrooms	177 g	410	17.00	19.00			
Tombstone® light	116 g	250	14.00	8.00			
Totinos® slices	1 slice	100	7.00	10.00	4.4	1.26	4.28
microwave	119 g	320	11.00	16.00	7.1	2.02	6.85
pan	124 g	320	16.00	13.00			
party	150 g	390	14.00	21.00	9.1	2.57	8.7.

FOOD	CARBO-HYDRATES (mg)	FIBER (mg)	CALCIUM (mg)	IRON (mg)	POTAS-SIUM (mg)	SODIUM (mg)	CHOLES-TEROL (mg)	% OF CALORIES FROM FAT
PIZZA (continued)								
Pepperoni (continued)								
Pillsbury®								
French bread	46		250	2.70	340	940		40
microwave	29	2.08	200	1.44	210	790	30	45
Stouffer®	34	0.00	200	1.80	210	820	98	46
French bread	41		200	2.70	310	1120		44
French bread w/mushrooms	40	3.18	20	3.60	380	1340	35	46
Tombstone® original	17	1.32	158	1.53	156	470	21	46
light	30	1.96	235	2.28	263	682	18	33
single thin	21	2.01	241	2.34	243	728	37	53
thin	12	1.13	135	1.31	135	406	21	53
Totinos® slices	20	1.29	80	1.08	85	530	19	43
microwave	34	1.96	100	1.80	310	880	29	39
my classic deluxe	23	1.73	200	1.44	170	630	25	45
pan	34	2.31	250	1.44	210	730	22	38
party	35	2.52	200	2.70	180	1310	37	49
Pepperoni & sausage								
Fox Deluxe®	26	1.77	100	1.80	150	640	26	45
Jenos® crisp	27	1.93	150	1.80	170	840	28	48
rolls, baked	22	1.57	40	2.70	110	380	19	51
Stouffer®	33	2.31	150	1.80	240	860	34	50
French bread	40		200	3.60	400	1350		46
Tombstone® light	30	2.01	241	2.34	270	610	15	35
Totinos®								
microwave	31	2.07	150	1.80	350	970	30	44
pan	34		250	1.80	210	720		40
Sausage								
Fox Deluxe®	26	1.77	100	1.80	150	630	26	45
Healthy Choice® Italian turkey sausage, French bread	48		250	4.50	350	390	25	14
Jenos®	17	1.18	100	1.44	115	460	17	45
crisp & tasty	28	1.93	150	1.80	170	850	28	48
rolls	24	1.57	60	2.70	180	440	19	47
Lean Cuisine®	40		250	4.50	390	960	45	28
Mr. P®	26	1.77	100	1.80	150	630	26	45
Pappalos® thin crust	28	1.81	200	1.08	180	490	26	32
French bread	41		250	1.80	290	1000		40
pan	34		200	1.44	190	550		45
Pillsbury®								
French bread	48		250	4.50	390	860		35
microwave	29	2.15	200	1.44	180	680	32	42
Stouffer®	32	2.31	200	1.80	250	830	34	45
French bread	41		200	2.70	330	1110		43
French bread, w/mushrooms	42		200	2.70	330	1050		42
Tombstone® light	29	2.01	241	2.34	270	570	10	29
Totinos® slices	20	1.31	80	1.08	115	540	19	90
microwave	33	2.07	100	1.44	340	870	30	45
pan	34		250	1.80	190	630		37
party	35	2.61	200	2.70	250	1180	38	48

FAST FOODS

FOOD	AMOUNT	CALO-RIES (kcal)	PROTEIN (g)	FAT (g)	MONO-UN-SATURATED FAT (g)	POLY-UN-SATURATED FAT (g)	SATU-RATED FAT (g)
PIZZA (continued)							
Supreme, Tombstone®							
light	130 g	261	16.00	9.00	4.0	1.87	3.00
single	130 g	308	15.00	18.00	6.0	2.00	7.00
thin	72 g	169	8.00	10.00	4.0	1.00	4.00
Vegetable							
w/onion, tomato, green pepper, mushroom	28.3 g	45.4	3.49	0.57			
Stouffer® French bread, deluxe	181 g	420	18.00	20.00	6.6	2.39	6.33
Tombstone® light	125 g	249	14.00	8.00	3.0	1.37	3.00
Totinos® party	152 g	300	11.00	13.00	5.1	1.67	5.07
SALADS							
Bacon bits only, McDonald's®	3 g	15	1.00	1.00	0.2	0.50	0.30
Caesar, dry, Suddenly Salad®	54.4 g	220	8.00	2.00			
Carrot/raisin, home recipe	1 cup	306	3.80	11.60			
Chef, w/ham & cheese	200 g	196	13.40	12.70			
Arby's®	411 g	205	18.50	9.50	1.4	1.00	3.90
Long John Silver's® ocean	234 g	110	12.00	1.00	0.4	0.20	0.40
McDonald's®	265 g	170	17.00	9.00	1.0	4.00	4.00
Chicken salad	1 cup	502	26.00	36.20			
Arby's® roast chicken	400 g	204	24.00	7.20	0.9	0.90	3.30
McDonald's® chunky chicken	255 g	150	25.00	4.00	1.0	1.00	2.00
Wendy's®	17.5 g	35	2.00	2.50		1.00	0.50
Coleslaw	1tbsp	5.52	0.10	0.21			
Croutons only, McDonald's®	11 g	50	1.00	2.00	1.0	0.50	1.30
Fruit							
canned, juice pack	1 cup	125	1.28	0.06			
canned, water pack	1 cup	73.5	0.86	0.17			
Green, tossed	207 g	32	2.60	0.16			
Lobster, w/tomato & egg	1 cup	211	13.20	13.00			
Macaroni	28.4 g	50.7	0.70	3.00			
Mandarin orange gelatin	28.4 g	22.7	0.40	0.00			
Pasta salad							
Hardees® w/chicken	414 g	230	27.00	3.00	1.0	1.00	1.00
Suddenly Salad® tortellini Italian	59.6 g	240	8.00	4.00			
Potato	1 cup	358	6.70	20.50			
Salad dressing							
Kraft®							
creamy dill	1 cup	400	8.00	22.00			
garden primavera	1 cup	340	10.00	14.00			
herb & garlic	1 cup	420	10.00	24.00			
homestyle	1 cup	480	8.00	32.00			
rancher's choice	1 cup	480	10.00	32.00			
McDonald's®							
peppercorn	1 oz	160	0.00	18.00	4.0	10.00	2.00
red French	1 oz	80	0.00	4.00	2.0	2.00	0.00
Subway®							
buttermilk ranch	56.7 g	348	1.00	37.00	7.0	24.00	5.00
lite Italian	56.7 g	23	1.00	1.00			

FOOD	CARBO-HYDRATES (mg)	FIBER (mg)	CALCIUM (mg)	IRON (mg)	POTAS-SIUM (mg)	SODIUM (mg)	CHOLES-TEROL (mg)	% OF CALORIES FROM FAT
PIZZA (continued)								
Supreme, Tombstone®								
light	29	2.37	222	2.43	306	691	16	31
single	22	2.61	242	2.41	286	713	39	53
thin	12	1.86	108	1.54	157	387	21	53
Vegetable								
w/onion, tomato, green pepper, mushroom	7	0.23	25	0.23	42.8	136		11
Stouffer® French bread, deluxe	41	4.67	350	2.70	230	830	20	43
Tombstone® light	30	2.51	233	2.32	278	498	7	29
Totinos® party	36	3.06	200	2.70	200	910	17	39
SALADS								
Bacon bits only, McDonald's®	0	0.00	0	0.00	4	95	1	60
Caesar, dry, Suddenly Salad®	40	0.35	80	1.44	200	900	49	8
Carrot/raisin, home recipe	56	16.70	96	3.00	928	377	33	34
Chef, w/ham & cheese	7	2.39	227	1.17	415	567	46	58
Arby's®	13		170	5.04	819	796	126	42
Long John Silver's® ocean	13		100	3.60	95	730	40	8
McDonald's®	8		150	1.51		400	111	48
Chicken salad	17	2.18	128	3.69	521	1395	67	65
Arby's® roast chicken	12		170	1.98	877	508	43	32
McDonald's® chunky chicken	7	0.96	34	1.02	436	230	78	24
Wendy's®	1	0.21			20	68	0	64
Coleslaw	1	0.30	4	0.05	15	2	1	34
Croutons only, McDonald's®	7	0.52	6	0.35	20	140	0	36
Fruit								
canned, juice pack	33	1.64	28	0.62	288	13	0	0
canned, water pack	19	4.50	17	0.74	191	7	0	2
Green, tossed	7	1.39	26	1.30	356	53	0	5
Lobster, w/tomato & egg	11	2.10	65	1.71	468	637	176	55
Macaroni	5	0.29	5	0.27	21	148	1	53
Mandarin orange gelatin	6	0.57			9	14	0	0
Pasta salad								
Hardees® w/chicken	23			9.00	620	380	55	12
Suddenly Salad® tortellini Italian	42		40	2.16	150	900		15
Potato	28		48	1.63	635	1323	171	52
Salad dressing								
Kraft®								
creamy dill	42	0.92	14	0.79	260	560	20	50
garden primavera	42	0.79	20	0.83	160	900	10	37
herb & garlic	42	1.01	15	0.88	200	600	20	51
homestyle	82	1.85	27	1.60	300	940	20	60
rancher's choice	42	1.01	15	0.88	260	1080	20	60
McDonald's®								
peppercorn	2	0.00	3	0.11	22	170	14	101
red French	10	0.00	3	0.11	22	220	0	45
Subway®								
buttermilk ranch	2	0.00	8	0.11	17	492	6	96
lite Italian	4	0.00	6	0.11	13	952	0	39

FAST FOODS

FOOD	AMOUNT	CALO-RIES (kcal)	PROTEIN (g)	FAT (g)	MONO-UN-SATURATED FAT (g)	POLY-UN-SATURATED FAT (g)	SATU-RATED FAT (g)
SALADS (continued)							
Seafood salad							
Long John Silver's®	337 g	270	16.00	7.00	2.0	3.00	1.00
seafood salad, scoop	142 g	210	14.00	5.00	1.6	2.50	0.83
Wendy's®	37 g	70	3.00	4.00		2.00	1.00
Three bean salad							
Alex®	28.4 g	33.2	1.3	0.2			
Del Monte® canned	28.4 g	22.4	0.71	0.06			
Tuna salad, w/celery, mayonnaise, pickle, egg	1 cup	350	30	22			
Wendy's®	52 g	100	7.00	6.00		3.00	1.00
Vegetable, tossed, w/out dressing							
plain	1½ cup	32	2.60	0.16	0.0	0.07	0.02
w/added cheese & egg	1½ cup	102	8.76	5.79	1.7	0.48	2.98
w/added chicken	1½ cup	105	17.44	2.18	0.6	0.56	0.58
w/added pasta & seafood	1½ cup	380	16.44	20.85	4.8	9.08	2.57
w/added shrimp	1½ cup	107	14.51	2.48	0.8	0.48	0.65
w/added turkey, ham, & cheese (chef style)	1½ cup	267	26.03	16.07	5.1	1.44	8.18
jellied	1 cup	121	3.22	0.11			
Long John Silver's® garden salad	246 g	170	9.00	9.00	1.0	0.78	0.85
McDonald's® garden salad	189 g	50	4.00	2.00	0.4	0.60	1.00
side salad	106 g	30	2.00	1.00	0.2	0.30	0.50
Waldorf gelatin	28.4 g	26.7	1.50	0.10			
SOUPS							
Arby's®							
roast beef & vegetable	227 g	96	5.00	3.00	1.0	1.00	1.00
Boston clam chowder	227 g	193	8.30	10.00	3.2	2.20	4.50
cream of broccoli	227 g	166	7.70	7.20	0.7	2.70	3.80
French onion	227 g	67	2.00	3.00	1.5	0.75	0.75
lumberjack mixed vegetable	227 g	89	2.30	3.60	1.4	0.20	1.70
old fashioned chicken noodle	227 g	99	6.00	1.80	0.5	0.30	0.50
pilgrim clam chowder	227 g	193	10.00	11.00	5.0	2.00	4.00
split pea & ham	227 g	200	8.00	10.00	1.0	1.00	5.00
tomato Florentine	227 g	84	3.00	2.00	0.6	0.67	0.67
Wisconsin cheese	227 g	281	9.00	18.00	4.5	4.50	9.00
Long John Silver's®							
seafood chowder w/cod	198 g	140	11.00	6.00	2.5	1.70	1.80
seafood gumbo w/cod	198 g	120	9.00	8.00	2.6	3.20	2.10
MEXICAN FOODS							
Burrito							
w/beans	2 burritos	448	14.07	13.50	4.7	1.20	6.89
w/beans & cheese	2 burritos	377	15.07	11.70	2.4	1.78	6.85
w/beans & chili peppers	2 burritos	413	16.38	14.67	5.3	0.96	7.61
w/beans & meat	2 burritos	508	22.48	17.80	7.0	1.22	8.32
w/beans, cheese, & beef	2 burritos	331	14.58	13.29	4.4	1.02	7.15
w/beans, cheese, & chili peppers	2 burritos	663	33.29	22.98	8.4	1.27	11.20
w/beef	2 burritos	523	26.59	20.80	7.4	0.85	10.46
w/beef & chili peppers	2 burritos	426	21.51	16.54	6.0	0.98	8.00

FOOD	CARBO-HYDRATES (mg)	FIBER (mg)	CALCIUM (mg)	IRON (mg)	POTAS-SIUM (mg)	SODIUM (mg)	CHOLES-TEROL (mg)	% OF CALORIES FROM FAT
SALADS (continued)								
Seafood salad								
Long John Silver's®	36	1.33	148	3.22	100	670	90	23
seafood salad, scoop	26	0.56	63	1.36	100	570	90	21
Wendy's®	5		150		25	300	0	51
Three bean salad								
Alex®	7	2.07			63	107		5
Del Monte® canned	5	1.52	10	0.28	38	101		2
Tuna salad, w/celery, mayonnaise, pickle, egg	7	1.03	41	2.7		434	68	57
Wendy's®	4	0.31		0.36	80	270	0	54
Vegetable, tossed, w/out dressing								
plain	7	1.39	26	1.30	356	53	0	5
w/added cheese & egg	5	1.00	100	0.68	371	119	98	51
w/added chicken	4	0.96	37	1.09	447	209	72	19
w/added pasta & seafood	32	1.63	73	3.16	600	1572	50	49
w/added shrimp	7	1.42	60	0.91	404	487	180	21
w/added turkey, ham, & cheese (chef style)	5	1.14	235	1.96	402	744	139	54
jellied	29		13	0.27	112	85	0	1
Long John Silver's® garden salad	13	2.07	42	1.73	20	380	5	48
McDonald's® garden salad	6	1.80	40	1.26	450	70	65	36
side salad	4	1.23	20	0.67	219	35	33	30
Waldorf gelatin	5	0.26	5	0.11	14	16	0	3
SOUPS								
Arby's®								
roast beef & vegetable	14	0.45	16	1.04	211	996	10	28
Boston clam chowder	18	1.36	150	1.44	318	1032	26	47
cream of broccoli	18	1.75	270	0.54	404	1050	24	39
French onion	7	0.91	25	0.64	106	1248	0	40
lumberjack mixed vegetable	13	1.25	41	1.87	268	1075	4	36
old fashioned chicken noodle	15	0.68	16	0.73	78	929	25	16
pilgrim clam chowder	18	1.92	134	1.95	379	1157	28	51
split pea & ham	21	3.86	32	2.02	272	1029	30	45
tomato Florentine	15	0.45	45	1.64	221	910	2	21
Wisconsin cheese	20	1.82	252	1.32	447	1084	32	58
Long John Silver's®								
seafood chowder w/cod	10		200	1.70	380	590	20	39
seafood gumbo w/cod	4		100	1.80	310	740	25	60
MEXICAN FOODS								
Burrito								
w/beans	71	4.71	113	4.52	653	986	5	27
w/beans & cheese	55	2.04	214	2.27	496	1166	27	28
w/beans & chili peppers	58	3.10	100	4.54	580	1043	33	32
w/beans & meat	66	3.66	105	4.89	656	1335	48	32
w/beans, cheese, & beef	40	2.36	131	3.73	410	990	125	36
w/beans, cheese, & chili peppers	85	5.09	288	7.68	810	2060	158	31
w/beef	59	1.71	84	6.09	739	1492	65	36
w/beef & chili peppers	49	1.34	87	4.43	499	1116	54	35

FAST FOODS

FOOD	AMOUNT	CALO-RIES (kcal)	PROTEIN (g)	FAT (g)	MONO-UN-SATURATED FAT (g)	POLY-UN-SATURATED FAT (g)	SATU-RATED FAT (g)
MEXICAN FOODS (continued)							
Burrito (continued)							
w/beef, cheese, & chili peppers	2 burritos	634	40.90	24.79	9.9	2.23	10.40
w/fruit (apple or cherry)	1 lg burrito	484	5.24	19.94	7.1	2.21	9.57
Healthy Choice® quick meal							
beef/bean, mild	1 burrito	270	12.00	7.00		3.00	3.00
beef/bean, medium	1 burrito	270	12.00	7.00		3.00	3.00
chicken con queso	1 burrito	280	15.00	8.00		3.00	2.00
Taco Bell® bean	1 burrito	387	15.00	14.00		2.00	4.00
w/beef	1 burrito	431	25.00	21.00		2.00	8.00
burrito supreme	1 burrito	440	20.00	22.00		2.00	8.00
double beef supreme	1 burrito	457	23.60	21.80	12.2	1.65	7.98
Chimichanga							
w/beef	1 item	425	19.62	19.67	8.0	1.14	8.51
w/beef & cheese	1 item	443	20.05	23.45	9.4	0.73	11.18
w/beef & red chili peppers	1 item	424	18.10	19.13	7.8	1.11	8.27
w/beef, cheese, & red chili peppers	1 item	364	14.67	17.55	7.0	0.55	8.37
Enchanadas, beef & bean, Lean Cuisine®	262 g	280	15.00	10.00	7.0	0.97	1.94
Enchilada							
w/cheese	1 item	320	9.64	18.85	6.3	0.82	10.59
w/cheese & beef	1 item	324	11.92	17.64	6.1	1.39	9.05
Stouffer® cheese	287 g	590	23.00	40.00	11.0	5.10	18.20
Swanson® beef	1 oz	34.9	1.24	1.53	0.6	0.43	0.46
Enchirito w/cheese, beef, & beans	1 item	344	17.90	16.08	6.5	0.33	7.95
Fajitas							
beef	1 fajita	244	11.00	10.30			
chicken	1 fajita	170	9.43	2.84			
Taco Bell®	1 fajita	382	19.80	19.70		1.51	9.32
Frijoles w/cheese	8 oz cup	226	11.37	7.78	2.6	0.70	4.08
Nachos							
w/cheese	6-8 nachos	345	9.09	18.95	7.9	2.23	7.78
w/cheese & jalapeno peppers	6-8 nachos	607	16.81	34.15	14.4	4.02	14.02
w/cheese, beans, ground beef, & peppers	6-8 nachos	568	19.78	30.69	10.9	5.69	12.49
w/cinnamon & sugar	6-8 nachos	592	7.19	35.98	11.8	4.13	18.21
Taco Bell®	106 g	346	7.49	18.50		1.55	5.74
Bellgrande	287 g	649	21.60	35.30		2.61	12.30
Pintos & cheese, Taco Bell®	1 serving	190	8.97	8.72		0.81	3.60
Taco	1 lg taco	569	31.77	31.60	10.1	1.48	17.48
Taco Bell®	1 taco	183	10.00	11.00		1.00	5.00
Bellgrande	1 taco	355	18.30	23.10	6.5	1.32	10.90
light	1 taco	410	19.00	28.80		5.36	11.60
soft	1 taco	228	11.80	11.80	3.7	1.21	5.37
La Choy® frozen snack rolls	1 item	32.7	1.13	1.43			

FOOD	CARBO-HYDRATES (mg)	FIBER (mg)	CALCIUM (mg)	IRON (mg)	POTAS-SIUM (mg)	SODIUM (mg)	CHOLES-TEROL (mg)	% OF CALORIES FROM FAT
MEXICAN FOODS (continued)								
Burrito (continued)								
w/beef, cheese, & chili peppers	64	1.79	223	7.81	667	2091	170	35
w/fruit (apple or cherry)	73	0.75	32	2.24	218	443	7	37
Healthy Choice® quick meal								
beef/bean, mild	42		60	2.70	270	520	15	23
beef/bean, medium	42		60	2.70	270	520	15	23
chicken con queso	40		100	2.70	260	500	20	26
Taco Bell® bean	63	3.00	190	4.00	495	1148	9	33
w/beef	48	2.00	150	4.00	380	1311	57	44
burrito supreme	55	3.00	190	4.00	501	1181	33	45
double beef supreme	42	5.68	145	3.95	431	1053	57	43
Chimichanga								
w/beef	43	2.25	63	4.55	587	910	9	42
w/beef & cheese	39	2.12	238	3.84	203	956	51	48
w/beef & red chili peppers	46	1.51	71	4.18	613	1169	9	41
w/beef, cheese, & red chili peppers	38	1.05	218	3.14	330	895	50	43
Enchanadas, beef & bean, Lean Cuisine®	32	3.88	150	2.70	460	890	60	32
Enchilada								
w/cheese	29	2.72	324	1.31	240	784	44	53
w/cheese & beef	30	3.00	228	3.08	574	1320	40	49
Stouffer® cheese	34	7.84	600	1.44	440	880	84	61
Swanson® beef	4	0.42	15	0.20	37	98	3	39
Enchirito w/cheese, beef, & beans	34	1.97	217	2.39	560	1251	49	42
Fajitas								
beef	28	2.15	69	2.32	296	247	26	38
chicken	28	2.15	67	1.68	302	328	13	15
Taco Bell®	31		269	2.84		1243	54	46
Frijoles w/cheese	29	3.89	188	2.24	605	882	36	31
Nachos								
w/cheese	36	1.95	272	1.27	172	816	18	49
w/cheese & jalapeno peppers	60	4.74	620	2.45	293	1736	83	51
w/cheese, beans, ground beef, & peppers	56	4.30	384	2.78	451	1800	21	49
w/cinnamon & sugar	63	1.37	85	2.89	79	439	39	55
Taco Bell®	38	1.39	191	0.93	159	399	9	48
Bellgrande	61		297	3.48	674	997	36	49
Pintos & cheese, Taco Bell®	19	4.87	156	1.42	399	642	16	41
Taco	41	3.21	339	3.72	728	1234	87	50
Taco Bell®	11	1.00	84	1.00	159	276	32	54
Bellgrande	18	4.54	182	1.92	334	472	56	59
light	18		155	2.44	316	594	56	63
soft	18	2.56	116	2.27	196	554	32	47
La Choy® frozen snack rolls	4	0.14	6			40	0	39

FAST FOODS

FOOD	AMOUNT	CALO-RIES (kcal)	PROTEIN (g)	FAT (g)	MONO-UN-SATURATED FAT (g)	POLY-UN-SATURATED FAT (g)	SATU-RATED FAT (g)
MEXICAN FOODS (continued)							
Taco salad	1½ cup	279	13.23	14.77	5.1	1.75	6.82
Taco Bell®	530 g	502	29.50	31.30	17.0	1.51	12.80
w/salsa	530 g	520	30.60	31.40	17.1	1.51	12.80
w/salsa & shell	595 g	941	36.00	61.30	21.6	12.10	18.70
Wendy's® w/taco chips	791 g	660	40.00	37.00			
Taco salad w/chili con carne	1½ cup	288	17.40	13.13	4.5	1.54	6.00
Tamales w/beef, Gebhardt®	1 tamale	112	3.00	8.00			
Tortilla grande, Stouffer®	273 g	530	24.00	33.00			
Tostada							
w/beans & cheese	1 tostada	223	9.60	9.86	3.0	0.75	5.37
w/beans, beef, & cheese	1 tostada	334	16.09	16.94	3.5	0.60	11.48
w/beef & cheese	1 tostada	315	18.99	16.35	3.3	0.97	10.40
w/guacamole	1 tostada	360	12.48	23.25	8.4	3.05	9.87
Taco Bell® regular	1 tostada	243	9.00	11.00		1.00	4.00
beefy	1 tostada	334	16.10	16.90	3.5	0.54	11.50
SANDWICHES & BURGERS							
BMT sandwich							
Subway® on honey wheat roll	1 sand-wich	1011	45.00	57.00	25.0	7.00	20.00
on Italian roll	1 sand-wich	982	44.00	55.00	24.0	7.00	20.00
BLT w/mayonnaise	1 sand-wich	282	6.80	15.60			
Cheeseburger, regular, single meat patty							
plain	1 burger	320	14.77	15.15	5.7	1.54	6.47
w/condiments	1 burger	295	15.96	14.14	5.3	1.09	6.31
w/condiments & bacon	1 burger	609	32.00	36.80			
w/condiments & vegetables	1 burger	359	17.84	19.79	7.1	1.47	9.19
Hardees® mushroom & Swiss	1 burger	490	30.00	27.00	12.0	2.00	13.00
McDonald's®	1 burger	305	15.00	13.00	1.0	5.00	7.00
Wendy's® single cheeseburger, everything	1 burger	490	29.00	27.00			
Cheeseburger, regular, double meat patty							
plain	1 burger	457	27.66	28.48	11.0	1.91	13.00
w/condiments & vegetables	1 burger	416	21.24	21.08	7.8	2.66	8.72
double-decker bun, plain	1 burger	461	22.12	21.62	8.3	1.83	9.51
double-decker bun, w/condiments & vegetables	1 burger	649	29.74	35.26	12.6	6.37	12.77
Burger King® double cheeseburger	1 burger	483	30.00	27.00	11.0	2.00	13.00
bacon double cheese deluxe	1 burger	592	33.00	39.00	14.0	8.00	16.00
Cheeseburger, large, single meat patty							
plain	1 burger	608	30.13	32.99	12.7	2.44	14.84
w/bacon & condiments	1 burger	609	32.00	36.76	14.5	2.71	16.25
w/condiments & vegetables	1 burger	564	28.19	32.94	12.6	2.03	15.04
w/ham, condiments, & vegetables	1 burger	745	39.51	48.18	18.8	3.85	21.13

FOOD	CARBO-HYDRATES (mg)	FIBER (mg)	CALCIUM (mg)	IRON (mg)	POTAS-SIUM (mg)	SODIUM (mg)	CHOLES-TEROL (mg)	% OF CALORIES FROM FAT
MEXICAN FOODS (continued)								
Taco salad	24	2.48	192	2.28	416	763	44	48
Taco Bell®	26	7.04	331	4.54	988	1056	80	56
w/salsa	30	7.04	367	5.14	1151	1431	80	54
w/salsa & shell	63	7.91	398	7.10	1212	1662	80	59
Wendy's® w/taco chips	46	10.50	532	9.23	1330	1110	35	50
Taco salad w/chili con carne	27	5.16	246	2.67	393	886	4	41
Tamales w/beef, Gebhardt®	8	2.22	9	0.60	65	542	22	64
Tortilla grande, Stouffer®	34		400	2.70	730	910		56
Tostada								
w/beans & cheese	27	3.75	211	1.88	403	543	30	40
w/beans, beef, & cheese	30	3.59	190	2.45	490	870	75	46
w/beef & cheese	23	2.47	217	2.86	572	896	41	47
w/guacamole	32	4.06	424	1.63	649	798	39	58
Taco Bell® regular	27	2.00	180	2.00	401	596	16	41
beefy	30	5.19	190	2.45	490	870	75	46
SANDWICHES & BURGERS								
BMT sandwich								
Subway® on honey wheat roll	88	6.00			1002	3199	133	51
on Italian roll	83	.5.00	64	4.26	917	3139	133	50
BLT w/mayonnaise	29	2.88	53	1.50	274	1222	44	50
Cheeseburger, regular, single meat patty								
plain	32	0.12	140	2.44	165	500	50	43
w/condiments	27	0.26	111	2.43	223	616	37	43
w/condiments & bacon	37		162	4.73	331	1044	112	54
w/condiments & vegetables	28	0.62	182	2.65	229	976	52	50
Hardees® mushroom & Swiss	33				370	940	70	50
McDonald's®	30		199	2.30	223	725	50	38
Wendy's® single cheeseburger, everything	35	2.69	234	4.31	495	1155	90	50
Cheeseburger, regular, double meat patty								
plain	22	0.11	232	3.41	308	635	110	56
w/condiments & vegetables	35	0.50	171	3.42	335	1051	60	46
double-decker bun, plain	44	0.16	224	3.70	285	892	80	42
double-decker bun, w/condiments & vegetables	53	1.24	169	4.71	389	920	94	49
Burger King® double cheeseburger	29	1.44	189	2.95	344	851	100	50
bacon double cheese deluxe	28	1.06	156	3.95	463	804	111	59
Cheeseburger, large, single meat patty								
plain	47	0.15	91	5.47	644	1589	96	49
w/bacon & condiments	37	0.78	162	4.73	331	1044	112	54
w/condiments & vegetables	38	0.83	205	4.66	445	1107	88	53
w/ham, condiments, & vegetables	38	0.63	301	5.04	539	1713	122	58

FAST FOODS

FOOD	AMOUNT	CALO-RIES (kcal)	PROTEIN (g)	FAT (g)	MONO-UN-SATURATED FAT (g)	POLY-UN-SATURATED FAT (g)	SATU-RATED FAT (g)
SANDWICHES & BURGERS (continued)							
Cheeseburger, large, single meat patty (continued)							
Jack in the Box® Jumbo Jack cheeseburger	1 burger	677	32.00	40.00	15.0	9.00	14.00
McDonald's® quarter pound cheesburger	1 burger	510	28.00	28.00	1.0	11.00	16.00
Cheeseburger, large, double meat patty, w/condiments & vegetables	1 burger	706	37.99	43.65	17.3	4.70	17.67
Burger King®							
barbecue bacon double cheeseburger	1 burger	536	32.00	31.00	13.0	2.00	14.00
mushroom Swiss double cheeseburger	1 burger	473	31.00	27.00	11.0	2.00	12.00
Cheeseburger, large, triple meat patty, plain	1 burger	796	56.06	50.97	21.5	3.15	21.71
Chicken fillet sandwich							
plain	1 sand-wich	515	24.11	29.45	10.4	8.38	8.53
w/cheese	1 sand-wich	632	29.40	38.76	13.6	9.95	12.45
Arby's ®	1 sand-wich	445	22.20	22.50	9.5	9.97	2.96
chicken cordon bleu	1 sand-wich	518	30.00	27.10	11.7	10.20	5.24
grilled chicken barbecue	1 sand-wich	386	23.40	13.10	5.2	4.40	3.60
grilled chicken deluxe	1 sand-wich	430	23.60	19.90	5.1	4.40	3.50
light roast chicken deluxe	1 sand-wich	276	24.00	7.00			
light roast chicken deluxe w/cheese	1 sand-wich	632	29.40	38.76			
Arthur Treacher®	1 sand-wich	413	16.20	19.20		6.70	
Burger King® BK broiler	1 sand-wich	379	24.00	18.00	7.9	3.84	3.00
BK broiler sauce	14 g	90	0.00	10.00	2.0	5.00	1.00
Hardees® grilled	1 sand-wich	310	24.00	9.00	3.0	5.00	1.00
Kentucky Fried Chicken®	1 sand-wich	482	21.00	27.00	3.9	9.00	6.00
McDonald's® McChicken sandwich	1 sand-wich	415	19.00	19.00	6.6	3.80	8.55
Rax® grilled chicken sandwich	1 sand-wich	440	24.00	19.00	4.4	5.37	2.92
Club sandwich	1 sand-wich	590	35.6	20.8			
Arby's®	1 sand-wich	560	30	30	9.2	8.4	11.6

FOOD	CARBO-HYDRATES (mg)	FIBER (mg)	CALCIUM (mg)	IRON (mg)	POTAS-SIUM (mg)	SODIUM (mg)	CHOLES-TEROL (mg)	% OF CALORIES FROM FAT
SANDWICHES & BURGERS (continued)								
Cheeseburger, large, single meat patty (continued)								
Jack in the Box® Jumbo Jack cheeseburger	46		273	4.60	499	1090	102	53
McDonald's® quarter pound cheesburger	34		295	3.72	341	1110	115	49
Cheeseburger, large, double meat patty, w/condiments & vegetables	40	1.03	240	5.91	596	1149	141	56
Burger King®								
barbecue bacon double cheeseburger	31	0.80	158	3.96	429	795	103	52
mushroom Swiss double cheeseburger	27			4.14		746	95	51
Cheeseburger, large, triple meat patty, plain	27	1.22	282	8.30	821	1211	161	58
Chicken fillet sandwich								
plain	39	0.36	60	4.68	353	957	60	51
w/cheese	42	0.32	258	3.63	334	1238	76	55
Arby's ®	52	1.56	60	2.88	403	958	45	46
chicken cordon bleu	52		170	3.06	464	1463	92	47
grilled chicken barbecue	47		70	3.96	596	1002	43	31
grilled chicken deluxe	42	0.00	70	2.52	659	901	44	42
light roast chicken deluxe	33		130	2.88	432	777	33	23
light roast chicken deluxe w/cheese	42	0.32	258	3.63	334	1238	76	55
Arthur Treacher®	44		59	1.70	279	708		42
Burger King® BK broiler	31	1.80	74	3.23	324	764	53	43
BK broiler sauce	0	0.00				95	7	100
Hardees® grilled	34	2.21	542	3.00	410	890	60	26
Kentucky Fried Chicken®	39	1.41	100	3.11	297	1060	47	50
McDonald's® McChicken sandwich	39	1.61	143	2.61	340	830	50	41
Rax® grilled chicken sandwich	36	1.61	114	3.56	340	1050	88	39
Club sandwich	42	4.17	103	4.3	583	2601	93	32
Arby's®	43	2.27	200	3.6	466	1610	100	48

FAST FOODS

FOOD	AMOUNT	CALO-RIES (kcal)	PROTEIN (g)	FAT (g)	MONO-UN-SATURATED FAT (g)	POLY-UN-SATURATED FAT (g)	SATU-RATED FAT (g)
SANDWICHES & BURGERS (continued)							
Club sandwich (continued)							
Subway® on Italian roll	1 sandwich	693	46	22		4	7
on honey wheat	1 sandwich	722	47	23		4	7
Wendy's® chicken club	1 sandwich	520	30	25		9	6
Chicken salad							
mayonnaise	1 oz	81.1	6.44	4.68			
cheese/potato	1 oz	55	5.13	1.59			
Cold cut combo, on wheat, Subway®	1 sandwich	883	48	41	1	10	12
on Italian	1 sandwich	853	46	40	1	10	12
Egg & cheese sandwich	1 sandwich	340	15.61	19.42	8.2	2.58	6.63
Fish sandwich							
w/tartar sauce	1 sandwich	431	16.94	22.77	7.6	8.25	5.24
w/tartar sauce & cheese	1 sandwich	524	20.60	28.60	8.9	9.43	8.14
Arby's® fish fillet	1 serving	526	23.00	27.00	9.2	10.60	7.00
Long John Silver's® batter dip	1 serving	350	19.00	3.70	2.4	0.34	0.90
McDonald's® Fillet o Fish	1 sandwich	370	14.00	18.00	6.0	4.00	8.00
Hamburger, regular, single meat patty							
plain	1 burger	275	12.32	11.81	5.4	0.92	4.14
w/condiments	1 burger	275	13.60	10.23	3.7	1.77	3.51
w/condiments & vegetables	1 burger	279	12.92	13.48	5.2	2.58	4.13
McDonald's® plain	1 burger	255	12.00	9.00	1.0	3.00	5.00
Wendy's® plain	1 burger	350	25.00	15.00	7.0	2.00	6.00
w/everything	1 burger	440	26.00	23.00			
kid's meal hamburger	1 burger	270	15.00	9.00			
Hamburger, regular, double meat patty							
plain	1 burger	544	29.92	27.90	12.1	2.34	10.38
w/condiments	1 burger	576	31.81	32.46	14.1	2.77	12.00
McDonald's® Big Mac	1 burger	560	25.00	26.00	1.0	9.00	16.00
Wendy's®	1 burger	540	34.30	26.60	10.3	2.80	10.50
Hamburger, large, single meat patty							
plain	1 burger	400	22.50	22.92	9.8	2.14	8.39
w/condiments & vegetables	1 burger	511	25.70	27.35	11.4	2.20	10.42
Burger King® Whopper	1 burger	630	26.00	36.00	13.8	2.22	16.50
Jack in the Box® Jumbo Jack hamburger	1 burger	584	26.00	34.00	13.0	8.00	11.00
McDonald's® quarter pound hamburger	1 burger	410	23.10	20.70	11.4	1.21	8.00
McDLT	1 burger	580	26.30	36.80	16.7	8.50	11.50

FOOD	CARBO-HYDRATES (mg)	FIBER (mg)	CALCIUM (mg)	IRON (mg)	POTAS-SIUM (mg)	SODIUM (mg)	CHOLES-TEROL (mg)	% OF CALORIES FROM FAT
SANDWICHES & BURGERS (continued)								
Club sandwich (continued)								
Subway® on Italian roll	83	5	57.5	3.09	971	2717	84	29
on honey wheat	89	6	96.3	3.18	1055	2777	84	29
Wendy's® chicken club	44	2.3	100	14.4	470	980	75	43
Chicken salad								
mayonnaise	3	0.425	6.8	0.255	27.2	75.4	9	52
cheese/potato	5	0.822	34.3	0.198	47.1	155	9	26
Cold cut combo, on wheat, Subway®	88	6	235	2.97	1010	2278	166	42
on Italian	83	5	227	2.86	876	2218	166	42
Egg & cheese sandwich	26	0.22	225	2.99	188	804	291	51
Fish sandwich								
w/tartar sauce	41	0.60	84	2.60	339	615	55	48
w/tartar sauce & cheese	48	0.37	185	3.50	353	939	68	49
Arby's® fish fillet	50		90	3.78	450	872	44	46
Long John Silver's® batter dip	39		150	1.80	310	740	25	10
McDonald's® Fillet o Fish	38	1.11	165	1.83	150	730	50	44
Hamburger, regular, single meat patty								
plain	31	0.12	63	2.41	145	387	36	39
w/condiments	33	0.34	52	2.46	215	564	43	33
w/condiments & vegetables	27	0.33	63	2.62	227	504	26	43
McDonald's® plain	30		100	2.70	215	490	37	32
Wendy's® plain	31	2.76	100	5.40	280	510	70	39
w/everything	36	2.73	100	5.40	430	850	75	47
kid's meal hamburger	33	1.32	100	3.60	210	590	35	30
Hamburger, regular, double meat patty								
plain	43	0.16	87	4.55	363	554	99	46
w/condiments	39	0.26	92	5.55	527	742	102	51
McDonald's® Big Mac	42		256	4.00	237	890	100	42
Wendy's®	40	2.27	102	5.95	565	791	122	44
Hamburger, large, single meat patty								
plain	25	0.14	74	3.57	268	474	71	52
w/condiments & vegetables	40	0.99	96	4.92	479	825	86	48
Burger King® Whopper	50	2.53	104	6.00	520	990	104	51
Jack in the Box® Jumbo Jack hamburger	42		134	4.50	492	733	73	52
McDonald's® quarter pound hamburger	34		142	3.68	322	660	86	45
McDLT	36		225	3.91		990	109	57

FAST FOODS

FOOD	AMOUNT	CALO-RIES (kcal)	PROTEIN (g)	FAT (g)	MONO-UN-SATURATED FAT (g)	POLY-UN-SATURATED FAT (g)	SATU-RATED FAT (g)
SANDWICHES & BURGERS (continued)							
McLean deluxe	1 burger	320	22.00	10.00	1.0	4.00	5.00
Wendy's® Big classic, quarter pound burger	1 burger	480	27.00	23.00	8.0	7.00	7.00
Hamburger, large, double meat patty	1 burger	540	34.27	26.57	10.3	2.80	10.52
Hardees® Big twin hamburger	1 burger	450	23.00	25.00	9.0	5.00	11.00
Hamburger, large, triple meat patty, w/condiments	1 burger	693	49.99	41.46	18.2	2.74	15.92
Wendy's® triple hamburger	1 burger	693	50.00	41.50	18.2	2.74	15.90
Ham & cheese sandwich	1 sand-wich	353	20.69	15.48	6.7	1.38	6.44
Arby's®	1 sand-wich	355	24.60	14.20	5.6	3.67	4.93
Subway® on wheat bread	1 sand-wich	673	39.00	22.00	8.0	4.00	7.00
on Italian bread	1 sand-wich	643	38.00	18.00	7.5	3.79	6.63
Ham, egg, & cheese sandwich	1 sand-wich	348	19.25	16.30	5.7	1.69	7.40
Hotdog							
plain	1 hotdog	242	10.39	14.54	6.8	1.71	5.11
w/chili	1 hotdog	297	13.51	13.44	6.6	1.19	4.86
w/corn flour coating (corndog)	1 hotdog	460	16.80	18.90	9.1	3.50	5.16
Italian, spicy, on Italian, Subway®	1 sand-wich	1043	42.00	63.00	28.0	7.00	23.00
Meatball, on honey wheat roll, Subway®	1 sand-wich	947	44.00	45.00	18.0	4.00	17.00
on Italian roll	1 sand-wich	918	42.00	44.00	17.0	4.00	17.00
Roast beef	1 sand-wich	346	21.50	13.80	6.8	1.70	3.6
w/cheese	1 sand-wich	474	32.20	18.00	3.6	3.51	9.0
Arby's® w/cheese	1 sand-wich	508	24.60	26.50	12.0	6.80	7.7
French dip	1 serving	368	22.00	15.40	7.5	2.37	5.5
giant	1 serving	544	33.20	26.30	12.6	2.80	10.9
junior	1 serving	233	11.50	10.80	4.7	2.29	3.7
light roast beef deluxe	1 serving	294	18.00	10.00	4.5	2.04	3.4
Philly beef 'n Swiss	1 serving	467	24.10	25.30	10.7	5.10	9.7
super	1 sand-wich	552	23.70	28.30	12.2	8.40	7.6
Hardees® regular	1 sand-wich	260	15.00	9.00	3.6	1.80	3.6
large	1 sand-wich	300	18.00	11.00	4.5	1.83	4.5
Subway® on Italian roll	1 sand-wich	689	42.00	23.00	9.0	4.00	8.0
on wheat roll	1 sand-wich	717	41.00	24.00	9.0	4.00	8.0

FOOD	CARBO-HYDRATES (mg)	FIBER (mg)	CALCIUM (mg)	IRON (mg)	POTAS-SIUM (mg)	SODIUM (mg)	CHOLES-TEROL (mg)	% OF CALORIES FROM FAT
SANDWICHES & BURGERS (continued)								
McLean deluxe	35	2.40	93	3.78	290	670	60	28
Wendy's® Big classic, quarter pound burger	44	2.32	150	6.30	500	850	75	43
Hamburger, large, double meat patty	40	0.68	102	5.85	569	791	122	44
Hardees® Big twin hamburger	34	1.74	80	4.00	280	580	55	50
Hamburger, large, triple meat patty, w/condiments	29	0.78	65	8.33	785	713	142	54
Wendy's® triple hamburger	29		65	8.33	785	713	142	54
Ham & cheese sandwich	33	0.13	130	3.25	290	772	58	39
Arby's®	35	1.04	170	2.70	382	1400	55	36
Subway® on wheat bread	86	6.00			918	2508	73	29
on Italian bread	81	5.00	304	2.17	834	1710	73	25
Ham, egg, & cheese sandwich	31	0.14	212	3.11	209	1005	245	42
Hotdog								
plain	18	0.29	24	2.31	143	671	44	54
w/chili	31	0.22	19	3.29	166	480	51	41
w/corn flour coating (corndog)	56	0.30	101	6.18	262	972	79	37
Italian, spicy, on Italian, Subway®	83	5.00			880	2282	137	54
Meatball, on honey wheat roll, Subway®	101				1498	2082	88	43
on Italian roll	96	3.02	78	4.97	1210	2022	88	43
Roast beef	34	0.70	54	4.23	316	792	52	36
w/cheese	27		183	5.05	345	1634	77	34
Arby's®								
w/cheese	43	1.06	150	6.12	321	1166	52	47
French dip	35		50	4.14	367	1018	43	38
giant	46		90	7.92	599	1433	72	44
junior	23		40	2.70	201	519	22	42
light roast beef deluxe	33		130	4.50	392	826	42	31
Philly beef 'n Swiss	38		290	4.14	409	1144	53	49
super	54	1.64	90	6.48	533	1174	43	46
Hardees® regular	31	0.80	56	3.11	260	730	35	31
large	32	0.94	66	3.65	320	880	45	33
Subway® on Italian roll	84	5.00	55	3.68	910	2288	83	30
on wheat roll	89	6.00	56	3.78	994	2348	75	30

FAST FOODS

FOOD	AMOUNT	CALO-RIES (kcal)	PROTEIN (g)	FAT (g)	MONO-UN-SATURATED FAT (g)	POLY-UN-SATURATED FAT (g)	SATU-RATED FAT (g)
SANDWICHES & BURGERS (continued)							
Seafood/crab on Italian, Subway®	1 sand-wich	986	29.00	57.00	15.0	28.00	11.00
on wheat	1 sand-wich	1015	31.00	58.00	16.0	28.00	11.00
Spread, canned, La Loma®	1 tbsp	23.3	1.33	1.33			
Steak sandwich	1 sand-wich	459	30.34	14.08	5.3	3.35	3.82
Subway® w/cheese	1 sand-wich	765	43.00	32.00	12.0	4.00	12.00
Submarine sandwich							
w/cold cuts	1 sub	456	21.85	18.62	8.2	2.28	6.81
w/roast beef	1 sub	411	28.64	12.96	1.8	2.61	7.09
w/tuna salad	1 sub	584	29.69	27.99	13.4	7.30	5.33
Subway® Italian	1 serving	671	34.10	38.80	15.7	8.50	12.80
roast beef	1 serving	623	37.70	32.00	13.0	6.80	11.50
tuna	1 serving	663	74.00	37.00	11.8	17.00	8.20
turkey	1 serving	486	32.80	19.00	6.0	7.00	5.30
Tuna salad, w/mayonnaise	1 oz	64.1	4.79	2.64			
Turkey sandwich							
Arby's® turkey deluxe	1 sand-wich	510	28.00	24.00			
roast, light	1 serving	260	20.00	6.00	2.1	2.29	1.5
Subway® turkey breast on wheat roll	1 sand-wich	674	42.00	20.00	7.0	7.00	6.00
SEAFOOD ENTREES							
Clam dinner, Long John Silver's®	1 serving	990	24.00	52.00	31.4	9.90	10.9
Fish							
Burger King® fish tenders	99 g	267	12.00	16.00	7.0	4.00	3.0
Long John Silver's®							
catfish fillet	1 serving	860	28.00	42.00	26.0	6.00	10.0
fish & chicken entree	1 serving	950	36.00	49.00	28.8	9.50	10.6
fish & fries-2 piece	1 serving	610	27.00	37.00	23.5	5.30	7.9
fish & more entree	1 serving	890	31.00	48.00	28.6	9.50	10.1
fish/lemon entree	1 serving	570	39.00	12.00	3.7	5.20	2.1
fish sandwich platter	1 serving	870	26.00	38.00	22.0	7.00	8.0
homestyle fish-6 piece	1 serving	1260	49.00	64.00	43.0	6.00	14.0
light fish/paprika	1 serving	300	24.00	2.00	0.6	0.67	0.6
light fish/lemon crumb	1 serving	270	23.00	5.00	1.4	1.10	0.8
Scallops, breaded & fried	6 scallops	386	15.75	19.40	12.5	0.60	4.8
Seafood platter, Long John Silver's®	1 serving	970	30.00	46.00	30.0	6.00	10.0
Shrimp, breaded & fried	6-8 shrimp	454	18.88	24.90	17.3	0.65	5.3
Long John Silver's®							
batter dipped shrimp	1 serving	30	1.00	2.00	1.5	0.00	0.
shrimp entree	1 serving	840	18.00	47.00	27.2	9.10	9.
shrimp & fish dinner	1 serving	1140	40.00	65.00	40.6	9.50	14.
shrimp, fish & chicken	1 serving	1160	45.00	65.00	40.3	9.60	14.
shrimp scampi	1 serving	610	25.00	18.00	6.0	7.00	3.

FOOD	CARBO-HYDRATES (mg)	FIBER (mg)	CALCIUM (mg)	IRON (mg)	POTAS-SIUM (mg)	SODIUM (mg)	CHOLES-TEROL (mg)	% OF CALORIES FROM FAT
SANDWICHES & BURGERS (continued)								
Seafood/crab on Italian, Subway®	94				557	1967	56	52
on wheat	100	2.49	230	4.41	641	2027	56	51
Spread, canned, La Loma®	1		7	0.24	53	100		51
Steak sandwich	52	0.41	91	5.17	525	798	73	28
Subway® w/cheese	83	6.00	231	4.22	909	1556	82	38
submarine sandwich								
w/cold cuts	51	0.68	189	2.51	394	1650	35	37
w/roast beef	44	0.65	41	2.81	330	845	73	28
w/tuna salad	55	0.60	74	2.65	335	1294	47	43
Subway® Italian	47		410	4.32	565	2062	69	52
roast beef	47		410	7.74	708	1847	73	46
tuna	50		420	5.58	530	1342	43	50
turkey	47		400	4.68	500	2033	51	35
tuna salad, w/mayonnaise	5	0.28	10	1.39	31	93	3	37
turkey sandwich								
Arby's® turkey deluxe	46		80	2.70		1220	70	42
roast, light	33		130	3.42	353	1262	33	21
Subway® turkey breast on wheat roll	88	7.00			605	2520	67	27
SEAFOOD ENTREES								
Clam dinner, Long John Silver's®	114		200	4.50	910	1830	75	47
fish								
Burger King® fish tenders	18	1.12	60	1.70	176	870	28	54
Long John Silver's®								
catfish fillet	90	0.07	200	4.63	1180	990	65	44
fish & chicken entree	102		200	4.50	1280	2090	75	46
fish & fries-2 piece	52		40	0.18	900	1480	60	55
fish & more entree	92	1.69	200	3.60	1230	1790	75	49
fish/lemon entree	80	2.02	200	5.40	1010	1470	125	19
fish sandwich platter	108	4.06	238	6.39	1050	1110	55	39
homestyle fish-6 piece	124	2.27	179	4.38	1660	1590	130	46
light fish/paprika	45	1.26	99	2.43	460	650	70	6
light fish/lemon crumb	37	2.43	60	2.70	460	680	75	17
scallops, breaded & fried	38	0.16	18	2.04	294	919	107	45
seafood platter, Long John Silver's®	109	5.33	109	4.13	1100	1540	70	43
shrimp, breaded & fried	40	0.13	84	2.94	184	1447	201	49
Long John Silver's®								
batter dipped shrimp	2				15	80	10	60
shrimp entree	88		200	3.60	840	1630	100	50
shrimp & fish dinner	108		200	4.50	1340	2440	145	51
shrimp, fish & chicken	113		200	4.50	1450	2590	135	50
shrimp scampi	87	0.00	299	13.60	560	2120	220	27

FAST FOODS

FOOD	AMOUNT	CALO-RIES (kcal)	PROTEIN (g)	FAT (g)	MONO-UN-SATURATED FAT (g)	POLY-UN-SATURATED FAT (g)	SATU-RATED FAT (g)
SIDE DISHES							
Coleslaw	¾ cup	147	1.45	10.97	2.4	6.40	1.61
Long John Silver's®	98 g	140	1.00	6.00	1.5	3.50	1.00
Corn-on-the-cob w/butter	1 ear	155	4.47	3.43	1.0	0.61	1.64
Hush puppies	5 hush puppies	256	4.88	11.59	7.8	0.39	2.69
Long John Silver's®	1 piece	70	2.00	2.00	1.3	0.20	0.40
Mixed vegetables, Long John Silver's®	113 g	60	2.00	2.00	0.6	0.67	0.67
Onion rings, breaded & fried	8-9 rings	275	3.70	15.51	6.6	0.67	6.95
Jack in the Box®	1 bag	380	5.00	23.00	15.2		5.50
Potato, baked							
topped w/cheese sauce	1 potato	475	14.62	28.74	10.7	6.04	10.56
topped w/cheese sauce & bacon	1 potato	451	18.40	25.89	9.7	4.75	10.13
topped w/cheese sauce & broccoli	1 potato	402	13.65	21.44	7.6	4.18	8.51
topped w/cheese sauce & chili	1 potato	481	23.22	21.86	6.8	0.90	13.04
topped w/sour cream & chives	1 potato	394	6.69	22.32	7.8	3.32	10.01
Arby's® deluxe	1 potato	621	17.20	36.40	11.1	3.90	18.10
mushroom 'n' cheese	1 potato	515	15.00	26.70	10.7	8.70	5.80
topped w/cheddar & broccoli	1 potato	417	10.50	17.90	6.6	3.90	6.90
Wendy's® w/cheese	1 potato	550	14.00	24.00	6.0	7.00	8.00
topped w/cheese & bacon	1 potato	510	17.00	17.00	3.0	8.00	4.00
topped w/cheese & broccoli	1 potato	450	9.00	14.00	3.0	7.00	2.00
cheese sauce only	35 g	40	1.00	2.00	1.0	0.50	0.50
Potato, french fried							
in beef tallow	76 g	237	3.03	12.23	5.3	0.61	5.6
in vegetable oil	76 g	235	3.03	12.23	6.0	1.88	3.7
Arby's® curly fries	99 g	337	4.20	17.70	7.6	1.50	7.4
cheddar fries	142 g	399	6.20	21.90	10.0	1.70	9.0
Burger King® Tater tenders	71 g	213	2.00	12.00	6.0	3.00	3.0
Long John Silver's®	85 g	250	3.00	15.00	7.4	5.10	2.5
McDonald's® regular order	68 g	220	3.00	12.00	1.0	2.50	8.0
medium order	97 g	320	4.00	17.00	1.5	3.50	12.0
large order	122 g	400	6.00	22.00	2.0	5.00	15.0
Wendy's®	136 g	360	5.00	17.00	12.0	1.00	4.0
Potato, mashed	⅓ cup	66	1.85	0.97	0.2	0.23	0.1
Potato cakes, Arby's®	85 g	204	1.80	12.00	5.5	4.30	2.2
Potato chips	1 oz	148	1.82	10.05	1.7	5.16	2.5
Potato salad	⅓ cup	108	1.46	5.73	1.6	2.87	0.5
Refried beans, Wendy's®	54 g	70	3.00	2.00	0.5	0.50	1.0
Rice, Spanish, Wendy's®	56 g	70	2.00	1.00	0.2	0.71	0.
Rice pilaf, Long John Silver's®	1 serving	160	3.00	3.00	1.3	1.00	0.
DESSERTS							
Apple pie, McDonald's®	1 pie	260	2.20	14.80	0.9	3.95	9.
Brownie	1 brownie	243	2.74	10.10	3.8	2.64	3.
Cookies							
Animal crackers	1 box	299	4.14	9.00	3.7	1.04	3.
chocolate chip	1 box	233	2.89	12.15	5.0	1.03	5

FOOD	CARBO-HYDRATES (mg)	FIBER (mg)	CALCIUM (mg)	IRON (mg)	POTAS-SIUM (mg)	SODIUM (mg)	CHOLES-TEROL (mg)	% OF CALORIES FROM FAT
SIDE DISHES								
Coleslaw	13	0.63	34	0.73	177	267	5	67
Long John Silver's®	20		60	0.72	190	260	15	39
Corn-on-the-cob w/butter	32	0.93	5	0.88	360	30	6	20
Hush puppies	35	0.39	69	1.43	188	965	135	41
Long John Silver's®	10		40	0.72	65	25	4	26
Mixed vegetables, Long John Silver's®	9	5.90	29	0.90	120	330	0	30
Onion rings, breaded & fried	31	0.33	73	0.85	129	430	14	51
Jack in the Box®	38	1.33	73	0.85	129	451	0	54
Potato, baked								
topped w/cheese sauce	47	1.33	310	3.02	1167	381	19	54
topped w/cheese sauce & bacon	44	1.34	309	3.15	1179	973	30	52
topped w/cheese sauce & broccoli	47	2.00	334	3.33	1440	484	20	48
topped w/cheese sauce & chili	56	3.20	409	6.13	1570	701	31	41
topped w/sour cream & chives	50	1.54	105	3.13	1383	182	23	51
Arby's® deluxe	59		700	2.70	1520	605	58	53
mushroom 'n' cheese	58		250	2.70	1445	923	47	47
topped w/cheddar & broccoli	55		100	2.70	1455	361	22	39
Wendy's® w/cheese	74	3.59	300	3.60	1210	640	30	39
topped w/cheese & bacon	75	9.85	100	4.50	1370	1170	15	30
topped w/cheese & broccoli	77		100	4.50	1310	450	0	28
cheese sauce only	5		60		75	310	0	45
Potato, french fried								
in beef tallow	29	0.62	12	1.02	541	124	13	46
in vegetable oil	29	0.62	12	1.02	541	124	0	47
Arby's® curly fries	43		20	1.44	724	167		47
cheddar fries	46		80	1.44	742	443	9	49
Burger King® Tater tenders	25					318	3	51
Long John Silver's®	28		200	0.72	370	500	0	54
McDonald's® regular order	26		10	0.52	484	110	0	49
medium order	36	3.35	14	0.73	692	150	0	48
large order	46	4.21	18	0.93	866	200	0	50
Wendy's®	50	4.62	20	1.08	760	220	0	43
Potato, mashed	13	0.66	17	0.37	236	182	2	13
Potato cakes, Arby's®	20			1.44	289	397		53
Potato chips	15	0.40	7	0.34	369.	133	0	61
Potato salad	13	0.34	13	0.69	256	312	57	48
Refried beans, Wendy's®	9	3.00		1.08	20	200	0	26
Rice, Spanish, Wendy's®	13	0.74	15	0.69	130	440	0	13
Rice pilaf, Long John Silver's®	30		20	1.80	125	340	0	17
DESSERTS								
Apple pie, McDonald's®	30	1.13	11	0.71	50	240	6	51
Brownie	39	0.54	25	1.29	83	153	9	37
Cookies								
Animal crackers	50	0.17	11	1.47	57	274	11	27
chocolate chip	36	0.32	20	1.47	82	188	12	47

FAST FOODS

FOOD	AMOUNT	CALO-RIES (kcal)	PROTEIN (g)	FAT (g)	MONO-UN-SATURATED FAT (g)	POLY-UN-SATURATED FAT (g)	SATU-RATED FAT (g)
SIDE DISHES (continued)							
Cookies (continued)							
McDonald's®							
Chocolaty	1 box	330	4.20	15.60	1.0	4.00	10.0
McDonaldland	1 box	290	4.20	9.20	1.0	1.00	7.0
Float, Dairy Queen®	397 g	330	6.00	8.00			
Fried pie, fruit (apple, cherry, or lemon)	1 pie	266	2.42	14.37	5.8	1.16	6.5
Frozen yogurt, vanilla, McDonald's®	80 g	105	4.00	1.00	0.2	0.50	0.3
Ice milk, vanilla, soft-serve, w/cone	1 cone	164	3.89	6.12	1.8	0.36	3.5
Ice cream cone, regular, Dairy Queen®	1 cone	230	6.00	7.00	1.0	1.00	5.0
dip	1 cone	330	6.00	16.00	4.0	3.00	8.0
Malt, Dairy Queen®	418 g	610	13.00	14.00	2.0	2.00	8.0
Milkshake, fast food							
chocolate	226 g	288	7.68	8.40	2.4	0.32	5.2
strawberry	226 g	255	7.60	6.40	1.9	0.25	4.2
vanilla	226 g	251	7.84	6.72	1.9	0.25	4.2
Arby's® jamoca	326 g	368	9.30	10.50	6.4	1.60	2.5
McDonald's® lowfat							
chocolate	293 g	320	11.60	1.70	0.1	0.70	0.9
strawberry	293g	320	10.70	1.30	0.1	0.60	0.6
vanilla	293 g	290	10.80	1.30	0.1	0.60	0.6
Polar swirl, Arby's®							
butterfinger	329 g	457	12.10	18.10	6.1	3.60	8.4
heath	329 g	543	10.60	21.80	13.3	2.60	5.2
oreo	329 g	482	10.50	19.70	7.2	2.17	10.4
peanut butter cup	329 g	517	14.00	24.00	11.0	4.80	8.
snickers	329 g	511	12.20	18.80	8.5	3.72	6.
Sundae							
caramel	1 sundae	303	7.30	9.27	3.0	1.01	4.
hot fudge	1 sundae	284	5.64	8.63	2.3	0.81	5.
strawberry	1 sundae	269	6.25	7.85	2.6	1.02	3.
Dairy Queen® regular	1 sundae	300	6.00	7.00	1.0	1.00	5.
banana split	1 sundae	510	9.00	11.00	2.9	0.39	7.
McDonald's®							
hot caramel	1 sundae	270	6.60	2.80	0.4	1.40	0.
hot fudge	1 sundae	240	7.30	3.20	0.5	0.20	0.
strawberry	1 sundae	210	5.70	1.10	0.2	0.50	0.

FOOD	CARBO-HYDRATES (mg)	FIBER (mg)	CALCIUM (mg)	IRON (mg)	POTAS-SIUM (mg)	SODIUM (mg)	CHOLES-TEROL (mg)	% OF CALORIES FROM FAT
SIDE DISHES (continued)								
Cookies (continued)								
McDonald's®								
Chocolaty	42	1.12	24	2.18	72	280	4	43
McDonaldland	47	0.56	9	2.07	38	300	0	29
Float, Dairy Queen®	59		200	0.00			20	22
Fried pie, fruit (apple, cherry, or lemon)	33	0.31	12	0.89	51	325	13	49
Frozen yogurt, vanilla, McDonald's®	22		112	0.23		80	3	9
Ice milk, vanilla, soft-serve, w/cone	24	0.10	153	0.15	169	92	28	34
Ice cream cone, regular, Dairy Queen®	36		150	0.72	260	95	20	27
dip	40		300	1.08	290	100	20	44
Malt, Dairy Queen®	106		400	1.44	570	230	45	21
Milkshake, fast food								
chocolate	46	0.40	255	0.70	454	218	30	26
strawberry	43	0.54	256	0.24	413	187	25	23
vanilla	41	0.54	275	0.21	394	186	26	24
Arby's® jamoca	59		250		525	262	35	26
McDonald's® lowfat								
chocolate	66		332	0.84		240	10	5
strawberry	67		327	0.09		170	10	4
vanilla	60		327	0.10		170	10	4
Polar swirl, Arby's®								
butterfinger	62		250	0.36	690	318	28	36
heath	76		250		520	346	39	36
oreo	66		250	0.72	666	521	35	37
peanut butter cup	61		250		612	385	34	42
snickers	73		250		610	351	33	33
Sundae								
caramel	49	0.15	189	0.22	318	195	25	28
hot fudge	48	0.16	207	0.58	395	182	21	27
strawberry	45	0.23	161	0.32	270	92	21	26
Dairy Queen® regular	54	2.19	150	1.08	290	140	20	21
banana split	93		300	3.60	860	250	30	19
McDonald's®								
hot caramel	59	1.04	222	0.08	414	180	13	9
hot fudge	51	1.25	235	0.48	274	170	6	12
strawberry	49	0.69	190	0.16	263	95	4	5

FATS & OILS

FOOD	AMOUNT	CALORIES (kcal)	FAT (g)	MONO-UN-SATURATED FAT (g)	POLY-UN-SATURATED FAT (g)	SATURATED FAT (g)
Butter, regular						
almond, honey & cinammon, salt	1 cup	1505	130	84.7	27.4	12.4
almond, plain	1 tbsp	101	9	6.1	2.0	0.9
almond, plain, salt added	1 cup	1582	148	95.9	31.0	14.0
cashew, plain, salt added	1 cup	94	8	4.7	1.3	1.6
pat	1 item	36	4	1.2	0.2	2.5
stick	1 item	813	92	26.6	3.4	57.3
sunflower seed, salt	1 cup	1481	122	23.3	80.6	12.8
tablespoon	1 tbsp	100	11	3.3	0.4	7.1
unsalted, pat	1 item	36	4	1.2	0.2	2.5
Heart Beat® Nucoa	1 tbsp	25	3	1.9	0.5	0.5
Country Morning Blend® Light	1 tsp	35	4	2.0	1.0	1.0
Land O Lakes® Stick, lightly salted	1 tsp	35	4	2.0	1.0	1.0
Butter, whipped						
pat	1 item	27	3	0.9	0.1	1.9
stick	1 item	542	61	17.7	2.3	38.2
tablespoon	1 tbsp	65	7	2.1	0.3	4.5
unsalted, pat	1 item	27	3	0.9	0.1	1.9
Butter Buds® Substitute, granules	1 fl oz	12	0	0.0	0.0	0.0
Cocunut cream	1 oz	208	20	0.2	0.1	4.5
Ghee	28.3 g	250	28	8.1	1.1	17.5
Fat, animal						
beef tallow	1 cup	1849	205	85.6	8.2	102.0
butter	1 cup	1627	184	53.2	6.8	115.0
butter oil	1 cup	1795	204	58.9	7.6	127.0
chicken, for cooking	1 tbsp	115	13	5.7	2.7	3.8
duck	1 cup	1846	205	101.0	26.5	68.1
goose	1 cup	1846	205	116.0	22.5	56.8
lard, pork	1 cup	1849	205	92.5	23.0	80.4
mutton tallow	1 cup	1849	205	83.2	15.9	96.9
turkey	1 tbsp	115	13	5.5	3.0	3.8
Grease, eulachon, Alaska	1 tbsp	900	100	62.9	2.4	27.6
Margarine						
cannola, soft	14 g	100	11	6.0	3.0	1.0
cocunut/safflower, hydrogenated	1 tsp	34	4	0.4	0.6	2.7
corn, regular, hydrogenated, hard	1 tsp	34	4	2.2	0.8	0.6
corn, regular, soft	1 tsp	34	4	1.5	1.5	0.7
corn/soybean, unsalted	1 tsp	34	4	1.7	1.2	0.7
corn, tub	1 cup	1549	174	69.4	62.8	33.9
imitation, 40% fat	1 tsp	17	2	0.8	0.7	0.4
imitatation spread, 60% fat	1 tsp	26	3	1.5	0.7	0.6
lard, hydrogenated	1 tsp	35	4	1.8	0.4	1.5
liquid, regular, soybean	1 tsp	34	4	1.3	1.7	0.6
liquid, vegetable oils	1 cup	1637	183	75.6	69.5	34.4
olive, tub	1 cup	1647	174	112.0	17.1	36.9
regular, hard, unsalted	1 tsp	34	4	1.7	1.2	0.7
regular, soft, unsalted	1 tsp	34	4	1.8	1.2	0.6
safflower, regular, soft, tub	1 tsp	34	4	1.1	2.1	0.4
safflower/soybean, hydrogenated	1 tsp	34	4	1.5	1.5	0.6
soybean, soft, tub, unsalted	1 tsp	34	4	1.7	1.3	0.6

FOOD	OLEIC FAT (g)	CARBO-HYDRATES (g)	CHOLES-TEROL (mg)	OMEGA 3 (g)	SODIUM (mg)	% OF CALORIES FROM FAT
Butter, regular						
almond, honey & cinammon, salt		67.40			425	78
almond, plain	6.0	3.3	0.0	0.00	2	84
almond, plain, salt added		53.00	0.0		1125	84
cashew, plain, salt added		4.40	0.0		98	76
pat	1.0	0.00	11.0	0.00	41	100
stick	23.1	0.0	248.0	0.00	937	100
sunflower seed, salt		70.10			1330	74
tablespoon	2.9	0.0	30.7	0.00	116	100
unsalted, pat	1.0	0.0	11.0		1	100
Heart Beat® Nucoa		0.00	0.0		110	100
Country Morning Blend® Light		0.00	5.0		35	100
Land O Lakes® Stick, lightly salted		0.00	5.0		35	100
Butter, whipped						
pat	0.8	0.00	8.0	0.00	31	100
stick	15.4	0.0	165.0	0.00	625	100
tablespoon	1.8	0.0	19.7	0.00	74	100
unsalted, pat	0.8	0.00	8.0	0.00	0	100
Butter Buds® Substitute, granules	0.0	1.00	0.0	0.00	355	0
Cocunut cream		7.9	0.0		9	85
Ghee		0.2	72.4		9	100
Fat, animal						
beef tallow	73.8	0.00	223.0		0	100
butter		0.1	497.0		1876	100
butter oil	51.3	0.00	524.0			100
chicken, for cooking	4.8	0.00	11.0	0.00	0	100
duck	90.5	0.00	205.0			100
goose	110.0	0.00	205.0			100
lard, pork	84.5	0.00	195.0	0.00	0	100
mutton tallow	77.1	0.00	209.0			100
turkey	4.6	0.00	13.0			100
Grease, eulachon, Alaska		0.00	3.0			100
Margarine						
cannola, soft		0.00		1.00	95	99
cocunut/safflower, hydrogenated	0.4	0.00			44	100
corn, regular, hydrogenated, hard	1.4	0.00	0.0	0.00	44	100
corn, regular, soft	1.5	0.00	0.0	0.00	51	100
corn/soybean, unsalted	1.4	0.00	0.0	0.00	0	100
corn, tub		1.0	0.0		2333	100
imitation, 40% fat	0.7	0.00	0.0	0.00	46	100
imitatation spread, 60% fat	1.5	0.00	0.0	0.00	48	100
lard, hydrogenated	1.6	0.00	2.0		44	99
liquid, regular, soybean	1.3	0.00	0.0	0.00	37	100
liquid, vegetable oils		0.00	0.0		1773	100
olive, tub		1.0	0.0		2333	95
regular, hard, unsalted	1.7	0.00	0.0	0.00	0	100
regular, soft, unsalted	1.8	0.00	0.0	0.00	1	100
safflower, regular, soft, tub	1.1	0.00	0.0	0.00	51	100
safflower/soybean, hydrogenated	1.4	0.00	0.0	0.00	44	100
soybean, soft, tub, unsalted	1.4	0.00	0.0	0.00	1	100

FATS & OILS

FOOD	AMOUNT	CALORIES (kcal)	FAT (g)	MONO-UN-SATURATED FAT (g)	POLY-UN-SATURATED FAT (g)	SATURATED FAT (g)
Margarine (continued)						
soybean, tub	1 cup	1549	174	67.6	65.9	33.0
stick/brick, corn	1 cup	1653	185	90.4	57.5	29.0
stick, brick, soybean	1 cup	1581	177	100.0	28.3	40.6
stick/brick, vegetable & animal oils	1 cup	1581	177	124.0	16.8	29.0
stick/brick, vegetable oils	1 cup	1581	177	116.0	17.5	36.4
vegetable oils, unspecified, tub	1 cup	1549	174	102.0	38.9	25.7
vegetable oil, unspecified, low energy	1 cup	784	88	39.7	30.8	17.4
Fleischmanns® Extra light	1 tbsp	50	6	3.8	1.5	0.7
Heart Beat® Nucoa	1 tbsp	25	3	2.2	0.4	0.4
no salt	1 tbsp	50	6	3.5	1.3	1.3
I Can't Believe Its Not Butter®	14 g	90	10		5.0	2.0
light	14 g	60	7		3.0	1.0
Molly McButter®	5 g	8	0			
Move Over Butter®	14 g	90	10		3.0	2.0
Parkay® Tub, Golden Spread	1 tbsp	90	10	4.4	2.0	1.0
Promise® Extra Light	1 tbsp	50	6	2.1	2.9	1.0
Promise Ultra® Fat Free	14 g	5	0			
Smart Beat®	14 g	20	2	1.0	1.0	
Weight Watchers® Extra Light	14 g	45	4		2.0	1.0
Sunflower® Vegetable oil, interstrfied	1 cup	1647	174	30.4	90.6	46.9
Sunflower® Vegetable oils, tub	1 cup	1647	174	56.0	81.6	27.1
Margerine, regular, unspecified oils						
pat	1 item	36	4	1.8	1.3	0.8
soft	1 tbsp	100	11	4.0	4.8	1.9
soft, tub	1 cup	1626	183	64.7	78.6	31.3
stick	1 item	812	91	40.5	28.7	17.9
tablespoon	1 tbsp	101	11	5.0	3.6	2.2
whipped	1 tbsp	70	8	2.5	3.1	1.4
Mazola® diet/low calorie	1 tbsp	50	6	2.1	2.6	1.0
no stick, spray (1 serving)	.720 g	6	1	0.2	0.4	0.1
Mayonnaise						
imitation, milk cream	15 g	15	1	0.3	0.1	0.4
imitation, soybean	15 g	35	3	0.7	1.6	0.9
imitation, soybean, cholesterol free	1 tbsp	68	7	1.5	3.9	1.1
soybean, commercial	1 tbsp	99	11	3.1	5.7	1.6
Best Foods® cholesterol free	1 tbsp	50	5	1.6	2.0	1.0
Heart Beat® Nucoa, low calorie	1 tbsp	40	4	0.6	2.0	1.0
Kraft®	1 tbsp	100	12		7.0	2.0
cholesterol free	1 tbsp	90	10	1.1	6.0	1.0
fat free	1 tbsp	12	0			
light, low calorie	1 tbsp	40	4	0.6	1.4	0.5
Oil, Alaska						
beluga	1 tsp	900	100			
corn	1 tbsp	884	100	24.2	58.7	12.
oogruk	1 tbsp	900	100	57.1	26.8	15.
seal	1 cup	2007	227			

388

FOOD	OLEIC FAT (g)	CARBO-HYDRATES (g)	CHOLES-TEROL (mg)	OMEGA 3 (g)	SODIUM (mg)	% OF CALORIES FROM FAT
Margarine (continued)						
soybean, tub		1.0	0.0		2333	100
stick/brick, corn		2.0	0.0		2170	100
stick, brick, soybean		1.9	0.0		2076	100
stick/brick, vegetable & animal oils		1.9			2076	100
stick/brick, vegetable oils		1.9	0.0		2076	100
vegetable oils, unspecified, tub		1.0	0.0		2333	100
vegetable oil, unspecified, low energy		0.9	0.0		2178	100
Fleischmanns® Extra light		0.00	0.0		55	100
Heart Beat® Nucoa		0.00	0.0		110	100
no salt		0.00	0.0		0	100
I Can't Believe Its Not Butter®		0.00			95	100
light		0.00			110	100
Molly McButter®		2.00			120	0
Move Over Butter®		0.00			100	100
Parkay® Tub, Golden Spread		0.00	0.0		120	100
Promise® Extra Light		0.00	0.0		50	100
Promise Ultra® Fat Free		1.00			90	0
Smart Beat®		0.00			105	90
Weight Watchers® Extra Light		2.00			75	80
Sunflower® Vegetable oil, interstrfied		1.0	0.0		2333	95
Sunflower® Vegetable oils, tub		1.0	0.0		2333	95
Margarine, regular, unspecified oils						
pat	1.8	0.0	0.0	0.00	47	100
soft	4.0	0.0	0.0	0.00	151	100
soft, tub	64.7	1.20	0.0	0.00	2449	100
stick	40.5	1.0	0.0		1066	100
tablespoon	5.0	0.1	0.0	0.00	132	100
whipped	2.4	0.00	0.0	0.00	97	100
Mazola® diet/low calorie	1.6	0.00	0.0	0.00	130	100
no stick, spray (1 serving)	0.1	0.00	0.0	0.00	0	100
Mayonnaise						
imitation, milk cream	0.3	1.70	6.0	0.00	76	50
imitation, soybean	0.7	2.40	4.0	0.00	75	75
imitation, soybean, cholesterol free	1.5	2.20	0.0	0.00	49	89
soybean, commercial	3.1	0.40	8.0	0.00	78	100
Best Foods® cholesterol free		1.00	0.0		80	90
Heart Beat® Nucoa, low calorie		1.00	0.0		110	90
Kraft®		0.00	5.0		70	100
cholesterol free		0.00	0.0		75	100
fat free		3.00			190	0
light, low calorie		1.00	5.0	0.00	15	90
Oil, Alaska						
beluga		0.00				100
corn		0.00				100
oogruk		0.00				100
seal		0.00				100

FATS & OILS

FOOD	AMOUNT	CALORIES (kcal)	FAT (g)	MONO-UN-SATURATED FAT (g)	POLY-UN-SATURATED FAT (g)	SATURATED FAT (g)
Oil, Alaska (continued)						
seal, mixed species	1 tsp	854	98	56.2	28.2	12.9
walrus	1 tbsp	900	100			
whale	1 tbsp	900	100			
willow, leaves	1 cup	584	61			
Oil, fish						
cod liver	1 tbsp	123	14	6.4	3.1	3.1
herring	1 tbsp	123	14	7.7	2.1	2.9
menhaden	1 tbsp	123	14	3.6	4.7	4.1
menhaden, hydrogenated	1 tbsp	113	13	0.0	0.0	12.0
salmon	1 tbsp	123	14	4.0	5.5	2.7
sardine	1 tbsp	123	14	4.6	4.3	4.1
Oil, vegetable						
almond	1 tbsp	120	14	9.5	2.4	1.1
apricot kernel	1 cup	1927	218	131.0	63.9	13.7
avocado	1 cup	1927	218	154.0	29.4	25.2
babassu	1 cup	1927	218	24.9	3.5	177.0
blended	1 oz	255	28	12.2	10.6	4.2
canola, Heart Beat® Nucoa	1 tbsp	120	14		4.0	1.0
canola/rapeseed	1 cup	1927	218	128.0	64.5	15.5
cocoa/cacao butter	1 tbsp	120	14	4.5	0.4	8.1
coconut	1 tbsp	117	14	0.8	0.3	11.8
corn	1 cup	1927	218	52.7	128.0	27.7
cottonseed	1 cup	1927	218	38.9	113.0	56.4
cupu assu	1 cup	1927	218	84.4	8.3	116.0
grapeseed	1 cup	1927	218	35.2	152.0	20.9
hazelnut	1 cup	1927	218	170.0	22.1	16.2
mustard	1 cup	1927	218	129.0	46.3	25.2
nutmeg butter	1 tbsp	120	14	0.7	0.0	12.2
oat	1 tbsp	120	14	4.8	5.6	2.7
olive	1 tbsp	119	14	9.9	1.1	1.8
palm	1 tbsp	120	14	5.0	1.3	6.7
palm kernel	1 tbsp	117	14	1.6	0.2	11.1
peanut	1 cup	1909	216	99.9	69.2	36.4
poppyseed	1 cup	1927	218	42.9	136.0	29.4
rice bran	1 tbsp	120	14	5.3	4.8	2.7
safflower	1 cup	1927	218	26.3	162.0	20.5
safflower, oleic above 70%	1 cup	1927	218	164.0	31.0	13.3
sesame	1 tbsp	120	14	5.4	5.7	1.9
sheanut	1 cup	1927	218	95.8	11.4	102.0
soybean	1 cup	1927	218	93.8	82.0	31.8
soybean/cottonseed	1 cup	1927	218	64.4	105.0	38.2
soybean, glycine max	1 cup	1927	218	50.7	126.0	31.4
soybean lecithin	1 tbsp	104	14	1.5	6.2	2.0
sunflower	1 tbsp	120	14	6.2	5.5	1.4
sunflower, linoleic above 60%	1 cup	1927	218	42.6	143.0	22.5
sunflower, oleic above 70%	1 cup	1927	218	182.0	8.3	21.3
sunflower,hydrogenated	1 cup	1927	218	101.0	79.3	28.3
teaseed	1 cup	1927	218	112.0	50.1	46.1
tomatoseed	1 cup	1927	218	49.6	116.0	43.0

FOOD	OLEIC FAT (g)	CARBO-HYDRATES (g)	CHOLES-TEROL (mg)	OMEGA 3 (g)	SODIUM (mg)	% OF CALORIES FROM FAT
Oil, Alaska (continued)						
seal, mixed species		8.60	68.8		7	100
walrus		0.00	120.0			100
whale		0.00				100
willow, leaves		8.10				94
Oil, fish						
cod liver	2.8	0.00	78.0	0.94		100
herring	1.6	0.00	104.0	0.85		100
menhaden	2.0	0.00	71.0	1.79		100
menhaden, hydrogenated		0.00	63.0			100
salmon	2.3	0.00	66.0	1.77		100
sardine	2.0	0.00	97.0	1.38		100
Oil, vegetable						
almond	9.4	0.00				100
apricot kernel	128.0	0.00				100
avocado	148.0	0.00	0.0		0	100
babassu	24.9	0.00	0.0		0	100
blended		0.00	0.0		3	100
canola, Heart Beat® Nucoa		0.00	0.0		0	100
canola/rapeseed	122.0	0.00				100
cocoa/cacao butter	4.4	0.00				100
coconut	0.8	0.00				100
corn	52.7	0.00	0.0	0.00	0	100
cottonseed	37.1	0.00	0.0		0	100
cupu assu	84.4	0.00	0.0		0	100
grapeseed	34.4	0.00	0.0		0	100
hazelnut	170.0	0.00	0.0		0	100
mustard	25.3	0.00	0.0		0	100
nutmeg butter	0.7	0.00				100
oat	4.8	0.00				100
olive	9.8	0.00	0.0		0	100
palm	5.0	0.00				100
palm kernel	1.6	0.00				100
peanut	96.7	0.00	0.0	0.00	0	100
poppyseed	42.9	0.00	0.0		0	100
rice bran	5.3	0.00	0.0	0.00	0	100
safflower	25.5	0.00	0.0	0.00	0	100
safflower, oleic above 70%	164.0	0.00	0.0		0	100
sesame	5.3	0.00	0.0	0.00	0	100
sheanut	94.8	0.00	0.0		0	100
soybean	93.1	0.00	0.0	0.00	0	100
soybean/cottonseed	63.0	0.00	0.0	0.00	0	100
soybean, glycine max	49.7	0.00	0.0		0	100
soybean lecithin	1.4	0.00				100
sunflower	6.2	0.00				100
sunflower, linoleic above 60%	42.6	0.00	0.0		0	100
sunflower, oleic above 70%	180.0	0.00	0.0		0	100
sunflower, hydrogenated	100.0	0.00	0.0		0	100
teaseed	109.0	0.00	0.0		0	100
tomatoseed	47.6	0.00	0.0		0	100

FATS & OILS

FOOD	AMOUNT	CALORIES (kcal)	FAT (g)	MONO-UN-SATURATED FAT (g)	POLY-UN-SATURATED FAT (g)	SATURATED FAT (g)
Oil, vegetable (continued)						
ucuhuba butter	1 cup	1927	218	14.6	6.3	186.0
walnut	1 cup	1927	218	49.6	138.0	19.8
Peanut butter, Health Valley®						
Natural						
creamy	1 tbsp	85	7	3.4	2.04	1.4
chunky	1 tbsp	85	7	3.4	2.04	1.4
Pork, fat						
cooked	1 oz	183	19	8.8	2.02	6.9
raw	1 oz	194	21	9.7	2.21	7.6
Salad dressing						
blue cheese	1 tbsp	77	8	1.9	4.3	1.5
blue cheese, commercial	1 cup	1176	121	66.9	40.2	8.6
blue cheese & herbs, dry	1.28 g	4	0	0.0	0.0	0.0
blue cheese, low calorie	1 tbsp	10	1	0.3	0.0	0.5
bright day	1 tbsp	60	6	1.1	3.9	1.0
buttermilk farm, dry mix	1.31 g	4	0	0.0	0.0	0.0
Caesar	1 tbsp	70	7			
cheese garlic, dry mix	1.33 g	4	0	0.0	0.0	0.0
cheese italian, dry mix	1.37 g	4	0	0.0	0.0	0.0
French	1 tbsp	67	6	1.2	3.4	1.5
French-low calorie, CNF	1 cup	387	27	14.8	8.8	1.8
French-low calorie, USDA	1 tbsp	22	1	0.2	0.5	0.1
French, regular	1 cup	1005	99	55.0	33.0	7.0
garlic and herbs, dry mix	1.37 g	3	0	0.0	0.0	0.0
garlic, prepared from mix	1 tbsp	83	9		3.4	1.4
green goddess	1 tbsp	68	7	2.6	3.5	0.9
home recipe, cooked	1 tbsp	25	2	0.6	0.3	0.5
Italian	1 tbsp	69	7	1.7	4.1	1.0
Italian, dry mix	1.28 g	3	0	0.0	0.0	0.0
Italian, low calorie, CNF	1 cup	120	7	4.0	2.4	0.5
Italian, low calorie, USDA	1 tbsp	16	2	0.3	0.9	0.2
Italian, regular	1 cup	1466	162	90.0	54.0	11.5
lemon & herbs, dry mix	1.10 g	3	0	0.0	0.0	0.0
light Italian, dry mix	1.46 g	4	0	0.0	0.0	0.0
light ranch, dry mix	1.44 g	4	0	0.0	0.0	0.0
light zesty Italian, dry	1.28 g	3	0	0.0	0.0	0.0
lite cheese Italian, dry	1.46 g	4	0	0.0	0.0	0.0
mayonnaise, >35% oil	1 cup	1163	115	63.8	38.3	8.3
mayonnaise, >65% oil	1 cup	1610	177	98.2	58.9	16.7
mayonnaise, low calorie	1 tbsp	20	2	0.4	1.0	0.4
mayonnaise, reduced fat	1 cup	726	73	42.6	22.1	4.7
mayonnaise, safflower, soy	1 cup	1577	175	28.6	121.0	18.9
mayonnaise type	1 tbsp	57	5	1.3	2.6	0.7
mayonnaise type, low fat	1 cup	678	60	34.7	17.4	3.2
mild Italian, dry mix	1.83 g	5	0	0.0	0.0	0.0
No oil Italian, dry mix	1.83 g	6	0	0.0	0.0	0.0
oil/vinegar, home recipe	1 tbsp	70	8	2.3	3.8	1.4
ranch style	1 tbsp	54	6	1.4	2.7	0.7
Russian	1 tbsp	76	8	1.8	4.5	1.7

FOOD	OLEIC FAT (g)	CARBO-HYDRATES (g)	CHOLES-TEROL (mg)	OMEGA 3 (g)	SODIUM (mg)	% OF CALORIES FROM FAT
Oil, vegetable (continued)						
ucuhuba butter	14.6	0.00	14.3		2156	100
walnut	48.5	0.00	0.0		0	100
Peanut butter, Health Valley®						
Natural						
creamy		3.00	49.0		1	74
chunky		3.00	0.0		1	74
Pork, fat						
cooked		0.00	20.7		9	93
raw		0.00	20.2		5	96
Salad dressing						
blue cheese	1.8	1.10	9.0	0.00	167	93
blue cheese, commercial		23.50	41.6		2886	93
blue cheese & herbs, dry	0.0	1.00	0.3	0.00	148	0
blue cheese, low calorie	0.3	1.00	4.0	0.00	177	90
bright day		2.00	0.0		75	90
buttermilk farm, dry mix	0.0	1.00	0.1	0.00	94	0
Caesar		1.00		0.00		90
cheese garlic, dry mix	0.0	1.00	0.3	0.00	167	0
cheese italian, dry mix	0.0	1.00	0.2	0.00	127	0
French	1.1	2.70	2.0	0.00	214	86
French-low calorie, CNF		39.50	15.6		5039	62
French-low calorie, USDA	0.2	3.50	1.0	0.00	128	37
French, regular		34.20	145.0		3987	89
garlic and herbs, dry mix	0.0	1.00	0.0	0.00	187	0
garlic, prepared from mix		0.50	0.0	0.00	222	100
green goddess		1.20	0.0	0.00	150	93
home recipe, cooked	0.6	2.40	8.0	0.00	117	54
Italian	1.6	1.50	0.0	0.00	116	93
Italian, dry mix	0.0	1.00	0.0	0.00	172	0
Italian, low calorie, CNF		15.10	14.4		3381	54
Italian, low calorie, USDA	0.3	0.70	1.0	0.00	118	85
Italian, regular		12.20	157.0		3703	99
lemon & herbs, dry mix	0.0	1.00	0.0	0.00	143	0
light Italian, dry mix	0.0	1.00	0.0	0.00	176	0
light ranch, dry mix	0.0	1.00	0.1	0.00	96	0
light zesty Italian, dry	0.0	1.00	0.0	0.00	133	0
lite cheese Italian, dry	0.0	1.00	0.2	0.00	137	0
mayonnaise, >35% oil		30.30	61.1		1469	89
mayonnaise, >65% oil		2.4	130.0		1142	99
mayonnaise, low calorie	0.4	2.00	2.0	0.00	44	90
mayonnaise, reduced fat		20.50	0.0		1577	90
mayonnaise, safflower, soy	28.6	6.00	57.2		1250	100
mayonnaise type	1.3	3.50	4.0	0.00	104	77
mayonnaise type, low fat		36.30	0.0		1814	80
mild Italian, dry mix	0.0	1.00	0.0	0.00	192	0
No oil Italian, dry mix	0.0	1.70	0.0	0.00	32	0
oil/vinegar, home recipe	2.3	0.3	0.0	0.00	0	100
ranch style		0.60	3.9	0.00	97	95
Russian	1.8	1.60	0.0	0.00	133	92

FATS & OILS

FOOD	AMOUNT	CALORIES (kcal)	FAT (g)	MONO-UN-SATURATED FAT (g)	POLY-UN-SATURATED FAT (g)	SATURATED FAT (g)
Salad dressing (continued)						
Russian, low calorie, CNF	1 cup	368	10	5.7	3.4	0.8
Russian, low calorie, USDA	1 tbsp	23	1	0.19	0.4	0.1
Russian, regular	1 cup	1210	124	69.1	41.4	8.8
sesame seed	1 tbsp	68	7	1.8	3.8	0.9
sweet and sour	1 tbsp	29	0	0.0	0.0	0.0
thousand island	1 tbsp	59	6	1.3	3.1	0.9
thousand island, low calorie	1 tbsp	24	2	0.4	1.0	0.2
thousand island, low cal	1 cup	492	36	20.1	12.0	2.7
thousand island, regular	1 cup	997	88	48.7	29.2	6.0
zesty Italian, dry mix	1.10 g	3	0	0.0	0.0	0.0
Good Seasons® Ranch, dry	1.0 g	3	0	0.0	0.0	0.0
Hidden Valley® Ranch, lite	1 tbsp	30	3	0.7	1.4	0.4
Kraft®	1 tbsp	70	7		4.0	1.0
bacon and tomato	1 tbsp	70	7		4.0	1.0
creamy buttermilk	1 tbsp	80	8		5.0	1.0
creamy cucumber	1 tbsp	70	8		4.0	1.0
creamy garlic	1 tbsp	50	5		3.0	1.0
creamy Russian	1 tbsp	60	5		3.0	1.0
golden Caesar	1 tbsp	70	7		4.0	1.0
Italian/sour cream	1 tbsp	50	5		3.0	1.0
mayonnaise, light	1 tbsp	50	5		3.0	1.0
Miracle whip coleslaw	1 tbsp	70	6		4.0	1.0
Miracle whip free	1 tbsp	20	0	0.0	0.0	0.0
Miracle whip light	1 tbsp	45	4			
Kraft® Fat Free						
catalina	1 tbsp	16	0			
French	1 tbsp	20	0			
Italian	1 tbsp	6	0			
ranch	1 tbsp	16	0			
thousand island	1 tbsp	20	0			
Rancher's Choice®						
creamy	1 tbsp	90	10		6.0	1.0
7 Seas®						
buttermilk	1 tbsp	80	8		5.0	1.0
creamy French	1 tbsp	60	6		3.0	1.0
creamy Italian	1 tbsp	70	7		4.0	1.0
Viva, herb and spice	1 tbsp	60	6		4.0	1.0
Viva, ranch	1 tbsp	80	8		5.0	1.0
7 Seas® Fat Free						
ranch	1 tbsp	16	0			
wine vinegar	1 tbsp	6	0			
Viva, Italian	1 tbsp	4	0			
Sandwich spread						
commercial	1 tbsp	60	5	1.1	3.1	0.8
Kraft®	1 tbsp	50	5		3.0	1.0
Shortening						
baking, soy/palm/cottonseed	1 tbsp	113	13	3.8	4.8	3.2
bread, soy/cottonseed	1 tbsp	113	13	4.2	5.2	2.8
bread, soybean/cottonseed	1 cup	1812	205	67.6	83.3	45.

FOOD	OLEIC FAT (g)	CARBO-HYDRATES (g)	CHOLES-TEROL (mg)	OMEGA 3 (g)	SODIUM (mg)	% OF CALORIES FROM FAT
Salad dressing (continued)						
Russian, low calorie, CNF		71.80	15.6		2257	25
Russian, low calorie, USDA	0.1	4.50	1.0		141	26
Russian, regular		25.50	44.1		2127	92
sesame seed	1.8	1.30	0.0	0.00	153	92
sweet and sour		6.90	0.0	0.00	68	9
thousand island	1.2	2.40	4.9	0.00	109	86
thousand island, low calorie	0.4	2.50	2.0	0.00	153	59
thousand island, low cal		41.90	36.7		2457	67
thousand island, regular		43.20	65.0		1745	79
zesty Italian, dry mix	0.0	1.00	0.0	0.00	121	0
Good Seasons® Ranch, dry	0.0	1.00	0.1	0.00	70	0
Hidden Valley® Ranch, lite		1.00	0.0		130	90
Kraft®		2.00	5.0		85	90
bacon and tomato		1.00			130	90
creamy buttermilk		1.00	5.0		120	90
creamy cucumber		1.00			190	100
creamy garlic		1.00			170	90
creamy Russian		2.00	5.0		150	75
golden Caesar		1.00			180	90
Italian/sour cream		1.00			120	90
mayonnaise, light		1.00			110	90
Miracle whip coleslaw		3.00	˙5.0		105	77
Miracle whip free	0.0	5.00	0.0	0.00	210	0
Miracle whip light		2.00	5.0	0.00	95	80
Kraft® Fat Free						
catalina		3.00			120	0
French		4.00			120	0
Italian		1.00			210	0
ranch		3.00			150	0
thousand island		5.00			135	0
Rancher's Choice®						
creamy		1.00	5.0		140	100
7 Seas®						
buttermilk		1.00	5.0		130	90
creamy French		2.00			240	90
creamy Italian		1.00			240	90
Viva, herb and spice		1.00			170	90
Viva, ranch		1.00	5.0		135	90
7 Seas® Fat Free						
ranch		4.00			120	0
wine vinegar		1.00			190	0
Viva, Italian		1.00			220	0
Sandwich spread						
commercial	1.1	3.40	12.0	0.00	153	79
Kraft®		3.00	5.0		95	90
Shortening						
baking, soy/palm/cottonseed	3.8	0.00	0.0			100
bread, soy/cottonseed	4.2	0.00				99
bread, soybean/cottonseed	67.6	0.00				100

FATS & OILS

FOOD	AMOUNT	CALORIES (kcal)	FAT (g)	MONO-UN-SATURATED FAT (g)	POLY-UN-SATURATED FAT (g)	SATURATED FAT (g)
Shortening (continued)						
cakes/frosting, soy	1 tbsp	113	13	4.7	4.9	2.6
canola, industrial, baking cake	1 cup	1812	205	137.0	20.6	45.1
canola, industrial, baking pastry	1 cup	1812	205	138.0	20.8	43.3
canola, liquid, to fry, industrial	1 cup	1812	205	156.0	25.8	21.5
canola, solid, to fry, industrial	1 cup	1812	205	150.0	7.9	45.5
canola and palm, industrial	1 cup	1845	205	154.0	10.2	41.0
confection, coconut/palm	1 cup	1812	205	4.5	2.0	187.0
confection, fractionated palm	1 cup	1927	218	64.4	1.1	143.0
frying, beef tallow/cottonseed	1 cup	1845	205	78.9	18.0	92.0
frying, hydrogenated palm	1 cup	1812	205	83.3	15.3	97.4
frying, soybean, linoleic < 1%	1 cup	1812	205	151.0	0.8	43.3
frying, soybean, linoleic = 30	1 cup	1812	205	89.6	68.6	37.7
frying, soybean/cottonseed	1 cup	1812	205	119.0	45.1	31.6
household, lard/vegetable oil	1 cup	1845	205	91.0	22.3	82.6
household, soybean/palm	1 cup	1812	205	104.0	29.1	62.7
industrial, lard/vegetable oil	1 tbsp	115	13	5.2	2.5	4.6
industrial, soybean/cottonseed	1 cup	1812	205	119.0	24.6	52.5
multipurpose, soy/palm	1 tbsp	113	13	6.5	1.82	3.9
soybean, industrial, baking	1 cup	1812	205	101.0	44.7	59.2
soybean, industrial, baking pastry	1 cup	1812	205	95.9	50.2	58.4
soybean, liquid, to fry, industrial	1 cup	1812	205	95.1	71.3	37.7
soybean, solid, to fry, industrial	1 cup	1812	205	134.0	23.0	47.6
soy and palm, industrial	1 cup	1845	205	107.0	47.1	51.2
vegetable oil, household	1 cup	1823	203	86.5	42.8	52.9
vegetable & animal oils, household	1 cup	1823	203	88.1	11.8	92.0
vegetable, soybean/cottonseed	1 cup	1812	205	89.0	52.2	51.2
Sour cream, fat free, real dairy	12 g	8	0			
Spread						
20% butter, 80% margarine	1 cup	1599	179	105.0	17.8	48.0
50% Butter, 50% margarine	1 cup	1550	175	86.3	11.2	68.9
Vegetable spray, Pam®						
butter flavored	0.9 g	7	0.8	0.2	0.5	0.1
unflavored	0.9 g	7	0.8	0.2	0.5	0.1
cooking spray, olive oil flavor	1.0 g	2	1.0			
Whale, bowhead blubber, fat, Alaska	19 g	870	96.5			

FOOD	OLEIC FAT (g)	CARBO-HYDRATES (g)	CHOLES-TEROL (mg)	OMEGA 3 (g)	SODIUM (mg)	% OF CALORIES FROM FAT
Shortening (continued)						
cakes/frosting, soy	4.7	0.00	0.0			100
canola, industrial, baking cake		0.00				100
canola, industrial, baking pastry		0.00				100
canola, liquid, to fry, industrial		0.00				100
canola, solid, to fry, industrial		0.00				100
canola and palm, industrial		0.00	0.0		0	100
confection, coconut/palm	4.5	0.00	0.0		0	100
confection, fractionated palm	64.0	0.00	0.0		0	100
frying, beef tallow/cottonseed	70.1	0.00	195.0		0	100
frying, hydrogenated palm	83.3	0.00	0.0		0	100
frying, soybean, linoleic < 1%	151.0	0.00	0.0		0	100
frying, soybean, linoleic = 30	89.6	0.00	0.0		0	100
frying, soybean/cottonseed	119.0	0.00	0.0		0	100
household, lard/vegetable oil	83.9	0.00	0.0		0	100
household, soybean/palm	104.0	0.00	0.0		0	100
industrial, lard/vegetable oil	4.9	0.00				100
industrial, soybean/cottonseed	119.0	0.00	0.0		0	100
multipurpose, soy/palm	6.5	0.00	0.0			100
soybean, industrial, baking		0.00				100
soybean, industrial, baking pastry		0.00				100
soybean, liquid, to fry, industrial		0.00	0.0		0	100
soybean, solid, to fry, industrial		0.00				100
soy and palm, industrial		0.00	0.0			100
vegetable oil, household		0.00	0.0		0	100
vegetable & animal oils, household		0.00	0.0		0	100
vegetable, soybean/cottonseed	88.9	0.00	0.0	0.00	0	100
Sour cream, fat free, real dairy		0.50			15	0
Spread						
20% butter, 80% margarine		1.6	97.5		2048	100
50% Butter, 50% margarine		1.0	236.0		1911	100
Vegetable spray, Pam®						
butter flavored		0.00	0.0		0	97
unflavored		0.00	0.0		0	97
cooking spray, olive oil flavor		0.00	0.0		0	100
Whale, bowhead blubber, fat, Alaska		0.00	150.0			100

SNACKS & SWEETS

FOOD	AMOUNT	CALO-RIES (kcal)	PROTEIN (g)	FAT (g)	MONO-UN-SATURATED FAT (g)	POLY-UN-SATURATED FAT (g)	SATU-RATED FAT (g)
SNACKS							
Banana chips	1 oz	147	0.7	9.5	0.6	0.2	8.2
Beef jerky, chopped & formed	1 lg piece	67	7.9	2.6	1.1	0.1	1.2
Cheetos® lite cheese flavored snack chips	25 g	120	2.0	6.0			1.1
Chex mix®	2 oz	241	6.2	9.8			
Combos® snacks cheddar, pretzel	1 oz	136	2.8	5.5			
Corn cakes	1 cake	35	0.7	0.2	0.1	0.1	0.0
Corn-based, extruded							
chips, plain	7-oz bag	1067	13.0	66.1	19.1	32.6	9.0
chips, barbecue-flavor	7-oz bag	1036	13.8	64.8	18.8	32.0	8.8
cones, plain	6 oz	867	9.8	45.7	2.9	1.3	38.7
cones, nacho-flavor	6 oz	912	11.0	54.0	3.7	1.4	45.5
onion-flavor	1 oz	142	2.2	6.4	3.8	0.9	1.2
puffs or twists, cheese-flavor	8 oz bag	1256	17.2	78.1	46.1	10.8	15.0
Doritos® corn chips							
cool ranch	28 g	140	2.0	7.0			1.1
nacho cheese, light	25 g	110	2.0	4.0			0.7
salsa rio	28.4 g	140	1.0	7.0			1.3
toasted corn, light	28 g	150	2.0	7.0			0.4
Fritos® wild mild ranch	28.4 g	150	2.0	9.0			1.5
Keebler®							
Hooplas, original	28.4 g	140	2.0	8.0			1.0
Pizzaria Pizza Supreme	28.4 g	140	3.0	6.0			1.0
Cornnuts®							
plain	1 oz	124	2.4	4.0	2.1	0.9	0.7
barbecue-flavor	1 oz	123	2.6	4.1	2.1	0.9	0.7
nacho-flavor	1 oz	124	2.7	4.0	2.1	0.9	0.7
Crisped rice bar							
almond	1-oz bar	130	2.0	5.8	2.1	2.2	1.1
chocolate chip	1-oz bar	115	1.4	3.8	1.1	1.0	1.5
Doo Dads® snack mix, original flavor	½ cup	129	2.9	5.3			
Fruit leather							
bars	1 bar	81	0.4	1.2	0.1	0.0	0.9
bars, w/cream	1 bar	89	0.2	2.0	1.0	0.2	0.6
pieces	1 oz	97	0.3	2.0	0.9	0.8	0.3
rolls	1 roll	73	0.2	0.6	0.3	0.1	0.1
Granola bars, hard							
plain, includes common varieties	1-oz bar	134	2.8	5.6	1.2	3.4	0.7
almond	1-oz bar	140	2.2	7.2	2.2	1.1	3.6
chocolate chip	1 bar	103	1.7	3.9	0.6	0.3	2.7
peanut	1 bar	113	2.6	5.0	1.4	2.8	0.6
peanut butter	1 bar	114	2.3	5.6	1.7	2.9	0.8
Nature Valley®							
cinnamon	1 bar	120	2.0	5.0			1.0
oat bran	1 bar	110	2.0	4.0			0.8
oats n honey	1 bar	120	2.0	5.0			1.0
peanut butter	1 bar	120	2.0	6.0			1.0
rice & cinnamon	1 bar	90	1.0	4.0			1.0

FOOD	CARBO-HYDRATES (mg)	FIBER (mg)	CALCIUM (mg)	IRON (mg)	POTAS-SIUM (mg)	SODIUM (mg)	CHOLES-TEROL (mg)	% OF CALORIES FROM FAT
SNACKS								
Banana chips	16.6		5	0.35	152	2	0	58
Beef jerky, chopped & formed	2.9			1.09		569	22	35
Cheetos® lite cheese flavored snack chips	16.0	1.1	31	0.43	65	270	0	45
Chex mix®	36.9			14.00		577	0	37
Combos® snacks cheddar, pretzel	18.4	0.0	54	0.86	37	317		36
Corn cakes	7.5	0.1	2	0.13	14	44	0	5
Corn-based, extruded								
chips, plain	112.7	2.2	251	2.62	281	1248	0	56
chips, barbecue-flavor	111.3	2.1	259	3.05	468	1511	0	56
cones, plain	107.0	1.0	5	4.32	138	1737	0	47
cones, nacho-flavor	97.3	0.5	61	2.16	209	1618		53
onion-flavor	18.5	0.3	8	1.06	40	278	0	41
puffs or twists, cheese-flavor	122.2	0.8	131	5.33	376	2383	9	56
Doritos® corn chips								
cool ranch	18.0	1.8	43	0.42	75	180	0	45
nacho cheese, light	18.0	1.1	31	0.43	70	250	0	33
salsa rio	18.0	1.3	35	0.48	80	190	0	45
toasted corn, light	19.0	1.9	3	0.62	55	80	0	42
Fritos® wild mild ranch	16.0	1.3	35	0.48	60	230	0	54
Keebler®								
Hooplas, original	18.0	1.3	35	0.48	40	210	0	51
Pizzaria Pizza Supreme	18.0					200		39
Cornnuts®								
plain	20.8	0.6	2	0.47	79	156	0	29
barbecue-flavor	20.3	0.7	5	0.48	81	277	0	30
nacho-flavor	20.3	0.7	10	0.48	88	180	1	29
Crisped rice bar								
almond	18.3		21	1.80	65	66	0	40
chocolate chip	20.7	0.6	6	1.79	48	79	0	30
Doo Dads® snack mix, original flavor	18.2		21	0.71	79	360	0	37
Fruit leather								
bars	18.0	0.2	7	0.18	32	18	0	13
bars, w/cream	18.7	0.2	5	0.20	51	23		20
pieces	22.2	0.7	5	0.21	46	114	0	19
rolls	17.7	0.3	7	0.21	62	13	0	7
Granola bars, hard								
plain, includes common varieties	18.3	0.3	17	0.84	95	83	0	38
almond	17.6	0.2	9	0.71	77	73	0	46
chocolate chip	17.0	0.2	18	0.72	59	81	0	34
peanut	15.0	0.1	9	0.59	72	66	0	40
peanut butter	14.7	0.2	10	0.57	69	67	0	44
Nature Valley®								
cinnamon	17.0	1.0	0	0.72	60	70	0	38
oat bran	16.0	1.0	0	0.72	60	90	0	33
oats n honey	17.0	1.0	0	0.72	60	65	0	38
peanut butter	15.0	1.0	0	0.72	70	70	0	45
rice & cinnamon	13.0	1.0	0	0.36	55	75	0	40

SNACKS & SWEETS

FOOD	AMOUNT	CALO-RIES (kcal)	PROTEIN (g)	FAT (g)	MONO-UN-SATURATED FAT (g)	POLY-UN-SATURATED FAT (g)	SATU-RATED FAT (g)
SNACKS (continued)							
Granola bars, soft							
uncoated, plain	1-oz bar	126	2.1	4.9	1.1	1.5	2.1
uncoated, chocolate chip	1-oz bar	119	2.1	4.7	1.0	0.6	2.9
uncoated, chocolate chip, graham, & marshmallow	1-oz bar	121	1.7	4.4	0.8	0.7	2.6
uncoated, nut & raisin	1-oz bar	129	2.3	5.8	1.2	1.6	2.7
uncoated, peanut butter	1-oz bar	121	3.0	4.5	1.9	1.2	1.0
uncoated, peanut butter & chocolate chip	1-oz bar	122	2.8	5.7	2.4	1.3	1.6
uncoated, raisin	1-oz bar	127	2.2	5.0	0.8	0.9	2.7
milk chocolate coated, chocolate chip	1-oz bar	132	1.6	7.1	2.2	0.5	4.0
milk chocolate coated, peanut butter	1 bar	187	3.7	11.4	2.4	0.7	6.2
Health Valley®							
fat free blueberry	1 bar	140	3.0	1.0			
fat free date	1 bar	140	3.0	1.0	0.4	0.3	0.3
Granola clusters, Nature Valley®	34 g	150	2.0	3.0			
Meat-based sticks, smoked	1 stick	109	4.3	9.8	4.1	0.9	4.1
Oriental mix, rice-based	1 oz	155	5.7	11.5			
Popcorn							
air popped	1 cup	31	1.0	0.3	0.1	0.2	0.1
oil-popped	1 cup	55	1.0	3.1	0.9	1.5	0.5
cakes	1 cake	38	1.0	0.3	0.1	0.1	0.1
caramel-coated, w/peanuts	1 oz	114	1.8	2.2	0.8	0.9	0.3
caramel-coated, w/out peanuts	1 oz	122	1.1	3.6	0.8	1.3	1.0
cheese-flavor	1 oz	149	2.6	9.4	2.8	4.4	1.8
Keebler®							
honey caramel	1 cup	120	1.0	3.0			1.0
white cheddar	1 cup	70	0.5	5.0			0.9
Pillsbury®							
butter, frozen	1 cup	70	1.0	4.3			
butter, shelf stable	1 cup	70	1.0	4.3			2.1
original, frozen	1 cup	70	1.0	4.3			2.1
original, shelf stable	1 cup	70	1.0	4.3			2.1
salt free, frozen	1 cup	57	1.0	2.3			
Pop Qwiz® natural flavor	1 cup	33	0.7	2.0			0.6
butter flavor	1 cup	33	0.7	2.0			0.3
Pop Secret®							
butter flavor	1 cup	33	0.7	2.0			0.3
butter flavor, light	1 cup	23	0.7	1.0			0.3
butter flavor, no salt	1 cup	33	0.7	2.0			0.3
butter flavor, singles	1 cup	33	0.5	2.0			0.5
butter flavor, singles, light	1 cup	23	0.5	1.0			0.2
butter flavor, no salt	1 cup	33	0.7	2.0			0.3
natural flavor	1 cup	33	0.7	2.0			0.6
natural flavor, light	1 cup	23	0.7	1.0			0.3
natural flavor, singles, light	1 cup	25	0.7	1.0			0.2

FOOD	CARBO-HYDRATES (mg)	FIBER (mg)	CALCIUM (mg)	IRON (mg)	POTAS-SIUM (mg)	SODIUM (mg)	CHOLES-TEROL (mg)	% OF CALORIES FROM FAT
SNACKS (continued)								
Granola bars, soft								
uncoated, plain	19.1	0.3	30	0.73	92	79	0	35
uncoated, chocolate chip	19.6	0.3	26	0.72	96	77	0	36
uncoated, chocolate chip, graham, & marshmallow	20.1	0.3	25	0.73	78	90	0	33
uncoated, nut & raisin	18.0	0.6	24	0.62	111	72	0	40
uncoated, peanut butter	18.2	0.2	26	0.60	83	116	0	33
uncoated, peanut butter & chocolate chip	17.6	0.4	23	0.55	107	93	0	42
uncoated, raisin	18.8	0.2	29	0.69	103	80	0	35
milk chocolate coated, chocolate chip	18.1	0.3	29	0.66	89	57	1	48
milk chocolate coated, peanut butter	19.6	0.8	40	0.53	124	71	4	55
Health Valley®								
fat free blueberry	33.0	3.7	20	3.60		10	0	6
fat free date	33.0	3.7	20	3.60		10	0	6
Granola clusters, Nature Valley®	28.0	1.7	24	0.85		115	0	18
Meat-based sticks, smoked	1.1	0.1	13	0.67		293	26	81
Oriental mix, rice-based	9.4	1.0	22	0.78	147	235	0	67
Popcorn								
air popped	6.2	0.3	1	0.21	24	0	0	9
oil-popped	6.3	0.4	1	0.31	25	97	0	51
cakes	8.0	0.2	1	0.19	33	29	0	7
caramel-coated, w/peanuts	22.9	0.5	19	1.11	101	84	0	17
caramel-coated, w/out peanuts	22.4	0.5	12	0.49	31	58		27
cheese-flavor	14.6	0.5	32	0.64	74	252	3	57
Keebler®								
honey caramel	22.0	1.7	1	0.36	25	180	0	23
white cheddar	6.5	2.8	28	0.64	50	135	2.5	64
Pillsbury®								
butter, frozen	6.7		0	0.12	32	160		56
butter, shelf stable	6.7	4.0	0	0.12	32	137	0.97	56
original, frozen	6.7	4.0	0	0.12	32	140	0	56
original, shelf stable	6.7	4.0	0	0.12	32	137		56
salt free, frozen	7.7		0	0.24	37	0		37
Pop Qwiz® natural flavor	3.7	0.7	0	0.12	20	57	0	54
butter flavor	3.7	0.7	0	0.12	20	57	0	54
Pop Secret®								
butter flavor	3.7	0.7	0	0.12	20	57	0	54
butter flavor, light	4.0	0.7	0	0.12	23	38	0	39
butter flavor, no salt	3.7	0.7	0	0.12	20	52	0	54
butter flavor, singles	3.8	0.7	0	0.12	20	52	0	54
butter flavor, singles, light	3.8	0.7	0	0.12	23	32	0	39
butter flavor, no salt	3.7	0.7	0	0.00	18	2	0	54
natural flavor	3.7	0.7	0	0.12	20	57	0	55
natural flavor, light	4.0	0.7	0	0.12	13	53	0	39
natural flavor, singles, light	3.8	0.7	0	0.12	46	53	0	36

SNACKS & SWEETS

FOOD	AMOUNT	CALO-RIES (kcal)	PROTEIN (g)	FAT (g)	MONO-UN-SATURATED FAT (g)	POLY-UN-SATURATED FAT (g)	SATU-RATED FAT (g)
SNACKS (continued)							
Pork skins							
plain	1 oz	154	17.4	8.9	4.2	1.0	3.2
barbecue-flavor	1 oz	152	16.4	9.0	4.3	1.0	3.3
Potato chips							
plain	8-oz bag	1217	15.8	78.6	22.3	27.6	24.9
barbecue flavor	7-oz bag	971	15.3	64.1	13.0	32.4	15.9
cheese flavor	6-oz bag	842	14.4	46.2	13.1	16.3	14.6
light	6-oz bag	801	12.2	35.4	8.2	18.6	7.1
sour cream & onion flavor	7-oz bag	1051	16.0	67.2	12.1	34.5	17.6
made from dried potatoes, plain	7-oz can	1106	11.7	76.0	14.4	39.6	18.7
made from dried potatoes, cheese flavor	6-¾-oz can	1053	13.3	70.7	13.6	35.7	18.3
made from dried potatoes, light	6-oz can	852	9.5	43.6	10.1	22.9	8.7
made from dried potatoes, sour cream & onion flavor	6-¾-oz can	1046	12.5	70.7	13.6	35.9	18.1
Frito Lay Sun Chips® original	28.4 g	140	2.0	7.0			1.1
Potato sticks	1 oz	148	1.9	9.8	1.8	5.1	2.5
Pretzels							
hard, plain	1 oz	108	2.6	1.0	0.4	0.3	0.2
hard, chocolate-flavor confectioner's coating	1 oz	130	2.1	4.7	1.5	0.6	2.2
hard, whole-wheat	1 oz	103	3.1	0.7	0.3	0.2	0.2
Keebler®							
bulk mini	1 item	2	0.0	0.0			0.0
transport pack	1 item	3	0.0	0.0			0.0
Pennysticks® oat bran nuggets	1 item	111	3.0	2.0			
Puffs, Health Valley®							
caramel corn, apple	1 oz	100	1.0	1.0			
caramel corn, original	1 oz	100	1.0	1.0			0.1
caramel corn, peanut	1 oz	100	1.0	1.0			
carrot lites	1 oz	150	2.0	8.0			
cheddar lites	1 oz	160	4.0	8.0			
cheddar lites, green onion	1 oz	160	4.0	8.0			
cheese flavor, green onion	1 oz	100	3.0	1.0			0.1
cheese flavor, original	1 oz	100	3.0	1.0			0.1
cheese flavor, zesty chili	1 oz	100	3.0	1.0			0.
Rice cakes, brown rice							
plain	1 cake	35	0.7	0.3	0.1	0.1	0.1
buckwheat	1 cake	34	0.8	0.3	0.1	0.1	0.1
corn	1 cake	35	0.8	0.3	0.1	0.1	0.1
multigrain	1 cake	35	0.8	0.3	0.1	0.1	0.
rye	1 cake	35	0.7	0.3	0.1	0.1	0.
sesame seed	1 cake	35	0.7	0.3	0.1	0.1	0.
Rice Krispie® bar							
w/almonds	1 bar	130	2.0	5.8			1.
w/chocolate chips	1 bar	115	1.4	3.8			1.
Sesame sticks, wheat-based	1 oz	153	3.1	10.4	3.1	4.9	1.8
Snack mix, Pepperidge Farm®							
classic	1 oz	140	4.0	8.0			
lightly smoked	1 oz	150	4.0	9.0			

FOOD	CARBO-HYDRATES (mg)	FIBER (mg)	CALCIUM (mg)	IRON (mg)	POTAS-SIUM (mg)	SODIUM (mg)	CHOLES-TEROL (mg)	% OF CALORIES FROM FAT
SNACKS (continued)								
Pork skins								
plain	0.0	0.0	8	0.25	36	521	27	52
barbecue-flavor	0.5		12	0.30	51	756	33	53
Potato chips								
plain	120.1	3.9	54	3.70	2894	1347	0	58
barbecue flavor	104.5	3.4	98	3.85	2498	1486	0	59
cheese flavor	98.1	2.5	122	3.13	2597	1348		49
light	113.8		35	2.29	2965	836	0	40
sour cream & onion flavor	101.9	3.9	143	3.17	2634	1237	14	58
made from dried potatoes, plain	101.1	2.7	48	2.97	1997	1299	0	62
made from dried potatoes, cheese flavor	96.7	2.1	210	3.06		1442	8	60
made from dried potatoes, light	110.3	3.1	58	2.57	1708	727	0	46
made from dried potatoes, sour cream & onion flavor	98.1	2.3	122	2.67		1375	5	61
Frito Lay Sun Chips® original	18.0	1.9	44	0.43	45	110	0	45
Potato sticks	15.1	0.3	5	0.64	351	71	0	60
Pretzels								
hard, plain	22.5	0.1	10	1.23	42	486	0	8
hard, chocolate-flavor confectioner's coating	20.1	0.6	21	0.57				33
hard, whole-wheat	23.0	0.5	8	0.76	122	58	0	6
Keebler®								
bulk mini	0.3	0.0	0	0.02	1	10	0	0
transport pack	0.5	0.0	0	0.03	1	15	0	0
Pennysticks® oat bran nuggets	22.0					449	2	16
Puffs, Health Valley®								
caramel corn, apple	22.0		0	0.36	25	75	0	9
caramel corn, original	22.0	1.7	0	0.36	25	75	0	9
caramel corn, peanut	22.0		0	0.36	25	75	0	9
carrot lites	18.0	1.0			50	10	0	48
cheddar lites	16.0	0.5			180	140	0	45
cheddar lites, green onion	16.0	0.5			180	140	1.6	45
cheese flavor, green onion	21.0	2.8	0	0.36	35	75	0	9
cheese flavor, original	21.0	0.1	0	0.34	35	75	0	9
cheese flavor, zesty chili	21.0	0.1	0	0.36	35	75	0	9
Rice cakes, brown rice								
plain	7.3	0.2	1	0.13	26	29	0	8
buckwheat	7.2	0.1	1	0.10	27	10	0	8
corn	7.3	0.1	1	0.11	25	26	0	8
multigrain	7.2	0.2	2	0.18	26	23	0	8
rye	7.2	0.2	2	0.16	28	10	0	8
sesame seed	7.3	0.2	1	0.14	26	20	0	8
Rice Krispie® bar								
w/almonds	18.3		21	1.80	65	66	0	40
w/chocolate chips	20.7		6	1.79	48	79	0	30
Sesame sticks, wheat-based	13.2		48	0.21		422	0	61
Snack mix, Pepperidge Farm®								
classic	14.0		40	0.72		359	0	52
lightly smoked	13.0		40	0.36		349	0	54

403

SNACKS & SWEETS

FOOD	AMOUNT	CALO-RIES (kcal)	PROTEIN (g)	FAT (g)	MONO-UN-SATURATED FAT (g)	POLY-UN-SATURATED FAT (g)	SATU-RATED FAT (g)
SNACKS (continued)							
Snack mix, Pepperidge Farm® (continued)							
spicy	1 oz	140	4.0	8.0			
Taro chips	1 oz	141	0.7	7.1	1.3	3.7	1.8
Tortilla chips							
plain	7½-oz bag	1067	15.0	55.8	32.9	7.7	10.7
nacho-flavor	8-oz bag	1131	17.8	58.1	34.3	8.1	11.1
nacho-flavor, light	6-oz bag	757	14.8	25.8	15.2	3.6	4.9
ranch-flavor	7-oz bag	969	15.1	47.2	27.8	6.5	9.0
taco-flavor	8-oz bag	1089	18.0	55.0	32.4	7.6	10.5
Trail mix							
regular	1 cup	693	20.7	44.1	18.8	14.5	8.3
regular, w/chocolate chips	1 cup	707	20.7	46.6	19.8	16.5	8.9
tropical	1 cup	570	8.8	24.0	3.5	7.2	11.9
SWEETS, Candies							
After Eight® mints	2 pieces	29	0.2	1.1	0.4	0.0	0.7
Almond Joy® candy bar	1 bar	232	2.4	13.8	2.6	1.2	8.3
Alpine White® bar w/almonds	1 bar	197	3.5	12.9	4.8	0.9	6.7
Baby Ruth® bar	1 bar	277	5.6	13.3	3.8	2.1	6.9
Bar None® candy bar	1 bar	224	3.5	14.6			
Bit-o-Honey® candy chews	1 bar	186	1.4	3.8			
Butterfinger® bar	1 bar	266	4.7	11.3	3.8	1.8	5.2
Butterscotch	1 oz	112	0.0	1.0	0.1	0.0	0.3
Cadbury's Caramello® candy bar	1 bar	220	2.8	11.4			
Caramels	1 piece	31	0.4	0.6	0.1	0.0	0.5
Caramels, chocolate-flavor roll	1 piece	22	0.1	0.2	0.1	0.1	0.0
Carob	1 bar	453	10.9	28.0	16.1	3.4	7.2
Confectioner's coating							
butterscotch	1 oz	147	0.6	8.2	1.0	0.1	6.8
peanut butter	1 oz	141	5.2	8.4	2.7	1.5	3.2
white	1 bar	453	5.2	25.8	8.1	0.7	15.1
Chunky® bar	1 bar	173	3.1	10.2	0.1	1.5	8.1
Demet's Turtles® candy	1 piece	82	1.1	4.7	1.9	0.8	1.8
Divinity, prepared from recipe	1 piece	38	0.1	0.0			
5th Avenue® bar	1 bar	280	4.7	12.7			
Fondant, prepared from recipe	1 piece	57	0.0	0.0			
Fudge							
brown sugar, w/nuts, prepared from recipe	1 piece	56	0.4	1.4	0.3	0.8	0.1
chocolate, prepared from recipe	1 piece	65	0.3	1.4	0.4	0.1	0.4
chocolate, w/nuts, prepared from recipe	1 piece	81	0.6	3.1	0.8	1.0	1.
chocolate marshmallow, prepared from recipe	1 piece	84	0.5	3.4	1.1	0.1	2.
chocolate marshmallow, w/nuts, prepared from recipe	1 piece	96	0.7	4.3	1.3	0.7	2.
peanut butter, prepared from recipe	1 piece	59	0.6	1.0	0.5	0.3	0.
vanilla, prepared from recipe	1 piece	59	0.2	0.9	0.3	0.0	0.
vanilla, w/nuts, prepared from recipe	1 piece	62	0.4	2.0	0.5	0.8	0.

FOOD	CARBO-HYDRATES (mg)	FIBER (mg)	CALCIUM (mg)	IRON (mg)	POTAS-SIUM (mg)	SODIUM (mg)	CHOLES-TEROL (mg)	% OF CALORIES FROM FAT
SNACKS (continued)								
Snack mix, Pepperidge Farm® (continued)								
spicy	14.0		20	0.00		339	4.99	51
Taro chips	19.3	0.3	17	0.34	214	97	0	45
Tortilla chips								
plain	133.9	2.8	327	3.25	419	1124	0	47
nacho-flavor	141.5	3.2	334	3.24	491	1606	8	46
nacho-flavor, light	121.7		270	2.77	462	1705	4	31
ranch-flavor	128.0		280	2.90	483	1212	1	44
taco-flavor	143.2	2.9	352	4.59	492	1788		45
Trail mix								
regular	67.4	3.6	117	4.58	1028	343	0	57
regular, w/chocolate chips	65.6	3.7	159	4.95	946	177		59
tropical	91.8	2.4	79	3.69	993	14	0	38
SWEETS, Candies								
After Eight® mints	6.1		2	0.12	13	1		34
Almond Joy® candy bar	29.2		40	0.60		67	1	54
Alpine White® bar w/almonds	17.6		81	0.20	146	26	4	59
Baby Ruth® bar	37.2		24	0.49	129	133	14	43
Bar None® candy bar	22.4	0.6	62	0.52	168	45	7	59
Bit-o-Honey® candy chews	38.9		27	0.14	60	124		18
Butterfinger® bar	40.5		15	0.64	130	83		38
Butterscotch	27.0	0.0	1	0.02	1	12	3	8
Cadbury's Caramello® candy bar	29.7		89	0.49		55	11	47
Caramels	6.2		11	0.01	17	20	1	17
Caramels, chocolate-flavor roll	5.2						0	8
Carob	41.9		391		765			56
Confectioner's coating								
butterscotch	18.9		10		53	27		50
peanut butter	12.7	0.3	31	0.48	143	71		54
white	52.2		175	0.14	259	76		51
Chunky® bar	20.0		50	0.44	187	19	4	53
Demet's Turtles® candy	9.9		27	0.23	52	16	4	52
Divinity, prepared from recipe	9.8	0.0	0	0.01	2	5	0	0
5th Avenue® bar	40.8	0.5	42	0.60	197	112	2	41
Fondant, prepared from recipe	14.8	0.0	0	0.01	3	6	0	0
Fudge								
brown sugar, w/nuts, prepared from recipe	10.9	0.1	16	0.25	52	14	1	23
chocolate, prepared from recipe	13.5	0.0	7	0.08	17	10	2	19
chocolate, w/nuts, prepared from recipe	13.8	0.1	9	0.14	30	11	3	34
chocolate marshmallow, prepared from recipe	14.3	0.2	9	0.19	28	21	5	36
chocolate marshmallow, w/nuts, prepared from recipe	15.1	0.3	11	0.23	37	21	5	40
peanut butter, prepared from recipe	12.5	0.0	7	0.04	21	12	1	15
vanilla, prepared from recipe	13.2	0.0	6	0.01	8	11	3	14
vanilla, w/nuts, prepared from recipe	11.3	0.1	7	0.06	17	9	2	29

SNACKS & SWEETS

FOOD	AMOUNT	CALO-RIES (kcal)	PROTEIN (g)	FAT (g)	MONO-UN-SATURATED FAT (g)	POLY-UN-SATURATED FAT (g)	SATU-RATED FAT (g)
SWEETS, Candies (continued)							
Golden Almond® chocolate bar	1 bar	466	8.9	32.1			
Golden Almond Solitaires® chocolate w/almonds	1 bar	455	9.9	31.4			
Golden III® chocolate bar	1 bar	471	5.9	30.0			
Goobers® chocolate covered peanuts	39-g pkg	200	5.4	13.1	5.8	2.0	4.8
Gumdrops, starch jelly pieces	10 small	135	0.0	0.0			
Hard candies	1 lollipop	22	0.0	0.0			
Jellybeans	10 small	40	0.0	0.1			
Kit Kat® wafer bar	1 bar	235	3.1	13.1	3.6	0.2	7.7
Krackel® chocolate bar	1 bar	236	2.9	13.1	3.3	2.6	5.6
Mars® almond bar	1 bar	233	4.0	11.5			
Mars® Milky Way® bar	1 bar	251	2.7	9.1	3.3	0.3	4.7
Marshmallows	1 regular	23	0.1	0.0			
Milk chocolate coated peanuts	1 cup	773	19.4	49.9	19.3	6.5	21.8
Milk chocolate coated raisins	1 cup	741	7.7	28.1	9.0	1.0	16.7
Milk chocolate	1 bar	226	3.0	13.5	4.4	0.4	8.1
w/almonds	1 bar	215	3.7	14.1	5.5	0.9	7.0
w/rice cereal	1 bar	198	2.5	10.6	3.5	0.3	6.4
M&M's® peanut chocolate candies	49-g pkg	242	5.2	13.2			
M&M's® plain chocolate candies	48-g pkg	229	3.0	10.6			
Mounds® candy bar	1 pkg	195	1.9	11.7	3.6	0.4	6.2
Mr. Goodbar® chocolate bar	1 bar	257	6.3	16.1	5.7	0.8	9.0
Nestle Crunch® milk chocolate w/crisp rice	1 bar	198	2.5	10.4	3.8	0.4	5.7
Oh Henry!® bar	1 bar	246		9.6	3.8	1.6	3.8
100 Grand® bar	1 bar	195	1.5	8.5			
Peanut bar	1 bar	209	6.2	13.5	6.7	4.3	1.7
Peanut brittle, prepared from recipe	1 oz	128	2.1	5.4	2.4	1.3	1.4
Praline, prepared from recipe	1 piece	177	1.1	9.5	5.9	2.4	0.7
Raisinets® chocolate covered raisins	45-g pkg	186	2.1	7.1	2.7	0.9	3.3
Reese's® peanut butter cups	1 pkg	248	5.6	15.9	1.1	1.1	11.8
Reese's Pieces® candy	55-g pkg	258	7.2	11.4			
Rolo® caramels in milk chocolate	55-g pkg	261	2.7	12.0			
Semisweet chocolate	1 oz	135	1.2	8.4	2.8	0.3	5.0
Sesame crunch	1 oz	146	3.3	9.4	3.6	4.1	1.3
Skittles® bite size candies	65-g pkg	255	0.2	1.9			
Skor® toffee candy bar	1 bar	211	1.8	13.8			
Slim Fast® Dutch chocolate bar	34 g	130	6.0	4.0	0.6	0.6	2.8
Snickers® bar	1 bar	277	5.8	13.6	4.1	0.5	7.2
Special Dark® sweet chocolate bar	1 bar	195	1.9	12.4			
Starburst® fruit chews	59-g pkg	234	0.2	4.9			
Sweet chocolate	1 bar	207	1.6	14.0	4.6	0.4	8.
Sweet chocolate coated fondant	1 lg patty	128	0.8	3.2	1.1	0.1	1.
Symphony® milk chocolate bar	1 bar	209	3.1	13.0			
Taffy, prepared from recipe	1 piece	56	0.0	0.5	0.0	0.0	0.
3 Musketeers® bar	1 bar	249	1.9	7.7	2.6	0.3	3.
Toffee, prepared from recipe	1 piece	65	0.1	3.9	1.1	0.2	2.
Truffles, prepared from recipe	1 piece	59	0.7	4.1	1.2	0.1	2.

FOOD	CARBO-HYDRATES (mg)	FIBER (mg)	CALCIUM (mg)	IRON (mg)	POTAS-SIUM (mg)	SODIUM (mg)	CHOLES-TEROL (mg)	% OF CALORIES FROM FAT
SWEETS, Candies (continued)								
Golden Almond® chocolate bar	41.3	2.0	279	1.27	400	54	10	62
Golden Almond Solitaires® chocolate w/almonds	40.0		305	1.19	428	46	10	62
Golden III® chocolate bar	50.8		275	0.55	413	79	17	57
Goobers® chocolate covered peanuts	19.0		49	0.52	196	16	4	59
Gumdrops, starch jelly pieces	34.6	0.0	1	0.14	2	15	0	0
Hard candies	5.9	0.0	0	0.02	0	2	0	0
Jellybeans	10.2	0.0	0	0.12	4	3	0	2
Kit Kat® wafer bar	28.5	0.2	83	0.39	142	46	11	50
Krackel® chocolate bar	29.1		84	0.38	161	64	9	50
Mars® almond bar	31.4	0.8	84	0.55	162	85		44
Mars® Milky Way® bar	43.5	0.1	78	0.45	144	144		33
Marshmallows	5.9	0.0	0	0.02	0	3	0	0
Milk chocolate coated peanuts	73.7		155	1.95	748	61	13	58
Milk chocolate coated raisins	129.8		163	3.24	976	68	5	34
Milk chocolate	26.1	0.2	84	0.61	169	36	10	54
w/almonds	21.8	0.6	92	0.67	182	30	8	59
w/rice cereal	25.4	0.2	69	0.30	137	58	8	48
M&M's® peanut chocolate candies	28.9	0.7	65	0.73	191	45		49
M&M's® plain chocolate candies	32.7	0.2	81	0.73	187	49		42
Mounds® candy bar	31.3		12	2.03		67	0	54
Mr. Goodbar® chocolate bar	25.7	0.6	56	0.60	225	17	10	56
Nestle Crunch® milk chocolate w/crisp rice	25.7	0.1	68	0.26	138	59	8	47
Oh Henry!® bar	36.9		62	0.32	185	135	5	35
100 Grand® bar	30.9	0.1	50	0.29	107	80	4	39
Peanut bar	18.9	0.6	31	0.39	163	91		58
Peanut brittle, prepared from recipe	19.7	0.4	8	0.39	59	128	4	38
Praline, prepared from recipe	24.2	0.2	12	0.46	82	24	0	48
Raisinets® chocolate covered raisins	32.0		48	0.54	231	16	2	34
Reese's® peanut butter cups	24.4	0.5	40	0.56	204	148	8	58
Reese's Pieces® candy	34.1	0.4	73	0.82	242	82	2	40
Rolo® caramels in milk chocolate	38.3	0.3	74	0.27	143	93	13	41
Semisweet chocolate	18.0	1.1	9	0.89	104	3	0	56
Sesame crunch	14.3	3.7		1.21			0	58
Skittles® bite size candies	62.4		2	0.06	15	30		7
Skor® toffee candy bar	22.1		45	0.16	95	92	24	59
Slim Fast® Dutch chocolate bar	17.0	6.0	160	2.89		90	0	28
Snickers® bar	36.8	0.5	70	0.48	199	164		44
Special Dark® sweet chocolate bar	25.2	0.4	8	0.86	139	4	0	57
Starburst® fruit chews	49.9		2	0.08	1	33		19
Sweet chocolate	24.5	0.4	10	1.13	119	7	0	61
Sweet chocolate coated fondant	28.1	0.7	6	0.55	59	9	0	23
Symphony® milk chocolate bar	22.7		94	0.40	154	34	11	56
Taffy, prepared from recipe	13.7	0.0	0	0.01	1	13	1	8
3 Musketeers® bar	46.1	0.2	50	0.44	80	117	6	28
Toffee, prepared from recipe	7.7	0.0	4	0.01	6	22	13	54
Truffles, prepared from recipe	5.4	0.0	19	0.12	37	8	6	63

SNACKS & SWEETS

FOOD	AMOUNT	CALO-RIES (kcal)	PROTEIN (g)	FAT (g)	MONO-UN-SATURATED FAT (g)	POLY-UN-SATURATED FAT (g)	SATU-RATED FAT (g)
SNACKS (continued)							
Twix®							
caramel cookie bar	1 pkg	273	3.1	13.4			
peanut butter cookie bar	1 pkg	253	5.4	14.5			
Ultra Slim Fast® cocoa almond crunch bar	28 g	110	2.0	4.0	0.6	0.6	2.8
Ultra Slim Fast® cocoa raspberry crunch	28 g	100	2.0	3.0			
Whatchamacallit® candy bar	1 bar	256	4.8	13.2			
York® peppermint pattie	1 sm pattie	38	0.3	1.0			
Y&S Nibs® cherry candy	1 oz	106	0.8	0.7			
Y&S Twizzlers® strawberry candy	71-g pkg	263	2.3	1.1			
SWEETS, Desserts							
Apple crisp, prepared from recipe	½ cup	230	2.5	5.1	2.2	1.5	1.0
Pepperidge Farm® Berkshire	1 oz	53	0.4	1.7	0.4	0.3	0.2
Apple'n'spice bake, Pepperidge Farm®	1 oz	40	0.5	0.5			
Bread pudding, prepared from recipe	½ cup	212	6.6	7.4	2.7	1.2	2.9
Brownie							
Gold Medal Robin Hood® fudge, mix	18.1 g	70	1.0	1.0			
Pepperidge Farm® hot fudge, Newport	1 oz	123	1.2	6.1	2.0	1.4	1.1
Pillsbury®							
microwave fudge	33.4 g	130	2.0	3.0		0.0	1.0
microwave walnut	37.4 g	160	3.0	5.0	2.0	2.0	1.0
Cupcake, chocolate/cream, Hostess Lights®	42.5 g	130	2.0	2.0		1.0	1.0
Danish, apple, Sara Lee® light	57 g	130	2.0	0.0	0.0	0.0	0.0
Egg custards							
baked, prepared from recipe	½ cup	148	7.1	6.6	2.1	0.5	3.
dry mix	21 g	86	1.4	1.3	0.5	0.2	0.
dry mix, prepared w/lowfat (2%) milk	½ cup	148	5.5	3.7	1.2	0.3	1.
dry mix, prepared w/whole milk	½ cup	163	5.5	5.4	1.7	0.3	3.
Jello® golden egg, dry mix	21.3 g	85	1.0	1.0	0.2	0.0	0.
Flan, caramel custard							
prepared from recipe	½ cup	220	7.0	6.3	2.1	0.5	3.
dry mix	21 g	73	0.0	0.0			
dry mix, prepared w/lowfat (2%) milk	½ cup	135	4.1	2.3	0.7	0.1	1.
dry mix, prepared w/whole milk	½ cup	150	4.0	4.1	1.2	0.2	2.
Gelatins							
dry mix	21.3 g	81	1.7	0.0			
dry mix, prepared w/water	½ cup	80	1.6	0.0			
dry mix, w/fruit, prepared from recipe	½ cup	73	1.2	0.2			

FOOD	CARBO-HYDRATES (mg)	FIBER (mg)	CALCIUM (mg)	IRON (mg)	POTAS-SIUM (mg)	SODIUM (mg)	CHOLES-TEROL (mg)	% OF CALORIES FROM FAT
SNACKS (continued)								
Twix®								
caramel cookie bar	37.5	0.1	68	0.38	118	115		44
peanut butter cookie bar	28.5	0.3	59	1.06	158	148		52
Ultra Slim Fast® cocoa almond crunch bar	18.0	3.0	150	2.38		30	0	33
Ultra Slim Fast® cocoa raspberry crunch	21.0	3.0	150	2.38		30	0	27
Whatchamacallit® candy bar	30.0	0.2	62	0.46	177	116	11	46
York® peppermint pattie	8.6		2	0.16		4	0	24
Y&S Nibs® cherry candy	26.2		18	0.17	18	67	0	6
Y&S Twizzlers® strawberry candy	65.9		25	0.35		197	0	4
SWEETS, Desserts								
Apple crisp, prepared from recipe	45.5	0.7	40	1.06	137	257	0	20
Pepperidge Farm® Berkshire	9.0	0.5	8	0.23		27	8.405	29
Apple'n'spice bake, Pepperidge Farm®	8.7		14	0.00		25	2.346	11
Bread pudding, prepared from recipe	30.9	0.3	143	1.38	282	291	83	31
Brownie								
Gold Medal Robin Hood® fudge, mix	15.0		0	0.36		65		13
Pepperidge Farm® hot fudge, Newport	15.4	0.9	12	0.33		49	24.56	45
Pillsbury®								
microwave fudge	25.0		0	1.08		110	0	21
microwave walnut	26.0	1.1	0	1.08		110	0	28
Cupcake, chocolate/cream, Hostess Lights®	26.0					190	0	14
Danish, apple, Sara Lee® light	30.0					120	0	0
Egg custards								
baked, prepared from recipe	15.1	0.0	158	0.43	216	109	123	40
dry mix	17.4	0.0	48	0.41	98	136	64	14
dry mix, prepared w/lowfat (2%) milk	23.6	0.0	197	0.34	287	200	74	23
dry mix, prepared w/whole milk	23.4		194	0.34				30
Jello® golden egg, dry mix	17.0	0.0	53	0.30		138	64.3	11
Flan, caramel custard								
prepared from recipe	34.9	0.0	132	0.50	185	86	140	26
dry mix	19.3	0.0	5	0.02	32	91	0	0
dry mix, prepared w/lowfat (2%) milk	25.6	0.0	153	0.08	194	66	9	15
dry mix, prepared w/whole milk	25.4	0.0	150	0.08	191	65	17	25
Gelatins								
dry mix	19.3	0.0	1		1	54	0	0
dry mix, prepared w/water	18.9	0.0	3		1	57	0	0
dry mix, w/fruit, prepared from recipe	17.9	0.2	5		110	30	0	2

FOOD	AMOUNT	CALO-RIES (kcal)	PROTEIN (g)	FAT (g)	MONO-UN-SATURATED FAT (g)	POLY-UN-SATURATED FAT (g)	SATU-RATED FAT (g)
SWEETS, Desserts (continued)							
Gelatins (continued)							
dry mix, reduced-calorie, aspartame-sweetened	2.5 g	8	1.4	0.0			
dry mix, reduced-calorie, aspartame-sweetened, prepared w/water	½ cup	8	1.3	0.0			
dry powder, unsweetened	1 envelope	23	6.0	0.0	0.0	0.0	0.0
Mousse, chocolate, prepared from recipe	½ cup	447	8.6	32.9	10.3	1.7	18.6
Puddings, banana							
dry mix, instant	25 g	92	0.0	0.2	0.0	0.1	0.0
dry mix, instant, prepared w/lowfat (2%) milk	½ cup	152	4.1	2.5	0.7	0.2	1.5
dry mix, instant, prepared w/whole milk	½ cup	167	4.0	4.2	1.2	0.3	2.6
dry mix, regular	22 g	83	0.0	0.1	0.0	0.0	0.0
dry mix, regular, prepared w/lowfat (2%) milk	½ cup	142	4.1	2.4	0.7	0.1	1.5
dry mix, regular, prepared w/whole milk	½ cup	157	4.0	4.2	1.2	0.2	2.6
ready to eat	5-oz can	180	3.4	5.1	0.4	0.4	0.2
Puddings, butterscotch							
Jello® instant mix	1 oz	105	0.0	0.0	0.0	0.0	0.0
Swiss Miss®	1 oz	37	0.5	1.5			
Puddings, chocolate							
prepared from recipe, w/lowfat (2%) milk	½ cup	206	4.9	3.9	1.3	0.4	2.0
prepared from recipe, w/whole milk	½ cup	221	4.9	5.6	1.8	0.5	3.1
dry mix, instant	25 g	89	0.6	0.5	0.2	0.1	0.2
dry mix, instant, prepared w/lowfat (2%) milk	½ cup	149	4.6	2.8	0.9	0.2	1.6
dry mix, instant, prepared w/whole milk	½ cup	164	4.6	4.5	1.4	0.3	2.2
dry mix, regular	24.8 g	90	0.6	0.5	0.2	0.0	0.
dry mix, regular, prepared w/lowfat (2%) milk	½ cup	150	4.7	2.9	0.8	0.1	1.
dry mix, regular, prepared w/whole milk	½ cup	158	4.6	4.8	1.4	0.2	3.
ready to eat	5-oz can	189	3.8	5.7	2.4	2.0	1.
Jello®							
instant, dry mix	28.4 g	101	0.0	0.0	0.0	0.0	0.
ready to eat, lite chocolate/vanilla, ready to eat	113 g	104	3.0	2.0	0.6	0.1	1.
Swiss Miss® chocolate parfait	1 oz	42	0.8	1.5	0.2	0.0	0.
Puddings, chocolate fudge, instant, dry mix	28.4 g	100	1.0	1.0			
Jello®							
ready to eat	113 g	171	3.0	6.0	2.2	0.2	3
ready to eat, lite	113 g	101	3.0	1.0	0.3	0.0	0

FOOD	CARBO-HYDRATES (mg)	FIBER (mg)	CALCIUM (mg)	IRON (mg)	POTAS-SIUM (mg)	SODIUM (mg)	CHOLES-TEROL (mg)	% OF CALORIES FROM FAT
SWEETS, Desserts (continued)								
Gelatins (continued)								
dry mix, reduced-calorie, aspartame-sweetened	0.1	0.0	0		0	54	0	0
dry mix, reduced-calorie, aspartame-sweetened, prepared w/water	0.1	0.0	2		0	56	0	0
dry powder, unsweetened	0.0	0.0	4	0.08	1	14		0
Mousse, chocolate, prepared from recipe	33.2	0.2	202	1.29	296	87	299	66
Puddings, banana								
dry mix, instant	23.2		1	0.03	4	375	0	2
dry mix, instant, prepared w/lowfat (2%) milk	29.0		150	0.09	192	435	9	15
dry mix, instant, prepared w/whole milk	28.9		147	0.09	189	434	17	23
dry mix, regular	19.9	0.0	4	0.01	4	173	0	1
dry mix, regular, prepared w/lowfat (2%) milk	25.5	0.0	154	0.07	193	232	9	15
dry mix, regular, prepared w/whole milk	25.3	0.0	151	0.07	189	231	17	24
ready to eat	30.1		120	0.18	156	278		26
Puddings, butterscotch								
Jello® instant mix	26.7	0.0	1	0.03		244	0	0
Swiss Miss®	5.7		20	0.00		52	0.25	36
Puddings, chocolate								
prepared from recipe, w/lowfat (2%) milk	40.5		155	0.71	256	137	9	17
prepared from recipe, w/whole milk	40.4		152	0.71	252	137	17	23
dry mix, instant	21.9	0.1	5	0.36	59	357	0	5
dry mix, instant, prepared w/lowfat (2%) milk	27.8	0.1	153	0.42	247	418	9	17
dry mix, instant, prepared w/whole milk	27.6	0.1	151	0.42	244	417	17	25
dry mix, regular	22.1	0.2	13	0.45	52	88	0	5
dry mix, regular, prepared w/lowfat (2%) milk	28.0	0.2	161	0.51	240	148	9	17
dry mix, regular, prepared w/whole milk	25.5	0.2	158	0.51	232	147	17	27
ready to eat	32.4		128	0.72	256	183	5	27
Jello®								
instant, dry mix	25.0		3	0.30		416	0	0
ready to eat, lite chocolate/vanilla, ready to eat	21.0	0.1	82	0.40		113	4.9	17
Swiss Miss® chocolate parfait	6.7	0.0	20	0.09		50	0.25	32
Puddings, chocolate fudge, instant, dry mix	25.0		4	0.50		380	0	9
Jello®								
ready to eat	28.0	0.0	104	0.50		121	1.4	32
ready to eat, lite	22.0	0.1	82	0.40		113	2.9	9

SNACKS & SWEETS

FOOD	AMOUNT	CALO-RIES (kcal)	PROTEIN (g)	FAT (g)	MONO-UN-SATURATED FAT (g)	POLY-UN-SATURATED FAT (g)	SATU-RATED FAT (g)
SWEETS, Desserts (continued)							
Puddings, coconut cream							
dry mix, instant	25 g	97	0.2	1.0	0.2	0.2	0.6
dry mix, instant, prepared w/lowfat (2%) milk	½ cup	157	4.3	3.4	0.9	0.3	2.0
dry mix, instant, prepared w/whole milk	½ cup	172	4.2	5.1	1.4	0.4	3.1
dry mix, regular	22 g	86	0.2	1.2	0.1	0.0	1.1
dry mix, regular, prepared w/lowfat (2%) milk	½ cup	146	4.3	3.5	0.7	0.1	2.5
dry mix, regular, prepared w/whole milk	½ cup	160	4.3	5.3	1.2	0.2	3.6
Jello® dry mix	14.8 g	61	0.0	2.0	0.1	0.0	0.3
instant	1 oz	117	0.3	2.9	0.2	0.0	0.6
Pudding, egg custard, Swiss Miss®	1 oz	47	3.2	1.5			
Pudding, French vanilla, dry mix, Jello®	25.7 g	94	0.0	0.0	0.0	0.0	0.0
Puddings, lemon							
dry mix, instant	25 g	94	0.0	0.2	0.1	0.1	0.0
dry mix, instant, prepared w/lowfat (2%) milk	½ cup	155	4.1	2.5	0.7	0.2	1.
dry mix, instant, prepared w/whole milk	½ cup	169	4.0	4.2	1.2	0.2	2.
dry mix, regular	21.2 g	77	0.0	0.1	0.1	0.1	0.
dry mix, regular, prepared w/sugar, egg yolk, & water	½ cup	163	1.0	2.0	0.8	0.4	0
ready to eat	5-oz can	177	0.1	4.3	1.8	1.6	0.
Jello® dry mix	14.2 g	52	0.0	0.0	0.0	0.0	0
instant	28.35 g	105	0.0	0.2	0.0	0.0	0
Puddings, milk chocolate							
Jello® ready to eat	113 g	173	4.0	6.0	1.0	0.1	1
milk chocolate/fudge, ready to eat	113 g	172	3.0	6.0	1.0	0.1	1
Yoplait®	113 g	180	6.0	4.0			
Puddings, rice							
prepared from recipe	½ cup	217	5.5	4.2	1.2	0.2	2
dry mix	27 g	102	0.7	0.0	0.8	5.1	2
dry mix, prepared w/lowfat (2%) milk	½ cup	161	4.8	2.4	1.5	5.1	4
dry mix, prepared w/whole milk	½ cup	175	4.7	4.1	2.0	5.2	5
ready to eat	5-oz can	231	2.8	10.7	4.6	4.0	1
Puddings, tapioca							
prepared from recipe	½ cup	189	7.2	6.6			
dry mix	23 g	85	0.0	0.0	0.1	0.1	0
dry mix, prepared w/lowfat (2%) milk	½ cup	147	4.1	2.4	0.8	0.2	1
dry mix, prepared w/whole milk	½ cup	161	4.1	4.1	1.3	0.3	2
ready to eat	5-oz can	169	2.9	5.3	2.3	1.9	
Jello®							
ready to eat	113 g	167	3.0	4.0	1.4	0.2	
tapioca/chocolate, dry mix	24.8 g	94	1.0	1.0	0.2	0.0	

FOOD	CARBO-HYDRATES (mg)	FIBER (mg)	CALCIUM (mg)	IRON (mg)	POTAS-SIUM (mg)	SODIUM (mg)	CHOLES-TEROL (mg)	% OF CALORIES FROM FAT
SWEETS, Desserts (continued)								
Puddings, coconut cream								
dry mix, instant	22.3	0.1	2	0.16	5	302	0	9
dry mix, instant, prepared w/lowfat (2%) milk	28.2	0.1	150	0.22	194	362	9	19
dry mix, instant, prepared w/whole milk	28.0	0.1	148	0.22	190	361	17	27
dry mix, regular	19.3	0.2	9	0.23	34	169	0	13
dry mix, regular, prepared w/lowfat (2%) milk	24.9	0.2	158	0.28	223	228	9	22
dry mix, regular, prepared w/whole milk	24.7	0.2	155	0.28	219	227	17	30
Jello® dry mix	12.0	0.0	6	0.10		100	0	30
instant	23.2	0.5	9	0.17		186	3.115	23
Pudding, egg custard, Swiss Miss®	5.2		37	0.36		47	0.998	28
Pudding, French vanilla, dry mix, Jello®	24.0	0.0	3	0.00		126	0	0
Puddings, lemon								
dry mix, instant	23.8		1	0.02	2	333	0	2
dry mix, instant, prepared w/lowfat (2%) milk	29.7		149	0.08	190	394	9	15
dry mix, instant, prepared w/whole milk	29.5		146	0.08	187	393	17	22
dry mix, regular	19.5		1	0.04	1	107	0	1
dry mix, regular, prepared w/sugar, egg yolk, & water	36.3		11	0.26	7	94	77	11
ready to eat	35.6	0.0	3		1	199	0	22
Jello® dry mix	13.0	0.0	1	0.00		72	0	0
instant	26.7	0.3	1	0.03		190	0	1
Puddings, milk chocolate								
Jello® ready to eat	29.0	0.1	115	0.40		126	1.6	31
milk chocolate/fudge, ready to eat	29.0	0.1	111	0.40		124	1.6	31
Yoplait®	30.0		150	0.36		105	10	20
Puddings, rice								
prepared from recipe	40.1	0.2	155	1.01	268	85	17	17
dry mix	24.6	0.0	4	0.48	1	99	0	0
dry mix, prepared w/lowfat (2%) milk	30.2	0.0	152	0.54	189	159	9	13
dry mix, prepared w/whole milk	30.0	0.0	149	0.54	186	158	17	21
ready to eat	31.3		73		85	121		42
Puddings, tapioca								
prepared from recipe	25.8	0.0	159	0.49	216	288	124	31
dry mix	21.7	0.0	1	0.03	1	110	0	0
dry mix, prepared w/lowfat (2%) milk	27.8	0.0	149	0.09	190	172	9	15
dry mix, prepared w/whole milk	27.6	0.0	147	0.09	186	171	17	23
ready to eat	27.5		119	0.33	148	168		28
Jello®								
ready to eat	29.0	0.1	114	0.10		135	1.6	22
tapioca/chocolate, dry mix	22.0	0.0	4	0.40		109	0	10

SNACKS & SWEETS

FOOD	AMOUNT	CALO-RIES (kcal)	PROTEIN (g)	FAT (g)	MONO-UN-SATURATED FAT (g)	POLY-UN-SATURATED FAT (g)	SATU-RATED FAT (g)
SWEETS, Desserts (continued)							
Puddings, tapioca (continued)							
tapioca/vanilla, dry mix	23 g	85	0.0	0.0	0.0	0.0	0.0
Swiss Miss®	28.35 g	37	0.5	1.5	0.4	0.1	0.6
Puddings, vanilla							
prepared from recipe	½ cup	130	4.0	4.1	1.2	0.2	2.5
dry mix, instant	25 g	92	0.0	0.2	0.1	0.1	0.0
dry mix, instant, prepared w/lowfat (2%) milk	½ cup	147	3.9	2.4	0.7	0.1	1.4
dry mix, instant, prepared w/whole milk	½ cup	161	3.9	4.1	1.2	0.2	2.5
dry mix, regular	22 g	81	0.1	0.1	0.0	0.0	0.0
dry mix, regular, prepared w/lowfat (2%) milk	½ cup	141	4.1	2.4	0.7	0.1	1.5
dry mix, regular, prepared w/whole milk	½ cup	155	4.1	4.2	1.2	0.2	2.6
ready to eat	½ cup	146	2.6	4.1	1.7	0.4	0.6
Jello® instant, dry mix	24.8 g	93	0.0	0.0	0.0	0.0	0.6
Pudding, York peppermint patty, Hershey®	113 g	180	3.0	6.0	2.2	0.2	3.6
Rennin, chocolate							
dry mix	2-oz pkg	207	1.4	1.9	0.6	0.1	1.
dry mix, prepared w/lowfat (2%) milk	½ cup	110	4.4	2.8	0.8	0.1	1.
dry mix, prepared w/whole milk	½ cup	125	4.4	4.5	1.3	0.2	2.
Rennin, vanilla							
prepared from recipe	½ cup	112	4.0	4.1	1.2	0.2	2.
dry mix	1 tbsp	41	0.0	0.0			
dry mix, prepared w/lowfat (2%) milk	½ cup	102	4.1	2.3	0.7	0.1	1.
dry mix, prepared w/whole milk	½ cup	116	4.0	4.1	1.2	0.2	2.
Rennin, tablets, unsweetened	1 tablet	1	0.0	0.0			
Rolls, Pillsbury®							
cinnamon danish w/icing	38.9 g	160	2.0	8.0	1.9	1.0	2
cinnamon w/icing	33.6 g	110	1.0	5.0	1.6	1.0	1
orange danish w/icing	38.9 g	150	2.0	7.0	1.7	1.0	2
raisin danish w/icing	38.9 g	150	2.0	7.0		1.0	2
Snack bar, Health Valley®							
apple bakes	42.5 g	100	2.0	3.0			
fruit & fitness	42.5 g	100	2.0	2.5			
Toaster streudel, Pillsbury®							
apple/spice	54.3 g	200	3.0	9.0		2.0	2
blueberry	54.3 g	190	3.0	9.0		2.0	2
cinnamon	54.3 g	200	5.0	10.0		2.0	2
strawberry	54.3 g	190	3.0	9.0		2.0	2
Turnover, Pillsbury®							
apple	56.6 g	170	2.0	8.0	4.5	1.0	2
cherry	56.6 g	170	2.0	8.0	3.7	1.0	2
Twinkie, Hostess® light	35.4 g	110	2.0	2.0		1.0	1

FOOD	CARBO-HYDRATES (mg)	FIBER (mg)	CALCIUM (mg)	IRON (mg)	POTAS-SIUM (mg)	SODIUM (mg)	CHOLES-TEROL (mg)	% OF CALORIES FROM FAT
SWEETS, Desserts (continued)								
Puddings, tapioca (continued)								
tapioca/vanilla, dry mix	22.0	0.0	1	0.00		110	0	0
Swiss Miss®	6.5	0.0	20	0.00		47	0.25	36
Puddings, vanilla								
prepared from recipe	19.6	0.0	145	0.09	185	113	17	28
dry mix, instant	23.2	0.1	3	0.04	3	360	0	2
dry mix, instant, prepared w/lowfat (2%) milk	28.1	0.1	146	0.10	185	407	9	15
dry mix, instant, prepared w/whole milk	27.9	0.1	144	0.10	182	406	16	23
dry mix, regular	20.6	0.0	3	0.01	4	166	0	1
dry mix, regular, prepared w/lowfat (2%) milk	26.1	0.0	153	0.07	194	224	9	15
dry mix, regular, prepared w/whole milk	26.0	0.0	150	0.07	190	223	17	24
ready to eat	24.8	0.0	99	0.15	128	153	8	25
Jello® instant, dry mix	23.0	0.0	1	0.00		347	0	0
Pudding, York peppermint patty, Hershey®	29.0	0.8	100	0.93		210	4.52	30
Rennin, chocolate								
dry mix	52.2	0.5	95			40		8
dry mix, prepared w/lowfat (2%) milk	18.3	0.1	171			71		23
dry mix, prepared w/whole milk	18.1	0.1	169			69	17	32
Rennin, vanilla								
prepared from recipe	15.3	0.0	151	0.08	185	95	17	33
dry mix	10.7		13			1		0
dry mix, prepared w/lowfat (2%) milk	16.4		161			62		20
dry mix, prepared w/whole milk	16.2					61		32
Rennin, tablets, unsweetened	0.2	0.0	34	0.06	3	234		0
Rolls, Pillsbury®								
cinnamon danish w/icing	19.0	0.5	0	0.72		240	0	45
cinnamon w/icing	17.0	0.4	0	0.36		260	0	41
orange danish w/icing	19.0	0.6	0	0.72		250	0	42
raisin danish w/icing	20.0		0	0.36		230	0	42
Snack bar, Health Valley®								
apple bakes	16.0	2.8	0	1.44		25	0	27
fruit & fitness	17.5	2.4	20	0.90		13	0	23
Toaster streudel, Pillsbury®								
apple/spice	26.0		0	0.36		190	5	41
blueberry	26.0		0	0.36		210	5	43
cinnamon	23.0		0	0.36		200	5	45
strawberry	26.0		0	0.36		200	5	43
Turnover, Pillsbury®								
apple	23.0	0.9	0	0.72		330	0	42
cherry	23.0	0.7	0	0.72		320	0	42
Twinkie, Hostess® light	21.0					160	0	16

SNACKS & SWEETS

FOOD	AMOUNT	CALO-RIES (kcal)	PROTEIN (g)	FAT (g)	MONO-UN-SATURATED FAT (g)	POLY-UN-SATURATED FAT (g)	SATU-RATED FAT (g)
SWEETS, Desserts (continued)							
Whipped topping, cool whip, extra creamy	4.45 g	13	0.0	1.0			
Bird's Eye®	4.05 g	13	0.1	1.0	0.1	0.0	0.9
lite	4.07 g	9	0.0	0.6			
Yogurt dessert, strawberry, light, Sara Lee®	64 g	120	2.0	1.0			
SWEETS, Cakes							
Banana, Pillsbury Plus® mix	43.7 g	190	3.0	4.0	1.3	0.0	1.0
Boston creme, Pepperidge Farm® supreme	1 oz	101	1.0	4.9	1.6	0.8	1.3
Butter, Pillsbury Plus® mix	43.1 g	170	2.0	3.0	2.1	0.0	0.5
Carrot							
Pepperidge Farm®							
classic	1 oz	104	0.8	6.4	1.5	3.0	1.
old fashion, w/icing	1 oz	100	0.7	6.0	1.5	3.0	1.
Pillsbury Plus® mix	44.3 g	180	2.0	5.0	2.3	0.0	1.
Cheesecake							
Jello®							
dry mix	39 g	164	3.0	4.0			
New York style	42.6 g	175	4.0	3.0			
Pepperidge Farm® strawberry	1 oz	70	1.4	2.1	0.8	0.4	0.
Cherries supreme, Pepperidge Farm®	1 oz	52	0.0	0.6			
Chocolate butter, Pillsbury Plus® mix	43.1 g	170	2.0	4.0	2.2	0.0	1
Chocolate chip, Pillsbury Plus® mix	44.8 g	190	3.0	5.0	1.8	0.0	2
Chocolate fudge layer, Pepperidge Farm®	1 oz	111	0.6	6.1	1.9	0.9	1
Chocolate mousse, Pepperidge Farm®	1 oz	76	1.2	3.6	0.0	0.0	1
light	71 g	190	3.0	9.0	3.6	2.0	3
Chocolate stripe layer, Pepperidge Farm®	1 oz	105	1.2	5.5	2.4	1.4	1
Chocolate, Sara Lee® free & light	48 g	110	2.0	0.0	0.0	0.0	0
Chocolate supreme, Pepperidge Farm®	1 oz	104	1.0	5.6	0.0	0.0	0
Coconut classic, Pepperidge Farm®	1 oz	102	0.9	4.9			
Coconut layer, Pepperidge Farm®	1 oz	111	0.6	4.9			
Coffee cinnamon swirl, Pillsbury®	44.3 g	180	2.0	9.0	1.5	1.0	2
Coffee pecan streusel, Pillsbury®	44.3 g	180	2.0	9.0	1.5	1.0	2
Dark chocolate, Pillsbury Plus® mix	43.1 g	180	3.0	5.0	1.7	0.0	
Devil's food							
Pepperidge Farm® layer	1 oz	111	0.6	5.5	1.1	0.7	0
Pillsbury Plus® mix	43.1	170	2.0	4.0	1.7	0.0	1
Fudge marble, Pillsbury Plus® mix	46.6 g	200	3.0	5.0	1.8	1.0	2
Funfetti, Pillsbury Plus® mix	45.3 g	190	3.0	4.0	2.1	1.0	
German chocolate							
Pepperidge Farm® classic	1 oz	111	0.9	5.8	2.4	1.3	
layer	1 oz	111	0.6	6.1	2.4	1.3	

FOOD	CARBO-HYDRATES (mg)	FIBER (mg)	CALCIUM (mg)	IRON (mg)	POTAS-SIUM (mg)	SODIUM (mg)	CHOLES-TEROL (mg)	% OF CALORIES FROM FAT
SWEETS, Desserts (continued)								
Whipped topping, cool whip, extra creamy	1.0	0.0	1	0.00		3	0.2	69
Bird's Eye®	0.9	0.0	0	0.01		1	0	70
lite	1.0	0.0	3	0.00		3	0.1	55
Yogurt dessert, strawberry, light, Sara Lee®	26.0					90	0	8
SWEETS, Cakes								
Banana, Pillsbury Plus® mix	35.0	0.4	20	0.36		280	0	19
Boston creme, Pepperidge Farm® supreme	13.6	0.2	14	0.25		66	17.37	43
Butter, Pillsbury Plus® mix	35.0	0.5	60	0.36		270	0	16
Carrot								
Pepperidge Farm®								
classic	12.8	0.3	0	0.14		112	19.97	55
old fashion, w/icing	12.7	0.3	0	0.24		107	9.982	54
Pillsbury Plus® mix	33.0	0.5	40	0.72		280	0	25
Cheesecake								
Jello®								
dry mix	30.0		85	0.30		248	0.7	22
New York style	33.0	0.3	95	0.40		320	1.2	15
Pepperidge Farm® strawberry	11.5	0.1	14	0.17		59	35.24	27
Cherries supreme, Pepperidge Farm®	11.7		12	0.22		11	24.56	11
Chocolate butter, Pillsbury Plus® mix	32.0	0.5	100	1.08		330	0	21
Chocolate chip, Pillsbury Plus® mix	35.0	0.9	60	0.72		270	0	24
Chocolate fudge layer, Pepperidge Farm®	14.2	0.5	0	0.44		86	12.28	50
Chocolate mousse, Pepperidge Farm®	10.0	0.0	8	0.43		104	1.996	43
light	25.0	0.4	71	0.40		30	5	43
Chocolate stripe layer, Pepperidge Farm®	12.3	0.5	0	0.44		86	12.28	47
Chocolate, Sara Lee® free & light	26.0	2.4	42	1.38		140	0	0
Chocolate supreme, Pepperidge Farm®	12.9	0.0	14	0.50		49	8.685	48
Coconut classic, Pepperidge Farm®	13.8		0	0.00		71	8.874	43
Coconut layer, Pepperidge Farm®	14.8		12	0.22		74	12.28	40
Coffee cinnamon swirl, Pillsbury®	22.0	0.1	0	0.72		170	0	45
Coffee pecan streusel, Pillsbury®	21.0	0.1	0	0.72		170	0	45
Dark chocolate, Pillsbury Plus® mix	33.0	0.8	100	0.72		340	0	25
Devil's food								
Pepperidge Farm® layer	14.8	0.5	0	0.22		83	12.28	45
Pillsbury Plus® mix	32.0	0.8	100	1.08		330	0	21
Fudge marble, Pillsbury Plus® mix	37.0	0.9	60	0.72		290	0	23
Funfetti, Pillsbury Plus® mix	36.0	0.6	20	0.36		280	0	19
German chocolate								
Pepperidge Farm® classic	12.9	0.3	0	0.00		102	19.97	47
layer	13.5	0.3	12	0.22		105	12.28	50

FOOD	AMOUNT	CALO-RIES (kcal)	PROTEIN (g)	FAT (g)	MONO-UN-SATURATED FAT (g)	POLY-UN-SATURATED FAT (g)	SATU-RATED FAT (g)
SWEETS, Cakes (continued)							
German chocolate (continued)							
Pillsbury Plus® mix	43.1 g	180	3.0	4.0	3.1	0.0	0.9
Golden, Pepperidge Farm® layer	1 oz	111	0.6	5.5	1.4	0.5	0.7
Lemon coconut, Pepperidge Farm® supreme	1 oz	93	1.0	4.3	1.4	0.7	0.7
Lemon supreme, Pepperidge Farm®	1 oz	62	1.4	1.8	0.9	0.5	0.4
Lemon, Pillsbury Plus® mix	43.1 g	170	2.0	3.0	2.0	0.0	1.0
Pound							
Pepperidge Farm® old fashion	1 oz	110	1.0	6.0	1.9	1.3	1.0
Sara Lee® free & light	28 g	70	1.0	0.0	0.0	0.0	0.0
Strawberry short, Pepperidge Farm®	1 oz	57	0.7	1.7	0.0	0.2	0.1
Strawberry stripe layer, Pepperidge Farm®	1 oz	107	0.7	5.3			
Strawberry, Pillsbury Plus® mix	44.3 g	180	2.0	4.0	2.1	0.0	1.0
Sunshine vanilla, Pillsbury Plus® mix	43.7 g	180	2.0	5.0	2.1	1.0	2.0
Vanilla fudge classic, Pepperidge Farm®	1 oz	111	0.9	4.9	0.9	0.0	2.1
Vanilla							
Hostess® lights	42.5 g	140	2.0	1.0		0.0	0.0
Pepperidge Farm® layer	1 oz	117	0.6	4.9	1.7	2.1	1.1
White, Pillsbury Plus® mix	43.7 g	180	2.0	4.0	2.0	1.0	1.0
Yellow, Pillsbury Plus® mix	43.7 g	180	2.0	5.0	2.1	1.0	2.0
SWEETS, Cookies							
Amaranth, Health Valley®	15.6 g	60	1.0	2.0			
Apple cinnamon oat bran, Frookie®	11 g	45	0.0	2.0	1.5	0.5	0.0
Arrowroot	2.5 g	11	0.2	0.3	0.2	0.0	0.1
Buttercup, Keebler®	5 g	23	0.3	1.0		0.0	0.0
Chocolate chip							
Keebler®	16 g	80	0.0	4.0	1.4	0.0	1.0
w/fiber	14.5 g	70	0.0	4.0	1.3	0.0	0.0
Pillsbury®	15.8 g	70	1.0	3.0	1.2	0.9	0.9
Chocolate fudge sandwich, Keebler®	17 g	80	0.0	4.0	2.2	0.0	1.0
Chocolate/cinnamon, Teddy Graham®	14.2 g	70	1.0	3.0	1.3	0.9	0.9
Commodore, Keebler®	13 g	60	1.0	2.0		0.0	0.0
Double fudge, Keebler®	16 g	80	0.0	4.0	1.0	0.0	1.0
Fancy fruit, Health Valley®							
apricot	15.6 g	45	1.0	1.5			
date pecan	15.6 g	45	1.0	1.5	0.7	0.4	0.
raisin oat	15.6 g	45	1.0	1.5	0.7	0.4	0.
Fancy peanut chunk, Health Valley®	15.6 g	45	1.0	1.5	0.7	0.4	0.
Fat free, Health Valley®							
apple centers	15.6 g	70	2.0	1.0			

FOOD	CARBO-HYDRATES (mg)	FIBER (mg)	CALCIUM (mg)	IRON (mg)	POTAS-SIUM (mg)	SODIUM (mg)	CHOLES-TEROL (mg)	% OF CALORIES FROM FAT
SWEETS, Cakes (continued)								
German chocolate (continued)								
Pillsbury Plus® mix	34.0	0.5	20	0.72		280	0	20
Golden, Pepperidge Farm® layer	14.8	0.2	12	0.22		68	12.28	45
Lemon coconut, Pepperidge Farm® supreme	12.7	0.1	7	0.24		73	9.982	42
Lemon supreme, Pepperidge Farm®	9.4	0.1	0	0.13		36	18.17	27
Lemon, Pillsbury Plus® mix	34.0	0.2	60	0.36		260	0	16
Pound								
Pepperidge Farm® old fashion	13.0	0.2	0	0.00		85	0	49
Sara Lee® free & light	17.0	0.2	36	0.35		105	0	0
Strawberry short, Pepperidge Farm®	10.0	1.4	13	0.24		17	23.26	27
Strawberry stripe layer, Pepperidge Farm®	14.0		0	0.24		80	13.28	45
Strawberry, Pillsbury Plus® mix	35.0	0.5	60	0.36		290	0	20
Sunshine vanilla, Pillsbury Plus® mix	33.0	0.6	60	0.36		280	0	25
Vanilla fudge classic, Pepperidge Farm®	14.7	0.0	0	0.00		71	15.57	40
Vanilla								
Hostess® lights	30.0		100	0.72		160	0	6
Pepperidge Farm® layer	15.4	0.2	0	0.00		74	12.28	38
White, Pillsbury Plus® mix	34.0	0.6	20	0.36		270	0	20
Yellow, Pillsbury Plus® mix	34.0	0.6	60	0.36		280	0	25
SWEETS, Cookies								
Amaranth, Health Valley®	9.5	2.2	0	0.36		23	0	30
Apple cinnamon oat bran, Frookie®	7.0	1.0	5	0.44		40	0	40
Arrowroot	1.9		1	0.07		10		25
Buttercup, Keebler®	3.7		0	0.12		37	0	39
Chocolate chip								
Keebler®	11.0	0.4	0	0.00		75	0	45
w/fiber	8.0	1.3	0			50	0	51
Pillsbury®	9.0	0.4	0	0.00		55	5	39
Chocolate fudge sandwich, Keebler®	12.0	0.3	0	0.36		70	0	45
Chocolate/cinnamon, Teddy Graham®	10.0	0.3	20	0.17		60	0	39
Commodore, Keebler®	10.0		0	0.14		65	0	30
Double fudge, Keebler®	11.0	0.3	0	0.36		65	0	45
Fancy fruit, Health Valley®								
apricot	6.0	0.9	0			23	0	30
date pecan	6.5	0.9	10	0.36		23	0	30
raisin oat	6.5	0.8	0	0.36		48	0	30
Fancy peanut chunk, Health Valley®	6.0	1.2	0	0.36		28	0	30
Fat free, Health Valley®								
apple centers	16.0	3.5	20	0.72		35	0	13

SNACKS & SWEETS

FOOD	AMOUNT	CALO-RIES (kcal)	PROTEIN (g)	FAT (g)	MONO-UN-SATURATED FAT (g)	POLY-UN-SATURATED FAT (g)	SATU-RATED FAT (g)
SWEETS, Cookies (continued)							
Fat free, Health Valley® (continued)							
apple spice	7.4 g	25	0.7	0.3	0.1	0.0	0.2
jumbo raisin	25.2 g	70	2.0	1.0			
raisin oatmeal	7.4 g	25	0.7	0.3	0.2	0.1	0.1
raspberry	15.6 g	70	2.0	1.0			
Fortune, La Choy®	6 g	15	0.2	0.1	0.0	0.1	0.0
French vanilla creme, Keebler®	17 g	80	0.0	4.0	1.4	0.0	0.0
Healthy graham cinnamon, Health Valley®	28.4 g	110	2.0	3.0			
Homeplate, Keebler®	13 g	60	1.0	2.0		0.0	1.0
Keebies, Keebler®	18 g	80	1.0	3.0		0.0	0.0
Oat bran fruit jumbos, Health Valley®	25.2 g	60	1.5	1.5	0.4	0.9	0.2
Oat bran, apple fiber, Keebler®	14.5 g	70	0.0	3.0	2.0	0.0	0.0
Oatmeal raisin, Pillsbury®	15.8 g	60	1.0	2.0	0.7	0.7	0.7
Oatmeal, fiber enriched, Keebler®	14.5 g	70	0.0	3.0		0.0	0.0
Oatmeal, Keebler®	18 g	80	1.0	4.0	1.6	0.0	1.0
Peanut butter							
Keebler®	17 g	80	1.0	4.0	2.0	0.0	1.0
Pillsbury®	15.8 g	70	1.0	3.0	1.5	0.8	0.8
Suddenly 'Smores, Nabisco®	21.3 g	100	1.0	4.0		1.0	2.0
Sugar							
Keebler®							
fiber enriched	14.5 g	70	0.0	3.0	0.8	0.0	0.0
old fashion	18 g	80	1.0	3.0	0.9	0.0	1.0
Pillsbury®	15.8 g	70	1.0	3.0	0.9	1.0	1.0
Vanilla wafer, Keebler®	3.75 g	20	0.0	1.0	0.3	0.0	0.3
Vanilla, Teddy Graham® Bearwich	14 g	60	1.0	2.0	1.2	0.2	0.5
Wafer, Keebler Krisp Kreem®	4.8 g	25	0.0	1.5	0.4	0.0	0.5
SWEETS, Frozen desserts							
Fruit & juice bars	1 bar	63	0.9	0.1			
Gelatin pops	1 pop	31	0.5	0.0			
Ice cream							
chocolate	½ cup	143	2.5	7.3	2.1	0.3	4.5
French vanilla, soft-serve	½ cup	185	3.5	11.2	3.0	0.4	6.4
strawberry	½ cup	127	2.1	5.6			
vanilla	½ cup	132	2.3	7.3	2.1	0.3	4.5
vanilla, rich	½ cup	178	2.6	12.0	3.5	0.5	7.4
Ice milk							
vanilla	½ cup	92	2.5	2.8	0.8	0.1	1.7
vanilla, soft-serve	½ cup	111	4.3	2.3	0.7	0.1	1.4
Ice pops	1 bar	42	0.0	0.0			
Ices, water							
lime	½ cup	75	0.4				
pineapple-coconut	½ cup	85	0.0	2.5			
fruit, reduced-calorie, aspartame-sweetened	1 bar	12	0.3	0.0			
Pudding pops							
chocolate	1 pop	72	1.9	2.2			

FOOD	CARBO-HYDRATES (mg)	FIBER (mg)	CALCIUM (mg)	IRON (mg)	POTAS-SIUM (mg)	SODIUM (mg)	CHOLES-TEROL (mg)	% OF CALORIES FROM FAT
SWEETS, Cookies (continued)								
Fat free, Health Valley® (continued)								
apple spice	5.7	1.0	7	0.24		13	0	12
jumbo raisin	16.0	3.5	20	0.72		35	0	13
raisin oatmeal	5.7	1.0	7	0.24		13	0	12
raspberry	16.0	3.5	20	0.72		35	0	13
Fortune, La Choy®	3.5	0.1	0	0.09		1	0	6
French vanilla creme, Keebler®	12.0	0.1	0	0.36		80	0	45
Healthy graham cinnamon, Health Valley®	17.0	3.0	0	0.72		50	0	25
Homeplate, Keebler®	10.0		0	0.00		130	0	30
Keebies, Keebler®	12.0		0	0.36		80	0	34
Oat bran fruit jumbos, Health Valley®	10.0	1.6	0	0.72		40	0	23
Oat bran, apple fiber, Keebler®	9.0	1.1	0	0.36		60	0	39
Oatmeal raisin, Pillsbury®	10.0	0.4	0	0.36		55	0	30
Oatmeal, fiber enriched, Keebler®	9.0	1.1	0	0.36		60	0	39
Oatmeal, Keebler®	13.0	0.4	0	0.36		110	0	45
Peanut butter								
Keebler®	10.0	0.4	0	0.72		100	0	45
Pillsbury®	9.0	0.3	0	0.00		75	5	39
Suddenly 'Smores, Nabisco®	15.0					90	0	36
Sugar								
Keebler®								
fiber enriched	9.0	1.1	0	0.36		60	0	39
old fashion	13.0	0.6	0	0.36		70	0	34
Pillsbury®	9.0	0.2	0	0.00		70	5	39
Vanilla wafer, Keebler®	2.5	0.0	0	0.09		15	0	45
Vanilla, Teddy Graham® Bearwich	10.0	0.2	4	0.28		75	0	30
Wafer, Keebler Krisp Kreem®	3.5	0.0	0	0.00		10	0	54
SWEETS, Frozen desserts								
Fruit & juice bars	15.6	0.0	4	0.15	40	3	0	1
Gelatin pops	7.3	0.0			1	20	0	0
Ice cream								
chocolate	18.6	0.2	72	0.61	164	50	22	46
French vanilla, soft-serve	19.1	0.0	113	0.18	152	52	78	54
strawberry	18.2	0.1	79	0.14	124	40	19	40
vanilla	15.5	0.4	85	0.06	131	53	29	50
vanilla, rich	16.5	0.0	87	0.04	118	41	45	61
Ice milk								
vanilla	15.0	0.0	92	0.07	139	56	9	27
vanilla, soft-serve	19.2	0.0	138	0.05	194	62	10	19
Ice pops	11.2	0.0	0	0.00	2	7	0	0
Ices, water								
lime	31.3				3		0	0
pineapple-coconut	16.9		0	3.39		34		26
fruit, reduced-calorie, aspartame-sweetened	3.2		1	0.07	13	3	0	0
Pudding pops								
chocolate	11.9	0.1	66	0.21	105	77	1	28

SNACKS & SWEETS

FOOD	AMOUNT	CALO-RIES (kcal)	PROTEIN (g)	FAT (g)	MONO-UN-SATURATED FAT (g)	POLY-UN-SATURATED FAT (g)	SATU-RATED FAT (g)
SWEETS, Frozen desserts (continued)							
Pudding pops (continued)							
vanilla	1 pop	75	1.9	2.1			
Jello®							
chocolate	47.2 g	79	2.0	2.0	0.1	0.0	1.8
chocolate/caramel	47.2 g	74	2.0	2.0	0.1	0.0	1.8
chocolate fudge	47.2 g	79	2.0	2.0	0.1	0.0	1.8
milk chocolate	47.2 g	80	2.0	2.0	0.1	0.0	1.8
vanilla	47.2 g	77	2.0	2.0	0.1	0.0	1.8
Sherbet, orange	½ cup	132	1.1	1.9	0.5	0.1	1.1
Yogurt							
chocolate	½ cup	115	2.9	4.3	1.3	0.2	2.6
vanilla	½ cup	114	2.8	4.0	1.1	0.2	2.5
SWEETS, Frostings							
Chocolate, creamy							
prepared from recipe, prepared w/butter	602 g	2409	7.9	69.3	20.1	2.5	42.7
prepared from recipe, prepared w/margarine	602 g	2411	8.0	68.9	29.7	20.1	15.5
dry mix	1 pkg	1510	5.1	20.2			
dry mix, prepared w/butter	1 pkg	1908	5.6	65.2			
dry mix, prepared w/margarine	1 pkg	1909	5.6	64.8			
ready to eat	16-oz pkg	1834	4.9	81.1	41.7	9.9	25.6
Coconut-nut, ready to eat	16-oz pkg	1903	6.8	110.7	56.4	15.8	32.5
Cream cheese-flavor, ready to eat	16-oz pkg	1906	0.3	79.9	41.7	10.8	23.3
Glaze, prepared from recipe	327 g	1173	2.1	25.7	11.0	7.5	5.7
Seven minute, prepared from recipe	387 g	1231	6.4	0.0			
Sour cream-flavor, ready to eat	16-oz pkg	1904	0.5	79.5	41.5	10.8	23.2
Vanilla, creamy							
prepared from recipe, prepared w/butter	574 g	1972	3.6	23.7	6.7	0.9	14.4
prepared from recipe, prepared w/margarine	574 g	2326	2.2	62.0	27.1	19.0	12.6
dry mix	1 pkg	1685	1.1	20.2			
dry mix, prepared w/butter	1 pkg	2188	1.3	86.2			
dry mix, prepared w/margarine	1 pkg	2190	1.3	85.8			
ready to eat	16-oz pkg	1936	0.6	77.6	40.5	10.5	22.6
White, fluffy							
dry mix	1 pkg	767	4.8	0.0			
dry mix, prepared w/water	1 pkg	770	4.9	0.0			
SWEETS							
Baking chocolate, unsweetened							
liquid	1-oz pkt	134	3.4	13.5	2.6	3.0	7.2
squares	1-oz square	148	2.9	15.7	5.2	0.5	9.2
Chewing gum	1 stick	10	0.0	0.0			
Cocoa, dry powder, unsweetened	1 tbsp	11	1.0	0.7	0.2	0.0	0.4
processed w/alkali	1 tbsp	11	0.9	0.7			

FOOD	CARBO-HYDRATES (mg)	FIBER (mg)	CALCIUM (mg)	IRON (mg)	POTAS-SIUM (mg)	SODIUM (mg)	CHOLES-TEROL (mg)	% OF CALORIES FROM FAT
SWEETS, Frozen desserts (continued)								
Pudding pops (continued)								
vanilla	12.6	0.0	61	0.03	65	50	1	25
Jello®								
chocolate	13.0	0.4	73	0.30		82	1	23
chocolate/caramel	12.0	0.4	64	0.20		63	0.8	24
chocolate fudge	13.0	0.4	73	0.30		82	1	23
milk chocolate	13.0	0.4	73	0.20		83	1.1	23
vanilla	13.0	0.0	70	0.10		50	0.9	23
Sherbet, orange	29.2	0.3	52	0.14	92	44	5	13
Yogurt								
chocolate	17.9	0.1	106		188	71	3	34
vanilla	17.4	0.1	103	0.22	152	63	2	32
SWEETS, Frostings								
Chocolate, creamy								
prepared from recipe, prepared w/butter	467.3	1.6	104	4.59	544	1144	176	26
prepared from recipe, prepared w/margarine	468.0	1.6	106	4.51	557	1235	5	26
dry mix	357.1			4.62	698	294	0	12
dry mix, prepared w/butter	357.3			4.71	713	754	121	31
dry mix, prepared w/margarine	357.7			4.66	722	819	0	31
ready to eat	291.9	1.7	37	6.55	905	845	0	40
Coconut-nut, ready to eat	243.9	12.3	62	2.52	858	899	0	52
Cream cheese-flavor, ready to eat	308.1	2.3	15	0.72	163	1094	0	38
Glaze, prepared from recipe	240.2	0.0	73	0.19	97	307	7	20
Seven minute, prepared from recipe	311.5	0.0	9	0.25	246	659	0	0
Sour cream-flavor, ready to eat	312.4		11	0.31	896	943		38
Vanilla, creamy								
prepared from recipe, prepared w/butter	448.4	0.0	128	0.36	166	366	67	11
prepared from recipe, prepared w/margarine	453.7	0.0	75	0.34	103	1175	5	24
dry mix	385.5	1.6	14	0.00	30	54	0	11
dry mix, prepared w/butter	365.6	0.9	45	1.27	102	1082	126	35
dry mix, prepared w/margarine	366.0	0.9	49	1.21	112	1149	0	35
ready to eat	320.5	0.7	14	0.50	169	418	0	36
White, fluffy								
dry mix	196.4	0.2	9		242	484		0
dry mix, prepared w/water	197.1	0.2	11		243	490		0
SWEETS								
Baking chocolate, unsweetened								
liquid	9.6	0.9	15	1.18	331	3	0	91
squares	8.0	0.7	21	1.79	236	4	0	95
Chewing gum	2.9				0	0	0	0
Cocoa, dry powder, unsweetened	2.7	0.3	6	0.69	76	1	0	57
processed w/alkali	2.7	0.3	6	0.78	125	1	0	57

SNACKS & SWEETS

FOOD	AMOUNT	CALORIES (kcal)	PROTEIN (g)	FAT (g)	MONO-UN-SATURATED FAT (g)	POLY-UN-SATURATED FAT (g)	SATU-RATED FAT (g)
SWEETS, Frozen desserts (continued)							
Cocoa, dry powder, unsweetened (continued)							
Hershey's® European style cocoa	1 tbsp	10	1.0	0.5			
Fruit butters, apple	1 tbsp	33	0.0	0.1			
Honey, strained or extracted	1 tbsp	64	0.1	0.0			
Jams & preserves	1 tbsp	48	0.1	0.0	0.0	0.0	0.0
Kraft® strawberry, local	1 tsp	6	0.0	0.0			
Jellies	1 tbsp	52	0.1	0.0			
Kraft® reduced calorie grape	1 tsp	6	0.0	0.0			
Marmalade, orange	1 tbsp	49	0.1	0.0			
Molasses	1 tbsp	53	0.0	0.0			
Molasses, blackstrap	1 tbsp	47	0.0	0.0			
Pectin, unsweetened, dry mix	1.75-oz pkg	163	0.1	0.1			
Pie fillings, canned							
apple	21-oz can	599	0.6	0.6	0.0	0.2	0.1
cherry	21-oz can	683	2.8	1.2	0.3	0.4	0.3
Sugars							
brown	1 cup	828	0.0	0.0			
granulated	1 cup	773	0.0	0.0			
powdered	1 cup	467	0.1	0.1			
maple	1-oz piece	100	0.0	0.1			
Syrups							
chocolate, thin-type, w/out added nutrients	2 tbsp	82	0.7	0.3	0.1	0.0	0.2
chocolate, thin-type, w/added nutrients	1 tbsp	46	0.3	0.2	0.1	0.0	0.1
chocolate, fudge-type	1 tbsp	73	0.9	2.8	0.8	0.7	1.2
corn, dark	1 tbsp	56	0.0	0.0			
corn, light	1 tbsp	56	0.0	0.0			
corn, high-fructose	1 tbsp	53	0.0	0.0			
malt	1 tbsp	76	1.5	0.0			
maple	1 tbsp	52	0.0	0.0			
sorghum	1 tbsp	61	0.0	0.0			
table blends, cane & 15% maple	1 tbsp	56	0.0	0.0			
table blends, corn, refiners, & sugar	1 tbsp	64	0.0	0.0			
table blends, pancake	1 tbsp	57	0.0	0.0			
table blends, pancake, w/butter	1 tbsp	59	0.0	0.3	0.1	0.0	0.2
table blends, pancake, w/2% maple	1 tbsp	53	0.0	0.0			
table blends, pancake, reduced-calorie	1 oz	46	0.0	0.0			
Toppings							
butterscotch or caramel	2 tbsp	103	0.6	0.1	0.0	0.0	0.1
marshmallow cream	1 oz	88	0.5	0.1			
nuts in syrup	2 tbsp	167	1.8	9.0	2.0	5.6	0.8
pineapple	2 tbsp	106	0.1				
strawberry	2 tbsp	107	0.1	0.1			

FOOD	CARBO-HYDRATES (mg)	FIBER (mg)	CALCIUM (mg)	IRON (mg)	POTAS-SIUM (mg)	SODIUM (mg)	CHOLES-TEROL (mg)	% OF CALORIES FROM FAT
SWEETS, Frozen desserts (continued)								
Cocoa, dry powder, unsweetened (continued)								
Hershey's® European style cocoa	2.8		7	1.73	256	3	0	45
Fruit butters, apple	8.6	0.1	1	0.02	16	0	0	3
Honey, strained or extracted	17.3		1	0.09	11	1	0	0
Jams & preserves	12.9	0.1	4	0.10	15	8	0	0
Kraft® strawberry, local	2.0				10	5	0	0
Jellies	13.5	0.1	2	0.04	12	7	0	0
Kraft® reduced calorie grape	2.0				10	5	0	0
Marmalade, orange	13.3		8	0.03	7	11	0	0
Molasses	13.8		41	0.94	293	7	0	0
Molasses, blackstrap	12.2		172	3.50	498	11	0	0
Pectin, unsweetened, dry mix	45.2		4	1.36	4	100	0	1
Pie fillings, canned								
apple	155.8		27	1.73	268	259	0	1
cherry	174.6		65	1.43	625	54	0	2
Sugars								
brown	214.0	0.0	187	4.19	762	86	0	0
granulated	199.8	0.0	2	0.12	4	3	0	0
powdered	119.4	0.0	1	0.07	3	2	0	0
maple	25.8	0.0	26	0.46	78	3	0	1
Syrups								
chocolate, thin-type, w/out added nutrients	22.1	0.1	5	0.79	84	36	0	3
chocolate, thin-type, w/added nutrients	12.4	0.1		2.55	90	29	0	4
chocolate, fudge-type	12.4	0.5	21	0.25	45	27	0	35
corn, dark	15.3	0.0	4	0.07	9	31	0	0
corn, light	15.3	0.0	1	0.01	1	24	0	0
corn, high-fructose	14.4	0.0	0	0.01	0	0	0	0
malt	17.1		15	0.23	77	8	0	0
maple	13.4	0.0	13	0.24	41	2	0	0
sorghum	15.7	0.0	31	0.80	210	2	0	0
table blends, cane & 15% maple	15.0	0.0	3	0.16	7	21	0	0
table blends, corn, refiners, & sugar	16.8	0.0	5	0.15	13	14	0	0
table blends, pancake	15.1	0.0	0	0.02	0	17	0	0
table blends, pancake, w/butter	14.8	0.0	0	0.02	1	20	1	5
table blends, pancake, w/2% maple	13.9	0.0	1	0.01	1	12	0	0
table blends, pancake, reduced-calorie	12.5	0.1	0	0.00	1	57	0	0
Toppings								
butterscotch or caramel	27.0		22	0.08		143		1
marshmallow cream	22.5	0.0	1	0.06	1	13	0	1
nuts in syrup	21.9			0.43			0	49
pineapple	27.9	0.0	9	0.20	133	26	0	0
strawberry	27.8	0.2	10	0.41	31	9	0	1

YOUR NUTRITIONAL NOTES

YOUR NUTRITIONAL NOTES

YOUR NUTRITIONAL NOTES

YOUR NUTRITIONAL NOTES

YOUR NUTRITIONAL NOTES

YOUR NUTRITIONAL NOTES

General Cooking and Nutrient Ingredient Measurements

U.S. SYSTEM OF MEASUREMENTS

grain (gr)	=	.03435 drams
dram (dr)	=	27¹¹/₃₂ grains or ¹/₁₆ ounce
ounce (oz)	=	16 drams or ¹/₁₆ pound
pound (lb)	=	16 ounces or 256 drams
pinch or dash	=	less than ⅛ Teaspoon or 2 to 3 drops
teaspoon (tsp)	=	⅓ tablespoon or 60 drops
tablespoon (tbl)	=	½ ounce, 3 teaspoons or ¹/₁₆ cup
gill	=	½ cup or 4 fluid ounces
cup	=	½ pint or 8 fluid ounces
pint (pt)	=	2 cups or 16 fluid ounces
quart (qt)	=	2 pints, 4 cups or 32 fluid ounces
gallon (gal)	=	4 quarts, 16 cups or 128 fluid ounces
peck (pk)	=	2 gallons or 8 quarts
bushel (bu)	=	4 pecks or 8 gallons

METRIC SYSTEM OF MEASUREMENTS

1 milliliters (ml)	=	¹/₁₀ centiliters
1 centiliter (cl)	=	10 milliliters or ¹/₁₀₀ liter
1 liter (l)	=	100 centiliter or 1000 milliliters
1 milligram	=	¹/₁₀ centigram
1 centigram (cg)	=	10 milligrams or ¹/₁₀₀ gram
1 gram (g)	=	100 centigrams or 1000 milligrams
1 kilogram (kg)	≐	1000 grams
1 kilocalorie (kcal or Cal)	=	A measure of heat energy representing the amount of heat needed to raise the temperature of 1 kilogram of water 1 degree Celsius

CONVERSION EQUIVALENTS

U.S. to Metric

1 grain	=	64.80 milligrams
1 dram	=	1.772 grams
1 ounce	=	28.35 grams
1 pound	=	.4536 kilograms
1 teaspoon	=	5 milliliters
1 tablespoon	=	15 milliliters
1 gill	=	⅑ liters
1 cup	=	.24 liters
1 pint	=	.473 liters
1 quart	=	.946 liters
1 gallon	=	3.785 liters

Metric to U.S.

1 milligram	=	.0154 grains
1 gram	=	.0353 ounces
1 kilogram	=	2.2046 pounds
1 milliliter	=	.034 ounces
1 centiliter	=	2 teaspoons
1 liter	=	2.113 pints or 1.056 quarts or .0264 gallon

COMPARATIVE WEIGHTS AND MEASURES

Some U.S. and English units for liquid and dry measurements have different values. Below a the most common variations.

UNITED STATES		ENGLISH (IMPERIAL) LIQUID MEASURE
1 teaspoon	=	⅘ teaspoon
1 tablespoon	=	⅘ tablespoon
1 gill	=	⅚ teacup
1 cup	=	⅚ breakfast cup
1 pint	=	⅚ pint
1 quart	=	⅚ quart
1 gallon	=	⅚ gallon

Please note that in dry measurement pints, quarts, pecks and bushels are equivalent one to one in American and English measuremen